1994
YEAR BOOK OF
SURGERY®

Statement of Purpose

The YEAR BOOK Service

The YEAR BOOK series was devised in 1901 by practicing health professionals who observed that the literature of medicine and related disciplines had become so voluminous that no one individual could read and place in perspective every potential advance in a major specialty. In the final decade of the 20th century, this recognition is more acutely true than it was in 1901.

More than merely a series of books, YEAR BOOK volumes are the tangible results of a unique service designed to accomplish the following:

- to *survey* a wide range of journals of proven value
- to *select* from those journals papers representing significant advances and statements of important clinical principles
- to provide *abstracts* of those articles that are readable, convenient summaries of their key points
- to provide *commentary* about those articles to place them in perspective

These publications grow out of a unique process that calls on the talents of outstanding authorities in clinical and fundamental disciplines, trained literature specialists, and professional writers, all supported by the resources of Mosby, the world's preeminent publisher for the health professions.

The Literature Base

Mosby subscribes to nearly 1,000 journals published worldwide, covering the full range of the health professions. On an annual basis, the publisher examines usage patterns and polls its expert authorities to add new journals to the literature base and to delete journals that are no longer useful as potential YEAR BOOK sources.

The Literature Survey

The publisher's team of literature specialists, all of whom are trained and experienced health professionals, examines every original, peer-reviewed article in each journal issue. More than 250,000 articles per year are scanned systematically, including title, text, illustrations, tables, and references. Each scan is compared, article by article, to the search strategies that the publisher has developed in consultation with the 270 outside experts who form the pool of YEAR BOOK editors. A given article may be reviewed by any number of editors, from one to a dozen or more, regardless of the discipline for which the paper was originally published. In turn, each editor who receives the article reviews it to determine whether or not the article should be included in the YEAR BOOK. This decision is based on the article's inherent quality, its probable usefulness to readers of that YEAR BOOK, and the editor's goal to represent a balanced picture of a given field in each volume of the YEAR BOOK. In addition, the editor indicates when to include figures and tables from the article to help the YEAR BOOK reader better understand the information.

Of the quarter million articles scanned each year, only 5% are selected for detailed analysis within the YEAR BOOK series, thereby assuring readers of the high value of every selection.

The Abstract

The publisher's abstracting staff is headed by a physician-writer and includes individuals with training in the life sciences, medicine, and other areas, plus extensive experience in writing for the health professions and related industries. Each selected article is assigned to a specific writer on this abstracting staff. The abstracter, guided in many cases by notations supplied by the expert editor, writes a structured, condensed summary designed so that the reader can rapidly acquire the essential information contained in the article.

The Commentary

The YEAR BOOK editorial boards, sometimes assisted by guest commentators, write comments that place each article in perspective for the reader. This provides the reader with the equivalent of a personal consultation with a leading international authority—an opportunity to better understand the value of the article and to benefit from the authority's thought processes in assessing the article.

Additional Editorial Features

The editorial boards of each YEAR BOOK organize the abstracts and comments to provide a logical and satisfying sequence of information. To enhance the organization, editors also provide introductions to sections or individual chapters, comments linking a number of abstracts, citations to additional literature, and other features.

The published YEAR BOOK contains enhanced bibliographic citations for each selected article, including extended listings of multiple authors and identification of author affiliations. Each YEAR BOOK contains a Table of Contents specific to that year's volume. From year to year, the Table of Contents for a given YEAR BOOK will vary depending on developments within the field.

Every YEAR BOOK contains a list of the journals from which papers have been selected. This list represents a subset of the nearly 1,000 journals surveyed by the publisher and occasionally reflects a particularly pertinent article from a journal that is not surveyed on a routine basis.

Finally, each volume contains a comprehensive subject index and an index to authors of each selected paper.

The 1994 Year Book Series

Year Book of Allergy and Clinical Immunology: Drs. Rosenwasser, Borish, Gelfand, Leung, Nelson, and Szefler

Year Book of Anesthesia and Pain Management: Drs. Tinker, Abram, Kirby, Ostheimer, Roizen, and Stoelting

Year Book of Cardiology®: Drs. Schlant, Collins, Engle, Gersh, Kaplan, and Waldo

Year Book of Chiropractic: Dr. Lawrence

Year Book of Critical Care Medicine®: Drs. Rogers and Parrillo

Year Book of Dentistry®: Drs. Meskin, Currier, Kennedy, Leinfelder, Berry, and Roser

Year Book of Dermatologic Surgery: Drs. Swanson, Glogau, and Salasche

Year Book of Dermatology®: Drs. Sober and Fitzpatrick

Year Book of Diagnostic Radiology®: Drs. Federle, Clark, Gross, Madewell, Maynard, Sackett, and Young

Year Book of Digestive Diseases®: Drs. Greenberger and Moody

Year Book of Drug Therapy®: Drs. Lasagna and Weintraub

Year Book of Emergency Medicine®: Drs. Wagner, Burdick, Davidson, McNamara, and Roberts

Year Book of Endocrinology®: Drs. Bagdade, Braverman, Poehlman, Kannan, Landsberg, Molitch, Morley, Odell, Rogol, Ryan and Nathan

Year Book of Family Practice®: Drs. Berg, Bowman, Davidson, Dietrich, and Scherger

Year Book of Geriatrics and Gerontology®: Drs. Beck, Reuben, Burton, Small, Whitehouse, and Goldstein

Year Book of Hand Surgery®: Drs. Amadio and Hentz

Year Book of Hematology®: Drs. Spivak, Bell, Ness, Quesenberry, and Wiernik

Year Book of Infectious Diseases®: Drs. Keusch, Wolff, Barza, Bennish, Gelfand, Klempner, and Snydman

Year Book of Infertility and Reproductive Endocrinology®: Drs. Mishell, Lobo, and Sokol

Year Book of Medicine®: Drs. Bone, Cline, Epstein, Greenberger, Malawista, Mandell, O'Rourke, and Utiger

Year Book of Neonatal and Perinatal Medicine®: Drs. Klaus and Fanaroff

Year Book of Nephrology®: Drs. Coe, Favus, Henderson, Kashgarian, Luke, Myers, and Curtis

Year Book of Neurology and Neurosurgery®: Drs. Bradley and Crowell

Year Book of Neuroradiology: Drs. Osborn, Eskridge, Grossman, and Harnsberger

Year Book of Nuclear Medicine®: Drs. Hoffer, Gore, Gottschalk, Rattner, Zaret, and Zubal

Year Book of Obstetrics and Gynecology®: Drs. Mishell, Kirschbaum, and Morrow

Year Book of Occupational and Environmental Medicine: Drs. Emmett, Frank, Gochfeld, and Hessl

Year Book of Oncology®: Drs. Simone, Longo, Ozols, Steele, Glatstein, and Bosl

Year Book of Ophthalmology®: Drs. Laibson, Adams, Augsburger, Benson, Cohen, Eagle, Flanagan, Nelson, Rapuano, Reinecke, Sergott, and Wilson

Year Book of Orthopedics®: Drs. Sledge, Poss, Cofield, Frymoyer, Griffin, Hansen, Johnson, Simmons, and Springfield

Year Book of Otolaryngology–Head and Neck Surgery®: Drs. Paparella and Holt

Year Book of Pain: Drs. Gebhart, Haddox, Jacox, Payne, Rudy, and Shapiro

Year Book of Pathology and Clinical Pathology®: Drs. Gardner, Bennett, Cousar, Garvin, and Worsham

Year Book of Pediatrics®: Dr. Stockman

Year Book of Plastic, Reconstructive, and Aesthetic Surgery: Drs. Miller, Cohen, McKinney, Robson, Ruberg, and Whitaker

Year Book of Podiatric Medicine and Surgery®: Dr. Kominsky

Year Book of Psychiatry and Applied Mental Health®: Drs. Talbott, Frances, Breier, Meltzer, Perry, Schowalter, and Yudofsky

Year Book of Pulmonary Disease®: Drs. Bone and Petty

Year Book of Rheumatology: Drs. Sergent, LeRoy, Meenan, Panush, and Reichlin

Year Book of Sports Medicine®: Drs. Shephard, Drinkwater, Eichner, Sutton, Torg, Col. Anderson, and Mr. George

Year Book of Surgery®: Drs. Copeland, Deitch, Eberlein, Howard, Luce, Ritchie, Seeger, Souba, and Sugarbaker

Year Book of Thoracic and Cardiovascular Surgery: Drs. Ginsberg, Lofland, and Wechsler

Year Book of Transplantation: Drs. Sollinger, Eckhoff, Hullett, Knechtle, Longo, Mentzer, and Pirsch

Year Book of Ultrasound: Drs. Merritt, Babcock, Carroll, Goldstein, and Mittelstaedt

Year Book of Urology®: Drs. Gillenwater and Howards

Year Book of Vascular Surgery®: Dr. Porter

1994

The Year Book of SURGERY®

Editor-in-Chief
Edward M. Copeland, III, M.D.

Editorial Board
Edwin A. Deitch, M.D.
Timothy J. Eberlein, M.D.
Richard J. Howard, M.D., Ph.D.
Edward A. Luce, M.D.
Wallace P. Ritchie, Jr., M.D., Ph.D.
James M. Seeger, M.D., F.A.C.S.
Wiley W. Souba, M.D., Sc.D.
David J. Sugarbaker, M.D.

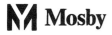 **Mosby**

St. Louis Baltimore Boston Chicago London Madrid Philadelphia Sydney Toronto

Vice President and Publisher, Continuity Publishing: Kenneth H. Killion
Director, Editorial Development: Gretchen C. Murphy
Developmental Editor: Diana Dodge
Acquisitions Editor: Karen Taeyaerts
Illustrations and Permissions Coordinator: Maureen Livengood
Director of Editorial Services: Edith M. Podrazik, R.N.
Senior Information Specialist: Terri Santo, R.N.
Information Specialist: Nancy Dunne, R.N.
Senior Medical Writer: David A. Cramer, M.D.
Senior Project Manager: Max F. Perez
Project Supervisor: Tamara L. Smith
Senior Production Editor: Wendi Schnaufer
Production Coordinator: Sandra Rogers
Editing Coordinator: Rebecca Nordbrock
Proofroom Supervisor: Barbara M. Kelly
Vice President, Professional Sales and Marketing: George M. Parker
Marketing and Circulation Manager: Barry J. Bowlus
Marketing Coordinator: Lynn Stevenson

1994 EDITION
Copyright © December 1994 by Mosby-Year Book, Inc.

Printed in the United States of America
Composition by International Computaprint Corporation
Printing/binding by Maple-Vail

Mosby-Year Book, Inc.
11830 Westline Industrial Drive
St. Louis, MO 63146

Editorial Office:
Mosby-Year Book, Inc.
200 North LaSalle St.
Chicago, IL 60601
International Standard Serial Number: 0090-3671
International Standard Book Number: 0-8151-7793-3

Table of Contents

Mosby Document Express

Copies of the full text of the original source documents of articles abstracted or referenced in this publication are available by calling Mosby Document Express, toll-free, at 1 (800) 55-MOSBY.

With Mosby Document Express, you have convenient, 24-hour-a-day access to literally every article on which this publication is based. In fact, through Mosby Document Express, virtually any medical or scientific article can be located and delivered by FAX, overnight delivery service, international airmail, electronic transmission of bitmapped images (via Internet), or regular mail. The average cost of a complete, delivered copy of an article, including up to $4 in copyright clearance charges and first-class mail delivery, is $12.

For inquiries and pricing information, please call the toll-free number shown above. To expedite your order for material appearing in this publication, please be prepared with the code shown next to the bibliographic citation for each abstract.

Journals Represented

Mosby subscribes to and surveys nearly 1,000 U.S. and foreign medical and allied health journals. From these journals, the Editors select the articles to be abstracted. Journals represented in this YEAR BOOK are listed below.

Academic Medicine
American Heart Journal
American Industrial Hygiene Association Journal
American Journal of Infection Control
American Journal of Pathology
American Journal of Physiology
American Journal of Roentgenology
American Journal of Surgery
American Journal of Surgical Pathology
American Surgeon
Anesthesiology
Annals of Plastic Surgery
Annals of Surgery
Annals of Thoracic Surgery
Archives of Surgery
British Journal of Cancer
British Journal of Surgery
British Medical Journal
Burns
Canadian Journal of Surgery
Canadian Medical Association Journal
Cancer
Cancer Research
Cardiovascular and Interventional Radiology
Chest
Circulation
Circulatory Shock
Critical Care Medicine
Digestive Diseases and Sciences
Diseases of the Colon and Rectum
European Journal of Cancer
European Journal of Surgery
Gastroenterology
Head and Neck
Human Pathology
Inquiry: The Journal of Health Care Organization, Provision, and Financing
Intensive Care Medicine
International Journal of Cancer
International Journal of Radiation, Oncology, Biology, and Physics
Journal of Burn Care and Rehabilitation
Journal of Clinical Investigation
Journal of Clinical Oncology
Journal of Experimental Medicine
Journal of Heart and Lung Transplantation
Journal of Immunology
Journal of Infectious Diseases
Journal of Interventional Radiology
Journal of Laboratory and Clinical Medicine
Journal of Nuclear Medicine
Journal of Pediatric Orthopedics

Journal of Pediatric Surgery
Journal of Surgical Oncology
Journal of Surgical Research
Journal of Thoracic and Cardiovascular Surgery
Journal of Trauma
Journal of Vascular Surgery
Journal of the American Medical Association
Journal of the National Cancer Institute
Lancet
Laryngoscope
Metabolism
Microsurgery
New England Journal of Medicine
Nutrition
Otolaryngology - Head and Neck Surgery
Pediatric Radiology
Plastic and Reconstructive Surgery
Radiology
S.A.M.J./S.A.M.T. - South African Medical Journal
Southern Medical Journal
Surgery
Surgery, Gynecology and Obstetrics
Thorax
Transplantation
Transplantation Proceedings
World Journal of Surgery
Wound Repair and Regeneration

STANDARD ABBREVIATIONS

The following terms are abbreviated in this edition: acquired immunodeficiency syndrome (AIDS), the central nervous system (CNS), cerebrospinal fluid (CSF), computed tomography (CT), electrocardiography (ECG), human immunodeficiency virus (HIV), and magnetic resonance (MR) imaging (MRI).

Introduction

The Editorial Board would like to thank Martin C. Robson, M.D., for his participation in the YEAR BOOK OF SURGERY and to welcome Edward A. Luce, M.D., from the University of Kentucky, to the Editorial Board. Also, James M. Seeger, M.D., from the University of Florida, joins the Editorial Board and expands the coverage of vascular surgery.

The disciplines of molecular biology and genetic engineering have rapidly moved to the forefront in virtually all aspects of surgical research, and clinical application is no longer "around the corner." It is here. Many of the recent advances in these disciplines are covered in this YEAR BOOK.

Health care reform and choice of medical career are topics that are becoming ever more frequent in the surgical literature. The number of individuals annually certified by the American Board of Surgery has changed very little during the past 10 years, and the number of chief resident slots in surgery has actually decreased. Primary care residency positions, as defined by positions in family practice, internal medicine and pediatrics, have increased dramatically. In fact, 49% of all certificates awarded between 1982 and 1992 were in these 3 primary care specialties. The Health Security Act, if passed, mandates that 55% of each graduating class of medical students enter a primary care discipline that includes obstetrics and gynecology. Had the physicians who were certified in a primary care discipline during the past 10 years actually practiced primary care, the 55% mandate would have already been met. The reality, of course, is that 75% of these individuals chose to subspecialize.

"Choice" of a medical career may be less of an option in the future, because federal funding may dictate the number of residency positions available. Any attempt by an institution to augment funding with additional monies may result in withdrawal of federal funding. The Surgical Residency Review Committee and the American Board of Surgery have applied stringent criteria to accreditation and certification, and they have attempted to keep the number of surgeons commensurate with the incidence of surgical illness. Nevertheless, the outcome of funding for surgical manpower remains unpredictable and will be a hotly debated topic.

Edward M. Copeland, III, M.D.

1 General Considerations

What Does the American Board of Surgery In-Training/Surgical Basic Science Examination Tell Us About Graduate Surgical Education?
DaRosa DA, Shuck JM, Biester TW, Folse R (Southern Illinois Univ, Springfield; Case Western Reserve Univ, Cleveland, Ohio; American Board of Surgery, Philadelphia)
Surgery 113:8–13, 1993   140-94-1-1

Background.—Surgeons need a complete understanding of all disease processes in which surgical involvement and management are indicated. The strengths and weaknesses in residents' basic science knowledge were assessed, as was their ability to progressively improve in their abilities to recall basic science information and clinical management facts, to analyze cause-and-effect relationships, and to solve clinical problems.

Methods.—Residents' knowledge of basic science was assessed using the results of the January 1990 American Board of Surgery's In-Training/Surgical Basic Science Exam (IT/SBSE). This examination included 142 basic science items and 97 clinical management questions. The scores of residents in postgraduate year 1 were compared with those of residents in postgraduate year 5. Content was considered known if 67% or more of the residents in each group answered the question correctly.

Findings.—New and graduating residents did not know 44% of the content tested in the basic science questions. The new residents did not demonstrate a basic science knowledge better than that of graduating residents. Residents performed better on basic science questions related to the cardiovascular–respiratory system. Only 20% of the endocrine-related questions were known at the beginning and end of training. Residents in postgraduate year 1 knew 38% of the basic science questions. Only 29% of the 63% of the basic science questions that were unknown on entry were known at the end of training. Fifty-two percent of the 71% of clinical management items unknown at entry were known at the end. Residents in postgraduate year 5 correctly answered more recall, analysis, and inference level questions than did residents between years 1 and 4.

Conclusion.—The American Board of Surgery's in-service examinations are useful for objectively measuring residents' knowledge and provide critical feedback to faculty, program directors, and residents. The findings should enable program directors to assess the strengths and weaknesses in residency training curricula.

▶ The assumption has often been made that new, incoming residents have a better basic science knowledge than graduating chief residents, because the new residents have more recently studied the basic sciences in medical school. This study disproves this assumption. The basic science portion of the IT/SBSE was instituted by The American Board of Surgery to improve the basic science knowledge of surgical residents during their training. The failure of graduating residents to answer correctly basic science questions that were unknown to new residents indicates that this goal has not been achieved and provides support for the insistence of the General Surgical Residency Review Committee that a strong basic science curriculum be put in place in all accredited general surgery programs.—E.M. Copeland, III, M.D.

Evaluations of Surgery Resident Performance Correlate With Success in Board Examinations
Wade TP, Andrus CH, Kaminski DL (St Louis Univ, Mo)
Surgery 113:644–648, 1993   140-94-1–2

Objective.—In most surgical residency programs, the assessment system includes objective measures of surgical knowledge, usually based on the In-Service Training Examination of the American Board of Surgery (ABSITE) and faculty members' subjective evaluations in both narrative and standardized formats. Although ABSITE scores have been shown to predict success on the qualifying (written) examination, for certification, the subjective evaluations have shown an inconsistent relationship to objective measures of competence. The relationship between both ABSITE scores and faculty evaluations of resident skills and future performance, was examined at St. Louis University.

Methods.—Objective and subjective evaluations made during the previous 15 years in a columnar university program in general surgery were reviewed. Both types of evaluations were assessed for their ability to predict success on the written (qualifying) and oral (certifying) American Board of Surgery (ABS) examinations.

Findings.—Of 40 residents taking the qualifying examination, 36 passed on the first attempt, 2 passed on the second or third attempt, and 2 failed on all 3 attempts. Of the 38 residents who passed, 28 passed the certifying examination on the first attempt, 8 on the second attempt, and 2 on the third attempt. A significant correlation was noted between ABSITE scores and success on the qualifying examination. The subjective assessments were not correlated with either ABSITE or qualifying scores. However, above-average subjective assessments did predict success on the certifying examination. Success on the certifying examination was also predicted by chief-year ABSITE total percentile score and the score on the first qualifying examination. The attrition rate in the St. Louis

University program was 23%, with more than half of the departures being voluntary.

Conclusions.—Subjective evaluations of surgical residents do predict later success on the Board's examination for certification. These findings suggest that the Board's certifying examination is an effective test of a candidate's knowledge of surgical facts and his or her ability to communicate them.

▶ At its best, the certifying examination of the American Board of Surgery would differentiate between qualified and nonqualified surgeons. If this were so, the examination could be uniformly used as a credentialing mechanism for surgical privileges in hospitals. The argument is often made that a series of oral examinations given on a single day cannot determine quality among candidates for hospital credentialing. This study refutes this argument. Observation of the clinical expertise of surgical residents by multiple faculty members over extended periods had a strong positive correlation with passing scores on the American Board of Surgery certifying examination. At least for the residents at this one institution, quality of clinical behavior was appropriately tested by the certifying examination.—E.M. Copeland, III, M.D.

Comparison of Housestaff's Estimates of Their Workday Activities With Results of a Random Work-Sampling Study
Oddone E, Guarisco S, Simel D (Veterans Affairs Med Ctr, Durham, NC; Duke Univ, Durham, NC)
Acad Med 68:859–861, 1993   140-94-1–3

Objective.—A formal time-analysis study based on random work sampling was performed to quantify a housestaff's workday activities. Previous studies in this area have been of limited validity because they depended on traditional techniques based on observers' records or the housestaff's recall.

Methods.—The 2 methods of quantifying workday activities were compared in a 3-month study of 18 interns and 18 residents rotating on the general medicine service at Duke University Medical Center. Twenty-six members of the housestaff first provided estimates of how they spent their workdays, using a list of 20 specific work activities and 13 work contacts. All 36 study participants then wore random reminder beepers and recorded what they were doing (activity) and with whom (contact) at each beep. Beepers were worn during on-call and off-call days, weekdays, and weekends.

Results.—The housestaff estimated that they spent 27% of their day performing histories and physical examinations; the actual proportion of time was 17%. They also overestimated the proportion of time spent teaching others (3.6% vs. 1.1%) and the time spent reading textbooks or journals (8.4% vs. 2.3%). There were considerable overestimates of the amount of time spent by housestaff with patients (19.9% vs. 13.4%), with attending physicians (7.7% vs. 16.9%), and with nurses (6.2% vs. 1.6%). The proportion of time spent alone was significantly underestimated (18.3% vs. 30%).

Conclusion.—Random work sampling performed throughout the housestaff's day revealed that interns and residents were inaccurate in their estimates of workday times. Assessments of the impacts of administrative changes and educational reforms are likely to be less accurate when based on the estimates of the housestaff or observers than on the results of random work sampling. The latter method reduces bias and gives quantifiable results.

▶ There is a need for quantifiable data on housestaff workday activities, because some states are legislating the length of residents' workweek. Observer error could be even greater than resident error. The Residency Review Committee also passes judgment on training programs, based on resident interpretation of the workday as transmitted to the site visitor (observer). Thus, observer bias may compound resident bias.

This study did not evaluate resident interpretation of the educational value of the workday. It is possible that the more work-intensive services are of more practical clinical value than the "easier" services, because the amount of time spent in independent study or in teaching others was grossly overestimated. At the University of Florida, our residents' excellent grades on the American Board of Surgery's In-Training Examination correlate with the more work-intensive services.—E.M. Copeland, III, M.D.

The Ivory Tower From Outside and In: A Survey of Minnesota Surgeons
Ward HB, Macauley MK, Foker JE (Univ of Minnesota, Minneapolis)
Surgery 114:436–441, 1993   140-94-1–4

Introduction.—Increasing competition from private hospitals has eroded the patient base of many university hospitals and may cause problems for their teaching programs. For example, during the past 10 years, the proportion of operations performed by residents at the University of Minnesota has decreased compared with procedures performed by residents at private hospitals. Therefore, a questionnaire was prepared to examine the attitudes of surgeons regarding the role of private surgeons in education and the relationship of the university to the private practice community.

Methods.—Questionnaires were mailed to all private surgeons (PS), university surgeons (US), and resident surgeons (RS) in Minnesota. Chi-square analysis was used.

Findings.—Responses were received from 71% of PS, 29% of US, and 64% of RS. The majority of PS, US, and RS believed that (1) teaching hospitals are the best way to educate surgeons; (2) surgery residencies should be based at university hospitals; and (3) complicated clinical cases should be referred for teaching purposes. There was less agreement on whether the university should take the lead in guaranteeing the quality of surgical care in the state and in deciding whether PS are better teachers than US. Resident surgeons were the only group in which the majority did not believe that practicing surgeons had any obligation to the state university or to society for their education.

Conclusions.—Most private surgeons continue to support the leadership of the university in medical education. However, those currently in RS positions believe they have less obligation to the university and society than do either US or PS. This difference may reflect a reaction to the rigors of their current program. However, if it reflects a true change in values, future support for university-based residency programs may be eroding.

▶ The implications from this study are ominous if RS in all programs nationwide believe they are less responsible (or loyal) to their institutions. Surgeons delay short-term goals to attain long-term ones, and they classically have taken on the traits and personalities of their professors—thus, the proliferation of surgical societies bearing the names of surgical chairmen. The professional self-discipline required of surgeons is contained within this gestalt.

Managed-care philosophies could further erode the bond between residents, faculty, and institutions as the requirement for appropriate case mix and volume dictates that surgical training be diffused into multiple hospital settings and the outpatient arena, thus limiting resident contact with dedicated surgical instructors. Also, the increasing administrative demands on senior faculty distances them from surgical practice and the training environment.

Those of us who are responsible for resident education and the propagation of surgical mores must be aware of our trainees' already shrinking dedication to the traditional centers of leadership, and we must preserve the moral attitudes established in the past century and a half, which are the fabric of our profession.—E.M. Copeland, III, M.D.

Factors Affecting Quality of Informed Consent
Lavelle-Jones C, Byrne DJ, Rice P, Cuschieri A (Univ of Dundee, Scotland)
BMJ 306:885–890, 1993   140-94-1–5

Background.—Although informed consent is a legal requirement for all surgical procedures, many patients are unaware of important details about their operations. The factors influencing the quality of informed consent were investigated.

Methods.—Two hundred sixty-five patients undergoing intrathoracic, intraperitoneal, and vascular operations were included in the study. One

Recall of Information by Patients at Various Assessment Points
Before and After Surgery

Assessment point	Poorly informed (score 0-3)	Well informed (score 4-6)
Admission (n=256)	153 (60)	103 (40)
Immediately after consent (n=253)	49 (19)	204 (81)
Day of discharge (n=242)	102 (42)	140 (58)
Outpatient review at 4-6 weeks (n=223)	133 (60)	90 (40)
At 6 months after discharge (n=192)	161 (84)	31 (16)

Values are numbers (percentages) of patients
(Courtesy of Lavelle-Jones C, Byrne DJ, Rice P, et al: *BMJ* 306:885–890, 1993.)

hundred ninety-two were followed up for 6 months. Patients completed standard questionnaires.

Findings.—Patients displayed the best recall of information immediately after signing the consent form. Thereafter, recall deteriorated (table). Sixty-nine percent of the patients said they had not read the consent form before signing it. Advanced age had an adverse effect on information recall at all assessment times. Impaired cognitive function decreased information recall only during the hospital stay. Patients with intelligence quotients (IQs) above average were better able to handle the information than patients with lower IQs, except for immediately after signing the consent form. Patients who believed that matters concerning their health were under their control were better informed than patients with an external locus of control. Cards containing information about surgery improved recall only on the day of discharge.

Conclusions.—Poor information recall was associated with advanced age, below average IQs, impaired cognitive function, and an external locus of health control. Written information may be more useful if provided before patients are admitted.

▶ From the medicolegal point of view, the results of this study are a bit frightening. On 2 different occasions preoperatively, patients were counseled about their surgical procedures and possible complications. However, only 32% of the best informed patients had significant recall of the explanation of the operation 6 months later. In an environment of the study of operative consent, 69% of patients admitted to not reading the consent form before signing it. Because most lawsuits are not settled until several years after the alleged event, those involving a physician's failure to explain an operative procedure adequately would seem to be possibly unfounded.—E.M. Copeland, III, M.D.

Factors Influencing the Specialty Choices of 1993 Medical School Graduates

Kassebaum DG, Szenas PL (Assoc of American Med Colleges, Washington, DC)

Acad Med 69:164–170, 1994   140-94-1–6

Introduction.—Increasing concern over how many physicians will be available in the future and what they will be practicing has prompted studies of what determines the career choices that medical school graduates make.

Data Source.—Students completing the 1993 Medical School Graduation Questionnaire of the Association of American Medical Colleges rated the factors that impinged on their medical career choices. Nearly all of the 8,128 senior students who indicated a specialty goal rated most or all of the 36 factors, using a 0-to-4 Likert-type scale to reflect the degree of influence of a given factor on the choice of a specialty. The choices were grouped as generalist, medical, surgical, and support specialties.

Findings.—The most influential factors related to the types of patient problems encountered, the student's own personality, and the chance of making a difference in individuals' lives. There were significant differences in factor ratings between specialty groups. For instance, future generalists rated patient contact factors higher than did those favoring other specialties.

Implications.—Current medical school graduates heavily base their career choices on their sense of the content and quality of a given discipline; the chance it affords to help others; and how well their own personality, ability, and skills fit in with the field that is chosen. If educators know what considerations are most important to medical graduates, it will be easier to determine what experiences and perceptions must change to achieve a desired mix of specialty decisions.

▶ If current health care reform tends to level out income for the various medical disciplines, one positive benefit will be the preservation of the altruistic reasons why individuals enter medical school in the first place. Why they select certain specialties is determined by this questionnaire (e.g., making a difference in individuals' lives, helping others, and studying disease processes). Income prospects, length of residency, and debt are probably becoming determinants of specialty choices as residents become more "worldly" and realize that medicine can be entrepreneurial. I am not opposed to the entrepreneurial spirit, but in my career, I have been disappointed to see individuals who could have had an enormous impact on the lives of others (patients, colleagues, residents, and students) select an area of medicine on the basis of what appeared to be financial motivation. As a result, such individuals often remove themselves from a major leadership or role model environment.—E.M. Copeland, III, M.D.

Explaining the Association Between Surgeon Supply and Utilization

Escarce JJ (Univ of Pennsylvania, Philadelphia)
Inquiry 29:403–415, 1992   140-94-1–7

Background.—Researchers have found a positive association between the supply of surgeons and the rate of use of individual operations, total surgery rate, and aggregate measures of use. One possible explanation is that a high supply of surgeons enables individuals to obtain care. A high supply may also reduce both the length of time that individuals must wait for an appointment and the travel time necessary to see a surgeon. Alternatively, surgeons in high-supply areas may "induce" demand for financial gain. Medicare enrollment and physician claims data were used to determine the effect of surgeon supply on demand for surgical services.

Methods.—Data were obtained by merging the Health Care Financing Administration's 1986 Part B Medicare Annual Data Beneficiary File and its 1986 Health Insurance Skeleton Eligibility Write-Off File. Ophthalmology, general surgery, orthopedic surgery, and urology were studied.

Findings.—These 4 specialties accounted for nearly one third of Medicare payments to physicians and for more than four fifths of payments to surgeons. Surgeon supply significantly and positively affected demand for services per enrollee in ophthalmology. Supply had a positive but nonsignificant effect on demand for services per enrollee in the other 3 specialties. The effect of surgeon supply on first-occurrences demand was significant and positive for all specialties but general surgery. By contrast, point estimates of the effect of supply on intensity-of-care demand were negative in general surgery, orthopedic surgery, and urology. These findings are consistent with the notions that higher surgeon supply reduces the time price of care and that patients or the referring physicians in high-supply areas more strongly prefer referrals to surgeons. An analysis of the effects of other variables suggested that the role of primary care physicians as an alternative source of care is more important than their role as a source of referrals to surgeons. The effect of primary care physicians reducing the use of surgical services may have been primarily caused by a decrease in the number of patients receiving care from surgeons.

Conclusions.—Higher surgeon supply increases the demand for initial contacts with surgeons, but it does not increase the demand for services among surgeons' patients. A high supply of surgeons may therefore improve access or be associated with stronger preferences for referrals to surgeons. These findings do not support the notion that demand for surgical service is induced in areas with a high supply of surgeons.

▶ General surgeons are not designated primary care physicians by the Health Care Financing Agency, yet this study by J.J. Escarce, Assistant Professor of Internal Medicine, University of Pennsylvania, indicates that an increase in primary care physicians in a geographic locale will decrease surgical visits by replacing the surgeon as the doctor rather than by eliminating the visit. Such a situation could result in an increase in cost, because a visit to a "cognitive" physician may be reimbursed at a higher rate than a surgical visit. This study also indicates that surgeons participate in the delivery of primary care. Whether "managed care" will be cost effective by interposing a primary care physician between the patient and a surgeon remains to be seen. This study did not confirm the widely held hypothesis that an increase in surgeons means an increase in surgical procedures.—E.M. Copeland, III, M.D.

Reforming Graduate Medical Education: Summary Report of the Physician Payment Review Commission
Schwartz A, Ginsburg PB, LeRoy LB (Physician Payment Review Commission, Washington, DC)
JAMA 270:1079–1082, 1993   140-94-1–8

Objective.—The Physician Payment Review System was created in 1986 to advise the United States Congress regarding reforms in the Medicare physician payment system. In recent years, the Commission has been concentrating on the areas of physician supply, specialty distribution, and financing of graduate medical education (GME). The Commission's recommendations for reform of the GME system were reviewed.

Context.—The recommendations were based on 3 working assumptions: (1) that there is, or soon will be, an oversupply of physicians in the United States; (2) that too many medical subspecialists and surgical specialists and too few primary care practitioners are being trained; and (3) that many physicians in all areas of practice are not prepared to work in ambulatory care settings. The recommendations are geared toward limiting further expansion in physician supply, rationalizing the allocation of residency positions, and making the entities that sponsor training programs more accountable to the nation's health care needs.

Recommendations.—The Commission's first recommendation is a congressional limit on the total number and mix of residencies funded. This need is not being met by the current residency approval process, which is primarily driven by the service needs of teaching institutions. The limit on the total number of residencies to be funded would be achieved by reducing the number of first-year positions to the number of United States medical graduates plus 10%. If implemented in 1992, such a policy would have required cutting about 2,500 positions. The commission also calls for bodies that accredit graduate training to assess educational quality and decide which specific positions in these fields should be funded. Presumably, funding would be denied to programs at the bottom of the list in educational quality. Some measures would be needed to prevent programs from financing positions beyond the statutory limit, such as accrediting only those positions from a national financing pool or making programs that fund outside the system ineligible for Medicare payments.

All payers, including self-insured employers, would contribute a percentage of premiums or payments to the national financing pool to cover the direct costs of GME in approved residencies. Medicare would be a contributor just like all other payers. Transitional relief funds would be allocated to teaching hospitals that lose residency slots, with preference given to hospitals with a high share of indigent patients. The loss of services previously provided by residents would be addressed by cutting services or using nonphysician practitioners or community physicians. If the Commission's recommendations had been fully implemented in 1992, $483 million in Medicare hospital payments would have been saved.

Discussion.—These recommendations can help in meeting the national goals of reducing resident supply, changing specialty mix, and providing additional training opportunities in ambulatory care. Because physicians have long working lives, the proposed changes in GME financing would not affect physician supply for many years. Faster achievement of policy goals may require retraining of some physicians already in practice.

▶ If the Health Security Act passes Congress in its present form, 55% of residency positions will be funded to train primary care physicians, as defined by positions in family practice, general internal medicine, general pediatrics, and obstetrics and gynecology. The total numbers of resident positions will be determined by the number of graduates of allopathic and osteopathic medical school plus 10%. Applying this formula to 1992 graduates, there would be a substantial increase (as much as 49%) in generalist positions and a decrease in specialists trained. For academic health centers, replacing the specialty resident workforce will be a challenge, because physician-extenders (e.g., physician assistants and nurse practitioners) command higher salaries than surgical residents and work fewer hours.

It has not been decided which governing body will distribute resident slots to training institutions. Residency Review Committees (RRCs) would seem most qualified, but the various RRCs do not have standardized special requirements for limiting (or expanding) resident complements. This lack of standardization among RRCs may result in the formation of another accrediting entity through the proposed National Council on Graduate Medical Education, which would be set up by the passing of the Health Security Act.—E.M. Copeland, III, M.D.

The Health Security Act and Academic Medicine
Clinton HR, First Lady of the United States
Acad Med 69:93–96, 1994   140-94-1-9

Purposes.—It is clear that the president will insist on health reform legislation that assures universal coverage with comprehensive benefits.

Educational Funding.—The current intent is to provide a funding stream for academic medical centers which, in the first 5 years, will total more than would be available under current formulas for graduate medical education within the Medicare system ($50 billion as opposed to $46 billion). Capping the rate of growth of Medicare and Medicaid with the goal of further reducing the deficit—but without establishing health care reform—would lower Medicare income through both indirect and direct medical education grants. Disproportionate payments will continue, so that the uncompensated care that remains after achieving universal coverage will be provided for.

Basic Principles.—Of foremost urgency is the providing of severe coverage with comprehensive benefits. Savings will be realized if efficiency becomes a high priority throughout the system. A single-claim system has the virtue of simplicity. Choice is a most important principle. It is important to recognize that choice is decreasing today, and that the proposed plan will reverse this decline. Finally, quality will be assured by using the expertise of academic and other medical centers throughout the country. Individuals must be accountable for their own health care, and health plans must critically monitor the services they provide.

Financing Universal Coverage.—Careful consideration of the alternative ways of financing universal health care ended in rejecting both a single-payer system, which entails a very broad-based tax that might amount to $500 billion, and mandating all individuals to purchase health insurance. Instead, it was decided to build on the employer–employee system that presently works for 90% of insured Americans. It is expected that 70% of the insured will pay no more for the same or better benefits when participating in purchasing cooperatives.

▶ This manuscript is an address given by Hillary Rodham Clinton before the annual meeting of the Association of American Medical Colleges in 1993. Although it had been written to solicit the potential support of the academic community for Clinton's Health Security Act, it shows a better understanding of the academic mission than its proposers had at the outset of the reform campaign. Consequently, all of the effort put forth by members of the academic community to preserve the quality of the American medical education process and research base has had a positive effect. I am cautiously optimistic. Reform is no doubt necessary because of escalating medical costs; however, the United States should not abdicate its premier position in medical education and research to a rapidly improving European system.—E.M. Copeland, III, M.D.

Female Surgeons in the 1990s: Academic Role Models

Neumayer L, Konishi G, L'Archeveque D, Choi R, Ferrario T, McGrath J, Nakawatase T, Freischlag J, Levinson W (Univ of Utah, Salt Lake City; Univ of California, Los Angeles; Med College of Wisconsin, Milwaukee; et al)
Arch Surg 128:669–672, 1993   140-94-1-10

Background.—Surgery has been a predominantly male profession, and the issue of available female mentors and role models for women who are interested in it has not been explored. The attitudes of female surgeons, who may serve in these roles, toward their careers and professional environment have not previously been characterized.

Methods.—Data were collected to characterize the participation of women in academic surgery and surgical education. As part of a larger survey, the 1,500 members of the Association of Women Surgeons were mailed questionnaires. The response rate was 45%. The mean age of those responding was 39.6 years.

Findings.—Three hundred eighteen of the 676 respondents held a faculty position. Two hundred thirty-nine of the respondents' practices were based in a university or university-affiliated hospital. The sample was biased toward more academically motivated surgeons. Two hundred thirty-six respondents said that tenure policies were unfair to women. However, women continued to participate in the academic process. Four hundred sixty-four respondents said they would encourage women medical students to pursue a career in surgery. Less than one fifth had a female mentor (Fig 1–1). Slightly more than half had a role model or mentor of either sex at some point in their career. Only 204 still had access to these mentors, however.

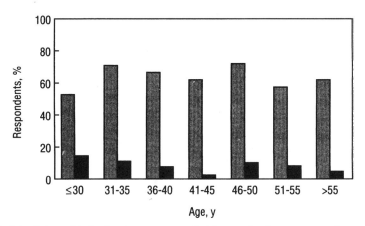

Fig 1–1.—Role models for female surgeons stratified by age, showing percentage of respondents who had any role model (*hatched bars*) and percentage who had female surgeon as role model (*filled bars*). (Courtesy of Neumayer L, Konishi G, L'Archeveque D, et al: *Arch Surg* 128:669–672, 1993.)

Conclusions.—Although the professional environment of surgery is sometimes perceived as antagonistic, more than two thirds of the respondents to this survey said they would encourage women in medical school to pursue the profession. The women in this survey had a strong commitment to surgical education as well as to their personal career, providing a solid system of support for women interested in becoming surgeons.

Women as Leaders in Organized Surgery and Surgical Education: Has the Time Come?
Jonasson O (American College of Surgeons, Chicago)
Arch Surg 128:618–621, 1993   140-94-1–11

Introduction.—Today, more than one third of medical school graduates and some 40% of entering students are women. By the turn of the century, 1 in 5 physicians in the United States will be women, compared to only 5% a few decades ago. However, few women enter the surgical specialties. When ophthalmology and gynecology are excluded, just 6% of female residents are in surgery, compared to 28% in internal medicine and 15% in pediatrics. Of female surgeons, very few hold senior roles in organized surgery or are found in high academic ranks. The reasons and possible solutions for the lack of female surgical leaders were reviewed.

Reasons.—Nationwide, just 44 women chair medical school clinical departments. Although most pediatrics residents are now women, only 10 women chair departments of pediatrics. Twenty-two percent of clinical faculty are women, but fewer than 8% of female faculty members are full professors. In contrast, 30% of male faculty members are full professors. No women head surgical departments other than obstetrics and gynecology.

Although it is argued that women simply have not had enough time in the field to reach the higher positions, the issue is more complex than that. Certainly, the conflict between family and career is stronger for women. Another problem is the lack of high-ranking female surgeons to provide the sponsorship and personal support needed for younger women to build their surgical careers.

Solutions.—Encouraging female students to choose a surgical career requires a high number of female faculty members and residents on the surgical staff. Active recruitment of women for surgical—and especially academic surgical—careers will provide much-needed role models and a core for future leadership. Sexism is better addressed by encouraging mutual respect and professionalism than by more legalistic and strident approaches. Women in the academic setting must be treated equally and should not devote more than the average amount of time teaching, counseling, or serving on committees. The rigid tenure timetables of many medical schools will have to be adjusted to assist women who are trying to raise a family during their early years on the faculty.

Discussion.—Although a generation or so will be needed before the number of women filling these roles is adequate, women represent an important source of talent and intellect that will serve the future of surgery well.

▶ The mean age of responders to a questionnaire sent to members of the Association of Women Surgeons was 39.6 years, which possibly indicates that the entry of women into academic surgery is a recent event. This would account, in part, for aspiring female surgeons' lack of role models on medical school faculties. This deficiency should soon be corrected, however, because most surgical programs have several matriculating female residents. Surgical chairpersons need to stimulate these women to enter academic surgery so that female residents of the future can be mentored by surgeons of both sexes.

Women physicians should demand to be treated equal to their male counterparts. Promotion, tenure, and salary should be periodically reviewed to insure equality. Clearly, reimbursement for women should be equal to that for men. If one segment of the surgical workforce is willing to work for lesser pay, third-party payers will soon insist that everyone work for this lesser pay scale.—E.M. Copeland, III, M.D.

Women Surgeons: Results of the Canadian Population Study
Mizgala CL, Mackinnon SE, Walters BC, Ferris LE, McNeill IY, Knighton T (Univ of Toronto; Washington Univ, St Louis, Mo; Statistics Canada, Ottawa, Ont)
Ann Surg 218:37–46, 1993   140-94-1–12

Purpose.—More and more women are entering medical training programs, but there has been no corresponding increase in the proportion of women entering the surgical specialties. There are few data on those women who do choose surgical careers, which would be very useful in efforts to increase enrollment by women in surgical training programs. A national survey of all practicing female surgeons in Canada was examined.

Methods.—The study sample comprised all practicing Canadian female surgeons identified from the membership rolls of 2 professional societies; all Canadian surgical specialists must be certified by examination. Of the 506 female surgeons so identified, 459 could be located, and all were sent a 93-item questionnaire designed to assess their ability to balance their careers with their personal and family life. The response rate was 91.3%. A modified Dillman 5-step computerized method was used in conducting the survey.

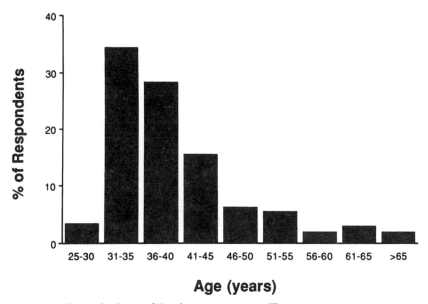

Age (years)

Fig 1–2.—The age distribution of Canadian women surgeons. The surgeons represent a young population, with 78% between ages 30 and 45 years and only 19% aged older than 45 years. (Courtesy of Mizgala CL, Mackinnon SE, Walters BC, et al: *Ann Surg* 218:37–46, 1993.)

Findings.—The respondents were a young group, with fewer than 20% older than age 45 years (Fig 1-2). About two thirds of the respondents were married, whereas only approximately 7% were separated or divorced. More than 90% of them were married to another professional, and one fourth were married to another surgeon. The husband's career did not take priority over the respondent's in most cases; however, when it did, it was a limiting factor. More than 70% of the respondents who had ever married had at least 1 child, most of them having delayed childbearing until after they had finished their surgical training. Eighty-two percent of the respondents were in full-time surgical practice, and another 6% were in part-time practice. Forty-one percent were in the subspecialty of obstetrics and gynecology, 21.2% were in ophthalmology, and 12.1% were in general surgery. Life satisfaction in areas (e.g., career and marriage) was high, and 88.3% were happy that they had chosen a surgical career. Eighty-two percent of the surgeons said that it was important to have a successful female faculty member as a role model, but only 20% had such a mentor.

Conclusions.—Female practicing surgeons in Canada appear able to combine a productive surgical career with a rewarding family life. Although compromises are necessary to achieve this goal, the women appear satisfied with their decision to pursue a surgical career.

▶ This is an important study because it indicates that women can combine a home-life and motherhood with a successful surgical career. Only 12% of women in this study, however, were general surgeons, once again reflecting the low percentage of women in this specialty compared with obstetrics and gynecology. Some program directors in general surgery find it difficult to recruit competitive female applicants to their programs. No doubt, those programs that provide female faculty role models and a safe training environment are most popular with female candidates. Female role models are not plentiful; only 20% of the respondents in this survey had such a mentor. Many of the best candidates for surgical residency training programs are women, particularly now that class distribution is equalizing. It behooves all surgical chairmen to recruit female faculty members, if possible, and/or to aid women physicians in other disciplines to create a proper institutional environment in which women are as comfortable as men.—E.M. Copeland, III, M.D.

The Risk of Exposure of Third-Year Surgical Clerks to Human Immunodeficiency Virus in the Operating Room

Vergilio J-A, Roberts RB, Davis JM (Cornell Univ, New York)
Arch Surg 128:36–39, 1993   140-94-1–13

Purpose.—The human immunodeficiency virus can be transmitted to health care personnel by exposure to blood and body fluids. Education in universal precautions can significantly decrease exposure to blood products, yet there have been few studies of the risk to third-year medical students when they assume clinical duties. This risk was examined in third-year students completing their 3-month surgical rotation.

Methods.—After their rotation, 101 students were anonymously surveyed about their exposure to blood and the mechanism of exposure, contact with HIV-positive patients, and knowledge of universal precautions. The response rate was 97%.

Results.—Sixty-eight percent of respondents were exposed to blood or blood products during their surgical rotation. Fifty percent sustained a splash to their mucous membranes; 45% were stuck with a needle; and 30% were exposed in some other way, including 3% who were cut by a scalpel. From the first to the fourth quarter, the number of exposures per student decreased from 3 to 1. This decrease was significantly related to increasing knowledge of universal precautions. Of the 48% of students who were cut or stuck in the operating room, two thirds were injured by someone else, usually the surgeon or assistant.

Conclusions.—Third-year medical students report significant exposure to blood and blood products during the surgical clerkship. The number of exposures decreases as the academic year progresses. The reasons for this decrease include inexperience at the beginning of the year, increasing awareness of universal precautions, and the distribution of goggles at the beginning of the surgical rotation. Most cut or stick injuries are not self-inflicted, suggesting that students are placed in the path of instrument transfer or injured when their hands are in the surgical field and not within their vision.

▶ During a surgical rotation, the almost 50% rate of exposure to fluids potentially containing HIV is much too high, especially when the exposure decreases in direct proportion to the length of time spent on the clinical services. An in-depth explanation of universal precautions plus a demonstration of practical applications should precede the third-year rotation and should be repeated before each surgical rotation to eliminate the length of time on clinical services as a variable affecting the rate of exposure. Educational programs, positioning of the students at the superior end of the operating room table (out of the path of sharp instruments), self-retaining retractors, and liberal use of the electrocautery have reduced sharp injuries to students at our institution.—E.M. Copeland, III, M.D.

Aerosol Penetration and Leakage Characteristics of Masks Used in the Health Care Industry
Weber A, Willeke K, Marchioni R, Myojo T, McKay R, Donnelly J, Liebhaber F (Univ of Cincinnati, Ohio)
Am J Infect Control 21:167–173, 1993   140-94-1–14

Background.—Health care workers are potentially exposed to a wide range of hazardous agents. Droplets less than 100 μm in diameter rapidly evaporate to form stable droplet nuclei 1–4 μm in size, which may remain airborne for long periods. Particles about 0.3 μm in diameter are generated during laser surgery, and carbon vaporization can lead to the emission of viable bacterial particles. Commonly used surgical power tools can produce blood-containing aerosols with particles less than 5 μm in size. Procedures used in patients with infectious tuberculosis also may pose a risk. Masks that offer protection against larger particles are not necessarily effective when particles less than 1 μm in diameter are present.

Method.—Eight surgical masks of varying shape, using different filter materials, were evaluated along with a dust-mist-fume (DMF) respirator. Penetration was examined by sealing the surgical mask or DMF respirator to the face of a mannequin with petroleum jelly.

Results.—The mask that performed least well had aerosol filter penetration approximating 100% for particles .2–1 μm in size (Fig 1–3). Penetration decreased as particle diameter increased. The two best performing masks exhibited 20% penetration at a particle size of .2 μm and about 1.5% penetration at 4 μm. The DMF provided the best protection

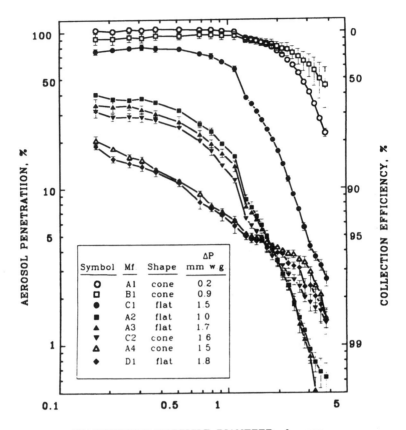

Fig 1–3.—*Abbreviations: Mf.,* manufacturer and model; *ΔP,* pressure drop. Aerosol penetration through the filter media of 8 surgical masks. (Courtesy of Weber A, Willeke K, Marchioni R, et al: *Am J Infect Control* 21:167–173, 1993.)

but increased the work of breathing to an unacceptable limit during long procedures.

Conclusion.—Surgical masks may fail to provide adequate protection where potentially hazardous submicrometer-sized aerosols are present.

Exposure to Blood-Containing Aerosols in the Operating Room: A Preliminary Study

Heinsohn P, Jewett DL (Univ of California, Berkeley; Abratech Corp, Mill Valley, Calif)
Am Ind Hyg Assoc J 54:446–453, 1993   140-94-1–15

Introduction.—Hepatitis B virus (HBV) and HIV are bloodborne pathogens that pose a significant risk to health care workers. Hepatitis B virus has been documented to have been transmitted oropharyngeally to persons wearing surgical masks. Particles measuring less than 5 μm are capable of being deposited in the gas-exchange region of the respiratory tract. In this region alveolar macrophages can be found, and these can be infected by HIV. It has previously been demonstrated that common surgical power tools are capable of generating inhalable blood-containing aerosols. The possibility of exposure to infective blood aerosols prompted a personal sampling study to assess exposure of operating room personnel to inhalable blood aerosols in the breathing zone of the operating room.

Methods.—Common procedures involving surgical power tools were analyzed. Primary and assistant surgeons were monitored via a personal cascade impactor worn beneath the surgical gown. The impactor was configured to monitor stage 2 (14.8 μm), stage 5 (3.5 μm), and stage 8 (.52 μm) effective cutoff aerodynamic diameters. Hemastix strips were used to detect blood in the samples collected.

Results.—The arithmetic mean exposure concentration for primary surgeons was 1.4 μg Hb/m^3; for assistant surgeons, the mean was 1.8 μg Hb/m^3. Hemoglobin was detected in impactor stage 2 in 90% of the samples, in stage 5 in 66% of the samples, and in stage 8 in 11% of the samples.

Conclusions.—These results demonstrate that operating room personnel are likely to be exposed to aerosolized blood in the breathing space of the operating room. At least until the ability of these aerosols to transmit disease is understood, respiratory protection equipment should replace surgical masks in the operating room, because masks do not provide adequate protection against potentially infectious blood aerosols.

▶ There was a 66% risk of aerosolized particles 3.5 μm in size and an 11% risk of particles 0.52 μm in size when measurements were done with a particle-collecting device worn around the neck of members of the operating room team. The mask that performed least effectively had a penetration rate of almost 100% for particle sizes under 1 μm. Therefore, operating room personnel who wear such a mask would have an 11% risk of exposing their upper respiratory tract to potentially infected droplets of blood or blood products when blood spatter occurs or power tools are used.

Mask manufacturers should be required to print the penetration rate of standard aerosol particles on a package insert. The safest situations are surgical power tools that do not produce aerosol particles smaller than 5 μm and masks that filter maximally, fit snugly, and allow easy passage of inhaled air without producing any noticeable work of respiration for members of the operating room team. It would appear that these circumstances are not uniformly met in operating rooms across the country; however, HIV infection and hepatitis infection resulting from aerosolized particles have not been identified as a major problem. Nevertheless, the potential for infection exists and should be minimized both for the patient and the operating room personnel.—E.M. Copeland, III, M.D.

Erythrocyte Viability in Postoperative Autotransfusion
Davis RJ, Agnew DK, Shealy CR, Friedman SE (Univ of South Carolina, Columbia; Baptist Med Ctr, Columbia, SC)
J Pediatr Orthop 13:781–783, 1993   140-94-1–16

Introduction.—In recent years, postoperative blood salvage has become popular as a means of minimizing the risks of disease transmission. The safety of postoperative blood salvage is established, but its efficacy has been questioned.

Methods.—The viability of postoperatively collected cells was determined in 10 consecutive patients undergoing the same surgical procedure: posterior spinal fusion with Cotrel-Dubousset instrumentation for idiopathic scoliosis. After surgery, a sample of blood was drawn, labeled with ^{51}Cr, and reinfused. The cells were then monitored at intervals up to 20 days postoperatively, and their activity was expressed as a percentage of postinfusion activity.

Results.—The labeled cells showed a mean survival of 76% of their initial activity by the fourth day and 75% by the seventh day. In all samples, plasma activity was less than 10% of cell activity. Spleen and sternum activity, measured with a Geiger counter, peaked early—suggesting destruction of a small percentage of mechanically damaged cells—but decreased by more than half by the fourth day.

Conclusions.—Survival of reinfused erythrocytes after postoperative collection in a suction drainage/reinfusion device was documented. The results are comparable to those reported for intraoperative and preoperative cell collection. Thus, postoperatively salvaged blood is as viable and effective as blood from other autologous and homologous sources.

▶ This important study documents that reinfusion of unwashed, filtered blood collected postoperatively results in erythrocyte cell viability equal to that of cells collected intraoperatively or preoperatively. Hemolysis of cells was also minimal in this study, because the plasma contained almost none of the radioactive tracer. Intraoperative autotransfusion reduces hemologous blood transfusion by 50% in patients undergoing cardiac procedures. Postoperative autotransfusion may do likewise for those procedures that are classically associated with an expected postoperative blood loss.—E.M. Copeland, III, M.D.

Exposure Rates to Patients' Blood for Surgical Personnel
Wright JG, McGeer AJ, Chyatte D, Ransohoff DF (Yale Univ, New Haven, Conn)
Surgery 114:897–901, 1993   140-94-1–17

Background.—Operating room personnel are at risk of acquiring HIV and other blood-borne infections via exposure to patients' blood. No previous studies have addressed the rates of exposure for the various surgical subspecialties.

Methods.—The rates of exposure to patients' blood were examined at a level I trauma center and tertiary care hospital. All cutaneous blood exposures or sharp injuries over a 3 months were studied. A study nurse interviewed the involved personnel immediately after the incident.

Findings.—A total of 2,292 surgical procedures were performed during the study. There were 168 cutaneous exposures and 70 sharp injuries. The exposed staff members completed an interview with the study nurse in 89% of cases and completed the questionnaire themselves in the remaining 11%. The rate of combined skin contact and sharp injury was 10.4 per 100 procedures. This rate was lowest (3.3) in pediatric surgery and highest (21.2) in general surgery. Rates also differed for different types of surgery, from 4.2 for craniotomy to 18.0 for laparotomy. The overall rate of sharp injury was 3.1 per 100 procedures and ranged from 1.3 in vascular surgery to 4.3 in general surgery.

Conclusions.—Exposure to patient blood seems to be highest in general surgical procedures. The reported rates vary significantly, perhaps as the result of varying surgical techniques, case-mix, or definitions of exposure.

▶ An exposure rate of 10.4 per 100 cases is impressively high. Fortunately, other studies have documented that the chance of seroconversion expected from such random exposure is quite low. Nevertheless, the prevalence of AIDS is increasing, and all hospital operating room personnel, especially those who work in high risk areas, should practice all preventative steps to reduce exposure. Wearing impenetrable gowns and face shields will reduce skin and mucous membrane exposure. The liberal use of the electrocautery for dissection, when safe, will reduce sharp injury, especially for the first assistant.—E.M. Copeland, III, M.D.

Comparison of Postoperative Mortality in VA and Private Hospitals
Stremple JF, Bross DS, Davis CL, McDonald GO (Veterans Affairs Med Ctr, Pittsburgh; VA Central Office, Washington, DC)
Ann Surg 217:277–285, 1993   140-94-1–18

Introduction.—As mandated by Congress in Public Law 96-166, Section 204, the Veterans Administration must compare postoperative morbidity and mortality rates for all surgical procedures with the prevailing national standard and analyze any deviation by individual medical record review. This study was undertaken to meet this requirement as well as to establish national standards for postoperative mortality rates.

Methods.—Hospital discharge data were obtained from the Hospital Cost Utilization Project, a database of more than 3 million discharges per year from 406 private short-term, general, and public hospitals. Also used was the VA Patient Treatment File database, which includes more than 1 million discharges per year from 132 VA Medical Centers. The list of procedures analyzed included all those accounting for at least 100 cases per year or at least 10 deaths in the VA system, for a total of 309 individual procedures in 113 comparison procedures or groups of procedures. A total of 830,000 discharges were considered, 507,000 from private hospitals and 323,000 from the VA. Thirteen potentially important comorbid conditions were identified and analyzed in a separate comparison. Adjustments for severity of illness were made with the Disease Staging method. Records from 1984 through 1986 were compared.

Results.—For all but 8 of the procedures or procedure groups analyzed, there were no significant differences in postoperative mortality rates between the VA and the private hospitals after adjustment for age, diagnosis, and comorbidity. The difference in mortality rates was significant for suture of ulcer, revision of gastric anastomosis, small-to-small intestinal anastomosis, appendectomy, and reclosure of postoperative disruption of the abdominal wall, all of which were higher in the VA; and for vascular bypass surgery, portal systemic venous shunt, and esophageal surgery, all of which were lower in the VA.

Conclusions.—Some of the differences in postoperative mortality may be related to the characteristics of veterans who use the VA hospitals, have lower income than other veterans, and are more likely to be retired for health reasons, to live alone, to have chronic health conditions that impair their usual activities, and to rate their health as poor. Statistically, there appear to be no differences in postoperative mortality between the VA and private medical care systems.

▶ This study will eliminate much of the speculation by government officials that the surgical care in VA hospitals is inferior to that in private hospitals as a result of resident education that occurs in university-affiliated VA hospitals. In fact, the presence of surgical residents may improve the mortality rate in VA hospitals, because of the 24-hour daily coverage that residents provide. It also is of interest that the results of procedures, such as portosystemic shunts, that were done more frequently in university-affiliated VA hospitals than in the university hospitals were significantly better in the VA hospitals. Veterans Administration surgeons have more experience with these procedures and, therefore, a better outcome.—E.M. Copeland, III, M.D.

Do the Poor Sue More?: A Case-Control Study of Malpractice Claims and Socioeconomic Status
Burstin HR, Johnson WG, Lipsitz SR, Brennan TA (Harvard Med School, Boston; Harvard School of Public Health, Boston; Arizona State Univ, Tempe)
JAMA 270:1697–1701, 1993   140-94-1-19

Introduction.—Some physicians—obstetricians in particular—believe that poor patients are more likely to sue. This may be a factor reducing

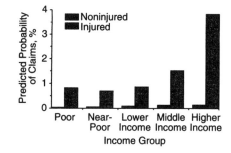

Fig 1-4.—Predicted probability of malpractice claims by income group and medical injury. (Courtesy of Burstin HR, Johnson WG, Lipsitz SR, et al: JAMA 270:1697-1701, 1993.)

the availability of physician care in poor neighborhoods. Associations between socioeconomic status and the filing of malpractice claims were examined.

Methods.—The analysis used data from the files of the New York State Department of Health, which mandates reporting of all malpractice claims. From a population of more than 2.6 million nonpsychiatric patients discharged from acute care hospitals in 1984, a random sample of 31,429 medical records was selected. These records were reviewed for adverse events caused by treatment that prolonged hospitalization and/or led to disability and then linked to the malpractice claim records. Each of 51 claimants so identified was matched to 5 nonclaimant controls. For 29 of the claimants, evidence of adverse events was not found in the medical record; these claimants were matched to uninjured controls for analysis. Variables compared included age, gender, race, insurance status, and income.

Findings.—After adjustment for severity of injury, poor patients and uninsured patients were both less likely to file malpractice claims. The poor were less likely to sue in both the injured and uninjured groups (Fig 1-4). Patients younger than 16 and older than 65 years were also less likely to file claims. No independent associations were noted between gender and race and the likelihood of filing a claim.

Conclusion.—Contrary to the perception of many physicians, poor and uninsured patients are significantly less likely to file malpractice claims. The risk of lawsuits should not play a role in physicians' decisions to serve the poor, and tort reforms to protect against lawsuits by the medically indigent may not be warranted. The elderly are also less likely to sue.

▶ This study is well designed and contains enough patients (31,429) to produce meaningful data. The poor were less likely to sue regardless of whether they were injured. I have always suspected that quality of care and communication reduces malpractice claims. A possible hidden result of this study is that, for the medical schools selected, there was no difference in quality of medical care and/or communication of the physicians with the poor and more affluent patients. If I am correct, I would hope a similar study of hospitals not affiliated with medical schools would show the same thing.—E.M. Copeland, III, M.D.

2 Critical Care

Introduction

Because *Science* recently voted nitric oxide the molecule of the year, it is only fitting that this year's selection of abstracts begins with nitric oxide. Nonetheless, it is somewhat ironic that nitric oxide, a molecule whose major claim to fame was as an industrial pollutant, a destroyer of ozone, and a potential carcinogen, should receive this award for medical and biological importance. However, to quote from a recent review on the L-arginine-nitric oxide pathway, "the discovery that mammalian cells generate nitric oxide, a gas previously considered to be merely an atmospheric pollutant, is providing information about many biologic processes" (1).

One of the most exciting potential therapeutic uses of nitric oxide is in the treatment of adult respiratory distress syndrome, because in patients with this syndrome, inhaled nitric oxide reduced pulmonary hypertension, improved ventilation-perfusion matching, and decreased the shunt fraction. This improvement in pulmonary function appears to be related to the fact that inhaled nitric oxide selectively dilates the vasculature of ventilated lung regions only, in contrast to systemically administered vasodilators, which dilate both ventilated and nonventilated vessels. Although localized increases in nitric oxide can be beneficial, excessive induction of systemic nitric oxide production by endotoxin and certain cytokines can lead to systemic vasodilation that is refractory to vasoconstrictor therapy. An example of this phenomenon is septic shock. In patients with septic shock that is refractory to standard therapy, administration of low doses of the nitric oxide synthase inhibitor N^G-monomethyl-L-arginine reversed the hypotension. However, caution must be exercised in using nitric oxide antagonists or inhibitors, because animal studies clearly show that excessive inhibition of nitric oxide can lead to severe vasoconstriction, organ damage, and rapid death.

Several other interesting advances in the prevention and treatment of adult respiratory distress syndrome have appeared during the past year. One of these is a prospective randomized controlled clinical trial documenting that prophylactic ketoconazole treatment decreases the incidence of adult respiratory distress syndrome and improves survival in septic patients. Additionally, encouraging preclinical studies investigating the usefulness of a new mode of ventilatory support (liquid ventilation) to treat respiratory therapy failure are appearing with increased frequency. Last, the role of extracorporeal membrane oxygenation in the treatment of respiratory failure continues to be defined.

Clinical trials evaluating the efficacy of resuscitative therapies directed at achieving supranormal levels of oxygen delivery continue to document that patients who manifest these levels have an improved survival rate. However, it is unknown to what extent this increased survival rate in patients who have a supranormal response develop is the result of the self-selection of healthier patients vs. the therapy used to increase oxygen delivery. On the other hand, it is clear that the routine transfusion of blood purely to increase the oxygen-carrying capacity in patients in intensive care units is neither necessary nor clinically beneficial. In contrast, the use of tonometrically measured gastric mucosal pH as an indicator of splanchnic perfusion and as a prognostic factor for survival is becoming more established each year. Similarly, data continue to accrue supporting the hemodynamic benefits of hemofiltration therapy in critically ill patients with organ failure, whereas anecdotal studies indicate that hemofiltration with dialysis may be an effective method of removing cytokines from the plasma of septic patients (2).

As multiple organ failure is the most common cause of death in the intensive care unit, studies clarifying its pathogenesis are uniquely important. In this regard, one important, common thread that has emerged during the past several years is the relationship between inflammation, ischemia, and organ injury. As illustrated by several of the selected articles, studies investigating these relationships (by providing new mechanistic information) have led to novel therapeutic options, which are currently being evaluated in preclinical and clinical trials. Likewise, because of the clinical importance of immunity, infection, and endotoxemia, selected studies in these areas have been included as well.

Edwin A. Deitch, M.D.

References

1. Moncada S, Higgs A: The L-arginine-nitric oxide pathway. *New Engl J Med* 329:2002–2012, 1993.
2. Bellomo R, Tipping P, Boyce N: Continuous veno-venous hemofiltration with dialysis removes cytokines from the circulation of septic patients. *Crit Care Med* 21:522–526, 1993.

Inhaled Nitric Oxide for the Adult Respiratory Distress Syndrome
Rossaint R, Falke KJ, López F, Slama K. Pison U, Zapol WM (Freie Universität Berlin, Germany; Massachusetts Gen Hosp, Boston)
N Engl J Med 328:399–405, 1993   140-94-2–1

Introduction.—Patients with adult respiratory distress syndrome (ARDS) experience pulmonary hypertension and right-to-left shunting of venous blood. Although vasodilators can reduce the abnormally elevated pulmonary vascular resistance, they may lead to systemic arterial hypotension, right ventricular ischemia, and heart failure. Researchers tested the hypothesis that inhaled nitric acid would selectively improve perfusion of ventilated lung regions, thus improving gas exchange and reducing pulmonary hypertension.

Patients and Methods.—Ten consecutive patients with severe ARDS entered the study. The patients ranged in age from 17 to 46 years; none had a history of lung disease. Nitric oxide was inhaled in 2 concentrations for 40 minutes each. During the inhalation period, hemodynamic variables, gas exchange, and ventilation-perfusion distributions were measured with multiple inert-gas–elimination techniques. The results were compared with those obtained with an intravenous infusion of prostacyclin at a rate of 4 ng per kilogram of body weight per minute. Seven patients were treated with continuous inhalation of nitric oxide at a concentration of 5 to 20 ppm for 3 to 53 days.

Results.—Nitric oxide inhalation usually resulted in a prompt reduction in the pulmonary-artery pressure (PAP) and a concomitant increase in the arterial oxygenation efficiency. During inhalation of nitric acid at 18 ppm, PAP decreased by 6 mm Hg from baseline; no significant difference was noted between 18 and 36 ppm. Intrapulmonary shunting decreased from 36% to 31% at a concentration of 18 ppm. The mean arterial pressure and cardiac output remained unchanged during nitric oxide administration. The intravenous infusion of prostacyclin reduced PAP but increased intrapulmonary shunting and reduced the arterial oxygenation efficiency and systemic arterial pressure. Continuous inhalation of nitric oxide consistently reduced PAP and augmented the arterial oxygenation efficiency. During daily brief interruptions of continuous nitric oxide therapy, PAP consistently increased and arterial oxygenation efficiency was consistently decreased.

Conclusion.—Inhalation of nitric acid for 3 to 53 days remained effective in reducing pulmonary artery hypertension and improving oxygen exchange without causing tachyphylaxis. The impact of inhaled nitric acid on outcome in ARDS remains to be determined.

▶ This is a good idea. What could possibly be a better way of correcting ventilation-perfusion mismatches in patients with ARDS than the selective vasodilation of only those alveoli that are being ventilated?

The use of inhaled nitric oxide is based on 2 concepts. First, ARDS is characterized by increased intrapulmonary shunting related to widespread vasoconstriction and occlusion of the pulmonary microvasculature. Second, in contrast to intravenously administered vasodilators, inhaled nitric oxide would only reach—and thereby only dilate—the microvasculature of ventilated regions of the lung. As documented in this abstracted study, this strategy worked. By selectively dilating only ventilated microvasculature and by improving the matching of ventilation to perfusion, inhaled nitric oxide decreased intrapulmonary shunting and improved arterial oxygenation while reducing pulmonary artery pressure.—E.A. Deitch, M.D.

A New Approach in the Treatment of Hypotension in Human Septic Shock by N^G-Monomethyl-L-Arginine, an Inhibitor of the Nitric Oxide Synthetase

Schilling J, Cakmakci M, Bättig U, Geroulanos S (Univ Hosp Zürich, Switzerland)
Intensive Care Med 19:227–231, 1993   140-94-2-2

Background.—Nitric-oxide synthetase is inhibited by N^G-monomethyl-L-arginine (L-NMMA). Physiologic vascular tone, blood pressure, and tissue perfusion, via guanylate-cyclase and cyclic guanosine monophosphate, are all regulated by nitric oxide (NO). Overproduction of NO occurs in advanced therapy–resistant septic shock in response to inflammatory mediators, resulting in vasodilation, decreased systemic blood pressure, and decreased vasoconstriction response to sympathetic stimuli. The use of L-NMMA was successful in the treatment of severe, prolonged hypotension in a patient with sepsis.

Case Report.—Man, 29, was seen in the intensive care unit with necrotizing pancreatitis. He required ventilatory support throughout his stay, during which he underwent a total of 11 surgical interventions. He underwent hemofiltration for 54 days, during which he had several episodes of septicemia, which was managed by antibiotics. His condition began to improve on day 90, and hemofiltration was stopped; however, on day 119 it had to be reintroduced because of severe septic shock caused by multiresistant coagulase-negative staphylococcus. Despite antimicrobial therapy and massive fluid replacement, the patient's condition deteriorated and he was expected to die.

Given this desperate situation, L-NMMA was administered, the first time it had been used therapeutically. The patient was given an intravenous bolus of 100 mg, followed by 3 injections of 200 mg. Blood pressure increased after each injection, dropping again to normal a few minutes later. The use of L-NMMA ultimately allowed cessation of the continuous high doses of noradrenaline and dobutamine the patient had been receiving. There were no side effects, and the patient remained hemodynamically stable for 12 days. Four weeks later, another septic episode required another course of L-NMMA, with the same results as the first time. Despite the immediate blood pressure response, heart rate and central venous pressure remained stable. There was a 32% decrease in cardiac output and an increase in PaO$_2$.

Conclusions.—This clinical experience with L-NMMA suggests that nitric oxide-synthetase inhibitors may be a useful treatment for septic shock. Formal toxicologic studies will be needed before these agents are introduced into clinical use.

L-Arginine Pathway in the Sepsis Syndrome

Lorente JA, Landín L, De Pablo R, Renes E, Liste D (Hospital Universitario de Getafe, Madrid; Hospital Ramón y Cajal, Madrid; Hospital 12 de Octubre, Madrid)

Crit Care Med 21:1287–1295, 1993   140-94-2-3

Introduction.—Sepsis is characterized by systemic vasodilation, defective vascular reactivity to vasocontrictors, and an abnormality in microvascular regulation. Endothelial-derived relaxing factor has recently been identified as nitric oxide, which is synthesized from L-arginine by an enzyme present in the vascular endothelium. It has been hypothesized that increased release of nitric oxide may contribute to sepsis. However, the effects on sepsis of inhibiting nitric oxide synthesis or, conversely, of providing excess substrate for conversion to nitric oxide have not been studied. The systemic and pulmonary hemodynamic effects of inhibiting nitric oxide synthesis and providing excess L-arginine were examined.

Study Design.—In prospective study of 15 patients with a diagnosis of sepsis, 8 received N^{ω}-nitro-L-arginine, followed by L-arginine, and 7 received L-arginine alone. Data were recorded before and after administration.

Results.—The administration of N^{ω}-nitro-L-arginine was followed by hypertension, a decrease in the cardiac index (from 3.5 to 2.7 L/min/m^2), a doubling of the systemic vascular resistance (from 1,871 to 3,825 dyne·sec/cm^2 ·m^2), plus an increase in right atrial and pulmonary artery occlusion pressures. These changes were reversed by the administration of L-arginine. The administration of L-arginine alone caused transient hypotension, increased cardiac index, and a decrease in both systemic and pulmonary vascular resistance. The oxygen consumption index increased significantly 1 minute after administration of L-arginine.

Conclusions.—In patients with sepsis, a continuous basal release of nitric oxide plays a role in the regulation of systemic and pulmonary vascular tone. L-Arginine has systemic and pulmonary vasodilatory actions. Further studies are needed to investigate the role of inhibitors of nitric oxide synthesis or of L-arginine in the treatment of patients with the sepsis syndrome.

▶ The first of these 2 abstracts, Abstract 140-94-2-2, clearly describes the beneficial effects of inhibiting production of nitric oxide in a septic patient who has refractory shock and thus highlights the fact that overproduction of nitric oxide may be clinically deleterious. However, as shown in numerous animal studies, indiscriminate or excessive inhibition of nitric oxide can lead to major adverse effects, including severe vasoconstriction, organ injury, and death. Thus, there appears to be a physiologic fine line between the beneficial vs. the deleterious effects of inhibition of nitric oxide, which appears to be somewhat dose-dependent. Thus, from a therapeutic standpoint, it is still not known to what extent the inhibition of nitric oxide synthesis is beneficial in septic patients.

Consequently, the value of the second abstract, Abstract 140-94-2-3, is that it provides some of the first hemodynamic data on the effects of inhibiting, as well as augmenting, synthesis of nitric oxide in patients with the sepsis syndrome. This study clearly shows that inhibition of nitric oxide synthesis induces several potentially deleterious hemodynamic effects, including a decrease in cardiac output and oxygen delivery, plus an excessive increase in systemic vascular resistance, pulmonary vascular resistance, and pulmonary artery pressure. Therefore, at the current time, although it is exciting, the use of drugs to modulate systemic nitric oxide synthesis in septic patients must be considered experimental.—E.A. Deitch, M.D.

A Double-Blind, Prospective, Randomized Trial of Ketoconazole, a Thromboxane Synthetase Inhibitor, in the Prophylaxis of the Adult Respiratory Distress Syndrome

Yu M, Tomasa G (Univ of Hawaii, Honolulu)
Crit Care Med 21:1635–1642, 1993   140-94-2-4

Objective.—Several prospective studies have identified sepsis as the major risk factor for the development of adult respiratory distress syndrome (ARDS). Whether the thromboxane A_2 synthetase inhibitor ketoconazole could reduce the incidence of ARDS in septic patients was investigated in a prospective, randomized, double-blind, placebo-controlled study.

Study Plan.—Fifty-four consecutive patients admitted to a surgical intensive care unit with a diagnosis of sepsis were enrolled in the study. They received either 400 mg of ketoconazole or a placebo, either orally or via nasogastric tube, within 24 hours of admission to intensive care. Drug administration was continued for 21 days or until the patient left the intensive care unit.

Results.—The frequency of ARDS was reduced from 64% in placebo recipients to 15% in ketoconazole-treated patients. Active treatment also was associated with a decrease in mortality from 39% to 15%. Time in the intensive care unit and the need for ventilatory assistance were not significantly different in the treatment and placebo groups.

Conclusion.—Administration of ketoconazole early in the course of sepsis may prevent the development of ARDS and significantly reduce mortality in high-risk septic patients.

▶ The results of this randomized controlled trial that uses ketoconazole to prevent the development of ARDS in septic patients are truly impressive. These results are even more impressive when one considers the long list of promising therapeutic agents that have been founded on the shoals of clinical trials during the past decade. The only limitation of this study was the authors' failure to define the underlying diseases and causes of sepsis in the patients who were enrolled. Because of this limitation, it is not possible to know exactly which patient populations are most likely to benefit from prophylactic ketoconazole therapy. Nonetheless, the results of this study are exciting and, if these promising results are verified by other investigators, I would expect that ketoconazole will earn a place in the treatment of the septic patient.—E.A. Deitch, M.D.

Intratracheal Perfluorocarbon Administration Combined With Mechanical Ventilation in Experimental Respiratory Distress Syndrome: Dose-Dependent Improvement of Gas Exchange

Tütüncü AS, Faithfull NS, Lachmann B (Erasmus Univ Rotterdam, The Netherlands; Alliance Pharmaceutical Corp, San Diego, Calif)
Crit Care Med 21:962–969, 1993   140-94-2-5

Introduction.—Advances in conventional mechanical ventilation have improved survival in respiratory distress syndrome, but this complex syndrome remains a major problem in the intensive care unit. In surfactant-deficient lungs, oxygenated perfluorocarbon liquids have been used as an alternative respiratory medium because of their low surface tension and ability to dissolve large amounts of respiratory gases. Rabbits were studied to determine the efficacy of intratracheal perfluorocarbon plus conventional mechanical ventilation in acute respiratory failure.

Methods.—In a prospective study, adult male New Zealand rabbits underwent repeated lung lavage with saline to induce respiratory failure. One group of animals was randomized to receive perfluorocarbon treatment, consisting of intratracheal instillation of incremental doses of 3mL of each liquid per kg, to a total volume of 15 mL/kg, whereas the other group received placebo treatment.

Results.—After the first dose of perfluorocarbon, partial pressure of oxygen in alveolar gas increased from 75 to 420 torr, and partial pressure of carbon dioxide in alveolar gas decreased from 49 to 43 torr. Both values remained stable thereafter. Perfluorocarbon treatment also induced significant declines in airway pressures. Alveolar ventilation was well preserved, and alveolar dead-space decreased and remained stable. Perfluorocarbon treatment was well tolerated.

Conclusions.—There were dramatic improvements in the pulmonary parameters in perfluorocarbon-treated rabbits in acute respiratory failure. The type of ventilatory support used in this study may represent an effective and simple technique of clinical perfluorocarbon application.

▶ Hard to believe, isn't it? However, other investigators have also documented that liquid breathing with perfluorocarbon solutions improves lung function in experimental models of adult respiratory distress syndrome (1) and in neonates with respiratory distress syndrome (2). One advantage and a unique aspect of this study on liquid ventilation is that by using partial liquid ventilation in combination with gas exchange, the authors were able to use a conventional ventilatory apparatus rather than the complex ventilatory and extracorporeal oxygenation apparatus required for full liquid ventilation.

A basic concept of liquid ventilation is that the liquid-filled lung can be expanded at low pressures, thereby limiting both ventilator-induced barotrauma and alveolar collapse. Thus, liquid ventilation offers some benefits over traditional gas ventilation. For this reason, it will become important for clinicians to become familiar with this technique as it winds its way from the laboratory to the bedside.—E.A. Deitch, M.D.

References

1. Leach LW, et al: *Crit Care Med* 21:1270, 1993.
2. Greenspan JS, et al: *J Pediatr* 117:106, 1990.

Extracorporeal Membrane Oxygenation: Support for Overwhelming Pulmonary Failure in the Pediatric Population. Collective Experience From the Extracorporeal Life Support Organization
O'Rourke PP, Stolar CJH, Zwischenberger JB, Snedecor SM, Bartlett RH (Extracorporeal Life Support Org, Ann Arbor, Mich)
J Pediatr Surg 28:523–529, 1993   140-94-2-6

Introduction.—Extracorporeal membrane oxygenation (ECMO) is an established therapy for newborns with overwhelming cardiorespiratory failure. Its value in older pediatric patients with respiratory failure is less clear. The role of ECMO in this patient population was examined using

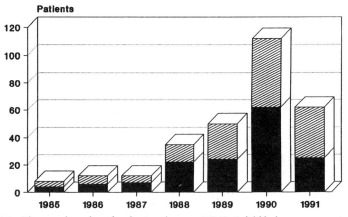

Fig 2-1.—The annual number of pediatric pulmonary ECMO. *Solid black* represents patients who died; *gray-shaded*, those who survived. Data from 1991 are incomplete. (Courtesy of O'Rourke PP, Stolar CJH, Zwischenberger JB, et al: *J Pediatr Surg* 28:523-529, 1993.)

data from the Extracorporeal Life Support Organization (ELSO), a multicenter registry.

Methods.—Pediatric patients were defined as older than 14 days and younger than 18 years of age. Between January 1982 and September 1991, 285 children in this age group were supported with ECMO at the participating centers. The therapeutic goal of ECMO support was to maintain adequate oxygen delivery and carbon dioxide removal while utilizing minimal mechanical ventilation and supplemental oxygen.

Results.—Seven of the 82 ECMO centers were responsible for 50% of the total registered cases. There was a ninefold increase in the annual number of treated patients between 1987 and 1990. The median age of the patients was 13 months; the most common diagnoses were viral pneumonia (32%) and adult respiratory distress syndrome (28%). Predicted mortality for the patients enrolled ranged from 85% to 100%. Overall survival was 47% (Fig 2-1). Survivors were significantly younger (mean age, 23 months) than nonsurvivors (mean age, 42 months). The nonsurvivors had a significantly higher mean airway pressure than the survivors (25.3 vs. 22.0 cm H_2O). The mean duration of ECMO was approximately 10 days. Mechanical complications directly related to the ECMO circuit occurred in 50% of the patients and were more frequent in nonsurvivors than in survivors. Survivors also experienced fewer medical complications than nonsurvivors.

Conclusion.—Most neonates treated with ECMO have intractable persistent pulmonary hypertension of the newborn, and ECMO is now considered the standard of care in these patients. Older pediatric patients have more heterogeneous diagnoses and present a spectrum of patient ages and lung development. Selection criteria for older children are poorly defined and nonspecific. Only a prospective randomized study can confirm the value of ECMO in this population.

▶ Although this article on ECMO is limited to pediatric patients, it does provide a good review of the current status of ECMO used as rescue therapy in patients with otherwise lethal respiratory failure. Furthermore, based on the higher-than-predicted survival rate in this group of patients with diverse diseases and advances in ECMO technology, reconsideration of the potential usefulness of ECMO in older patients seems to be in order.—E.A. Deitch, M.D.

Effect of Maximizing Oxygen Delivery on Morbidity and Mortality Rates in Critically Ill Patients: A Prospective, Randomized, Controlled Study

Yu M, Levy MM, Smith P, Takiguchi SA, Miyasaki A, Myers SA (Univ of Hawaii, Honolulu)

Crit Care Med 21:830–838, 1993   140-94-2-7

Background.—There is considerable disagreement about shock resuscitation. The effects on morbidity and mortality of optimizing oxygen delivery $\dot{D}o_2$) to supranormal levels in patients with sepsis, septic shock, and adult respiratory distress syndrome were studied.

Methods.—Sixty-seven patients were included in the prospective, randomized, controlled trial. All patients had pulmonary artery catheters and met the criteria for sepsis or septic shock, adult respiratory distress syndrome, or hypovolemic shock. Patients in the treatment group were assigned a therapeutic $\dot{D}o_2$ indexed ($\dot{D}o_2I$) goal of more than 600 mL/min/m². To achieve this goal, fluid boluses, blood products, and inotropes were used. The therapeutic goal in the control group was simply the "normal" $\dot{D}o_2I$ range of 450–550 mL/min/m². Attempts were made to achieve these goals within 24 hours of study entry.

Findings.—The treatment and control groups were comparable in mortality, development of organ failure, days in the intensive care unit, and days in the hospital. Clinically distinct subgroups emerged: those in the treatment group who achieved supranormal $\dot{D}o_2I$, those in the control group with normal $\dot{D}o_2I$, a treatment subgroup that failed to reach the target $\dot{D}o_2I$, a control group that self-generated to high $\dot{D}o_2I$ values, and a small number of patients who could not even reach a $\dot{D}o_2I$ of 450 mL/min/min². These subgroups were similar and matched. The death rate was significantly lower among patients in groups reaching supranormal values of $\dot{D}o_2I$, whether the patients were treated or self-generated, when compared with patients reaching normal $\dot{D}o_2I$ values.

Conclusions.—Subgroup analysis in this study showed a strong, significant difference between patients with supranormal values of oxygen transport and patients with normal levels of $\dot{D}o_2$. Supranormal values of $\dot{D}o_2I$ were associated with a significant reduction in death rates (14% vs. 56%; $P < .001$). Thus, the current standard of care of treating critically ill patients to normal $\dot{D}o_2I$ should be reconsidered. Maximizing to high $\dot{D}o_2I$ may be more appropriate.

▶ What is the chicken and what is the egg? In other words, is survival increased because of therapy directed to achieve supranormal, rather than normal, levels of oxygen delivery, or do the development and maintenance of a hyperdynamic response characterized by supranormal levels of oxygen delivery just identify those patients who are more likely to survive? This distinction is important both clinically and conceptually.

This study provides data that can be interpreted to support both options. On one hand, there was no difference in outcome between the patients randomized to normal vs. supranormal oxygen delivery. On the other hand, patients who had supranormal oxygen delivery develop, whether as a goal of therapy or spontaneously, had increased survival. Until studies evaluating the effect of increasing oxygen delivery from normal to supranormal levels are done in patients with normal oxygen delivery values after full-volume resuscitation, it will not be possible to determine whether the lower mortality rate in patients with supranormal oxygen delivery is secondary to self-selection of healthier patients or to active therapeutic interventions. Until these data become available, the question of what is the chicken and what is the egg must remain unanswered. Nonetheless, in the absence of convincing data that aggressive resuscitation is dangerous, I concur with the authors' recommendation to try to achieve supranormal levels of oxygen delivery.—E.A. Deitch, M.D.

Effects of Blood Transfusion on Oxygen Transport Variables in Severe Sepsis

Lorente JA, Landín L, De Pablo R, Renes E, Rodríguez-Díaz R, Liste D (Hosp Ramón y Cajal, Madrid; Hosp Universitario de Getafe, Madrid)
Crit Care Med 21:1312–1318, 1993   140-94-2–8

Purpose.—Previous studies have shown that sepsis is characterized by an abnormal relationship between oxygen delivery and oxygen uptake. Whether increasing oxygen delivery by means of a packed red cell transfusion would improve oxygen utilization in patients with sepsis was investigated in a prospective, randomized, interventional study.

Study Design.—Sixteen patients with severe sepsis and a hemoglobin concentration below 10 g/dL received, in random order, 800 mL of packed red cells transfused over 90 minutes and a dobutamine infusion, 10 μg/kg/min. Hemodynamic and oxygen transport variables were measured before and after each intervention. At least 20 minutes was allowed during dobutamine infusion to reach the steady state.

Results.—Dobutamine infusion increased oxygen delivery by a mean of 48.5% and oxygen uptake by a mean of 21.7%. Blood transfusion increased oxygen delivery by a mean of 21.4%, but oxygen uptake did not change significantly.

Conclusion.—The failure of blood transfusion to increase oxygen uptake in septic patients with an abnormal relationship between oxygen delivery and oxygen uptake illustrates that oxygen uptake in these patients depends more on blood flow than on global oxygen delivery.

▶ Blood transfusions are not without risk; they are immunosuppressive and are associated with the transmission of infectious agents. Hence, it is important to be sure that the indications for transfusion are well justified and will benefit the patient. Thus, the importance of this study, which further documents that prophylactic blood transfusions done purely to increase the oxygen carrying capacity in patients in the intensive care unit, is without measurable clinical benefit. One must always remember that it is more important to treat the patient than the doctor. In the case of blood transfusions done solely to increase oxygen carrying capacity, it appears that one is treating the doctor and not the patient.—E.A. Deitch, M.D.

Assessment of Splanchnic Oxygenation by Gastric Tonometry in Patients With Acute Circulatory Failure

Maynard N, Bihari D, Beale R, Smithies M, Baldock G, Mason R, McColl I
(Guy's Hosp, London; Lewisham Hosp, London)
JAMA 270:1203–1210, 1993   140-94-2–9

Introduction.—Up to 85% of deaths that occur in surgical intensive care units (ICUs) are associated with acute circulatory failure and progression to multiple organ failure (MOP). The clinical condition resulting from these events has been described as the sepsis syndrome or a state of nonbacterial clinical sepsis. Splanchnic ischemia may play a role in such cases leading to a reduction in gut barrier function. The importance of splanchnic ischemia in acute circulatory failure was investigated.

Patients and Methods.—The study subjects were 83 consecutive patients in 2 general ICUs in London. The group had a mean age of 60.7 years and a mean 24-hour Acute Physiology and Chronic Health Evaluation II (APACHE II) score of 20.3. All had acute circulatory failure in the first 24 hours after admission to the ICU and were receiving mechanical ventilation at the time of the study. Gastric intramucosal pH, systemic hemodynamics, oxygen transport, and metabolic variables were measured at admission and at 12 and 24 hours after admission.

Results.—The ICU mortality of the patients studied was 39.7%; the hospital mortality was 41%. Compared with survivors, nonsurvivors had a significantly higher heart rate and a significantly lower mean arterial pressure. Survivors and nonsurvivors showed no consistent differences in cardiac index, oxygen delivery, and oxygen uptake. The mean gastric intramucosal pH was 7.40 on admission and at 24 hours in survivors; corresponding findings for nonsurvivors, 7.28 and 7.24, differed significantly. Admission arterial pH was significantly lower in nonsurvivors, base exchange was more negative, and lactate concentration was higher. Of the variables studied, gastric intramucosal pH had a high sensitivity (88%) for the prediction of an ICU death. The likelihood ratio for gastric intramucosal pH was 2.32, higher than for any other variable.

Conclusion.—Gastric intramucosal pH as measured by tonometry was the most reliable indicator of adequacy of tissue oxygenation in these patients. Inadequate oxygenation of the gut is associated with a poor outcome, and attempts to improve splanchnic blood flow and gastric intramucosal pH may help increase survival in patients with MOF.

▶ The observation that gastric mucosal pH was the best predictor of survival is of potential importance for several reasons. First, it points out that compared with systemic measurements, assessment of regional (organ) oxygenation is likely to be a more accurate measure of adequate oxygen delivery and, hence, outcome. Second, a decrease in mucosal gastric pH may serve as an early warning that tissue perfusion is inadequate and therefore could identify patients in whom therapy directed at improving tissue perfusion would be warranted. Third, it may be possible to assess the efficacy of specific therapeutic maneuvers directed at improving organ blood flow by monitoring changes in gastric mucosal pH.

This discussion does not directly address the underlying reasons why patients with tonometrically documented intestinal ischemia have a worse outcome. For a discussion of how splanchnic hypoperfusion might promote distant organ injury, see the next abstract.—E.A. Deitch, M.D.

Intestinal Ischemia-Reperfusion Injury Causes Pulmonary Endothelial Cell ATP Depletion
Gerkin TM, Oldham KT, Guice KS, Hinshaw DB, Ryan US (Duke Univ, Durham, NC; Univ of Michigan, Ann Arbor; Washington Univ, St Louis, Mo)
Ann Surg 217:48–56, 1993   140-94-2-10

Background.—Intestinal ischemia–reperfusion can activate the endogenous inflammatory response that initiates multiple organ failure and associated morbidity, including adult respiratory distress syndrome. Previous studies have shown that cellular adenosine triphosphate (ATP) depletion is an early sign of endothelial cell dysfunction. Whether noncellular humoral factors associated with intestinal ischemia–reperfusion cause ATP depletion in pulmonary endothelial cells was tested.

Methods.—All experiments were done in Sprague-Dawley rats. After midline laparotomy, the superior mesenteric artery was occluded with a

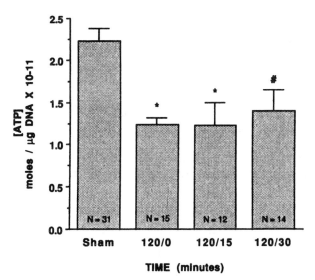

Fig 2–2.—Endothelial cell ATP levels after 4-hour incubation with intestinal ischemia–reperfusion plasma. Data are pooled from 5 individual experiments with sample size indicated. Time points on the *x-axis* represent minutes of intestinal ischemia/minutes of intestinal reperfusion. For example, 120/0 represents 120 minutes of ischemia and no reperfusion. (*P < .001 vs. sham; #P < .005 vs. sham). (Courtesy of Gerkin TM, Oldham KT, Guice KS, et al: *Ann Surg* 217:48–56, 1993.)

microvascular clip. Intestinal ischemia was maintained for 120 minutes, followed by clip removal and reperfusion. Plasma samples were obtained from the portal vein after ischemia and after reperfusion for 15 and 30 minutes. Monolayers of cultured rat pulmonary artery endothelial cells were then incubated with the plasma samples. Cytotoxicity was measured using a ^{51}Cr-release assay.

Results.—Pulmonary artery endothelial cells incubated for 4 hours in plasma from rats undergoing 120 minutes of intestinal ischemia showed a significant decrease in cellular ATP levels, whereas cells incubated for 4 hours in plasma from sham-operated animals had stable ATP levels (Fig 2-2). Incubation of endothelial cells with plasma from either sham animals or injured animals caused no significant cytotoxic injury.

Conclusion.—Humoral factors associated with intestinal ischemia-reperfusion injury cause depletion of pulmonary endothelial cell energy stores, which may predispose the cell to more severe injury by other mediators of the endogenous inflammatory response. The precise humoral factors responsible for the ATP depletion have not yet been identified.

▶ The prognostic importance of adequate intestinal perfusion was clearly documented in Abstract 140-94-2-9, which investigated the clinical utility of gastric tonometry. Why, however, is gut ischemia such a poor prognostic finding? The answer appears to be the result of intestinal injury predisposing to the development of a systemic inflammatory response, as well as to the translocation of bacteria and their products (endotoxin) from the gut to the systemic tissues, which thereby promotes distant organ injury.

In the lung, activation of the systemic inflammatory response leads to acute lung injury and clinical respiratory failure through alterations in endothelial cell function and the recruitment of neutrophils. Studies such as this one, which investigates the potential mechanisms by which intestinal injury leads to endothelial cell injury, are helping us to understand the pathogenesis of adult respiratory distress syndrome, as well as the role of the intestine in the development of multiple organ failure.—E.A. Deitch, M.D.

Improved Cardiovascular Stability During Continuous Modes of Renal Replacement Therapy in Critically Ill Patients With Acute Hepatic and Renal Failure
Davenport A, Will EJ, Davidson AM (St James's Univ Hosp, Leeds, England)
Crit Care Med 21:328–338, 1993   140-94-2-11

Background.—Studies have shown that when compared with standard hemodialysis, intermittent daily hemofiltration by machine results in greater cardiac stability, less change in intracranial pressure, and less cerebral edema. Whether continuous modes of renal replacement treatment result in improved cardiovascular stability compared with standard daily intermittent therapy in critically ill patients was investigated.

Methods.—Thirty-two consecutive, critically ill, mechanically ventilated patients were enrolled in a prospective, randomized, controlled trial. All patients had combined acute hepatic and renal failure. By random assignment, the patients were treated with either intermittent machine hemofiltration or 2 continuous modes of renal replacement therapy, continuous arteriovenous hemofiltration (CAVH) or arteriovenous hemofiltration with dialysis (CAVHD). Cardiac output, tissue oxygen delivery, and uptake were determined during 32 treatments with intermittent machine hemofiltration and during the first 5 hours of 25 continuous treatments.

Results.—In the first hour of therapy, the cardiac index was reduced by a mean of 15% during intermittent machine hemofiltration. No significant change occurred during the continuous modes of treatment. The decrease in cardiac output during intermittent machine hemofiltration was related to a maximum reduction in the mean arterial pressure from 82 to 66 mm Hg and a mean decrease in pulmonary artery occlusion pressure of 27%, tissue oxygen delivery of 15%, and tissue oxygen uptake of 12%. There was no significant change in systemic vascular resistance, and pulmonary vascular resistance increased by a mean of 50%. There also was a mean maximum increase in intracranial pressure of 45% in the first hour of intermittent machine hemofiltration. No significant changes occurred in the same time during continuous modes of renal replacement therapy.

Conclusions.—In critically ill patients with impairment of tissue oxygen delivery, the use of continuous modes of renal replacement therapy is preferred because of the better cardiovascular tolerance, compared with that of daily intermittent machine treatments.

▶ There is no doubt that hemofiltration is associated with better preservation of cardiovascular function than is standard hemodialysis, and this study indicates that continuous hemofiltration maintains cardiovascular function better than intermittent hemofiltration. Thus, this article was chosen to stress the clinical benefits of hemofiltration in critically ill patients with acute renal failure.—E.A. Deitch, M.D.

Impaired β-Adrenergic Receptor Stimulation of Cyclic Adenosine Monophosphate in Human Septic Shock: Association With Myocardial Hyporesponsiveness to Catecholamines
Silverman HJ, Penaranda R, Orens JB, Lee NH (Univ of Maryland, Baltimore)
Crit Care Med 21:31–39, 1993   140-94-2-12

Objective.—Several studies have identified myocardial hyporesponsiveness to administered catecholamines in human sepsis. Whether this phenomenon is caused by impaired β-adrenergic receptor stimulation of cyclic adenosine monophosphate (cAMP), the primary mediator of myocardial inotropy, was determined.

Dose Response to Dobutamine in Septic and Septic Shock Groups

	Sepsis (n = 7) Dobutamine Dose (µg/kg/min)			Septic Shock (n = 9) Dobutamine Dose (µg/kg/min)		
	0	5	10	0	5	10
HR (beats/min)	101 ± 9	107 ± 10	113 ± 10 *	125 ± 6	123 ± 5	128 ± 6
MAP (mm Hg)	92 ± 5	98 ± 5	101 ± 6	69 ± 5	74 ± 5	73 ± 5
PAOP (mm Hg)	13 ± 1	12 ± 1	12 ± 1	13 ± 2	13 ± 2	13 ± 2
CI (L/min·m²)	4.4 ± 0.3	5.5 ± 0.4†	6.1 ± 0.4†	3.1 ± 0.3	3.5 ± 0.4	3.8 ± 0.3
SVR (dyne·sec/cm⁵)	828 ± 108	704 ± 78	658 ± 77	1027 ± 161	984 ± 145	888 ± 121
LVSWI (g·m/m²)	51.5 ± 5.3	67.5 ± 10.0	74.1 ± 11.5 *	19.2 ± 2.3	23.1 ± 2.7	24.5 ± 2.8

Abbreviations: HR, heart rate; *MAP*, mean arterial pressure; *PAOP*, pulmonary artery occlusion pressure; *CI*, cardiac index; *SVR*, systemic vascular resistance; *LVSWI*, left ventricular stroke work index.

Analysis was performed between the respective means of the absolute changes from baseline.

* $P < .05$; † $P < .01$ compared with septic shock.

(Courtesy of Silverman HJ, Penaranda R, Orens JB, et al: *Crit Care Med* 21:31–39, 1993.)

Patients.—The study population consisted of 7 normal volunteers, 9 critically ill patients who were not septic, 16 patients who were septic and not in shock, and 17 patients who were septic and in shock. Hemodynamic monitoring data were obtained from patients who were nonshock septic and those who were in septic shock. To evaluate the integrity of the β-adrenergic receptor complex, isoproterenol- and sodium fluoride–stimulated cAMP accumulations were measured in circulating lymphocytes. To determine whether impaired β-adrenergic receptor complex functioning represents a physiologic defect, the heart rate responses to sequential infusions of dobutamine, 5 and 10 μg/kg/min, were obtained in patients who were nonshock septic and those who were in septic shock.

Results.—At 2 days after the onset of sepsis, patients in septic shock had significantly lower hemodynamic values than patients who were nonshock septic. Furthermore, patients in septic shock had significantly greater reductions in cAMP accumulations in response to stimulation with isoproterenol and sodium fluoride than did patients who were nonshock septic. Finally, patients in septic shock had significantly lower heart rate responses to administration of dobutamine than patients who were nonshock septic (table).

Conclusions.—The myocardial hyporesponsiveness to catecholamine administration in patients with septic shock appears to be attributable to impaired β-adrenergic receptor stimulation of cAMP.

▶ Why is it that patients in septic shock respond to pressor agents so poorly? Is it a result of ischemic damage, energetic failure of the cells, circulating antagonists, etc.? This study indicates that the answer is decreased β-adrenergic receptor function. Because myocardial depression and peripheral vascular dilatation that is unresponsive to catecholamines are major components of septic shock, studies investigating the basic biology of these phenomena are of importance. Consequently, this basic study was chosen for 2 reasons. First, because it helps clarify why patients in septic shock do not show a good response to exogenous catecholamines and, second, because good therapy follows good science, i.e., it is only through studies investigating the mechanisms of disease that we will be able to develop new and appropriate therapeutic options.—E.A. Deitch, M.D.

Blockade of Complement Activation Prevents Local and Pulmonary Albumin Leak After Lower Torso Ischemia-Reperfusion

Lindsay TF, Hill J, Ortiz F, Rudolph A, Valeri CR, Hechtman HB, Moore FD Jr (Harvard Med School, Boston; T Cell Sciences, Inc, Cambridge, Mass; Naval Blood Research Labs, Chelsea, Mass)
Ann Surg 216:677–683, 1992   140-94-2–13

Introduction.—Ischemia of the lower torso, followed by reperfusion, leads to both local muscle edema and necrosis and remote injury, as re-

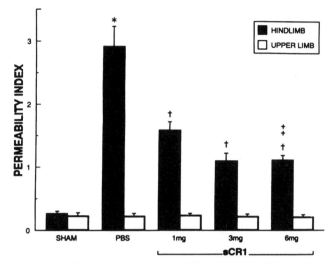

Fig 2–3.—Treatment with sCR1 reduced the permeability index in hindlimb muscle after 4 hours of bilateral hindlimb ischemia and 4 hours of reperfusion. The 6-mg dose was significantly better than the 1-mg dose. *P < .001 vs. sham; †P < .01 vs. PBS; ‡P < .05. The permeability index for the control upper limb muscle is shown to the right of each ischemic histogram. (Courtesy of Lindsay TF, Hill J, Ortiz, et al: *Ann Surg* 216:677–683, 1992.)

flected by increased permeability of small pulmonary vessels and neutrophil sequestration. Serum complement may help mediate the remote response to hindlimb ischemia, because skeletal muscle ischemia and reperfusion reportedly consume factor B, a component of the alternate complement pathway.

Objective and Methods.—Adult rats were subjected to 4 hours of bilateral hindlimb ischemia, produced by tourniquets above the trochanter and, later, to 4 hours of reperfusion. Either phosphate-buffered saline (PBS) alone or saline-containing soluble human complement receptor type 1 (sCR1) was infused at the end of the ischemic period, the latter in a dose of 1, 3, or 6 mg. Lung permeability was estimated using radioiodine, and neutrophil sequestration in the lungs and in skeletal muscle was determined by myeloperoxidase (MPO) content.

Results.—Muscle permeability increased with the duration of reperfusion after 4 hours of hindlimb ischemia. Muscle edema also progressed during reperfusion. Pulmonary MPO activity was significantly increased after 4 hours of reperfusion, as were levels of radioiodine in bronchoalveolar lavage fluid. The increase in the permeability index of ischemic muscle noted after reperfusion was inhibited by administering sCRI (Fig 2–3). Microvascular permeability in the lungs also decreased. The functional activity of the classical complement pathway was reduced after ischemia and declined further after administration of sCRI. Functional activity of the alternate pathway was not altered by ischemia and reperfusion.

Implications.—Complement is activated during tourniquet ischemia in the rat, mediating permeability changes in both ischemic muscle and the lungs during reperfusion. The complement dependence of both local and systemic responses to skeletal muscle ischemia may allow the development of new interventions.

▶ Abstract 140-94-2–10 documented that intestinal ischemia can lead to pulmonary endothelial cell injury and thereby predispose to the development of adult respiratory distress syndrome. This abstract documents that hindlimb ischemia can also lead to pulmonary injury, apparently through the activation of complement. Taken together, these 2 articles illustrate that ischemic injury of 2 different tissues can lead to pulmonary injury. As such, they highlight the important concept that severe ischemia of 1 tissue or organ can lead to injury of a second organ through the activation of systemic inflammatory mediators.

That the authors' results document that the use of sCR1 to inhibit complement activation prevented increased local muscle and distant lung permeability is also important. These findings clearly establish a role for complement activation in the pathogenesis of ischemia-mediated increases in microvascular permeability. These encouraging results with sCR1 are consistent with those from other studies showing that modulation of complement activation via the use of soluble complement receptors can ameliorate ischemic tissue damage (1). For those who are interested, the role of the complement system in shock and tissue injury has been recently reviewed (2).—E.A. Deitch, M.D.

References

1. Pemberton M, et al: *J Immunol* 150:5104, 1993.
2. Deitch EA, Mancini MC: *Arch Surg* 128:1222, 1993.

In Vivo Neutralization of P-Selectin Protects Feline Heart and Endothelium in Myocardial Ischemia and Reperfusion Injury
Weyrich AS, Ma X-l, Lefer DJ, Albertine KH, Lefer AM (Thomas Jefferson Univ, Philadelphia; Johns Hopkins Univ, Baltimore, Md)
J Clin Invest 91:2620–2629, 1993   140-94-2–14

Background.—Rapid P-selectin expression on endothelial cells may be partly responsible for the initial cascade of polymorphonuclear neutrophil (PMN)–mediated effects that ultimately cause myocardial tissue damage after ischemia reperfusion. However, no in vitro study has assessed the role of P-selectin in the regulation of PMN recruitment in an ischemic–reperfusion setting.

Methods and Results.—The cardioprotective effects of an mAb to P-selectin, mAb PB1.3, were assessed in cats subjected to myocardial ischemia and reperfusion. PB1.3, 1 mg/kg, given after 80 minutes of ischemia, significantly attenuated myocardial necrosis when compared with a nonblocking mAb, NBP1.6. Endothelial release of endothelium-derived relaxing factor was also significantly preserved in ischemic-reperfused coronary arteries isolated from animals given PB1.3 compared with NBP1.6. Endothelial preservation was directly associated with decreased endothelial adherence of PMNs in ischemic–reperfused coronary arteries. Immunohistochemical localization of P-selectin was significantly upregulated in the cytoplasm of endothelial cells lining coronary arteries and veins after 90 minutes of ischemia and 20 minutes of reperfusion. Venous vessels were the main site of intracytoplasmic expression. PB1.3 significantly reduced adherence of unstimulated PMNs to thrombin and histamine stimulated endothelial cells in vitro in a concentration-dependent fashion.

Conclusions.—Adherence of PMN to endothelium by P-selectin is an important early result of reperfusion injury. A specific monoclonal antibody to P-selectin produces significant endothelial preservation and cardioprotection in myocardial ischemia and reperfusion.

▶ That endothelial cells actively participate in the evolution of processes injurious to tissues and induced by a variety of insults has recently been recognized. In this paradigm, tissue injury is mediated by activated neutrophils that bind to activated endothelial cells through specific receptors. The exact signals that initiate this process may vary to some extent between different organs but, in general, they include endotoxin, oxidants, activated complement factors, cytokines, thrombin, and histamine. Regardless of the initiating factors, endothelial–leukocyte interactions appear to be a common pathway leading to microvascular and tissue injury.

As illustrated by this abstracted article on ischemia/reperfusion–mediated myocardial injury, the process involves an endothelial phenotype changing from a noninflammatory to a proinflammatory phenotype. These activate proinflammatory endothelial cells have lost their anticoagulant properties and now activate the extrinsic clotting pathway. Furthermore, these proinflammatory endothelial cells express surface receptors, such as P-selectin, E-selectin, and intercellular adhesion molecule-1, that promote leukocyte adherence. This shift in endothelial phenotype ultimately results in focal microvascular thrombosis and leukocyte-mediated endothelial injury.

Although this biology may be interesting, why is it important for clinicians to know? The answer is that this biology has led to the development of novel therapeutic approaches to the treatment of immune, ischemic, and inflammatory disorders in which leukocyte–endothelial interactions lead to tissue injury. The general term used to describe this therapeutic strategy is "anti-adhesion" therapy, and several pharmaceutical companies are preparing to or are considering testing various antiadhesion compounds in patients.—E.A. Deitch, M.D.

Influence of an Anti-Tumor Necrosis Factor Monoclonal Antibody on Cytokine Levels in Patients With Sepsis

Fisher CJ Jr, for the CB0006 Sepsis Syndrome Study Group (Cleveland Clinic Found, Ohio)
Crit Care Med 21:318–327, 1993   140-94-2–15

Introduction.—In sepsis syndrome, micro-organisms and/or their by-products stimulate the host to produce inflammatory cytokines that result in a systemic host response. The incidence of sepsis continues to increase in hospitalized patients, and mortality remains at approximately 40%. The safety, pharmacokinetics, and activity of an anti-tumor necrosis factor (TNF)-α monoclonal antibody in severe sepsis were determined. In animal studies, such therapy has reduced mortality caused by both gram-negative and gram-positive bacterial infections.

Methods.—An open-label, prospective, phase II multicenter trial began with escalating doses of a murine monoclonal antibody (CB0006). Eighty patients were enrolled from 7 academic medical centers in Europe and 5 in the United States. For intravenous administration of the anti–TNF-α antibody, patients were assigned to 1 of 4 dose groups: .1 mg/kg, 1 mg/kg, 10 mg/kg, or 2 doses of 1 mg/kg given 24 hours apart. All received standard supportive care and antimicrobial therapy as well.

Results.—Gram-negative infections were documented in 29 patients, and gram-positive infections were seen in 18. There were 12 mixed infections, and in 17 patients the causative micro-organisms were not clearly documented. The 4 treatment groups did not differ significantly in final outcome. The 28-day, all-cause mortality was 41%. Increased levels of interleukin-6, but not of TNF-α, predicted fatal outcome. The 33 patients who were in septic shock at study entry had higher TNF-α levels and a lower survival rate (41% vs. 71%) than patients who were not in shock at entry. Despite the development of antimurine antibodies in 98% of patients, the murine monoclonal anti–TNF-α antibody was well tolerated. No adverse clinical events were attributed to CB0006. The serum half-life of CB0006 averaged 40.1 hours. In all but the low-dose group, TNF-α levels rapidly decreased after the infusion of antibody and returned to baseline values within 12 hours.

Conclusion.—The use of the murine anti–TNF-α monoclonal antibody appears to be safe and may prove useful in patients with high circulating TNF levels. Whether this antibody will be effective and have a clinical role in the treatment of sepsis must await further clinical studies.

▶ Don't buy the stock, and be careful of the "spin" put on the results of these clinical trials. In essence, this is one more in an increasingly long list of studies failing to document an improvement in survival in septic patients receiving anticytokine therapy.—E.A. Deitch, M.D.

Effects of Dopamine on T-lymphocyte Proliferative Responses and Serum Prolactin Concentrations in Critically Ill Patients

Devins SS, Miller A, Herndon BL, O'Toole L, Reisz G (Univ of Missouri, Kansas City)

Crit Care Med 20:1644–1649, 1992   140-94-2-16

Introduction.—Intravenous dopamine is often given by infusion to patients in the intensive care unit (ICU) to maintain urine volume, cardiac output, and blood pressure. Recently, however, studies have suggested that infusion of dopamine may cause adverse endocrine and lymphocytic effects. The outcome of a prospective, controlled assessment of the effects of dopamine infusion on serum T cells and prolactin in ICU patients was reported.

Methods.—All patients in an ICU were considered for the nonblinded study assessing the effects of dopamine, more than 5 µg/kg/min, infused for more than 4 hours compared with control patients who did not receive the drug. The drug and control groups were compared for Acute Physiology and Chronic Health Evaluation II (APACHE II) scores, prolactin levels, and lymphocyte function.

Results.—Over 4 months, 149 blood samples were taken from 47 patients, 20 of whom became controls. Six patients received infusion of dopamine, at least 5 µg/kg/min, for more than 4 hours. Eight other potential subjects were eliminated from the study. After infusion of dopamine, the patients' serum prolactin levels fell precipitously (92% for males and 90% for females) and closely paralleled the dopamine dose. The concanavalin A–stimulated T-cell proliferation significantly fell for a brief period in those receiving the dopamine infusion compared with controls. The lymphocyte counts significantly decreased in the dopamine infusion group. The APACHE II scores did not differ significantly for the dopamine and the control patients.

Conclusion.—A significant decrease in serum prolactin levels occurs in patients receiving intravenous dopamine. In addition, a significant, but transitory, decrease in T-cell response to concanavalin A stimulation also appeared in the dopamine-treated patients. These results suggest an altered endocrine and immune function resulting from dopamine administration to critically ill individuals.

▶ This article documenting that dopamine has potentially profound effects on the endocrine and immune systems was chosen as a springboard for a discussion of the increasingly well-recognized interactions between the neuroendocrine and immune systems. It is well established that traditional neuroendocrine mediators and hormones, such as prolactin, cortisol, endorphins, and others, can exert profound effects on the immune system. It is equally well established that immune cell products, such as IL-1, TNF, and IL-6, can exert multiple modulatory effects on intermediary metabolism and/or CNS function. Because it is now clear that traditional hormones may exert regulatory effects on various immune functions, it is not surprising that changes in circulating hormone levels can result in alterations in immune function as illustrated in the current article. However, with the exception of cortisol, the relationship and contribution of hormone-induced inhibition of immune function to the development of infection in the ICU patient is unclear. Thus, at the present time, that dopamine reduces prolactin levels and impairs mitogen-induced T-cell proliferation should not deter us from using this drug. However, neither should we lose sight of the important fact that the drugs we use in our sickest patients frequently have actions that may not be beneficial.—E.A. Deitch, M.D.

Interleukin 10 Protects Mice From Lethal Endotoxemia
Howard M, Muchamuel T, Andrade S, Menon S (DNAX Research Inst, Palo Alto, Calif)
J Exp Med 177:1205–1208, 1993   140-94-2–17

Introduction.—Produced by immune activation of subpopulations of helper T cells, B cells, and macrophage/monocytes, interleukin-10 (IL-10) causes decreased production of IL-1, IL-6, and tumor necrosis factor-α (TNF-α) in vitro. Production of these monokines is increased in mice in which IL-10 is neutralized. Whether monokine suppression by IL-10 has the potential to protect against lipopolysaccharide-induced shock, which is a monokine-mediated inflammatory reaction, was determined.

Observations.—The investigators induced shock in BALB/c mice by intraperitoneal injection of endotoxin, in doses ranging from 250 to 425 μg. Mice were completely protected against the lethal effects of lipopolysaccharide by a single injection of recombinant murine IL-10. This was so at all doses of IL-10—0.5, 1.0, and 10.0 μg, regardless of whether it was given at the same time or 30 minutes after endotoxin injection. The protective effect of IL-10 correlated with a substantial decrease in endotoxin-induced release of TNF-α. In animals receiving a prior injection of neutralizing anti–IL-10 antibodies there was a reversal of the protective effects.

Conclusions.—These findings in mice suggest a possible use of IL-10 as a clinical treatment for bacterial sepsis. Unlike most other reagents tested, it has protective effects even when given after endotoxin. Interleukin-10 might also be useful as a general anti-inflammatory reagent.

▶ A lot of attention has been focused on the proinflammatory cytokines, IL-1, IL-6, and TNF-α. Less attention has been focused on the immunosuppressive or inhibitory cytokines IL-4, IL-10, IL-13, and transforming growth factor-β (TGF-β). This article was chose to acquaint the reader with one of these endogenous immunoregulatory cytokines.

Basically, this article illustrates that there is more than one way to skin a cat and more than one way to control an excessive cytokine response. It is too early to know whether this strategy of administering an inhibitory cytokine to control the production of proinflammatory cytokines will ultimately be clinically effective. Nonetheless, the idea is intellectually appealing.—E.A. Deitch, M.D.

A Controlled Trial of HA-1A in a Canine Model of Gram-Negative Septic Shock
Quezado ZMN, Natanson C, Alling DW, Banks SM, Koev CA, Elin RJ, Hosseini JM, Bacher JD, Danner RL, Hoffman WD (Natl Ctr for Research Resources, Bethesda, Md)
JAMA 269:2221–2227, 1993   140-94-2-18

Background.—There have been numerous attempts to decrease the harmful effects of endotoxin, the principal mediator of septic shock. The human IgM antibody HA-1A has been reported to react with the lipid A moiety of endotoxin. Animal studies of its protective effects against sepsis have given conflicting results.

Methods.—A canine model of gram-negative septic shock that simulated the cardiovascular abnormalities of human sepsis was used to explore the possible therapeutic effects of the HA-1A antibody. The blinded, placebo-controlled study included 27 purpose-bred beagles implanted with an intraperitoneal clot infected with *Escherichia coli* 0111:B4. When the clot was implanted, the dogs received HA-1A, 10 mg/kg^{-1}; human IgM antibody at the same dose, or human serum albumin. All 3 groups received antibiotic and fluid therapy.

Results.—Fifteen percent of the HA-1A group survived for the full 28-day study, compared with 57% of the 2 control groups (P = 0.05) (Fig 2-4). At 24 hours, the mean arterial pressure and cardiac index were lower and the lactate levels were higher in the HA-1A group than in the control groups. All 3 groups showed similar and significant increases in their levels of endotoxemia and bacteremia. Toxicity studies revealed that neither human IgM antibody in infected dogs nor HA-1A in noninfected dogs had any harmful effects.

Conclusions.—There was no effect of HA-1A on bacteremia or endotoxemia in this septic model, and the administration of HA-1A was associated with a decrease in survival. Serious consideration should be given to the restriction of the clinical use of HA-1A until its beneficial and deleterious effects are better defined.

▶ So, the Food and Drug Administration may have been right all along in not approving HA-1A for clinical use. Although we constantly bemoan the obstructionist nature of drug approval in the United States compared to that in some other countries, the results of this well-designed experimental study showing that HA-1A is harmful in a clinically relevant model of treated peritonitis should give us all pause.—E.A. Deitch, M.D.

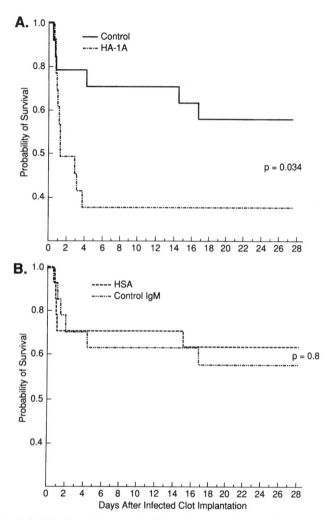

Fig 2–4.—Probability of survival vs. number of days after clot implantation for (**A**) infected animals given HA-1A ($n = 13$) or control therapy ($n = 14$; combined control human IgM antibody and control human serum albumin [HSA] groups); and (**B**) infected animals given control human IgM antibody ($n = 11$) or control HSA therapy ($n = 11$). (Courtesy of Quezado ZMN, Natanson C, Alling DW, et al: *JAMA* 269:2221–2227, 1993.)

Candiduria as an Early Marker of Disseminated Infection in Critically Ill Surgical Patients: The Role of Fluconazole Therapy

Nassoura Z, Ivatury RR, Simon RJ, Jabbour N, Stahl WM (New York Med College, Bronx, NY)
J Trauma 35:290–294, 1993   140-94-2-19

Introduction.—Critically ill surgical patients frequently have *Candida* in their urine, but the precise colony count that determines infection remains uncertain. The key is to distinguish between colonization and invasive infection. Some patients who were treated for candiduria by irrigating the bladder with amphotericin later were found to have systemic infection, prompting a study of the value of early systemic treatment.

Retrospective Series.—Twenty-seven patients with candiduria (colony count, greater than 100,000/mL) were studied. They had either incurred injuries or were general surgical or neurosurgical patients. All were receiving broad-spectrum antibiotics for bacterial infection. Seventeen of these patients had candidiasis. They had higher Acute Physiology and Chronic Health Evaluation II (APACHE II) scores at the time of admission and at the time candiduria was discovered than did those whose infection remained localized. Disseminated infection was detected a mean of 10 days after detection of candiduria. Ten of the 17 patients with dissemination (58.8%) had positive blood cultures. Nine patients (53%) died of multisystem organ failure and sepsis while receiving intravenous amphotericin therapy. None of the 10 patients without disseminated infection died of sepsis.

Prospective Series.—Twenty other patients with candiduria received systemic fluconazole at the time candiduria was detected. None of them had disseminated candidiasis, although they were as severely ill at admission as the patients in the retrospective group who had dissemination. Five percent of the prospectively studied patients died of sepsis.

Conclusions.—Candiduria may be an early indicator of systemic infection in trauma or surgical patients with persistent sepsis and organ failure. Appropriate treatment may be delayed if positive blood cultures or isolation of *Candida* at multiple sites is awaited. Intravenous administration of fluconazole at the time candiduria is noted may prevent dissemination.

▶ Distinguishing colonization from infection in patients with candiduria is notoriously difficult and inaccurate. Because of the potential toxic effects of systemic amphotericin-B therapy, it was customary to withhold systemic therapy in patients with candiduria in the absence of definite evidence of systemic infection. However, this approach of waiting to start antifungal therapy until definite evidence of systemic candidiasis is present was associated with a relatively high mortality. With the availability of fluconazole, as shown in this article, it is now better to treat than to wait.—E.A. Deitch, M.D.

The Failure of Conventional Methods to Promote Spontaneous Transpyloric Feeding Tube Passage and the Safety of Intragastric Feeding in the Critically Ill Ventilated Patient
Marian M, Rappaport W, Cunningham D, Thompson C, Esser M, Williams F,

Warneke J, Hunter G (Univ of Arizona, Tucson)
Surg Gynecol Obstet 176:475–479, 1993   140-94-2–20

Purpose.—Critically ill patients need aggressive nutritional support, preferably enteral support. It is commonly thought that transpyloric feeding reduces the incidence of pulmonary aspiration and is better tolerated than intragastric feeding. Conventional methods of placing nasoduodenal feeding tubes are often successful in ambulatory patients, but there are few data on their effectiveness in critically ill, ventilated patients. The success of conventional tube placement methods and the safety of intragastric feeding in the critically ill population were evaluated.

Methods.—The first part of the prospective study included 68 consecutive, critically ill, ventilated patients for whom nasoduodenal tube feeding was ordered. Weighted-tip tubes were placed with the patient on the right side, and metoclopramide was used to promote transpyloric passage. Successful transpyloric placement was confirmed by abdominal radiography within 72 hours of placement. In the second part of the study, 42 patients were fed by the gastric route. They were assigned to receive either continuous or bolus feeding, depending on their physician's preference.

Results.—In the first part of the study, successful duodenal intubation was achieved by 72 hours in only 10 of the 68 patients. Success in transpyloric passage was unrelated to age, gender, admitting diagnosis, or time of tube placement. In the second part of the study, 25 of the 42 patients achieved their enteral feeding goal rate by 72 hours, whereas 34 achieved their goal rate by 5 days. Total parenteral nutrition was required by 8 patients. Ten patients had a total of 11 complications develop, including 1 case of aspiration pneumonia.

Conclusions.—For most critically ill, ventilated patients, conventional methods of duodenal intubation are unsuccessful. For selected patients in the intensive care unit, nasogastric feeding appears to be safe. Elevating the head of the bed and checking gastric residuals is essential to reducing the incidence of aspiration. Patients must be watched closely for aspiration and/or intolerance of tube feedings.

▶ I agree. Just because nasogastric tube placement is technically easier than nasoduodenal placement does not mean it is bad. My experience with patients in the intensive care unit is similar to that of the authors. Thus, I, too, believe that nasogastric feeding can be a safe and effective route of enteral alimentation, especially when started early and monitored carefully.—E.A. Deitch, M.D.

Association of Hypomagnesemia and Mortality in Acutely Ill Medical Patients

Rubeiz GJ, Thill-Baharozian M, Hardie D, Carlson RW
Crit Care Med 21:203–209, 1993   140-94-2–21

Introduction.—Hypomagnesemia is a frequent finding in acutely ill hospitalized patients, both adults and infants. Chernow et al. reported increased mortality for postoperative patients who were hypomagnesemic, but limited data are available relating mortality to hypomagnesemia in acutely ill medical patients.

Study Plan.—Prospective observations were made in 381 consecutive acutely ill patients admitted from the emergency department to the medical ward or medical intensive care unit of a tertiary care hospital serving an inner city population. The serum magnesium level was estimated at admission, and Acute Physiology and Chronic Health Evaluation II (APACHE II) scores were calculated.

Findings.—Patients with hypomagnesemia and those with normal magnesium levels had comparable APACHE II scores, but the former patients had about twice the mortality of the normal-magnesium group. Among patients who died, those with hypomagnesemia did so 8 days sooner than the others. Other associated metabolic abnormalities (e.g., hypokalemia and hypocalcemia were frequent in both hypomagnesemic and normomagnesemic patients, but hypokalemia and azotemia were more frequent in the hypomagnesemic group.

Conclusion.—Acutely ill medical patients who are hypomagnesemic when admitted have increased mortality.

▶ This article was chosen because hypomagnesemia is one of the most common electrolyte abnormalities in hospitalized patients. Thus, prospective clinical studies indicating that hypomagnesemic patients in the intensive care unit have a worse prognosis are worthy of attention.—E.A. Deitch, M.D.

3   Burns

Introduction

Assessment of a major thermal injury includes an estimate of prognosis. For that reason, many formulae have been developed to predict the risk of death in patients with major thermal injuries. When variables, such as burn size, burn depth, patient age, preexistent disease, and the presence or absence of inhalation injury, are taken into consideration, these formulae provide relatively accurate assessments of a patient's chance of survival (e.g., 50% chance of survival vs. 20% chance of survival). Although they are good at assessing outcome in groups of patients, these prognostic formulae are less accurate in determining whether an individual patient will survive. Thus, what is needed is a simple diagnostic test that can be used to identify survivors and nonsurvivors in the relatively early postburn period. Based on a study indicating that patients whose rate of increase in body temperature after surgery was less than 1°C per hour died, body temperature returning to normal after surgery may be such a test. If further studies verify the prognostic accuracy of this metabolic stress test, then our ability to identify nonsurvivors and survivors accurately will be improved.

Our inability to adequately prevent or treat the early and late complications of smoke inhalation injury significantly contributes to the high mortality rate observed in burn patients with concomitant inhalation injuries. Consequently, it is of importance to develop and test improved methods of supporting pulmonary function, as well as therapeutic approaches directed at interrupting the disease process. Thus, 2 articles were selected to illustrate some of the promising work being done in clinically relevant animal models — work that has provided some insight into better ways of accomplishing these goals. Likewise, approaches to limit the depth of the burn wound, to facilitate burn wound coverage, and to understand and, hence, modulate burn scar formation continue to receive significant clinical and research attention. Consequently, experimental and clinical articles dealing with these topics were selected.

Although multiple organ failure (MOF) continues to be a major cause of death in burn patients, limited information is available on the natural history of MOF in burn patients compared with other surgical patient populations. Consequently, a recent publication reviewing the epidemiology of MOF in burn patients and describing a MOF scoring system for use in the burn patient was included in this years selection of papers. Based on this study, burn patients with MOF appear to share many clinical similarities with other patient populations with MOF. For example, infection appeared to contribute to the development of MOF in about two thirds of the burn patients and, thus, the relationship between infection and MOF appears to be similar between the burn and nonburn patient populations. Interest in the biology of infection, inflammation, and immune responsiveness continues to be high not only because of the potential relationships of these factors to MOF, but because the development of infections or alterations in the immunoinflammatory response correlates with a poor outcome. Consequently, clinical and basic science studies are being directed at improving our ability to understand and treat burn-induced infectious complications and alterations in host defense, which continues to be an area of active research. The selected articles cover a number of subjects and range from clinical studies directed at improving antibiotic dosing schedules to basic science studies directed at understanding the cytokine response.

Other topics covered include the erythropoietic response to thermal injury, care of the burned pregnant patient, and the effect of electrical injuries on neuropsychiatric behavior.

Edwin A. Deitch, M.D.

Recovery From Postoperative Hypothermia Predicts Survival in Extensively Burned Patients

Shiozaki T, Kishikawa M, Hiraide A, Shimazu T, Sugimoto H, Yoshioka T, Sugimoto T (Osaka Univ, Japan)
Am J Surg 165:326–330, 1993   140-94-3-1

Introduction.—Extensively burned patients who experience intraoperative hypothermia and have difficulty in rewarming often succumb to the burn injury. The factors affecting postoperative hypothermia were examined in 16 adult patients with a burn injury index greater than 35.

Methods.—All patients had been in good general health before the injury. Eight survived their burns, and 8 died after a mean survival of 58 days. The group had undergone a total of 74 débridements and/or skin graft operations. All had been rewarmed similarly during the postoperative period. Body temperature was monitored continuously in either the rectum or urinary bladder.

Results.—Hypothermia of less than 35°C had occurred in 89% of the 74 operations. The rate of temperature rise (RTR) was significantly lower in nonsurvivors than in survivors (Fig 3–1). Findings in 7 patients (4 survivors and 3 nonsurvivors) who were monitored by continuous indirect calorimetry demonstrated that RTR was primarily determined by heat production. The measured energy expenditure was 2.7 times the basal energy expenditure in survivors, but it reached only 1.7 times the

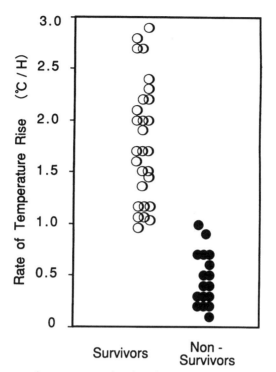

Fig 3–1.—The rate of temperature rise (RTR) in the 2 groups. Values of RTR were significantly lower in nonsurvivors than in survivors ($P < .001$). (Courtesy of Shiozaki T, Kishikawa M, Hiraide A, et al: *Am J Surg* 165:326–330, 1993.)

basal energy expenditure in nonsurvivors. In nonsurvivors, the RTR had already decreased significantly in the first 2 weeks after injury.

Conclusion.—Despite preventive measures, intraoperative hypothermia is an inevitable complication of any operation with general anesthesia. Patients who are unable to increase their heat production after postoperative hypothermia appear to be unable to produce the additional energy required to overcome other stresses.

▶ We all know how difficult but important it is to accurately identify which patients with major thermal injuries will survive and which will not. Consequently, numerous biochemical, metabolic, and immunologic variables have been examined during the past 2 decades in an attempt to identify early but accurate predictors of survival or death in these critically ill patients. In spite of the use of increasingly complex, sophisticated, time-consuming, and expensive methodology, the search for the prognostic holy grail has failed. Thus, the potential importance of this article is that it provides a simple and practical approach to determining the prognosis of an individual patient. Simply stated, the basic observation of this study is that patients whose RTR after surgery is less than 1°C per hour will not survive.—E.A. Deitch, M.D.

Heparin Improves Oxygenation and Minimizes Barotrauma After Severe Smoke Inhalation in an Ovine Model

Cox CS Jr, Zwischenberger JB, Traber DL, Traber LD, Haque AK, Herndon DN (Univ of Texas, Galveston)
Surg Gynecol Obstet 176:339–349, 1993   140-94-3-2

Background.—After inhalation injury, intraluminal casts of sloughed tracheobronchial endothelial cells and a protein-rich exudate often led to airway obstruction. Pulmonary edema caused by increased pulmonary microvascular permeability is mediated by the release of cationic proteases, including oxygen free radicals. Heparin may limit the protease-induced increase in microvascular permeability and scavenge oxygen free radicals. In a previous study, nebulized heparin and dimethyl sulfoxide reduced the increase in microvascular permeability associated with smoke inhalation injury. In a more recent study, the effects of continuous intravenous infusion of heparin on acute pulmonary injury were evaluated after smoke inhalation in sheep.

Methods.—Thirty minutes after standardized smoke inhalation injury, 12 ewes received either heparin or a saline solution vehicle intravenously.

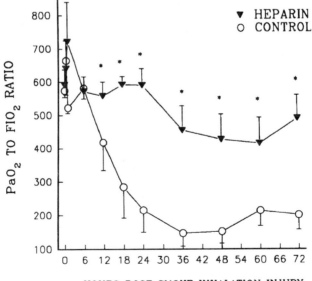

HOURS POST SMOKE INHALATION INJURY

Fig 3–2.—The PaO_2 to FIO_2 ratio represents the fall in arterial oxygenation relative to the fractional inspired concentration of oxygen. Both groups displayed decreases in oxygenation, but the control group had a greater decrease in the PaO_2 to FIO_2 ratio, as is commonly seen after smoke inhalation injury. The PaO_2 to FIO_2 ratio was significantly higher in the heparin group compared with the control group. *$P < .05$ at hours 12–72 postinjury. (Courtesy of Cox CS Jr, Zwischenberger JB, Traber DL, et al: *Surg Gynecol Obstet* 176:339–349, 1993.)

At 6-hour intervals, hemodynamics, blood gases, and conjugated dienes were assessed.

Results.—Although oxygenation, indicated by the PaO_2 to FIO_2 ratio, decreased in both groups, a greater decrease was observed in controls. The PaO_2 was significantly higher and peak airway pressures were lower in the heparin group compared with controls from 12 to 72 hours after injury (Fig 3–2). Histology revealed significantly fewer airway tracheobronchial casts in the heparin group compared with controls. Significantly higher pulmonary blood-free wet-to-dry weight ratios were found in controls than in the heparin group. Heparin had no effect on pulmonary-tissue or plasma-conjugated dienes or on pulmonary leukosequestration.

Conclusion.—In an ovine smoke inhalation model, intravenously administered heparin decreases the formation of tracheobronchial casts, improves oxygenation, minimizes barotrauma, and reduces pulmonary edema. However, heparin does not reduce postinjury oxygen free radical activity.

▶ With all the experimental studies being published each year on this subject, one can reasonably ask why this study was chosen. The answer is that heparin was effective when given after the injury. That is, heparin given 30 minutes *after* the sheep were exposed to smoke, at a dose that doubled the normal clotting time, significantly improved pulmonary function and reduced barotrauma. Although the cellular mechanisms remain to be determined, heparin undoubtedly exerted this protective effect by preventing pulmonary epithelial damage and the formation of tracheobronchial casts. The next step is to test the effectiveness of heparin therapy in an injury model combining surface burn and smoke inhalation; and if it is effective in this situation, we hopefully can move onto clinical trials.—E.A. Deitch, M.D.

Decreased Pulmonary Damage in Primates With Inhalation Injury Treated With High-Frequency Ventilation

Cioffi WG, deLemos RA, Coalson JJ, Gerstmann DA, Pruitt BA Jr (US Army Inst of Surgical Research, Fort Sam Houston, Tex; Univ of Texas Health Science Ctr, San Antonio)
Ann Surg 218:328–337, 1993   140-94-3–3

Objective.—It had previously been observed that mortality was significantly reduced by the prophylactic use of high-frequency flow interruption (HFFI) in patients with bronchoscopically diagnosed inhalation injury requiring ventilation. Using a primate model of inhalation injury, 2 forms of high-frequency ventilation were compared with conventional volume ventilation (CON) to determine the relationship between ventilatory mode and pulmonary damage.

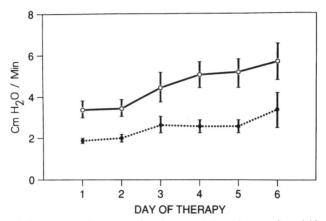

Fig 3–3.—The barotrauma index was significantly greater in CON (*open circles, solid lines*) than in HFFI (*solid circles, dashed lines*) at all time points. (Courtesy of Cioffi WG, deLemos RA, Coalson JJ, et al: *Ann Surg* 218:328–337, 1993.)

Methods.—Eighteen adult male baboons were randomized to 1 of 4 groups. Three animals served as controls and had no injury, no ventilatory support, and lung lavage only; 5 had positive pressure CON, 5 had HFFI, and 5 had high-frequency oscillatory ventilation (HFO) after moderate smoke injury. Ventilatory support was designed to achieve the same physiologic end points. Within 7 days—or sooner if irreversible cardiopulmonary failure was present—the animals were euthanized and the pulmonary pathologic changes scored and compared. Physiologic and repetitive biochemical data were analyzed between groups, using analysis of variance for repeated measures.

Results.—Two animals in the HFO group did not survive the study; all others were euthanized at the end of 154 hours. At all time points, CON-treated animals required significantly greater respiratory rates than HFFI-treated animals. Peak airway pressures were significantly greater in the HFO group than in the CON and HFFI groups. Physiologic end points were achieved in CON and HFFI, but not in HFO. There was no difference in hemodynamic variables between CON and HFFI. Despite similar values for partial pressure of oxygen, fraction of inspired oxygen, AA gradient, and partial pressure of carbon dioxide, the barotrauma index was greater in CON compared with HFFI (Fig 3-3). There was significantly less parenchymal damage in animals treated with HFFI than in those treated with CON.

Conclusion.—Progressive lung injury during treatment for smoke inhalation may result from ventilatory management itself. The prophylactic use of HFFI in smoke-injured primates appears to lead to a decrease in ventilator-induced pulmonary injury when compared to HFO and CON. During the study, normal arterial blood gases were maintained with CON and HFFI, but not with HFO. These findings offer an explanation for the lower mortality rate in patients treated for inhalation injury with HFFI.

▶ These authors have previously shown that the prophylactic use of one specific variant of high-frequency ventilatory support appeared to improve survival in burn patients with inhalation injuries (1). Why was this therapy effective, and are other modes of high-frequency ventilatory support equally or even more effective? These were the important questions asked, and in answering these questions the results of this study speak for themselves. Nonetheless, it is important to point out the basic similarity between this study and Abstract 140-94-3-2, which shows a beneficial effect of prophylactic heparin on the pathogenesis of smoke-induced pulmonary injury. The basic idea behind both types of therapy is that if small airway plugging secondary to the production of tracheobronchial casts can be reduced, then pulmonary function will be improved.—E.A. Deitch, M.D.

Reference

1. Cioffi WG, et al: *Ann Surg* 213:575, 1991.

U75412E, a Lazaroid, Prevents Progressive Burn Ischemia in a Rat Burn Model
Choi M, Ehrlich HP (Harvard Med School, Boston)
Am J Pathol 142:519–528, 1993   140-94-3–4

Background.—The immediate, irreversible injury resulting from a burn is followed by a delayed, reversible tissue loss in the surrounding area that is caused by progressive ischemia. The role of lipid peroxidation in the pathogenesis of progressive ischemia was investigated in a rat model.

Methods and Findings.—A row of four 10- × 20-mm burns was inflicted, separated by 3 unburned 5- × 20-mm skin bridges. These interspaces became ischemic and necrotic within 24 hours, resulting in a single wound with the merger of burn sites. A lipid peroxidation inhibitor, U75412E, was found to preserve vascular patency and restore blood flow. It also prevented an increase in tissue conjugated dienes and maintained tissue viability in the interspaces. Four separate burn wounds healed between viable strips of hair-bearing skin bridges. The treatment was efficacious when given systemically between 2 hours before and 1 hour after the burns were inflicted (Fig 3-4).

Conclusion.—The lipid peroxidation inhibitor used in this study was found to avert progressive burn ischemia. The lazaroid effect may be related to the preservation of the integrity of the endothelial cell membrane and restoration of vascular patency in the stasis zone through the

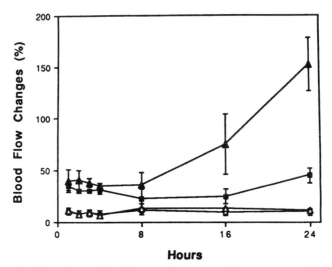

Fig 3–4.—Blood flow changes: blood flow in the burn sites and the interspaces was followed for 24 hours with a Laser Doppler Perfusion Scanner. Up to 4 hours, there was no significant difference between the untreated, vehicle-alone, and lazaroid-treated groups. Between 8 and 24 hours, the blood flow in the interspaces of the lazaroid-treated rats (*filled triangles*) increased. At 24 hours, the interspaces of the lazaroid-treated rats showed a threefold increase in blood flow compared with the vehicle-alone group (*filled squares*) (P < 0.001). No significant difference was noted between the burn sites of the vehicle-alone (*open squares*) and the lazaroid-treated (*open triangles*) groups. (Courtesy of Choi M, Ehrlich HP: *Am J Pathol* 142:519–528, 1993.)

inhibition of iron-dependent lipid peroxidation reaction and scavenging lipid peroxides.

▶ That burn injuries which appear to be of partial thickness shortly after injury may progress to full-thickness injuries during the next several days is a well-established and highly frustrating clinical observation. If this progression of dermal necrosis could be halted so that spontaneous wound healing would occur, many lives would potentially be saved. Thus, studies such as this one, which investigates the pathophysiology of burn wound necrosis and the potential ways of modulating this process, are of major importance.—E.A. Deitch, M.D.

Wound Closure and Outcome in Extensively Burned Patients Treated With Cultured Autologous Keratinocytes
Rue LW III, Cioffi WG, McManus WF, Pruitt BA Jr (US Army Inst of Surgical Research, Fort Sam Houston, Tex)
J Trauma 34:662–668, 1993   140-94-3–5

Introduction.—Several different techniques have been studied to achieve timely wound coverage in patients with massive burns. Several studies have reported success with cultured autologous keratinocytes

(CAK). An experience with CAK in patients with massive burns was reported.

Patients.—The experience compared 16 patients (mean age, 30 years) with major burns over a mean total body surface area of 68%. The patients were hospitalized for a mean of 132 days; 2 died. A total of 22 applications of CAK were made over a mean of 16% of body surface area. The mean cost per patient was nearly $44,000. The mean percentage engraftment at the time of discharge was 47%, but the mean body surface area of definitive wound coverage was just 5%. Patients having fascial incisions tended to have a smaller area of definitive wound coverage at higher cost. Patients with greater burn areas had a lesser extent of initial engraftment and less late graft loss than those with lesser burns, resulting in a similar extent of definitive coverage.

Conclusions.—This experience suggests that CAK does not reduce the time to closure of massive burn wounds and therefore has no important effect on the outcome for such patients. The technique is clearly more effective in some patients than in others; therefore, future studies should address specific causes of graft failure and techniques to optimize successful engraftment.

▶ Having built a better mousetrap does not always mean that one will catch the mouse. The development of sophisticated technology resulting in the commercial availability of in vitro cultured keratinocytes is one example of a better mousetrap. However, in spite of almost one decade of clinical experience, it remains to be proven whether this technology results in improved survival in patients with massive deep burn injuries. Thus, although commercially available, further technical improvements in the use of cultured autologous kerotinocytes appear to be necessary for this technology to reach its therapeutic potential.—E.A. Deitch, M.D.

Enhanced Expression of mRNA for Transforming Growth Factor-β, Type I and Type III Procollagen in Human Post-Burn Hypertrophic Scar Tissues

Ghahary A, Shen YJ, Scott PG, Gong Y, Tredget EE (Univ of Alberta, Edmonton, Canada; Univ of Manitoba, Winnipeg, Canada)
J Lab Clin Med 122:465–473, 1993   140-94-3–6

Background.—Hypertrophic scarring is a frequent sequel of extensive thermal injury, and it may lead to significant functional and cosmetic impairment. Excessive collagen formation underlies the condition. It remains uncertain how expression of the procollagen gene is regulated in fibrotic disorders.

Objective and Methods.—The possible role of locally synthesized transforming growth factor beta-1 (TGF-β1) and procollagen in post-burn hypertrophic scarring was examined by comparing levels of mRNAs for type I and type III procollagen and TGF-β1 in human scar tissue and in normal dermis from the same patients. Samples were taken from 6 patients who, within the past year, had received burn injuries that had culminated in the formation of hyperemic, elevated, thickened, noncompliant scars.

Findings.—Northern blot analysis of RNA from scar tissue and normal skin yielded 2 transcripts each for the pro-alpha 1(I) and pro-alpha 1(III) chains and 1 for TGF-β1. The average amount of pro-alpha 1(I) mRNA was 102% higher in hypertrophic scar tissue than in normal skin. Expression of pro-alpha 1(III) was increased 91%, and that of TGF-β1, 61%. On quantitative analysis of Northern blots, specific messages were increased by as much as 250% in scar samples compared with normal skin.

Interpretation.—It is possible that locally synthesized TGF-β1 regulates the expression of type I and type III procollagens in a paracrine or autocrine manner, or both, in postburn hypertrophic scars.

▶ Why does scarring occur, and how can we control this process? These questions are important, because most burn patients survive. In survivors, the cosmetic and functional sequelae associated with burn injuries significantly modify the patients' ultimate ability to make a full return to society. Thus, studies directed at clarifying the biology of hypertrophic scar formation are critical to evolving effective means of limiting burn scar formation.—E.A. Deitch, M.D.

Multiple Organ Failure in Patients With Thermal Injury

Saffle JR, Sullivan JJ, Tuohig GM, Larson CM (Univ of Utah Health Science Ctr, Salt Lake City)
Crit Care Med 21:1673–1683, 1993   140-94-3–7

Introduction.—The syndrome of multiple organ failure is the most frequent reason for admission and the most common cause of death in the surgical intensive care unit. The scoring systems used to quantify the severity of multiple organ failure have often excluded burn injury. The frequency and consequences of multiple organ failure were assessed in a sample of burn patients, and a system for scoring organ failure in thermal injury was developed.

Methods.—The Thermal Injury Organ Failure Score was designed to quantify organ failure systematically and to record the occurrence of specific clinical abnormalities. A total organ failure score was obtained for each patient by adding the scores from all organ systems. Scores ranged from 0 (normal) to 6 (severe dysfunction); the highest possible total score was 33 points. This system was developed in a review of 529 patients admitted for acute burn injury and was used for prospective assessment of 83 adult burn patients. The accuracy of the Thermal Injury Or-

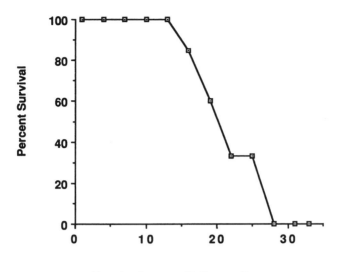

Total Organ Failure Score

Fig 3–5.—Patient survival according to total Thermal Injury Organ Failure Scores. (Courtesy of Saffle JR, Sullivan JJ, Tuohig GM, et al: *Crit Care Med* 21:1673-1683, 1993.)

gan Failure system was compared to that of Acute Physiologic and Chronic Health Evaluation II (APACHE II).

Results.—The 529 burn patients whose cases were reviewed had a mean age of 27.5 years. The mean burn size was 15% of the total body surface area, and the mean organ failure score was 4.62. Thirty-three patients (6.2%) died. Nonsurvivors had a significantly higher organ failure score (23.1) than did survivors (3.28). Only 1 patient whose total score was less than 15 died, whereas no patient with a score of more than 26 survived (Fig 3-5). A score greater than or equal to 15 indicated dysfunction of at least 3 organs. The mortality rate of patients with high (greater than or equal to 15) scores increased with age and burn size. Although pulmonary dysfunction was the most frequent form of organ failure, cardiovascular and neurologic scores were more closely correlated with outcome. Sepsis was present in 22 of the patients who died.

Conclusion.—Because burn injuries have generally been excluded from systems designed to predict outcome in intensive care unit patients, relatively little is known about multiple organ failure in burn victims. The Thermal Injury Organ Failure Score should be a valuable investigational tool in studies of thermally injured patients.

▶ To begin to predict whether therapy developed for use in nonburn patients with multiple organ failure will be effective in burn patients (and vice versa), it is important to determine, as was done in this study, whether multiple organ failure is similar between burn and nonburn patient populations. It is equally important to develop a reproducible quantifiable scoring system with which to assess organ function in thermally injuried patients, so that the response to new therapies can be compared between different burn units. The scoring system described in this report takes an important first-step in that direction.—E.A. Deitch, M.D.

Aminoglycoside Dosing in Burn Patients Using First-Dose Pharmacokinetics

Hollingsed TC, Harper DJ, Jennings JP, Morris SE, Saffle JR (Univ of Utah, Salt Lake City)
J Trauma 35:394–398, 1993   140-94-3-8

Purpose.—In burn patients, the development of gram-negative infections is an important cause of morbidity and mortality. Treatment is with aminoglycoside antibiotics, but aminoglycoside pharmacokinetics are altered in these patients, sometimes resulting in subtherapeutic serum drug concentrations. An initial experience with first-dose (FD) pharmacokinetic calculations was reviewed to ascertain the proper aminoglycoside dosing regimen in burn patients.

Methods.—Twelve burn patients treated with aminoglycoside antibiotics using FD pharmacokinetic calculations were compared with 14 patients treated with conventional dosing (CD) methods. In the FD group, a loading dose of either gentamicin, about 3 mg/kg, or amikacin, 10 mg/kg, was given. One to 5 hours later, blood samples were taken for measurement of drug levels. Information on the volume of distribution and the half-life of the antibiotic was used to calculate a patient-specific dosing regimen that would result in therapeutic peak and trough levels.

Results.—Therapeutic antibiotic levels were achieved in a mean of 44 hours in the FD group compared with 97 hours in the CD group. Sixty-seven percent of the FD group had therapeutic serum drug concentrations with the first set of steady-state levels, compared to just 11% of the CD group. First-dose patients required a mean of 2 dosing changes vs. 4 for the CD patients.

Conclusions.—First-dose pharmacokinetic calculations can improve maintenance of therapeutic serum aminoglycoside concentrations in burn patients. Routine use of FD calculations is recommended; these calculations can easily be made by computer, even at the bedside. It is still necessary to measure serum peak and trough levels twice a week to avoid toxicity and to adjust for intrapatient variability.

▶ Computers continue to change our lives. Because prompt attainment of therapeutic aminoglycoside levels is associated with improved survival in patients with gram-negative bacteremia, the ability to use the computer to derive patient-specific aminoglycoside dosing schedules is a major potential advance. This is especially true in burn patients, because of the extensive variability in their rate of drug metabolism. Thus, the approach of using FD pharmacokinetic calculations to determine optimal aminoglycoside dosing schedules appears to be of significant value. It is likewise important to remember that drug metabolism is frequently altered in other hypermetabolic states besides burn injury and, thus, the approach described by the authors is likely to benefit multiple patient populations.—E.A. Deitch, M.D.

Bone Marrow Toxicity by Silver Sulfadiazine
Gamelli RL, Paxton TP, O'Reilly M (Loyola Univ, Maywood, Ill; Mt Sinai Hosp, Chicago; Univ of Vermont, Burlington)
Surg Gynecol Obstet 177:115–120, 1993   140-94-3–9

Purpose.—For burn patients, topical silver sulfadiazine (SSD) is the mainstay of antimicrobial therapy for the prevention of sepsis. It is associated with a 3% to 5% incidence of leukopenia, which usually remits spontaneously, despite the continued use of SSD. The effects of SSD on the production of granulocytes and macrophages was studied in a mouse model of cutaneous injury.

Observations.—In mice with a full-thickness burn to 10% of their total body surface area, daily application of SSD caused no consistent bone marrow suppression. For those with a 10% full-thickness skin excision and daily application of SSD, total counts of peripheral blood leukocytes were decreased by nearly 50%, compared to counts of untreated controls (skin excision without SSD). On the first day after the skin-excision injury plus SSD, the absolute number of granulocytes was only 10% of that of controls. Mice receiving SSD after skin-excision injury had a marked reduction in nucleated bone marrow cells on assay of granulocyte-macrophage progenitor cells. Adding SSD to culture plates containing maximally stimulated normal mouse or human bone marrow cells resulted in dose-dependent depression of colony count.

Conclusions.—Silver sulfadiazine is cytotoxic to myelopoietic tissue in vitro and alters the myeloid cell compartment in vivo. These effects may explain the transient SSD-associated leukopenia observed in burn patients receiving topical SSD. Self-correction of this leukopenia, conceivably via early recovery of granulocyte-macrophage progenitor cells and marrow cellularity, should obviate the need for discontinuation of SSD therapy.

▶ If leukopenia develops in a burn patient receiving topical sulfadiazine, should the drug be stopped? Based on a review of the literature, the answers to this question include yes, no, and maybe. Thus, one can see the clinical relevance of this study. Additionally, based on my experience in burn patients, I concur with the authors' conclusion that leukopenia is not an indication to stop topical therapy with sulfadiazine.—E.A. Deitch, M.D.

Molecular Mechanisms of Decreased Interleukin-2 Production After Thermal Injury

O'Riordain DS, Mendez MV, O'Riordain MG, Molloy RG, Holzheimer RG, Collins K, Saporoschetz I, Mannick JA, Rodrick ML (Harvard Med School, Boston)
Surgery 114:407–415, 1993   140-94-3–10

Introduction.—Severe thermal or traumatic injury leads to alterations in T-cell activation, reduced lymphocyte interleukin-2 (IL-2) production, and associated depression of T-lymphocyte proliferation. The abnormalities of the T-lymphocyte signal transduction pathways that lead to abnormal production of IL-2 after thermal injury were investigated.

Methods.—One hundred fifty A/J mice, aged 7–8 weeks were used in the study. They were anesthetized, subjected to a 20% full-thickness scald burn injury or sham burn, and killed at intervals from 4 to 21 days later. The spleens were harvested, and splenocytes were prepared for in vitro studies. Cells were cultured with either concanavalin A or a combination of the phorbol ester PMA and the calcium inophore A23187 for measurement of IL-2 production. Expression of cytokine messenger RNA (mRNA) was measured by Northern blot analysis, and IL-2 production was measured by bioassay.

Results.—The production of IL-2 and the expression of IL-2 mRNA were both consistently suppressed in concanavalin A–stimulated cells from burned mice compared with the mice with sham burns. A similar suppression occurred when T cells were activated with PMA and A23187, bypassing the earlier stages of the signal transduction mechanism. Cells from the burned animals showed consistent increases in IL-1β and expression of tumor necrosis factor-α mRNA, suggesting that decreased expression of IL-2 mRNA was specific to IL-2 and not representative of a global decrease in expression of cytokine mRNA.

Conclusion.—The precise defects that lead to abnormal T-cell activation after thermal injury remain unclear. The findings of this study, however, confirm that abnormal IL-2 production by stimulated T cells occurs as a consequence of burn injury. The principal cellular abnormalities that result in these alterations appear to lie downstream of the initiating signal transduction events and before IL-2 gene transcription.

Administration of Dehydroepiandrosterone to Burned Mice Preserves Normal Immunologic Competence

Araneo BA, Shelby J, Li G-Z, Ku W, Daynes RA (Univ of Utah, Salt Lake City)
Arch Surg 128:318–325, 1993   140-94-3–11

Introduction.—Patients with burn injuries often experience a dysregulation of the lymphokine-monokine production resulting from the body's metabolic and neuroendocrine response to the thermal injury itself. In an animal model study, whether stress-induced changes in steroid hormones observed during thermal injury trauma mediate the immune function changes seen in burn patients was determined.

Methods.—Female and male mice with induced thermal injuries underwent treatment with 100 μg of dehydroepiandrosterone within 1 hour of injury to determine its effects on T-cell–derived lymphokines and the cellular immune response. Monoclonal antibody reagents were made to test these 2 response types.

Results.—After the thermal injury the injured animals demonstrated T-cell production of interleukin-2 and interferon-γ but at depressed levels that paralleled the reduction in contact hypersensitivity responsiveness. Comparing the injured mice and the control animals, thermal injury produced a decrease in the capacity of the activated T cells to secrete interleukin-2, interferon-γ, interleukin-3, and granulocyte/monocyte-colony-forming factor. Dehydroepiandrosterone treatment of the thermally injured animals promoted normal immune functions and cellular immune responses based on the results of the postmortem splenocyte lymphokine assays. The in vivo dehydroepiandrosterone treatment also promoted resistance to *Listeria monocytogenes* in thermally injured mice.

Conclusion.—The administration of a single steroid hormone, dehydroepiandrosterone, allowed the thermally injured animal to maintain its normal immunologic responsiveness. Dehydroepiandrosterone appears to promote immune function as well as inhibit immune dysfunction.

▶ The search for the mechanisms of burn and trauma-induced immune suppression has now reached the molecular level. Abstract 140-94-2–10 illustrates that after thermal injury, the ability to induce the production of the immune-enhancing cytokine interleukin-2 (IL-2) is impaired, whereas the ability to stimulate the synthesis of the proinflammatory cytokines interleukin-1 and tumor necrosis factor remains largely intact. Because IL-2 is important in maintaining cell-mediated immunity and aids in controlling bacterial infection, impaired production of IL-2 has been proposed as one of the major immune defects predisposing the burn patient to infection. Hence, one can see the importance of studies investigating the basic biology of IL-2 regulation after thermal injury.

Abstract 140-94-2–11 compliments Abstract 140-94-2–10 by illustrating that the administration of a weak androgen steroid, dehydroepiandrosterone, prevents the development of burn-induced alterations in production of IL-2 and improves T-cell function. Taken together, these 2 studies illustrate that thermal injury acts as a selective modulator of T-cell function, with the production of some cytokines being depressed and that of others being unaffected or even augmented.—E.A. Deitch, M.D.

Plasma Cytokines After Thermal Injury and Their Relationship to Infection

Drost AC, Burleson DG, Cioffi WG Jr, Mason AD Jr, Pruitt BA Jr (United States Army Inst of Surgical Research, Fort Sam Houston, Tex)
Ann Surg 218:74–78, 1993   140-94-3–12

Background.—In a previous study, it was reported that levels of the cytokines interleukin 1β (IL-1β) and interleukin 6 (IL-6) were significantly elevated in the plasma of patients with thermal injury compared with control subjects who were not burned. Both cytokines were highest during the first weeks after injury; IL-1β correlated with burn size and IL-6 correlated with mortality rate. To identify modalities useful for the early detection of infection in patients who were severely burned, researchers analyzed the relationship of IL-1β, IL-6, and tumor necrosis factor-α (TNF-α) to infection.

Methods.—Twenty-seven patients with an average age of 35.8 years agreed to participate in the study. The patients had burns covering 17.5% to 89% of their total body surface. During the study, there were 14 episodes of pneumonia, 1 case of fungal wound infection, 1 case of septicemia, and 6 episodes of tracheobronchitis. Blood was drawn from the patients 3 times a week for measurements of IL-1β (253 samples),

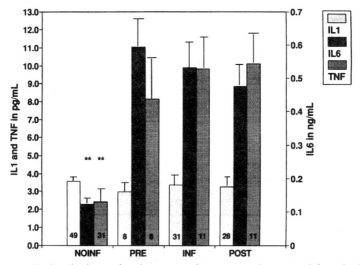

Fig 3–6.—Cytokine levels in infected patients and in patients who remained free of infection. *NOINF* represents detectable samples from patients who remained free of infection. These were compared to detectable samples from infected patients divided into 1 of 3 periods. *INF* is an 8-day period, with day 1 being 1 day before diagnosis of infection. *PRE* is the 8-day period before *INF*, and *POST* reflects an 8-day window after *INF*. All data are expressed in means ± standard errors of the means. **$P < .01$. *$P < .05$. *NOINF* is significantly different from any of the 3 infection periods. (Courtesy of Drost AC, Burleson DG, Cioffi WG Jr, et al: *Ann Surg* 218:74–78, 1993.)

IL-6 (419 samples), and TNF-α (409 samples) by enzyme-linked immunosorbent assay.

Results.—Detectable IL-1β levels were seen in 40% of samples from 7 patients who were infection-free and in 74.4% of samples from 14 patients who became infected. Detectable plasma IL-6 concentrations were also more common in patients who were infected than in patients who were infection-free (78.4% vs. 58%). The IL-6 level was higher in patients who were infected who died than in those who survived. Only 15.4% and 27% of plasma samples from 11 patients who were infection-free and 16 patients who were infected, respectively, were positive for TNF-α. An 8-day infection window, starting 1 day before the infection was diagnosed, was assigned to all surviving patients who were infected. The prior 8 days were called preinfection, and the recovery period of 8 days after the infection window was defined as "postinfection". During any of these 3 periods, the mean plasma IL-6 and TNF-α concentrations in patients who remained free of infection were significantly lower than those of patients who were infected (Fig 3–6).

Conclusion.—Plasma IL-6 and TNF-α levels are related to severe bacterial infection in patients who are burned. Postburn infection did not appear to alter IL-1β. Determination of cytokine levels may aid in the early diagnosis of systemic bacterial infection.

▶ I agree with the authors' results, but I disagree with their basic conclusion that determinations of cytokine levels will aid in the early diagnosis of infection. It is because I disagree with this conclusion that I chose this paper. Although it is true that plasma IL-6 and TNF levels of the infected patient group differed statistically from those observed in the noninfected group of patients, life is not that simple. For example, cytokines were not detected in the plasma of a relatively high percentage of the infected patients, and many of the uninfected patients had high plasma cytokine levels. Thus, considerable overlap existed between individuals of both groups, in spite of the fact that the average values of the 2 groups were different. It is important to remember that for a diagnostic test to accurately discriminate between patients with and without the disease process in question, there should be both a low false positive and a low false negative rate. Such does not appear to be the case in this study, and it highlights the aphorism of "reader beware".
—E.A. Deitch, M.D.

Correlation of the Local and Systemic Cytokine Response With Clinical Outcome Following Thermal Injury
Rodriguez JL, Miller CG, Garner WL, Till GO, Guerrero P, Moore NP, Corridore M, Normolle DP, Smith DJ, Remick DG (Univ of Michigan, Ann Arbor)
J Trauma 34:684–695, 1993   140-94-3–13

Background.—Previous studies have noted correlations between systemic underproduction of interleukin-2 and overproduction of interleukin-6 (IL-6), and poor clinical outcome in patients with major burns. Most recently, an association has been found between local upregulation of interleukin-8 (IL-8) in the lung and early pulmonary physiologic dysfunction. In a prospective study, the local and systemic production of tumor necrosis factor (TNF), IL-6, and IL-8 was examined after burns.

Methods.—The study sample comprised 88 patients with acute thermal injury. One group did not require admission to an intensive care unit, another group required intensive care unit admission but had no evidence of inhalation injury, and a third group required intensive care unit admission and had evidence of inhalation injury. A group of elective surgical patients was also studied. Specimens of bronchial secretions, blood, and skin were tested for the various cytokines.

Results.—Forty-eight hours after injury, the burn patients demonstrated significant amounts of TNF, IL-6, and IL-8 in the systemic circulation, the lung, and in normal as well as thermally injured skin. The finding of the 3 cytokines in lung and skin was associated with upregulation of TNF, IL-6, and IL-8 mRNA. On logistic regression analysis, and after adjustment for burn severity, IL-8 in the lung was associated with early pulmonary dysfunction and nosocomial pulmonary pneumonia.

Conclusions.—Patients with acute thermal injuries have an early systemic, lung, and skin response involving the cytokines TNF, IL-6, and IL-8. The cytokines found in the lung and skin after burn injury are produced locally and are not drawn from the systemic cytokine pool. Local organ failure may result from the lung IL-8 response.

▶ In my opinion, this is one of the best studies published to date on the effect of thermal injury on cytokine production. Not only have the authors performed these studies in patients, but they have also determined the contribution of the lung and skin to the cytokine response. By going beyond taking random blood samples, they have provided new and important information on the local levels and production of IL-6, IL-8, and TNF in thermally injured patients. Because cytokines act locally in the tissues, information on tissue and organ cytokine levels will be important in clarifying the true biological and clinical significance of the burn-induced cytokine response. Thus, this study is important for many reasons.—E.A. Deitch, M.D.

The Activation of Bone Marrow Macrophages 24 Hours After Thermal Injury
Ogle CK, Guo X, Alexander JW, Fukushima R, Ogle JD (Shriners Burns Inst, Cincinnati, Ohio; Univ of Cincinnati, Ohio)
Arch Surg 128:96–101, 1993   140-94-3-14

Objective.—Whether thermal injury can program the macrophages of bone marrow so that they could be stimulated to produce larger amounts of various mediators after release was determined.

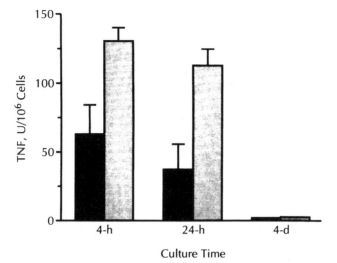

Fig 3–7.—The in vitro production of TNF by lipopolysaccharide-stimulated guinea pig bone marrow macrophages at different culture times. Macrophages from unburned (*black bars*) or burned (*gray bars*) animals, obtained 24 hours later, were incubated for the indicated times in M199 medium containing 10% heat-inactivated fetal bovine serum and 10 mg of lipopolysaccharide per L. Supernatants were assayed for TNF or other substances. *Bars* indicate means ± standard error of the mean (*n* = 6 in all figures). (Courtesy of Ogle CK, Guo X, Alexander JW, et al: *Arch Surg* 128:96–101, 1993.)

Methods.—Bone marrow macrophages were obtained from guinea pigs subjected to a 50% full-thickness flame burn. The animals were killed 24 hours after injury. Macrophages were stimulated by lipopolysaccharide, and the production of tumor necrosis factor (TNF), interleukin-1 (IL-1), prostaglandin E_2, and complement component C3 was monitored.

Findings.—Cells from burn-injured animals produced significantly more TNF than did those from control animals after incubation in vitro for 4 or 24 hours (Fig 3–7). No difference in the production of IL-1 was noted at these intervals, but after 4 days in culture, macrophages from burned animals produced significantly more IL-1 than those from normal animals. Cells from burn-injured animals produced larger amounts of prostaglandin E_2. They also produced more C3 than did cells from uninjured animals, but only after 4 days of culture. Marrow macrophages from burned animals were significantly more cytotoxic for target cells (L929 fibroblasts) than were cells from control animals.

Conclusion.—Thermal injury is able to prime bone marrow macrophages so that they may be stimulated to produce both immunoactive and immunosuppressive mediator substances. The same cells become much more cytotoxic after thermal injury of the host.

▶ This article was chosen, in part, because it illustrates a potentially important but relatively unrecognized phenomenon, i.e., the phenomenon of priming. In this phenomenon, immune and inflammatory cells that receive a specific stimulus are "primed" so that they respond to a second stimulus with an exaggerated response. The concept of priming leading to an excessive cytokine response upon restimulation serves as the basis for the 2-hit hypothesis of organ injury, in which the initial insult primes the cell and the subsequent insult detonates it.—E.A. Deitch, M.D.

Increased Gut Permeability Early After Burns Correlates With the Extent of Burn Injury

Ryan CM, Yarmush ML, Burke JF, Tompkins RG (Massachusetts Gen Hosp; Harvard Med School, Boston)
Crit Care Med 20:1508–1512, 1992   140-94-3–15

Background.—Increased gut permeability is observed after burn injuries. A better understanding of the events and mediators leading to this increased permeability is needed. The goal of this study was to test the hypothesis that intestinal permeability is increased early after thermal injury, and that an increase in gut permeability is related to the extent of injury.

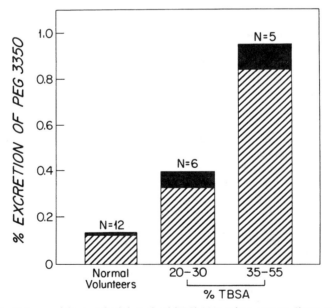

Fig 3–8.—Gut permeability to polyethylene glycol (PEG) 3350 in burn patients. Shown are the percentages of oral dosages that were excreted in the urine and those percentages found in control volunteers in a previously published study. Total body surface area (TBSA) burned; mean (*hatched area*) ± standard error measurement (*black area*). (Courtesy of Ryan CM, Yarmush ML, Burke JF, et al: *Crit Care Med* 20:1508–1512, 1992.)

Methods.—Fourteen patients were studied in a nonrandomized, controlled study. All had burns covering more than 20% of their body surface. Intestinal absorption and renal excretion of polyethylene glycol 3350 was used as the macromolecule to assess gut permeability. Polyethylene glycol 400 intestinal absorption was used as an internal control for abnormal motility and malabsorption.

Findings.—The burn victims excreted a mean 0.56% of polyethylene glycol 3350, compared with 0.12% in control volunteers previously reported (Fig 3–8). Excretion of polyethylene glycol 400 did not differ in patients and healthy volunteers. The percentage of polyethylene glycol 3350 excretion correlated with the percentage of body surface burned. Patients with smaller injuries excreted 0.32%, which was greater than normal and less than that excreted by patients with larger injuries.

Conclusion.—In this series, gut permeability was increased early after burn injury, confirming previous findings. The increased gut permeability to polyethylene glycol 3350 was correlated with burn injury extent.

▶ This article was chosen because of my interest in the gut and because it provides information indicating that large molecules that are normally excluded by the barrier function of the intestinal epithelium may reach the systemic circulation shortly after thermal injury. Because many of the substances found in the intestinal lumen, such as endotoxin, may "prime" the immunoinflammatory system, loss of intestinal barrier function may predispose the burn patient to an exaggerated cytokine response, as discussed in Abstract 140-94-3-14.—E.A. Deitch, M.D.

A Serial Study of the Erythropoietic Response to Thermal Injury
Deitch EA, Sittig KM (Louisiana State Univ, Shreveport)
Ann Surg 217:293–299, 1993   140-94-3-16

Objective.—Because of the risks associated with blood transfusion, the reduction of transfusion requirements in burn patients has become desirable. One potential approach is erythropoietin replacement therapy to bolster red cell production. However, it is not known whether erythropoietin levels are increased or decreased after thermal injury. Thus, a prospective study was done to characterize the erythropoietic response to thermal injury.

Methods.—During a 4-month period, 24 patients with burns covering 15% to 80% of their total body surface area (TBSA) and requiring excision and grafting of at least 10% of TBSA were studied. To assess the potential effect of burn wound size on the erythropoietic response, serum iron, total iron binding capacity (TIBC), ferritin, erythropoietin, transferrin saturation, hemoglobin, and reticulocyte counts were measured on burn days 1, 3, 5, 7, 10, 14, and weekly thereafter.

Results.—Hemoglobin levels, serum iron, TIBC, and transferrin saturation progressively decreased, whereas ferritin, reticulocyte counts, and erythropoietin levels gradually increased. There was an inverse correlation between the degree of anemia and the magnitude of the erythropoietin response, indicating that erythropoietin production remains intact after thermal injury. However, in spite of the increased erythropoietin production and increased reticulocyte counts, patients remained anemic, suggesting that the erythropoietic response is somehow impaired.

Conclusion.—Until the mechanisms underlying the anemia and the impaired erythropoietic response of thermal injury are better understood, the role of erythropoietin replacement therapy after burn injury remains speculative.

▶ Until the recent availability of recombinant human erythropoietin (rHuEPO), the therapeutic options for improving erythropoiesis in burn patients were quite limited. With the ready availability of rHuEPO, it would make sense to treat selected burn patients with this erythropoietic growth factor when endogenous production was impaired. However, based on the results of this study, which indicate that erythropoietin levels increased appropriately during anemia, it appears that the failure of these patients to correct their anemia was not primarily related to a failure of erythropoietin production.—E.A. Deitch, M.D.

Burns With Pregnancy: A Review of 25 Cases
Jain ML, Garg AK (JLN Hosp and Research Centre, Bhilai (MP), India)
Burns 19:166–167, 1993   140-94-3–17

Objective.—Burns during pregnancy can threaten the life of the mother and fetus. Although the prognosis has historically been regarded as poor, the mother's chance of survival has improved. A series of 25 pregnant burn patients treated over 6 years was studied.

Patients.—Seven patients had burns of 15% to 30% total body surface area (TBSA), 8 had burns of 31% to 49% TBSA, 8 had burns of 50% to 65% TBSA, and 2 had burns of 95% to 100% TBSA. Sixteen patients had full-term, normal delivery. Nine aborted, including 4 of 6 in the first trimester, 4 of 12 in the second trimester, and 1 of 7 in the third trimester. Three patients died after abortion, and the 2 patients with the most severe burns died as well. Eleven patients were managed by general anesthesia and split-thickness skin grafting; none of these patients died or aborted after surgery.

Conclusions.—With adequate treatment, a good maternal and fetal outcome can be achieved in pregnant burn patients. Fetal survival is related to gestational age, with abortion being most common in the first trimester. Abortion must commonly results from septicemia.

▶ This article was chosen to stress that the majority of pregnant burn patients spontaneously deliver healthy infants and to dispel the myth that emergency cesarean sections or induced abortions are mandatory to improve maternal or fetal survival.—E.A. Deitch, M.D.

Auditory and Neuropsychiatric Behavior Patterns After Electrical Injury

Grossman AR, Tempereau CE, Brones MF, Kulber HS, Pembrook LJ (Sherman Oaks Hosp and Med Ctr, Los Angeles)
J Burn Care Rehabil 14:169–175, 1993   140-94-3-18

Introduction.—Those who survive electrocution-type injury most often exhibit signs of CNS insult, including loss of consciousness, confusion, and amnesia. Recovery tends to be slow and incomplete, but in a given case it may be difficult to determine whether the symptoms represent a neurobehavioral condition or post-traumatic stress disorder (PTSD). Patients whose electric injuries were severe enough to produce symptoms, but not so marked as to produce obvious structural brain damage, were studied.

Patients.—Forty-eight patients admitted with electric current injuries and 53 others who had flash, contact, or arcing burns were studied. Sixteen patients with current injuries and 18 whose injuries were not ascribed to the passage of current underwent serial neurologic and auditory evaluations and received trauma-based psychiatric treatment.

Observations.—Twelve of the 16 (75%) patients with current injuries met criteria for persistent neurobehavioral disorder (PNBD), and 1 met *DSM III-R* criteria for PTSD. Four of the 18 (22%) patients with other forms of electric injury met the criteria for PTSD after 1 year of observation, but none received a diagnosis of PNBD. Eight patients with current injuries but none in the other group had persistent auditory abnormalities. The neurosensory hearing losses usually affected frequencies of 3,000 Hz or higher. Both patients with exit sites on the scalp had severe PNBD. Four patients with electric current injuries and 2 with other injuries had permanent peripheral nerve damage.

Conclusions.—The nervous system in general and the auditory system in particular are vulnerable to electric current injury. Multidisciplinary studies will nearly always distinguish between organic brain disorders and PTSD or other emotional disorders in the months after electric injury. Persistent auditory symptoms should suggest the possibility of permanent brain damage.

▶ This article stresses the important fact that the care of the burn patient does not end with closure of the burn wound. These patients must be carefully observed for late signs of injury. Failure to recognize or appropriately treat the neuropsychologic aspects of thermal injury is a relatively common problem that must be guarded against.—E.A. Deitch, M.D.

4 Trauma

Introduction

During the past year, progress in the field of trauma care has continued its rapid pace, and the efforts made in the past decade to educate society regarding the unique clinical demands of trauma care have borne fruit. For example, epidemiologic studies highlighting the importance of regionalized prehospital care systems and optimal transport policies, as well as the role of early diagnosis and definitive operative therapy of major injuries in reducing "preventable" deaths, have been a major factor in improving survival of the trauma patient. Nonetheless, because trauma remains the major cause of death in individuals younger than 44 years of age and accounts for more years of life lost than does either cancer or heart disease, more work is needed. Thus, attention continues to be focused on ways to improve the care of the trauma patient. The articles selected for inclusion in this section include topics that range from strategies to improve the prehospital phase of trauma care to the basic biology of injury.

Evidence that prehospital care policies and therapy improve outcome after major injury continues to increase. One example of this concept is a prehospital study indicating that a "scoop and run" policy may be superior to a "stay and stabilize" policy that delays transport from the field to the hospital. Likewise, encouraging results regarding survival have been reported in a prospective trial of small-volume resuscitation with hypertonic saline administered during transport from the field to the hospital.

Studies evaluating the accuracy and clinical value of an increasing array of diagnostic tests directed toward improving our ability to identify abdominal and thoracic injuries continue to appear. These include laparoscopy, ultrasonography, and transesophageal echocardiography. Based on the results of these clinical trials, there are new diagnostic algorithms that increase diagnostic accuracy and, thereby, improve patient care. In addition, as illustrated by a study using sequential CT scans to monitor the healing rate of hepatic injuries, noninvasive techniques are providing important information on the natural history of solid organ injuries. As we all know, having diagnosed an injury is not enough; we must successfully treat that injury. Thus, surgical technique, operative tricks, and surgical strategies remain of paramount importance. To that end, several articles that deal with these important topics have been included. The specific areas covered are the management of difficult liver injuries, surgical strategies in cold and coagulopathic patients, reoperation in the patient with postoperative bleeding, and the role and timing of intramedullary femoral fracture fixation in multitrauma patients with and without major thoracic injuries.

Because it is clear that the care of the trauma patient does not end with closure of the operative wounds, the development and use of physiologically based strategies to reduce postoperative complications, as well as the development of organ failure, continue to be major areas of investigation. To that end, controversy still exists regarding the best means of determining whether oxygen delivery has been optimized. Selected basic studies investigating the mechanisms and pathophysiology of impaired oxygen delivery, organ dysfunction, and sepsis in the trauma patient have been included to provide insight into potential future therapeutic options. Finally, the last article chosen deals with the financial aspects of trauma and the potential effects it may have on patient care.

Edwin A. Deitch, M.D.

Impact of On-Site Care, Prehospital Time, and Level of In-Hospital Care on Survival in Severely Injured Patients

Sampalis JS, Lavoie A, Williams JI, Mulder DS, Kalina M (McGill Univ, Montreal; Univ of Toronto; Urgences-santé, Montreal)
J Trauma 34:252–261, 1993   140-94-4-1

Background.—Trauma is the leading cause of death in North America for individuals younger than age 45 years. Half of these deaths occur instantaneously or within 1 hour of the time of injury. About 15% of trauma-related deaths occur more than 1 week after the injury, the result of complications or infections. Early deaths, which occur between the first hour and 1 week after the injury, may be reduced by prehospital trauma care. There is some concern that on-site advanced life support (ALS) increases the time between injury and definitive care. The impact of on-site care, total prehospital time, and the level of in-hospital care on short-term survival were tested in this study.

Methods.—A sample of 360 severely injured patients was selected from a cohort of 8,007 trauma victims. The patients had received prehospital care from Urgences-santé, an emergency medical system in Montreal that dispatches physicians to the scene to provide on-site care. Trauma victims are generally transferred to the nearest hospital with an emergency room; none of the hospitals in Montreal fulfills all criteria for a level I trauma center. The primary outcome of this case referent study was 6-day survival.

Results.—The odds of dying were significantly higher for patients with various comorbid conditions; those injured in motor vehicle crashes; those with penetrating injuries; and those with injuries to the head, chest, and abdomen. The mean response, scene, transport, and total hospital times were similar for cases and referents. In multiple logistic regression analysis, the use of ALS at the scene was not associated with survival. Treatment at a level I–compatible hospital, however, was associated with a 38% reduction in the odds of dying. The most significant association with the odds of dying was Injury Severity Score category, followed by a total prehospital time exceeding 60 minutes.

Conclusion.—Findings support the "golden hour" principle for prehospital management of trauma patients. Physician-provided on-site ALS did not improve short-term survival in these severely injured patients. Reduced prehospital time and high-level in-hospital care, the basic components of a regionalized trauma care system, are critical factors in improving survival.

▶ Based on an everincreasing number of studies, it is essentially uncontestable that the development of regionalized trauma systems, consisting of emergency prehospital trauma care systems and designated trauma hospitals, has improved survival of trauma patients with potentially life-threatening injuries. Nonetheless, controversy exists among experts regarding what constitutes optimal prehospital trauma care. To quote that famous modern philosopher Ross Perot, "The devil is in the details."

The major value of this paper is that the authors have examined the devilish controversy as to whether ALS manuevers done in the field are beneficial or detrimental. This controversy revolves around whether a "stay and stabilize" policy, in which transport from the field is delayed and ALS manuevers are done to limit physiologic deterioration during transport, is superior to a "scoop and run" policy, in which the time taken to transport the patient to the designated trauma hospital is minimized. The authors' results indicating that on-site ALS in the field—even when administered by physicians—did not improve survival in an urban trauma system, supports the "scoop and run" philosophy, as does their observation that a prehospital time exceeding 60 minutes was associated with a significantly increased risk of death. Although one of the limitations of this study is that predetermined protocols for ALS were not in place, it does emphasize that temporizing treatment in the field is no substitute for definitive treatment in the hospital.—E.A. Deitch, M.D.

A Multicenter Trial for Resuscitation of Injured Patients With 7.5% Sodium Chloride: The Effect of Added Dextran 70
Vassar MJ, Fischer RP, O'Brien PE, Bachulis BL, Chambers JA, Hoyt DB, Holcroft JW, and the Multicenter Group for the Study of Hypertonic Saline in Trauma Patients (Univ of California-Davis, Sacramento; Univ of Texas, Houston; Miami Valley Hosp, Dayton, Ohio; et al)
Arch Surg 128:1003–1013, 1993   140-94-4–2

Introduction.—Combining 7.5% sodium chloride with a colloid was found to be beneficial in an animal model of hemorrhagic shock, but it

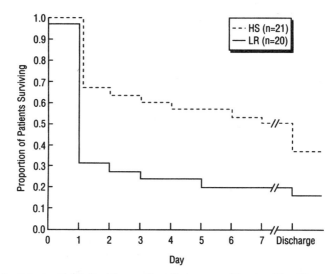

Fig 4–1.—Patients with baseline Glasgow Coma Scale scores of 8 or less. The difference in overall survival between patients in the hypertonic saline (HS) group and those in the lactated Ringer's (LR) solution group was not significant (34% vs. 12%, respectively). By logistic regression, the odds ratio for improvement in survival with administration of HS was 8. By Cox proportional-hazards analysis, it was 2.4. (Courtesy of Vassar MJ, Fischer RP, O'Brien PE, et al: *Arch Surg* 128:1003–1013, 1993.)

appeared to have no value with respect to blood pressure response and survival in a single-center clinical trial of hypotensive trauma patients. In multicenter trial, the use of 250 mL of a 7.5% sodium chloride solution, both with and without added dextran 70, was evaluated for prehospital resuscitation of injured patients.

Methods.—Patients from 6 trauma systems were enrolled in the study from March 1990 through June 1991. Those eligible had systolic blood pressures less than 90 mm Hg at any time in the field or during helicopter transport. The solutions, infused in a double-blind, randomized manner, were as follows: lactated Ringer's solution, 7.5% sodium chloride, 7.5% sodium chloride combined with 6% dextran 70, and 7.5% sodium chloride combined with 12% dextran 70.

Conventional fluids were also given as the patients' conditions required. Patients receiving less than 200 mL of the study solution were not included. Outcome measures were blood pressure response, survival to hospital discharge, and survival compared with that predicted by norms from the Major Trauma Outcome Study (MTOS).

Results.—The overall survival rate was 49% for the lactated Ringer's solution group, 60% for the hypertonic saline (7.5% sodium chloride) group, 56% for the group receiving 7.5% sodium chloride combined with 6% dextran 70, and 45% for the group receiving 7.5% sodium chloride combined with 12% dextran 70. The differences in survival among the groups were not statistically significant. Patients in the hypertonic saline solution group, however, did have a significantly higher rate of survival than that predicted by MTOS norms (60% vs. 48%). Also, the mean change in systolic blood pressure on arrival at the emergency department was significantly higher in these patients than in patients in the Ringer's solution group. Finally, in patients with baseline Glasgow Coma Scale scores of 8 or less, logistic regression analysis showed a survival advantage for the hypertonic saline solution group over the Ringer's solution group (Fig 4-1).

Conclusion.—Results confirmed that prehospital administration of 7.5% sodium chloride in hypotensive patients with trauma results in a clinically significant increase in blood pressure. Hypertonic saline solution without added dextran 70 was found to be as effective as the more expensive solutions containing the colloid.

▶ One's view of this paper can almost reflect one's basic philosophy, i.e., whether the glass is half full or half empty. By nature, I am a "half-full" person. Thus, although the overall survival rate of the patient groups receiving hypertonic saline was not significantly increased, that survival of many of the hypertonic saline–treated cohorts (but none of the patients treated with lactated Ringer's solution) was higher than predicted by TRISS methodology indicates to me that small-volume therapy done in the field with hypertonic saline may be beneficial. This is especially true when one considers previous clinical studies evaluating the therapeutic efficacy of hypertonic saline therapy in the field.—E.A. Deitch, M.D.

The Cost of Not Wearing Seat Belts: A Comparison of Outcome in 3,396 Patients
Rutledge R, Lalor A, Oller D, Hansen A, Thomason M, Meredith W, Foil MB, Baker C (Univ of North Carolina, Chapel Hill; Carolinas Med Ctr, Charlotte, NC; Bowman Gray School of Medicine, Salem, NC; et al)
Ann Surg 217:122–127, 1993   140-94-4–3

Objective.—In North Carolina, only 64% of drivers used seat belts 1 year after passage of a mandatory use law. Data from 8 trauma centers in the state were reviewed in an attempt to relate seat belt use to patient outcome. Data on belt use were available for 3,396 of 6,237 individuals involved in motor vehicle accidents. Of these, 1,480 wore belts and 1,916 did not.

Findings.—Crash victims, peaking at ages 10 to 39 years, had the lowest rate of seat belt use. A blood alcohol level higher than 100 mg/dL was found in 21% of the unbelted group and 9% in the belted group. Trauma scores at the scene and in the emergency department were comparable in the 2 groups, but Glasgow Coma Scale scores were significantly worse in the unbelted group. Head injury occurred in 44.5% of the unbelted and in 33% of the belted group. Unbelted individuals required more ventilator time and longer intensive care unit stays. Hospital charges, excluding professional fees, were nearly 50% higher for un-belted patients. The mortality rate was 7% in the unbelted group and 3% in those wearing seat belts.

Conclusion.—In motor vehicle accidents, wearing seat belts is associated with less severe injury, lower mortality, and less use of hospital resources.

▶ It is nice to see that seat belts work and that law-abiding citizens are rewarded. The results of this study should prompt lawmakers to consider the folly of repealing mandatory motorcycle helmet laws. The study also highlights the significant clinical value of epidemiologic studies directed at identifying the societal factors affecting injury outcome.—E.A. Deitch, M.D.

The Role of Diagnostic Laparoscopy in the Management of Trauma Patients: A Preliminary Assessment
Salvino CK, Esposito TJ, Marshall WJ, Dries DJ, Morris RC, Gamelli RL (Loyola Univ, Maywood, Ill)
J Trauma 34:506–515, 1993   140-94-4–4

Introduction.—The use of laparoscopy has been extended from gynecologic practice to a wide range of general surgical problems. Diagnostic laparoscopy (DL) was compared with diagnostic peritoneal lavage (DPL) in trauma patients acutely requiring evaluation of the abdomen.

Methods.—Seventy-five trauma patients were prospectively studied with DL followed by DPL. Fifty-nine of the patients had blunt injuries, and 16 had stab wounds. The average age of the group was 32 years, and the mean Injury Severity Score was 11. Ninety-three percent of the procedures were performed in the emergency department.

Results.—Forty-two (56%) of the patients had negative findings on both DPL and DL. Twenty of 23 patients with negative DPL findings had abnormal, but insignificant, findings on DL. All 20 were managed nonsurgically with no complication. The remaining 3 patients with DPL cell counts of less than 10,000 red blood cells underwent surgery solely on the basis of DL findings of diaphragmatic lacerations from stab wounds. Three patients had abnormal DL findings and positive DPL findings. All 7 patients with both positive DPL and significant DL findings had therapeutic laparotomies with no postoperative complications. Overall, management decisions based on DL rather than the results of DPL would have improved the care of 6 (8%) of these 75 patients.

Conclusion.—Although DL takes slightly longer to perform than DPL, the information obtained with DL is more specific. In cases of abdominal stab wounds, DL offers an advantage over DPL as a primary assessment tool. In this series of patients, the use of DL would have potentially improved care in 3 of 10 patients with positive DPL findings and in

3 of 65 patients with negative DPL findings. Diagnostic laparoscopy can be performed safely in stable patients under local anesthesia.

▶ Video games are fun, and an increasing number of studies using DL in trauma patients indicate that this technique may even be helpful. The rationale for using DL is that although DPL is accurate in identifying greater than 95% of patients with abdominal injuries, it has its limitations. Diagnostic peritoneal lavage does not identify the nature of the injury or the organs injured, and it is unreliable in patients with retroperitoneal or diaphragmatic injuries. Additionally, nontherapeutic laparotomy rates in patients with positive DPLs range from 10% to 25%. Many of these limitations of DPL—such as the identification of retroperitoneal injuries and the nature of solid organ injuries—can be obviated by abdominal contrast CT scans. However, CT scans also have their Achilles heel in that they miss diaphragmatic, hollow viscus, and mesenteric injuries. Because of the limitations of DPL and CT scans, the use of laparoscopy as a diagnostic test has been increasingly evaluated during the past 5 years.

Although many good studies of DL have appeared during the past year (1, 2), this prospective study was chosen because each patient underwent both DPL and DL. By using this study design, it was possible for the authors to compare directly the accuracy of DL to the gold-standard DPL. Consequently, their results showing that DL may be superior to DPL—especially in patients with thoracoabdominal stab wounds in which the risk of diaphragmatic injury is significant—is worthy of note.

Although the clinical role of DL is still in limbo, it is wise to remember that, although it is potentially dangerous to be among the first to adopt a new technique, it is equally bad to ignore the data.—E.A. Deitch, M.D.

References

1. Fabian TC, et al: *Ann Surg* 217:557, 1993.
2. Townsend MC, et al: *J Trauma* 35:647, 1993.

Prospective Evaluation of Surgeons' Use of Ultrasound in the Evaluation of Trauma Patients

Rozycki GS, Ochsner MG, Jaffin JH, Champion HR (Washington Hosp Ctr, Washington, DC; Uniformed Services Univ of the Health Sciences, Bethesda, Md)
J Trauma 34:516–527, 1993   140-94-4–5

Introduction.—Surgeons in Europe and Japan commonly use ultrasound in the evaluation of trauma patients. This practice is not widespread in the United States, however. Ultrasound may not be available in the trauma resuscitation area, technicians are not present around-the-clock, and surgeons lack experience with the technique. The ability of surgeons to master specific ultrasound techniques and apply the imaging method to the detection of intra-abdominal fluid or pericardial effusion in patients with blunt and penetrating injuries was investigated.

Methods.—Four attending trauma surgeons, 4 trauma fellows, and 25 surgical residents at a level I trauma center took part in the study. All successfully completed a 32-hour course in ultrasound that focused on the identification of fluid in 3 dependent abdominal areas and in the pericardial sac. All sonograms were obtained with the patient in the supine position and within 30 minutes of arrival in the trauma resuscitation area. Examinations were performed on 476 patients, 84% with blunt injuries and 16% with penetrating injuries.

Results.—The surgeons' ultrasound evaluations yielded 369 true negative, 71 true positive, 19 false negative, and 17 false positive results. In the detection of fluid, ultrasound had a sensitivity of 79% and a specificity of 95.6%. Reviewing sonologists confirmed the surgeons' interpretations of 90% of the scans.

Conclusion.—The results confirmed the surgeons' ability to master specific ultrasound techniques for identification of fluid in the abdomen and pericardial sac. With experience, the time required for examination decreased from an average of 4.7 minutes to 2.5 minutes per patient. Ultrasound is recommended for use by trauma surgeons because of its accuracy, noninvasive nature, speed, and modest cost.

▶ The use of ultrasound as a noninvasive, rapid diagnostic technique in trauma patients is gaining momentum in the United States (1), based on studies from other countries (2, 3) demonstrating its clinical utility. Thus, whether we want to or not, it appears likely that surgeons who care for trauma patients may have to learn to perform and interpret emergency room ultrasound evaluations. Based on this study, it appears that obtaining the necessary skill to accomplish this task may not be all that difficult. Time will tell.—E.A. Deitch, M.D.

References

1. Shackford SR: *J Trauma* 35:181, 1993.
2. Forster R, et al: *J Trauma* 34:264, 1992.
3. Liu M, et al: *J Trauma* 35:267, 1993.

Use of Transesophageal Echocardiography in the Evaluation of Traumatic Aortic Injury
Kearney PA, Smith DW, Johnson SB, Barker DE, Smith MD, Sapin PM (Univ of Kentucky, Lexington)
J Trauma 34:696–703, 1993   140-94-4-6

Objective.—Aortography is the "gold standard" for the diagnosis of thoracic artery injury. In patients with blunt chest trauma, aortography is widely used to avoid the potentially fatal outcome associated with diag-

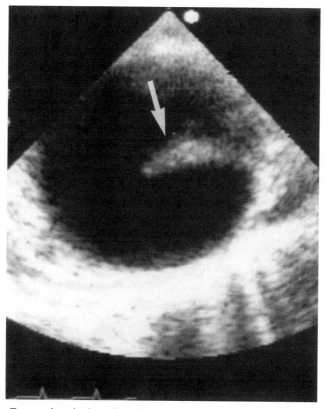

Fig 4–2.—Transesophageal echocardiographic image of ruptured thoracic aorta. *Arrow* points to intraluminal echogenic defects indicative of aortic wall disruption. (Courtesy of Kearney PA, Smith DW, Johnson SB, et al: *J Trauma* 34:696–703, 1993.)

nostic delay; as a result, the negativity rate is as high as 90%. Preliminary reports have suggested that transesophageal echocardiography (TEE) is useful in evaluating suspected rupture of the thoracic aorta. The role and predictive value of TEE in evaluating suspected aortic injury were prospectively examined.

Methods.—The study sample comprised 69 patients with blunt chest trauma and suspected injury to the thoracic aorta, based on the mechanism of injury and radiographic findings of the chest. All patients underwent both TEE and aortography, which were performed and interpreted by staff radiologists and cardiologists.

Results.—Transesophageal echocardiography took a mean of 27 minutes compared with 76 minutes for aortography; neither procedure resulted in any complications. Sixty-one patients were shown to have no sign of aortic injury by either technique. One patient had a false positive result on aortography. Four of the 7 aortic injuries detected by TEE were confirmed by aortography (Fig 4–2). Two patients had false negative aortograms, 1 detected at thoracotomy and the other not detected until autopsy. In all cases, TEE accurately predicted the presence or absence of aortic injury, with a sensitivity and specificity of 100%.

Conclusion.—These findings suggest that TEE can play an important role in the assessment of patients with suspected aortic injury. It is a safe and efficient diagnostic method for use in patients with multiple injuries. Further experience at more centers will be needed to fully define its role.

▶ As discussed in the paper, because of the lethality of a missed aortic injury, the indications for aortography in patients with blunt chest trauma are broad and ill defined. Although conceptually it is better to have a liberal policy of aortography and a high negative rate than to miss a thoracic aortic injury, practically speaking, the logistics and potential consequences of transporting the multiply injured patient to the radiology suite is not trivial. Thus, the availability of an accurate, noninvasive bedside modality for diagnosing aortic injury would be a major advance. Transesophageal echocardiography may be such an advance. Because it is performed at the bedside, TEE can be done in the emergency room, intensive care unit, or operating room. Like the authors of this study, my own personal experience with TEE has been good, and I believe as more experience with TEE is accumulated, it will replace aortography as the initial screening test for the diagnosis of aortic injury.—E.A. Deitch, M.D.

Hepatic Injury From Blunt Trauma in Children: Follow-Up Evaluation With CT
Bulas DI, Eichelberger MR, Sivit CJ, Wright CJ, Gotschall CS (George Washington Univ, Washington, DC)
AJR 160:347–351, 1993   140-94-4–7

Introduction.—Many children who undergo surgery for hepatic injuries from blunt trauma are found to have been candidates for conservative management. With the use of CT, nonsurgical treatment of children who are hemodynamically stable is often possible. A CT grading system was used to evaluate the frequency of complications and the time course of healing in children with hepatic injury.

Methods.—The patient group included 45 children with CT or surgical evidence of hepatic injury. In 43 cases, CT scans were obtained at the time of the initial injury. The remaining 2 children were hemodynamically unstable upon admission and were taken directly to surgery. Two radiologists independently reviewed the scans and classified hepatic injuries as mild (< 25% of 1 lobe injured), moderate (25% to 50% of 1 lobe injured), or severe (> 50% of 1 lobe injured), and as superficial or deep. Follow-up CT scans were performed at a mean of 4.1 months after injury. A second follow-up scan was obtained if the lesion had not yet resolved. Children were allowed to resume full activities only after complete resolution of the lesion.

Results.—The initial evaluation identified 12 mild, 19 moderate, and 14 severe hepatic injuries; 20 injuries were superficial and 25 were deep. Of the 20 cases of large hemoperitoneum, 10 involved children with injuries classified as severe. Associated abdominal injuries had occurred in 20 children. Thirty-seven patients were treated nonoperatively. All of the mild hepatic injuries appeared to have healed on follow-up studies 1 week to 11 months after the injury; 80% of the moderate injuries had resolved completely in between 3.5 and 6 months. Although residual lesions were seen in 7 of 11 children with severe injuries who were reexamined 9–15 months after injury, no delayed hepatic complications occurred.

Conclusion.—The use of CT to grade liver injuries in children can help to estimate the time course of healing. Because healing can be variable or delayed, follow-up scans are recommended at 3–6 months after moderate injuries and 9 months after severe injuries. Intravenous contrast material was useful in 4 studies but offered no additional information in 28 of 32 studies.

▶ This article was chosen because of the basic information it provides on the natural history of liver injuries and because follow-up information on hepatic injuries is limited. Thus, this article provides data that can be used to inform patients and their families of approximately how long a liver injury will take to heal. Because of their active life-styles, this is particularly important in children and adolescents. Unfortunately, however, major questions raised by this article, which are not answered, are whether restricting activities improves the rate of healing and whether partial healing is adequate for the child to resume full activity.—E.A. Deitch, M.D.

Balloon Tamponade for Bilobar Transfixing Hepatic Gunshot Wounds
Poggetti RS, Moore EE, Moore FA, Mitchell MB, Read RA (Denver Gen Hosp; Univ of Colorado, Denver; Univ of São Paulo, Brazil)
J Trauma 33:694–697, 1992   140-94-4-8

Background.—Because urgent hepatic lobectomy to treat life-threatening liver trauma has a high mortality rate, nonresectional alternatives are preferred. A balloon tamponade device that has proven very effective in treating penetrating hepatic gunshot wounds was described.

Technique.—The device is assembled by placing a 16-inch 12F catheter inside a Penrose drain, of which one end has been sutured closed. A second suture is placed at a distance approximately 6 cm greater than the anticipated hepatic wound to provide a water-tight barrier in the proximal end of the balloon. This device is then positioned in the liver via the gunshot wound track, leaving 2–3 cm of extra balloon at either side of the wound (Fig 4–3). The balloon is inflated

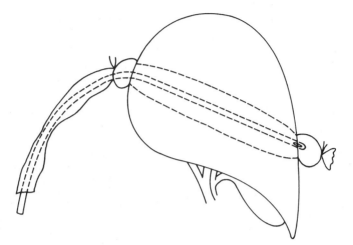

Fig 4–3.—The tamponade balloon positioned in a transfixing gunshot wound via both lobes of the liver. (Courtesy of Poggetti RS, Moore EE, Moore FA, et al: *J Trauma* 33:694-697, 1992.)

with normal saline mixed with contrast medium to allow postoperative radiographic evaluation. The abdomen is closed with towel clips. The balloon is left in place for 24–36 hours and then extracted.

Comment.—The balloon device has controlled the bleeding in 5 patients brought to Denver General Hospital with deep penetrating gunshot wounds to the liver. A similar device has been used successfully in Brazil.

▶ The concept that more is not always better, especially when it comes to treating major liver injuries, has become increasingly recognized during the past decade. The potential usefulness of this ingenious operative trick speaks for itself.—E.A. Deitch, M.D.

The Staged Celiotomy for Trauma: Issues in Unpacking and Reconstruction
Morris JA Jr, Eddy VA, Blinman TA, Rutherford EJ, Sharp KW (Vanderbilt Univ, Nashville, Tenn)
Ann Surg 217:576–586, 1993   140-94-4-9

Objective.—Trauma celiotomy is done under adverse conditions, mainly in that tissue damage has occurred hours before the patient comes to surgery. This has led to the concept of staged celiotomy for the trauma patient in extremis, consisting of initial damage control, restoration of physiologic reserve, and reoperation. The key clinical events and decisions taking place in the reconstruction/unpacking phase of staged trauma celiotomy were reviewed.

Patients.—Over an 8-year period, the investigators performed trauma celiotomies in 1,175 of 13,817 consecutive trauma patients. One hundred seven of these patients, representing about 9% of the celiotomy patients, had staged celiotomy with abdominal packing. Of the 58 patients who survived to the reoperative phase, 74% survived to be discharged from the hospital. Hemorrhage required a return to the operating room for 9 patients, and multiple packing procedures were needed for 13. The 117 complications encountered included abdominal compartment syndrome in 16 patients, positive blood cultures in 8, and abdominal abscesses in 6.

Discussion.—In trauma patients who are undergoing staged celiotomy, reoperation should be done only after correction of temperature, coagulopathy, and acidosis. This will usually be within 36 hours after the damage control phase. Normothermic patients with bleeding over 2 U of packed cells/hr should undergo emergency surgery. Abdominal compartment syndrome is a common complication, occurring in 15% of patients in this series and is characterized by high peak inspiratory pressure, carbon dioxide retention, and oliguria.

Delayed Gastrointestinal Reconstruction Following Massive Abdominal Trauma
Carrillo C, Fogler RJ, Shaftan GW (Brookdale Hosp Med Ctr, Brooklyn, NY)
J Trauma 34:233–235, 1993   140-94-4-10

Background.—The use of temporizing measures to control major exsanguinating injuries continues to gain in popularity. The principles of

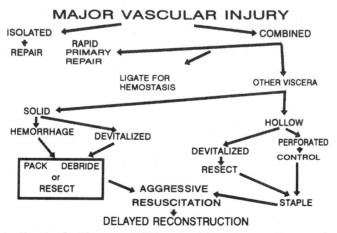

Fig 4-4.—Algorithm for "damage control" in major abdominal trauma. (Courtesy of Carrillo C, Fogler RJ, Shaftan GW: *J Trauma* 34:233-235, 1993.)

abdominal tamponade were used and definitive surgical repair delayed in patients with pancreaticoduodenal destruction.

Methods.—Management involved initial liver packing; aggressive volume restoration; a temporizing surgical procedure for "damage control"; secondary postoperative resuscitation and stabilization; delayed reexploration, usually after 48–96 hours; and late reconstruction (Fig 4–4).

Outcome.—Five of the 7 patients with pancreaticoduodenal destruction were discharged alive. Recently the same concepts have been applied to other types of critical abdominal injuries involving massive blood loss, hypothermia, and acidosis. Seven patients with other major penetrating abdominal injuries have been managed by temporization and delayed repair, and all of them have survived.

Conclusion.—Although primary intra-abdominal packing with delayed definitive reconstruction is associated with a high rate of complications, the method is superior to immediate reconstruction in an unstable trauma victim.

▶ Abstracts 140-94-4–9 and 140-94-4–10 illustrate the general concept of damage control at the initial operation, followed by definitive repair/reconstruction of hollow viscus and solid organ injuries at a subsequent laparotomy, at which time hemostatic packs are removed. This staged approach to the definitive repair and reconstruction of abdominal injuries has clearly resulted in the salvage of patients with otherwise lethal injuries. The concept to remember is that it is always better to live to fight another day. Additionally, in selected instances, this policy is also applicable for operatively stabilizing patients before transfer to a trauma center.—E.A. Deitch, M.D.

Primary Intramedullary Femur Fixation in Multiple Trauma Patients With Associated Lung Contusion: A Cause of Posttraumatic ARDS?
Pape H-C, Auf'm'Kolk M, Paffrath T, Regel G, Sturm JA, Tscherne H (Hannover Med School, Germany)
J Trauma 34:540–548, 1993   140-94-4–11

Background.—Primary stabilization of major fractures in patients with multiple trauma is thought to reduce complications, particularly the incidence of pulmonary infection and adult respiratory distress syndrome (ARDS). Although intramedullary nailing is considered especially advantageous, a number of severely injured patients have experienced a deterioration in pulmonary function and the development of lethal ARDS after intramedullary nailing. Consequently, the possible association of an increased incidence of ARDS with intramedullary stabilization of femoral shaft fractures was investigated in patients with multiple trauma.

Patients and Methods.—Patients admitted to the study had injury severity scores greater than 18, a femoral midshaft fracture treated by intramedullary nailing, and primary admission within 8 hours of injury. Patients who died of head injury or hemorrhagic shock were excluded. The group of 106 patients was divided into those with severe chest trauma (Abbreviated Injury Scale ≥ 2) and those without (Abbreviated Injury Scale < 2) and was further subdivided according to the time of femur stabilization: less than 24 hours after trauma (primary pulmonary nailing) or more than 24 hours after trauma (secondary reduction).

Results.—Patients without thoracic trauma who received early intramedullary nailing spent less time receiving ventilation and had shorter intensive care unit stays than the patients who underwent secondary stabilization. The patients without thoracic injuries who received delayed treatment had a higher incidence of pulmonary infections. However, when primary intramedullary fracture stabilization was done in patients with severe chest injuries, an increased incidence of post-traumatic ARDS and mortality was seen.

Conclusion.—In the absence of severe chest trauma, primary intramedullary femoral nailing appears to be beneficial. However, when multiple trauma is accompanied by thoracic trauma, the early fixation of fractures by intramedullary nailing increases the risk of the development of ARDS. In these cases, definite fracture reduction should be delayed and alternative methods, such as external fixation, should be used.

▶ The message of this article is clear. Early intramedullary fixation of femoral fractures is beneficial, except in those patients with severe thoracic injuries. The observation that the stay in the intensive care unit and the duration of intubation were reduced by greater than 50% by early fracture fixation in patients without severe thoracic injuries is consistent with results in a considerable body of recent literature. Thus, this observation, although important, is not new. In contrast, that early intramedullary fracture fixation was associated with an increased incidence of ARDS (21% vs. 4%) and overall mortality (33% vs. 7.7%) in patients with severe chest trauma is both new and important.

The mechanisms underlying the increased susceptibility of patients with thoracic injuries to the development of lethal ARDS after early intramedullary femoral nailing are not known. Nonetheless, based on this study and the absence of data to the contrary, it appears prudent to avoid early intramedullary femoral nailing in patients with severe thoracic trauma.—E.A. Deitch, M.D.

▶↓ The following article was chosen to illustrate one of the controversies involved in determining how to assess whether resuscitation is complete and optimal. It focuses on the prognostic importance of repaying the oxygen debt that occurs after major trauma.—E.A. Deitch, M.D.

Lactate Clearance and Survival Following Injury

Abramson D, Scalea TM, Hitchcock R, Trooskin SZ, Henry SM, Greenspan J
(State Univ of New York, Brooklyn)
J Trauma 35:584–588, 1993   140-94-4-12

Background.—Past studies of the resuscitative process in patients with serious injuries have stressed the optimization of oxygen delivery, oxygen consumption, and the cardiac index. It seems reasonable that the serum level of lactate, a marker of anaerobic metabolism, could be an important predictor of outcome.

Study Plan.—The value of monitoring the serum level of lactate was examined in a prospective series of 76 consecutive trauma patients who were admitted to the surgical intensive care unit (ICU) directly from the emergency department or the operating room and who lived at least 48 hours. Both the serum level of lactate and oxygen transport were measured at admission to the ICU and after 8, 16, 24, 36, and 48 hours. The criterion for normal lactate clearance was a level of 2 mmol/L or less by 24 hours and maintained at 48 hours.

Results.—Fifty-one of the 76 patients (67%) survived. On the basis of the Injury Severity Score, time in the ICU, or total hospital days, survivors could not be distinguished from those who died. Surviving patients required significantly fewer units of blood before admission to intensive care and during the 48-hour study. The cardiac indices did not differ significantly in the 2 groups, nor were there substantial differences in oxygen delivery or oxygen consumption. Serum levels of lactate were significantly lower in the surviving patients at all times except initially. All patients whose level of lactate was normal within 24 hours of admission to intensive care survived, as did 78% of those who were normalized between 24 and 48 hours; and 14% of those whose levels remained abnormal at 48 hours.

Conclusion.—In these seriously injured patients, achievement of a normal serum level of lactate within 24 hours of admission to intensive care predicted survival far better than the attainment of fixed levels of cardiac index, oxygen delivery, or oxygen consumption.

▶ This study says it is not the cardiovascular response that is important but, rather, it is the ability of the patient to clear lactate that is the major correlate of survival. To the extent that a persistently elevated serum lactate level in patients sustaining major blood loss reflects a shift from aerobic to anaerobic metabolism, it is a reasonable marker of inadequate oxygen delivery at the tissue level and a potential indicator of inadequate resuscitation. However, the physiology is not that simple. Serum lactate levels are based on 2 major factors. One factor is lactate's rate of production in the tissues; the second factor is its rate of clearance by the liver. Thus, inadequate hepatic clearance (i.e., liver injury) and increased peripheral tissue production can both result in increased serum lactate levels. At the current time, it is not possible to solve the controversy surrounding this subject. See reference 1 for a presentation of data indicating that the ability to develop specific cardiovascular parameters correlates with survival.—E.A. Deitch, M.D.

Reference

1. Bishop MH, et al: *Crit Care Med* 21:56, 1993.

Decreased Red Blood Cell Deformability and Impaired Oxygen Utilization During Human Sepsis
Powell RJ, Machiedo GW, Rush BF Jr (Univ of Medicine and Dentistry of New Jersey, Newark)
Am Surg 59:65–68, 1993   140-94-4-13

Background.—Sepsis remains a leading cause of delayed death in seriously injured patients. Altered microcirculatory flow appears to be a major event preceding organ dysfunction in septic patients. Red cell deformability (RCD) is reduced in the septic state, and this may affect the ability of erythrocytes to traverse the microcirculation and, consequently, impair oxygen delivery and utilization.

Patients and Methods.—The effect of altered RCD on hemodynamic status and oxygen use was examined in 10 patients admitted to surgical intensive care, all of whom had clinical sepsis, as evidenced by a white blood cell count of more than 12×10^9/L, a temperature of 38.6°C or higher (or persistently above 37.7°C), and positive cultures. Six of the 10 patients were septic at the outset, and in 4 patients, sepsis occurred later. Red cell deformability was estimated by passing diluted, washed red cells through a 4.7-μm polycarbonate filter at a pressure of -10 cm of water.

Findings.—Patients with an RCD index (DI) below .75 were more often septic than those with normal values (> .75), had a higher mixed venous oxygen saturation, and had lower values for arterial-venous oxygen difference. Only 20% of patients with a DI above .75 were septic. No significant association was found between RCD and the cardiac index, systemic vascular resistance, oxygen delivery, or oxygen consumption.

Conclusion.—These findings provide indirect evidence that decreased RCD contributes to impaired microcirculatory flow in septic patients and, therefore, to abnormal oxygen utilization.

▶ The primary observation of this study—that patients with stiff red blood cells have impaired oxygen utilization—is quite provocative and complements the findings from previous work by these authors. Basically, their hypothesis is that decreased RCD leading to impaired tissue microcirculatory blood flow results in impaired cellular oxygen delivery. If the hypothesis that impaired RCD plays a major role in the pathogenesis of impaired oxygen availability and, consequently, promotes organ dysfunction is correct, then it opens a whole new avenue of therapeutic options for improving tissue oxygen delivery and preventing or limiting the development of organ injury. Time and more work in this field will tell whether this concept is true. In the meantime, we should keep our eyes and minds open.—E.A. Deitch, M.D.

Trauma Causes Early Release of Soluble Receptors for Tumor Necrosis Factor

Tan LR, Waxman K, Scannell G, Ioli G, Granger GA (Univ of California, Irvine)

J Trauma 34:634–638, 1993   140-94-4–14

Background.—In patients with trauma and hemorrhagic shock, tumor necrosis factor (TNF) plays an unknown physiologic role. Its bioactivity may be regulated by soluble forms of the recently identified 55-kd and 75-kd membrane receptors (TNFR).

Methods.—An enzyme-linked immunosorbent assay was used to measure serum circulating TNF and TNFR in 9 patients within 2 hours of severe traumatic injury. The mean Injury Severity Score was 31, and the mean Revised Trauma Score was 6. Eight uninjured controls were also studied.

Results.—The TNFR levels were significantly higher in the trauma patients than in the controls—6.99 and .67 ng/mL, respectively. The trauma victims did not have increased TNF levels, however. In vitro, TNFR-containing serum inhibited the cytotoxicity of TNF. Higher cell survival was correlated with higher levels of 55-kd but not 75-kd TNFR.

Conclusion.—Tumor necrosis factor appears to be a potent releasing factor for TNFR. Higher TNFR levels were documented after trauma, which may provide indirect evidence of the presence of TNF. Tumor necrosis factor and its receptors may play an important pathophysiologic role in trauma and hemorrhagic shock.

▶ This article was chosen not so much for its specific content as for its reflection of an emerging approach to the problem of uncontrolled inflammation and inflammation-induced organ failure. The basic idea behind this approach is that if we can understand the way the body regulates the immunoinflammatory response, we can use these same regulatory systems to stimulate a suboptimal response and shut down an excessive response. In that light, evidence that serum levels of soluble receptors for many of the inflammatory cytokines (interleukin-1 and interleukin-6, in addition to TNF), as well as other proinflammatory factors, are increased during sepsis or after trauma is important. Because the biological activity of circulating cytokines is greatly reduced once they bind to their soluble receptors, these soluble receptors may be a natural defense that helps prevent the inflammatory response from getting out of control. Simply stated, the production and release of cytokine receptors may be one of the host's ways of modulating the response to injury and infection; in that regard, the release of cytokine receptors may function as an immunologic thermostat.—E.A. Deitch, M.D.

Bacterial Translocation Occurs in Humans After Traumatic Injury:
Evidence Using Immunofluorescence
Brathwaite CEM, Ross SE, Nagele R, Mure AJ, O'Malley KF, Garcia-Perez FA
(Univ of Medicine and Dentistry of New Jersey, Camden)
J Trauma 34:586–590, 1993   140-94-4-15

Introduction.—The concept of bacterial translocation—the passage of intestinal bacteria from the gut lumen into normally sterile tissue, causing systemic disease in the absence of anatomical alteration in the intestinal architecture—has been supported by animal experiments. The occurrence of bacterial translocation in trauma patients who have sustained

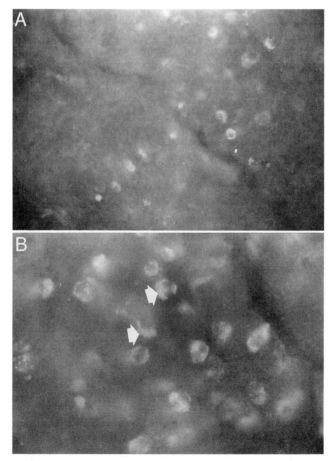

Fig 4–5.—Photomicrographs of mesenteric lymph node taken from a trauma patient. Immunofluorescence analysis reveals *Escherchia coli* beta-galactosidase in cytoplasmic granules of macrophages (*arrows*). **A,** original magnification, ×200; **B,** original magnification, ×500. (Courtesy of Brathwaite CEM, Ross SE, Nagele R, et al: *J Trauma* 34:586–590, 1993.)

hemorrhagic shock (HS) has been documented, and the effect of the presence or absence of HS on the occurrence of bacterial translocation was studied further.

Method.—During a 5-month period, patients at a level I trauma center who required celiotomy and had no abdominal hollow viscus injury were entered into a study. After surgical hemostasis, a distal ileal mesenteric lymph node was removed and a sample of portal venous blood was obtained. The Injury Severity Score, Trauma Score, and period of HS were recorded before the specimens were obtained.

Results.—Twenty-two of the 26 patients initially enrolled in the study were eligible for analysis. Fifteen were in HS; the mean period of HS was 69 minutes. This group had a mean Trauma Score of 10 and a mean Injury Severity Score of 29. Only 2 patients had positive results of portal venous blood cultures. The results of all but 1 of the mesenteric lymph node cultures were negative, but indirect immunofluorescence analysis of the mesenteric lymph node specimens produced different results. In all cases, the *Escherichia coli* beta-galactosidase enzyme was detected within the cytoplasm of macrophages (Fig 4–5). The findings were similar for the 7 patients not in HS. Three patients from the group initially in HS died within the first 24 hours after injury.

Conclusion.—Bacterial translocation occurs in humans after major trauma and may be independent of HS. The exact route of translocation remains unclear. Because organisms may have been phagocytized by macrophages, culture techniques may not detect bacterial translocation. The critical determinant of multiple organ failure has yet to be identified. Only 1 patient in this series had multiple organ failure, despite the finding of *E. coli* beta-galactosidase within macrophages in the mesenteric lymph nodes.

▶ One major controversy concerns the role of gut barrier failure in the pathogenesis of multiple organ failure. Does the gut leak after major trauma and thereby contribute to the septic response? Some say yes, and some say no. The basic idea behind the gut hypothesis of multiple organ failure is as follows: The loss of intestinal barrier function allows bacteria, endotoxin, and other potentially injurious factors from the intestinal lumen to reach the portal and systemic circulations and, thus, contribute to the development of systemic infection and multiple organ failure. Although this study indicates that bacterial translocation occurs in trauma patients, the data are not sufficient to resolve this controversy.—E.A. Deitch, M.D.

Granulocytes of Critically Ill Patients Spontaneously Express the 72 kD Heat Shock Protein

Kindås-Mügge I, Hammerle AH, Fröhlich I, Oismüller C, Micksche M, Traut-

inger F (Univ of Vienna)
Circ Shock 39:247–252, 1993   140-94-4–16

Background.—Heat shock proteins (HSPs) are synthesized in mammalian cells in response to a variety of stresses. The 70-kD HSP family is among the most prominent classes of HSPs in humans; the 73-kD constitutive HSP is readily apparent in all cells under physiologic conditions, and the 72-kD HSP (HSP72) is stress-inducible. Polymorphonuclear neutrophils (PMNs) appear to play a major role in the pathophysiology of severe tissue injury through their release of oxidants and proteases. Recent studies have considered whether HSPs have a role in the protection of tissues from oxidative injury. The expression of HSP72 in the PMNs of 20 patients with major tissue injury was analyzed.

Methods.—Sixteen of the patients had multiple trauma, and 4 had undergone major surgery; all were admitted to the intensive care unit. None had sepsis/septic syndrome or positive blood cultures. The expression of HSP72 was investigated in PMNs of the patients and 10 healthy donors by immunohistochemistry.

Results.—A spontaneous expression of HSP72 in PMNs was detected by immunohistochemistry in 12 patients (60%). Although no specific staining could be detected in the PMNs of healthy donors, HSP72 could be induced by heat treatment. An impairment of respiratory burst activity, compared to controls, was found in the PMNs of 50% of the patients expressing HSP72 without previous heat treatment. No correlation of HSP72 with body temperatures was established.

Conclusion.—The results of this study demonstrate for the first time that PMNs from a high percentage of patients with severe tissue injury express HSP72. Immunohistochemical data were confirmed by Western blot analysis from patient PMNs. These findings contribute to the evidence that induction of HSPs in patients with multiple organ failure may be a sign of autoregulatory protective mechanisms against cellular injury.

▶ Heat shock proteins. Why heat shock proteins? The answer is that these stress- and injury-induced proteins may prove to be critical regulators of whether a cell lives or dies. There is increasing evidence that HSPs are involved in cellular repair mechanisms and, clearly, as our cells go, so go we.—E.A. Deitch, M.D.

Medicare's Resource-Based Relative Value Scale Fee Schedule Portends a Gloomy Future for Trauma Surgery

Moore FA, Moore EE, Read RA, Ogunkeye JO (Denver Gen Hosp; Univ of Colorado, Denver)
J Trauma 34:900–907, 1993   140-94-4–17

Background.—The new Medicare resource-based relative value scale (RBRVS) is designed to redistribute payments across specialties to favor cognitive-based services, mainly evaluation and management services, rather than procedure-based services. This shift is of understandable concern to surgeons, with almost all surgical specialties expecting serious cuts in reimbursement. Trauma surgery would appear to be particularly vulnerable as a result of its clinical services and payer mix. To respond, all trauma surgeons should understand the impact of the new scale on Medicare revenues.

Implications.—The effects of the new system for trauma surgery in comparison to 4 other surgical specialties were calculated. Although plastic surgery can expect a 4% increase in revenue, all others will see reductions. The greatest will be a 14% reduction for trauma surgery, compared to 10% for cardiothoracic surgery, 5% for vascular surgery, and 4% for general surgery. Procedure reimbursement will decrease from 8% to 13% for these specialties, in line with the intention of the new scale. However, trauma surgery is the only specialty that can expect a reduction in reimbursement for cognitive services, a result of the fact that trauma cognitive services are inpatient based whereas other surgical cognitive services are outpatient based. Trauma surgeons will lose 17% in cognitive service fees, compared to increases of about 25% for general and vascular surgeons.

Conclusion.—The new Medicare RBRVS fee schedule poses a significant challenge to the economic stability of the trauma surgery specialty. This outcome is inequitable and appears to be in opposition to the goals of the new fee schedule. Other types of physician reimbursement will follow the lead of Medicare reform, so trauma system planners must take a proactive role in this evolving process.

▶ It seems almost paradoxical that at a time when the life-saving value of trauma systems and the societal contributions of hospitals and clinicians who care for trauma patients are just becoming better recognized by lawmakers and the public, the financial stability of this system is in such jeopardy. This article serves to remind us all that "He who pays the piper calls the tune." —E.A. Deitch, M.D.

5 Infection

Introduction

The 1990s are seeing the increasing dominance of medical practice by corporate medicine. The emphasis is on the cost and quality of medical care. Some of the indicators of quality of care in surgical practice that are easiest to measure are the incidence of wound infections and other nosocomial infections. Four articles (Abstracts 140-94-5-1 through 140-94-5-4) discuss subjects relating to the impact on hospital cost of patients with nosocomial infections and the prevention of nosocomial infections. Prophylactic antibiotics have long been a mainstay of the prevention of postoperative wound infections for patients having class II (clean-contaminated) operations. Abstract 140-94-5-1 suggests that prophylaxis for class I (clean) operations can also reduce the incidence of postoperative wound infections. The next 3 abstracts discuss the high cost of postoperative infections and the prevention and sources of these infections. Abstract 140-94-5-5 reports that catheter-related infections are not necessarily reduced by using central venous catheters with silver impregnated cuffs.

Intra-abdominal infections continue to provide a challenge for those treating surgical infections. It is difficult for one center to accumulate enough patients with intra-abdominal infection to perform a meaningful randomized study of therapy or to accumulate a large enough number of patients to study these infections with statistical validity. Abstract 140-94-5-6 reports on a cooperative trial by members of the Surgical Infection Society, who pooled their data and studied some patients with serious abdominal infections (Acute Physiology and Chronic Health Evaluation [APACHE] II score > 10). Abstract 140-94-5-7 from Europe discusses various scoring systems to evaluate patients with intra-abdominal infections. Patients with intra-abdominal infections stratified according to valid scoring systems will allow one to be sure comparable patients are being evaluated between groups or institutions. These patients are so complex and their diseases are so involved that scoring systems must be used to assure that patients with comparable levels of illness are being evaluated. One of the most difficult intra-abdominal infections to deal with is infected pancreatic necrosis or pancreatic abscess. Despite the use of innovative techniques to deal with this infection, the mortality rate continues to be high in most centers. The open-packing technique is advocated (Abstract 140-94-5-8) and is probably being used by most centers, because it is one way of providing continuous access to the retroperitoneum for continued removal of infected materials with reoperation.

Another source of infection in hospital patients, one not widely considered before the discovery of HIV, is the transmission of infection from hospital workers to patients. Although sporadic cases of transmission of infection were previously reported, especially regarding hepatitis B, it was not until HIV infection became a serious problem that serious investigations (which then often met with much resistance) were initiated. The possibility of transmission from health care workers to patients received widespread attention from the press with the reporting of the transmission of AIDS from a Florida dentist to his patients. Abstracts 140-94-5-9 and 140-94-5-10 discuss the prevalence of HIV infection in patients of 2 surgeons who died of AIDS. In none of the patients did HIV infection develop. These and other papers on the subject are relevant because of the pressure for all surgeons and other health care workers who perform invasive procedures to be tested for HIV and hepatitis.

Richard J. Howard, M.D., Ph.D.

Prophylaxis Against Wound Infection Following Herniorrhaphy or Breast Surgery

Platt R, Zucker JR, Zaleznik DF, Hopkins CC, Dellinger EP, Karchmer AW, Bryan CS, Burke JF, Wikler MA, Marino SK, Holbrook KF, Tosteson TD (Harvard Med School, Boston; Channing Lab, Boston; Brigham and Women's Hosp, Boston; et al)
J Infect Dis 166:556–560, 1992   140-94-5-1

Background.—Recent research shows that prophylaxis prevents about 50% of all postoperative infections after elective herniorrhaphy and certain types of breast surgery. However, no research has demonstrated the efficacy of prophylaxis for wound infection alone after such procedures. Data on several thousand patients would be needed to address this question.

Methods.—The effect of perioperative antibiotic prophylaxis on definite wound infection was determined using data from 3,202 herniorrhaphies or selected breast surgery procedures. Patients were identified before surgery and were monitored for 4 or more weeks. Thirty-four percent were given prophylaxis at the surgeon's discretion.

Findings.—Eighty-six definite wound infections occurred, for an incidence of 2.7%. The risk of infection was higher for prophylaxis recipients, with a higher proportion of mastectomies, longer procedures, and other factors. After adjustment for surgery duration and procedure type, prophylaxis recipients were found to have 41% fewer definite wound infections and 65% fewer definite wound infections that required parenteral antibiotic treatment. The magnitude of the effect was not meaningfully changed by further adjustment for age, body mass index, the presence of drains, diabetes, or exposure to corticosteroids.

Conclusion.—A protective role is indicated for perioperative antibiotic prophylaxis to prevent postoperative wound infection after breast or hernia surgery. Further research is needed to identify optimal clinical applications of these findings.

▶ In a smaller subset from this study (1), these authors showed that overall infections were reduced in patients receiving prophylactic antibiotics for herniorrhaphy or breast surgery compared with control patients who did not receive prophylactic antibiotics; however, there was no significant difference in wound infection rates. This study includes patients from the previous study, who were randomized, and, in addition, patients who were eligible but did not participate in the randomized study. Heretofore, antibiotic prophylaxis has only been advocated for clean-contaminated operations—not for clean operations (unless a foreign body was inserted as part of the operation). However, the great majority of operations done in the United States are clean operations. Thus, the cost of antibiotics would be greatly increased, and with their greater use there would be greater selective pressures in the facilities that use these antibiotics toward resistant organisms.—R.J. Howard, M.D., Ph.D.

Reference

1. Platt R, et al: N Engl J Med 322:153, 1990.

The Economic Impact of Infections: An Analysis of Hospital Costs and Charges in Surgical Patients With Cancer
Shulkin DJ, Kinosian B, Glick H, Glen-Puschett C, Daly J, Eisenberg JM (Univ of Pennsylvania, Philadelphia; Georgetown Univ, Washington, DC)
Arch Surg 128:449–452, 1993   140-94-5-2

Objective.—In an effort to determine the cost of surgical infections, researchers performed an economic analysis of the care provided to patients undergoing major abdominal operations. Because postoperative fever also results in increased hospital costs, they also calculated the economic impact of fever without documented infection.

Methods.—All patients studied were undergoing surgery for gastrointestinal malignancies and were part of a randomized, controlled trial evaluating the use of nutritional supplements to reduce postoperative complications. None had preoperative evidence of infection. Hospital bills and medical records were reviewed for the patients' clinical and demographic characteristics, use of medical care services, and hospital charges. Costs were determined by the use of Medicare cost-charge ratios obtained from the hospital's Medicare Cost Report.

Mean Costs and Charges by Category of Infection and Presence of Fever

	Infections		No Infection	
	Major	Minor	Febrile	Afebrile
No. of patients	13	8	13	51
Mean(±SD) costs, $*	58 067±65 841†	16 726±10 211	30 236±28 451‡	14 961±7950
Mean(±SD) charges, $ §	151 259±173 047†	41 721±25 724	75 094±68 642‡	37 512±21 012

* Analysis of variance (ANOVA) F Statistic, 8.50; $P \leq .0001$ using ANOVA.
† Student's t test significant at $P = .05$ comparing major infection with all other categories.
‡ Student's t test significant at $P = .01$ comparing febrile patients with no infection with afebrile patients with no infection.
§ ANOVA F statistic, 8.52; $P \leq .0001$ using ANOVA.
(Courtesy of Shulkin DJ, Kinosian B, Glick H, et al: Arch Surg 128:449-452, 1993.)

Results.—Twenty-seven postoperative infections occurred in 21 of the 85 patients. Patients with and without infection had no statistically significant differences in clinical and demographic characteristics. In the postoperative period, patients with infectious complications incurred higher total costs and charges than did patients without infection (table). Multivariate analysis indicated that a surgical infection added $12,542 to the cost of patient care; fever without documented infection added $9,145. Infected patients incurred higher costs for microbiology tests, radiology services, drugs, and room charges. Longer hospital stay accounted for 26% of additional charges, laboratory testing for 25%, radiology tests for 4%, pharmaceuticals for 10%, and other services for 35%.

Conclusion.—Postoperative surgical infections substantially add to the cost of patient care. These additional costs were principally found among patients with major infections; the increased costs of minor infections were not significant.

▶ Postoperative infection (an even fever without infection) greatly increases the cost of hospitalization. As we move into an era of corporate medicine, with large insurance companies and managed care providers being able to select physicians and hospitals that have low cost but high quality, minimizing postoperative infections (and other complications) will be important for maintaining one's patient base. Nosocomial infections (such as wound infections) are already being widely used by these providers as an indicator of quality of care. One problem with using quality of care as an indicator for selecting hospitals is that, over time, results of hospitals with high and low infection rates and differences in other indicators of quality tend to converge; therefore, cost may become the overriding or sole criterion for selecting health care providers.—R.J. Howard, M.D., Ph.D.

The Gastrointestinal Tract: The "Undrained Abscess" of Multiple Organ Failure
Marshall JC, Christou NV, Meakins JL (Univ of Toronto; McGill Univ, Montreal)
Ann Surg 218:111–119, 1993   140-94-5-3

Background.—Infection of patients in the intensive care unit (ICU) by ICU staff or visitors and by contaminated devices has been well documented. However, most infections acquired by patients in the ICU are caused by the patient's own flora after pathologic colonization of the gastrointestinal (GI) tract. This GI colonization may be an important precursor to the development of the multiple organ failure (MOF) syndrome. The association between proximal GI colonization and the development of ICU-acquired infection and multiple organ failure among an ICU population of critically ill surgical patients was investigated.

Patients and Methods.—A total of 41 ICU surgical patients were studied. Specimens were obtained from the stomach and upper small bowel for quantitative culture. The numeric score indicated the severity of the organ dysfunction.

Results.—At least one episode of an ICU-acquired infection developed in 33 patients and involved at least one organism simultaneously cultured from the upper GI tract in all but 3 of them. *Candida, Streptococcus faecalis, Pseudomonas,* and coagulase-negative staphylococci were the most common causes of the ICU-acquired infections, as well as the most common species colonizing the proximal GI tract. The GI colonizations correlated with the development of invasive infection within one week of culture for *Pseudomonas* (90% vs. 13% in noncolonized patients), and in *Staphylococcus epidermidis* (80% vs. 6% in noncolonized patients). A weaker association was found for colonization with *Candida.* Types of infections that occurred in patients as a result of colonization included 16 cases of pneumonia, 12 cases of wound infection, 11 cases of urinary tract infection, 11 cases of tertiary recurrent peritonitis, and 10 cases of bacteremia. *Pseudomonas* infections caused the highest mortality rate. *Candida, Pseudomonas,* or *Staphylococcus epidermidis* colonizations caused the most significant organ dysfunction in these patients.

Conclusion.—The GI tract is a major reservoir for organisms that trigger ICU-acquired infection. In the critically ill surgical patient, the pathologic GI colonization that occurs is associated with the development of multiple organ failure. The clinical challenge in affirming or denying the GI hypothesis lies in discovering an effective drainage method.

▶ Noting that infections are extremely common in patients in the ICU and that most of these infections result from organisms commonly found in the GI tract, the authors propose that the GI tract is the source of many, if not most, nosocomial infections occurring in the ICU. These infections may ultimately lead to multiple organ failure. The hypothesis certainly is rational, and bacterial translocation provides a mechanism by which these intestinal microflora gain access to the circulation. However, the role for bacterial translocation in human disease has never been clearly established.

Such thinking, however, has led to selective decontamination of the digestive tract (SDDT). The rationale is to reduce the bacterial load with the hope of reducing the likelihood of infectious complications in ICU patients. Although SDDT can reduce the risk of infection in ICU patients, no study has shown that it reduces the mortality of such patients; it is criticized for that reason. However, the purpose of SDDT is to reduce infection rates, and it does just that. Mortality rates may not be the best way of judging its efficacy.—R.J. Howard, M.D., Ph.D.

Postoperative Pneumonia: A Prospective Study of Risk Factors and Morbidity
Ephgrave KS, Kleiman-Wexler R, Pfaller M, Booth B, Werkmeister L, Young S

(Veterans Affairs Med Ctr, Iowa City, Iowa)
Surgery 114:815–821, 1993   140-94-5-4

Background.—Postoperative pneumonia (PP) has been associated with the microaspiration of pathogens from the gastrointestinal tract. The role of gastric bacterial aspiration in the development of this serious complication was investigated in a prospective study.

Methods.—One hundred forty veterans who were scheduled for major elective surgery requiring nasogastric tubes were included in the study. Cultures of the gastric contents and sputum were obtained twice a day after surgery.

Findings.—Twenty-six patients (18.6%) had PP. The only difference between those with and without PP was a history of chronic obstructive pulmonary disease, which was noted in 38.5% of those with PP and only 20% of those without. The type of operation significantly influenced the incidence of PP and the mean operating time (Fig 5-1). Increased postoperative morbidity was associated with PP. The length of stay in the surgical intensive care unit, days intubated, total postoperative days, and mortality were all higher in patients with PP. At study entry, 38% of the patients had gastric pathogens, and 32% of these patients had PP, compared with 13% of those whose initial gastric cultures were sterile. Colonization of sputum for more than 24 hours with gastric pathogens occurred in 28% of patients. These patients had a PP incidence of 40%, compared with 12% for patients without evidence of microaspiration.

Conclusion.—In this series, the incidence of PP was 18.6%. This pneumonia appears to be associated not only with chronic obstructive pulmonary disease but also with the presence of gastric bacteria during

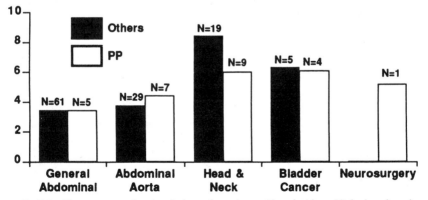

Fig 5–1.—The mean operating time in hours for patients with and without PP, broken down by surgical site. (Courtesy of Ephgrave KS, Kleiman-Wexler R, Pfaller M, et al: *Surgery* 114:815-821, 1993.)

surgery and transmission of gastric bacteria to the pulmonary tree after operation.

▶ This study again points out what has been known for a long time, i.e., nasal gastric tubes promote aspiration of gastric contents and gastric bacteria. These tubes are overused in many settings and are left in too long.—R.J. Howard, M.D., Ph.D.

A Prospective, Randomized Evaluation of the Effect of Silver Impregnated Subcutaneous Cuffs for Preventing Tunneled Chronic Venous Access Catheter Infections in Cancer Patients
Groeger JS, Lucas AB, Coit D, LaQuaglia M, Brown AE, Turnbull A, Exelby P
(Mem Sloan-Kettering Cancer Ctr, New York; Cornell Univ, New York)
Ann Surg 218:206–210, 1993   140-94-5-5

Background.—Tunneled chronic cuffed Silastic central venous access catheters in patients with cancer are often associated with infection, and this complication can be life threatening. Antimicrobial silver-impregnated cuffs placed on nontunneled percutaneously inserted central venous catheters may render a catheter less prone to infection.

Methods and Findings.—Two hundred patients with cancer were randomly assigned to receive a dual-lumen 10-French tunneled cuffed Silastic central venous access catheter or the same catheter with a second, more proximal subcutaneous silver-impregnated cuff. These 2 groups had a hazard rate for infections per day of .0022 and .0027, respectively. Comparison of infectious complications of patients with silver-cuffed catheters and those with control catheters disclosed no statistical difference in the number of catheter-related infections or median time to first infection (table). Regression analysis of the infection-free interval of both catheter types indicated no differences over the lifetime of the catheter or for the first 48 days after insertion.

Catheter-Related Tunnel Infections and Bacteremia-Fungemia

	Standard Catheter	Silver Impregnated Cuff
No. of devices	108	92
No. of tunnel infections (TI)	0	2
No. of catheter bacteremia/fungemia (CBF)	35	33
Total days at risk until first TI or CBF	16,044	13,029
Median infection-free time (days)	117	105
Hazard rate for infection/day (95% confidence limit)	0.0022 (0.0015–0.0030)	0.0027 (0.0019–0.0037)
Total days *in situ* (median)	143 ± 155 (103)	147 ± 163 (89)

(Courtesy of Groeger JS, Lucas AB, Coit D, et al: *Ann Surg* 218:206–210, 1993.)

Conclusion.—The silver-impregnated cuff used in this study did not reduce the incidence of catheter-related bacteremias-fungemias, tunnel infections, or the spectrum of causative micro-organisms in patients with cancer with tunneled chronic venous access catheters. The low incidence of infections in this series indicates that a much larger number of patients is needed to find a statistically significant difference between the groups.

▶ Silver-impregnated subcutaneous cuffs are promoted as reducing the incidence of tunnel infections in patients having long-term venous access catheters. The rationale for impregnated cuffs is that bacteria tracking down the outside of the catheter from the skin would be inhibited or killed by silver ions leaching out of the cuffs. These catheters are more expensive than catheters without silver-impregnated cuffs. This paper shows how a logical idea can be proved invalid by a well-done, randomized, controlled trial. In a study of 200 patients, there was no difference in catheter-related bacteremias, fungemias, tunnel infections, or the spectrum of causative micro-organisms in patients with cancer who had tunneled chronic venous access catheters, regardless of whether the catheters had silver-impregnated cuffs.—R.J. Howard, M.D., Ph.D.

Surgical Infection Society Intra-Abdominal Infection Study: Prospective Evaluation of Management Techniques and Outcome
Christou NV, Barie PS, Dellinger EP, Waymack JP, Stone HH (McGill Univ, Montreal; Cornell Univ, New York; Univ of Washington, Seattle; et al)
Arch Surg 128:193–199, 1993   140-94-5–6

Background.—In an attempt to reduce the high mortality rate of severe peritonitis, 3 alternatives to the conventional approach to therapy have been proposed in recent years. These treatments are radical peritoneal débridement, continuous postoperative peritoneal lavage, and the "open-abdomen" approach. Studies of the value of these management techniques have had conflicting results. In this evaluation of 239 patients with surgical infection in the abdomen and an Acute Physiology and Chronic Health Evaluation (APACHE) II score greater than 10, researchers sought to identify the best method for treatment of severe peritonitis.

Methods.—The study design was that of an open, consecutive, prospective, observational data-collection analysis. Data sheets were sent to all members of the Surgical Infection Societies of North America and Europe. Information on all cases was entered into a computer for statistical analysis.

Results.—The patient group consisted of 140 men with a mean age of 59 years and 99 women with a mean age of 69 years. Renal failure was present in 10% of the patients, a history of cancer in 22%, and diabetes in 27%. All patients reported abdominal pain. Tenderness was noted in

Logistic Regression Analysis Coefficients of Some Important
Variables Contributing to Overall Fit

Variable	Coefficient	SEM	Coefficient of the SEM
Death as the Dependent Variable			
Constant	−0.2928	0.983	−0.298
APACHE II score	0.126	0.032	3.93
Albumin level	−0.133	0.035	−3.74
NYHA cardiac function status of 1 or 2	1.019	0.640	1.59
NYHA cardiac function status of 3	2.182	0.984	2.22
NYHA cardiac function status of 4	2.288	0.951	2.41
Reoperation as the Dependent Variable			
Constant	0.814	0.987	0.825
Albumin level	−0.043	0.025	−1.700
Age	−0.019	0.011	−1.800
APACHE II score	0.046	0.025	1.770

Abbreviation: NYHA, New York Heart Association.
(Courtesy of Christou NV, Barie PS, Dellinger EP, et al: *Arch Surg* 128:193–199, 1993.)

79% of patients and distention in 50%. Seventy-seven patients (32%) died. The mortality rate was higher in patients who underwent reoperation (42%) than in those who did not (27%). The difference in mortality rate between patients treated with a "closed-abdomen" technique and those treated with an "open-abdomen" technique was not significant (31% vs. 44%, respectively). Interactions among the variables significantly related to mortality in univariate analysis were examined using logistic regression analysis. With death as the dependent variable, only APACHE II score, serum albumin level, and New York Heart Association cardiac function status were significantly and independently associated with mortality. With reoperation as the dependent variable, age, albumin level, and APACHE II score made significant and independent contributions (table).

Conclusion.—Despite advances in critical care and the availability of powerful antibiotics, the mortality rate associated with severe peritonitis remains high. These findings suggest that the host response to infection and the cardiovascular reserve of the patient, not the bacteria present, may be determinants of mortality in intra-abdominal infection. Strategies to reduce mortality may need to focus on means of controlling the host cytokine response to the initiating event.

▶ Only with cooperative data collection is one likely to accumulate a large enough number of patients with intra-abdominal infection to reach statistically valid conclusions. This large trial stratified patients with APACHE scores and studied those with scores greater than 10. Although it wasn't a randomized, prospective trial, it attempted to evaluate the open-abdomen technique and found that it was no better than the closed-abdomen technique for treating patients with peritonitis. It is unlikely that a prospective, randomized trial will ever be done because of the strong prejudices held by advocates of both open- and closed-abdomen techniques. Despite modern supportive therapy, the mortality rate of patients with intra-abdominal infection who have an APACHE score greater than 10 remains high. However, as pointed out in the discussion, most patients seen with peritonitis have low APACHE scores; therefore, the results of this paper are not reflective of many patients seen with peritonitis.—R.J. Howard, M.D., Ph.D.

Prospective Evaluation of Prognostic Scoring Systems in Peritonitis
Ohmann C, Wittmann DH, Wacha H, and the Peritonitis Study Group (Heinrich-Heine Univ, Düsseldorf, Germany; Med College of Wisconsin, Milwaukee; Hosp zum Heiligen Geist, Frankfurt, Germany)
Eur J Surg 159:267–274, 1993   140-94-5-7

Objective.—In a prospective multicenter trial, the comparative accuracy of 3 prognostic scoring systems was assessed in a group of 271 patients with surgically confirmed peritonitis. The systems examined included the Acute Physiology and Chronic Health Evaluation (APACHE) II score, the Mannheim Peritonitis Index (MPI), and the Peritonitis Index Altona (PIA) II.

Results.—The 30-day postoperative mortality rate was 21%; 79% of deaths resulted from infection. An analysis of the receiver operating characteristic curves indicated that the APACHE II discriminated better than the other scoring systems. For instance, at a fixed specificity of 80%, the APACHE II was 75% sensitive compared with 60% for the MPI and 55% for the PIA II. The APACHE II system did not generally yield sharp predictions compared with the other systems. Studies of reliability showed that only with the APACHE II were there no significant differences between observed and predicted death rates (Fig 5–2). Neither the MPI nor the PIA II was a reliable prognostic scoring system.

Conclusion.—Each of the prognostic scoring systems examined had at least 1 point of strength, and none of them performed satisfactorily in all respects. At present, the APACHE II remains the standard for assessing the severity of peritonitis.

▶ Prognostic scoring systems in patients with peritonitis are imprecise predictors of outcome, and as these authors point out, they are of no use in predicting outcome for individual patients. Nevertheless, they can be helpful in stratifying patients for clinical studies and in comparing results from 1 institu-

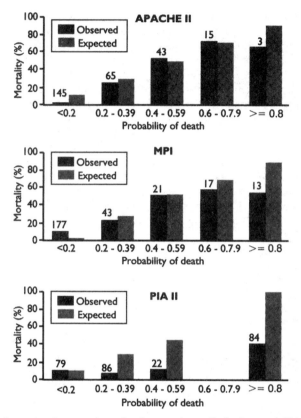

Fig 5–2.—Comparison between observed and expected mortality by 3 scores (which indicates reliability of calibration). There were significant differences between observed and expected mortality for MPI and PIA II but not for APACHE II (goodness of fit test). (Courtesy of Ohmann C, Wittmann DH, Wacha H, et al: *Eur J Surg* 159:267–274, 1993.)

tion to another. It is somewhat surprising that APACHE II was a better method for accessing these patients than 2 scoring systems specifically designed for patients with peritonitis. The APACHE II system was designed to evaluate patients in intensive care units, not patients with peritonitis.—R.J. Howard, M.D., Ph.D.

Techniques and Complications of Open Packing of Infected Pancreatic Necrosis
Orlando R III, Welch JP, Akbari CM, Bloom GP, Macaulay WP (Hartford Hosp, Conn; Univ of Connecticut, Hartford)
Surg Gynecol Obstet 177:65–71, 1993   140-94-5-8

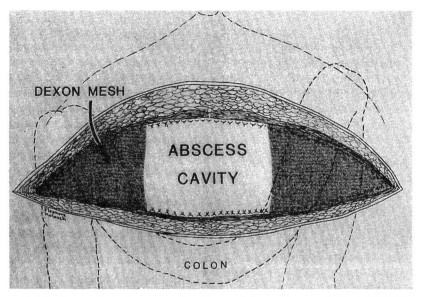

Fig 5–3.—Drawing illustrating mesh as adjunct to wound closure. (Courtesy of Orlando R III, Welch JP, Akbari CM, et al: *Surg Gynecol Obstet* 177:65-71, 1993.)

Background.—Acute pancreatitis continues to have an overall mortality rate of 10%. The results of open packing of infected pancreatic necrosis were reported.

Methods.—Fifteen patients with infected pancreatic necrosis were managed with open packing between 1982 and 1991. The underlying pancreatitis was caused by ethanol in 7 cases, gallstones in 4, drugs in 2, trauma in 1, and surgery in 1. Operative pancreatic debridement was done through a midline incision in 4 patients and a transverse incision in 11. All wounds were left open or were partially closed over gauze packing. Polyglycolic mesh was used as an adjunct to wound closure to prevent evisceration (Fig 5-3). Other procedures done at initial surgery were transverse colectomy in 2 cases, duodenal diverticulization in 1, jejunostomy in 6, and cholecystostomy in 4. A mean of 5 subsequent dressing changes was needed in the operating room; subsequent dressing changes were done in the intensive care unit.

Outcomes.—The survival rate was 80%. The mean time in intensive care was 26 days. Early complications were pulmonary insufficiency in 14 cases, bleeding in 4, intestinal fistulas in 4, and a pancreatic fistula in 1. Incisional hernia, occurring in 7 patients, was the most common late complication.

Conclusion.—Open packing is an effective treatment in patients with infected pancreatic necrosis. However, it is a labor-intensive treatment and requires a committed team of surgeons, interventional radiologists, and critical-care providers. Complications can be minimized by attending to specific technical aspects.

▶ Infected pancreatic necrosis has a high mortility rate. A variety of surgical treatments have been claimed to lower the mortality rate, usually by between 15% and 30%. All authors would agree that débridement of necrotic material and drainage of infected material is required. Open packing techniques permit débridement, either in the intensive care unit or in the operating room, without the necessity for completely reopening the abdomen. In the 1993, YEAR BOOK OF SURGERY (1), the retroperitoneal approach to the management of severe acute pancreatic necrosis was reviewed. Although that technique obviated the necessity of entering the peritoneal cavity, the mortality rate of patients so treated (22%) did not differ from transperitoneal approaches.—R.J. Howard, M.D., Ph.D.

Reference

1. 1993 YEAR BOOK OF SURGERY, p 116.

Absence of HIV Transmission From an Infected Orthopedic Surgeon: A 13-Year Look-Back Study

von Reyn CF, Gilbert TT, Shaw FE Jr, Parsonnet KC, Abramson JE, Smith MG (Dartmouth-Hitchcock Med Ctr, Lebanon, NH; Brown Univ, Providence, RI; New Hampshire Dept of Health and Human Services, Concord)

JAMA 269:1807–1811, 1993   140-94-5–9

Purpose.—Although occupational transmission of HIV from patients to health care workers is well recognized, there is only 1 known case of transmission from a health care worker to a patient. The "look-back" studies seeking evidence of HIV transmission from infected surgeons and other physicians to their patients have all been negative, but the studies have been small and have been conducted mainly in areas with a high background rate of HIV infection. The risk of HIV transmission from an HIV-infected surgeon to patients on whom he performed invasive procedures over a 13-year period, was examined in a retrospective epidemiologic follow-up study.

Methods.—The orthopedic surgeon had been practicing in the same community in New Hampshire, a state with a low background rate of HIV infection, for 16 years when his HIV infection was discovered. The surgeon's low CD4 cell count suggested a long-standing infection, and he voluntarily withdrew from practice. A mailing was sent to all 2,317 patients on whom the surgeon had performed an invasive procedure during his time in practice, advising them of the situation, stressing their low risk of HIV infection, and offering free and anonymous HIV counseling and testing. The infected surgeon's confidentiality was maintained throughout the study, in which he was an active participant. The surgeon's patient records were checked against state health records to identify deceased patients and possible HIV-related causes of death.

Findings.—A total of 1,174 patients were tested for HIV, for a response rate of 51%. The tested group included patients from every year of practice and every category of invasive procedure. An enzyme-linked immunosorbent assay was negative for HIV infection in every case. Two patients reported having HIV infection before their operation. Ninety-two of the 1,082 nonresponders were found to have died, but none apparently died of HIV infection, AIDS-defining opportunistic infections or tumors, or other conditions suggesting HIV infection. The total cost of patient notification and testing was about $158,500.

Conclusion.—This look-back study found no cases of HIV transmission from an infected surgeon to his patients. Assuming that the surgeon adheres to standard infection control practices, the risk of such transmission appears to be very low. When HIV infection is recognized in a health care worker, routine notification and testing of patients would appear to be unnecessary.

Investigation of Potential HIV Transmission to the Patients of an HIV-Infected Surgeon
Rogers AS, Froggatt JW III, Townsend T, Gordon T, Brown AJL, Holmes EC, Zhang LQ, Moses H III (Maryland State Dept of Health and Mental Hygiene, Baltimore; Johns Hopkins Univ, Baltimore, Md; Univ of Edinburgh, Scotland; et al)
JAMA 269:1795–1801, 1993   140-94-5-10

Background.—The risk of the transmission of HIV from an infected health care worker to a patient has not been thoroughly studied. Overall, about 16,000 patients treated by 32 infected health care workers have been tested for HIV infection. Eighty-four patients were seropositive, but it has not been demonstrated that any of these were infected by the health care worker involved. Further investigation of the patients of an HIV-infected surgeon was reported.

Methods.—From 1984 through 1990, the HIV-infected surgeon was the admitting or operating surgeon for 1,131 patients. Patients presumed to be living were contacted by mail. The AIDS case registries were also searched for the names of this surgeon's patients.

Findings.—One hundred one of the patients had died, 119 had no available address, 413 had known HIV test results, and 498 did not respond to the questionnaire. None of the study patients were found in AIDS case registries. One patient newly diagnosed as HIV-positive was thought to have been infected by a transfusion in 1985. No HIV transmission occurred in 369 person-hours of surgical exposure.

Conclusion.—The patients of publicly disclosed HIV-infected health care workers whose practice involves invasive procedures should be investigated when resources permit. The risk of HIV transmission during surgery may be so small that it can only be detected by pooling data from many studies.

▶ After the announcement in the public press that a dentist had transmitted HIV infection to 5 of his patients (a sixth patient was later shown to be infected), there was a cry for the testing of physicians and dentists. After a conference held by the Centers for Disease Control and Prevention (CDC), the CDC advocated testing for HIV and hepatitis B in all dentists and surgeons who perform "exposure-prone invasive procedures". Because of resistance from the medical community, there was no meeting held to define "exposure-prone" procedures, and the matter was left to the states to define. This issue has largely died. Abstracts 140-94-5–9 and 140-94-5–10 report that patients cared for by 2 surgeons were not infected with HIV. There have been several other publications reporting on investigations of patients cared for by surgeons or dentists who died of AIDS. In addition, the CDC has investigated more than 22,000 patients cared for by many HIV-infected health care workers. To date, not a single individual was found to have been infected or claims to have been infected by being cared for by an HIV-infected health care worker. Thus, except for the dentist who transmitted HIV to his patients (the likelihood of intentional transmission cannot be excluded), there is not a single individual who has been infected with HIV by being cared for by an infected health care worker. However, the risk is not zero. Hepatitis B has been transmitted to patients by infected surgeons, dentists, and other health care workers.—R.J. Howard, M.D., Ph.D.

Necrotizing Infections of the Perineum
Salvino C, Harford FJ, Dobrin PB (Hines Veterans Affairs Hosp, Ill; Loyola Univ, Maywood, Ill)
South Med J 86:908–911, 1993   140-94-5–11

Background.—Since its introduction, the term "Fournier's gangrene" has been generalized to encompass all necrotizing soft tissue infections of the perineum or genitalia. Just under 500 cases of perineal and genital gangrene have been reported worldwide. Data on 10 men with necrotizing perineal infections were reviewed.

Patients and Methods.—The patients were admitted to a veterans affairs hospital over a 6-year period with a diagnosis of Fournier's gangrene of the perineum. The average patient age was 60 years. Symptoms had been present for 2 to 5 days, when information on duration was available. Most patients had signs of localized infection at the initial examination—such as edema, erythema, or pain—which rapidly developed into spreading, full-thickness cutaneous gangrene within 24 hours. Each patient had at least 1 chronic, debilitating disease, including diabetes in 6. Aggressive initial débridement was undertaken quickly, usually within

24 hours of presentation, with an average of 2.6 débridements per patient.

Findings.—Signs of sepsis usually subsided within 48 hours of the initial débridement. Seven patients had a recognized nidus for the progressive, necrotizing infection: a perirectal abscess in 5 and urethral trauma because of suprapubic catheterization in 2. Two of the patients with perirectal abscess were managed with diverting colostomy. The bacteriologic flora were polymicrobial in all patients, with *Escherichia coli, Bacteroides* species, and staphylococci predominating. Treatment included broad-spectrum antibiotics and early nutritional supplementation. The average hospital stay was 4 weeks. One patient, who had been transferred from another institution with inadequate débridement, died of sepsis.

Discussion.—Successful treatment of necrotizing infections of the perineum (Fournier's gangrene) consists of quick recognition of the problem, aggressive nutritional supplementation, and early and repeated débridement. Even patients with a perirectal nidus of infection do not necessarily need diverting colostomy.

▶ This paper reviews treatment of necrotizing soft tissue infection of the peritoneum (Fournier's gangrene). As with other necrotizing soft tissue infections, early aggressive débridement is the mainstay of therapy. All patients should be evaluated after initial débridement for persistence or extension of the necrotizing infection.—R.J. Howard, M.D., Ph.D.

Comparison of Peripheral Blood Leukocyte Kinetics After Live *Escherichia coli,* Endotoxin, or Interleukin-1α Administration: Studies Using a Novel Interleukin-1 Receptor Antagonist
Hawes AS, Fischer E, Marano MA, Van Zee KJ, Rock CS, Lowry SF, Calvano SE, Moldawer LL (Cornell Univ, New York)
Ann Surg 218:79–90, 1993   140-94-5–12

Background.—The lipopolysaccharide (LPS) component of the outer membrane of gram-negative bacteria triggers a number of metabolic and immunologic responses in the host, including acute granulocytopenia followed by granulocytosis, lymphopenia, and transient monocytopenia. Interleukin-1 (IL-1) is a macrophage-derived cytokine that mediates host responses to infection and inflammation.

Objective.—Studies were done in baboons to determine whether the hematologic and immunologic effects of bacteremia and endotoxemia can be replicated by administering recombinant human interleukin-1α. A specific IL-1 receptor antagonist (IL-1ra) was used to determine whether endogenous IL-1 participates in the changes associated with endotoxemia or gram-negative septic shock.

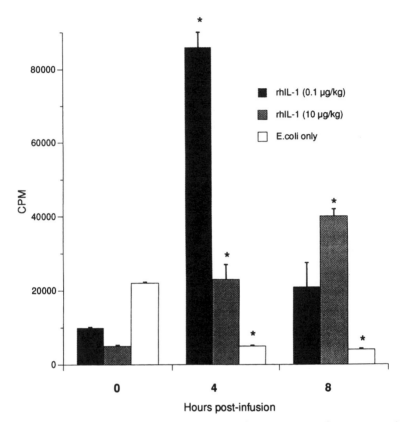

Fig 5–4.—In vitro mononuclear cell proliferative capacity after administration of in vivo IL-1α or live *Escherichia coli.* Animals were treated in vivo with either of 2 different doses of IL-1α (10 or .1 μg/kg) or LD₁₀₀ of live *E. coli;* PHA-stimulated (2 μg/mL) proliferative capacity was assessed at baseline and at 4 and 8 hours after infusion. The values are expressed as mean ± standard error of mean . *P < .01 vs. baseline. (Courtesy of Hawes AS, Fischer E, Marano MA, et al: *Ann Surg* 218:79–90, 1993.)

Methods.—Baboons were given recombinant human IL-1α, LPS derived from *Salmonella typhosa,* or live *Escherichia coli,* with or without IL-1ra. Blood was collected hourly and analyzed by using flow cytometric techniques.

Results.—Both endotoxin and *E. coli* bacteremia produced acute granulocytopenia, which gradually resolved in endotoxemic animals but persisted in those that were bacteremic. Both LPS and live *E. coli* led to early lymphopenia and monocytopenia, which persisted throughout the study. Administration of recombinant human IL-1α led to an early, transient fall in granulocytes followed by sustained granulocytosis. Lymphopenia and transient monocytopenia also were noted. Mononuclear cell proliferative capacity increased markedly after a higher dose of recombinant human IL-1α, but decreased even more after administration of *E. coli* (Fig 5–4). Administration of IL-1ra did not alter leukocyte kinetics in animals given live bacteria or LPS, but it significantly lessened the mono-cytopenia resulting from recombinant human IL-1α.

Conclusion.—Recombinant human IL-1α reproduces some of the hematologic changes seen in bacteremia and endotoxemia, but an endogenous IL-1 response is not required for these changes to occur. Other LPS-induced inflammatory mediators, such as tumor necrosis factor-α, may be involved.

▶ Despite an explosion of studies on cytokines and their modulating effects on the biological interactions involved in sepsis and bacteremia, the physiologic alterations of sepsis are still unclear. This paper follows kinetics of live *E. coli* endotoxin or recombinant IL-1α. Although LPS is thought to cause most of the biological effects of *E. coli,* live bacteria produce effects not found by administration of LPS alone, and these effects are not mediated solely by IL-1α. The continuing delineation of the physiologic basis of sepsis provides further evidence of how complex the mechanisms of sepsis and bacteria–host interactions are.—R.J. Howard, M.D., Ph.D.

Streptococcal Toxic Shock-Like Syndrome: The Importance of Surgical Intervention
Wood TF, Potter MA, Jonasson O (Ohio State Univ, Columbus)
Ann Surg 217:109–114, 1993   140-94-5-13

Background.—Streptococcal toxic shock–like syndrome (TSLS)—which has a rapid, fulminant course like that of staphylococcal toxic shock syndrome—is caused by the pyrogenic exotoxins A, B, and C produced by group A hemolytic streptococci. Features of TSLS include fever, rash, desquamation, hypotension, and multisystem organ dysfunction. Its recognition was probably preceded by the emergence of more virulent strains of streptococci that are more likely to produce potent exotoxins. Six cases of TSLS treated during the past 6 years were reported.

Patients.—Four patients were female and 2 were male, ranging in age from 13 to 67 years. In one patient with Hodgkin's disease and recent chemotherapy, TSLS developed in the throat with bilateral empyemas, which were managed with chest tubes. Another patient with multiple operations for recurrent oral cancer responded to débridement of the infected areas of the head and neck. The predisposing condition in 3 patients was obesity. One of these was a young girl with TSLS of the vagina, which was managed by hymenotomy and bilateral fasciotomy. The sites of disease in the other 2 patients were the breast and axilla in 1 and the leg in the other; both were successfully treated by débridement. Finally, buttock cellulitis and myonecrosis developed in a patient with systemic lupus erythematosus who was receiving immunosuppressive therapy. Débridement was performed for this patient, but he died of disseminated intravascular coagulation and profound anemia shortly after the operation.

Conclusion.—Six cases of streptococcal TSLS are described. This syndrome, commonly associated with streptococcal infection of the soft tissue and skin, leads to the development of a large bacterial inoculum with overwhelming exotoxin production and resistance to antibiotic treatment alone. Patients with streptococcal TSLS need early diagnosis, penicillin treatment, and radical operative débridement, together with prompt administration of penicillin or clindamycin.

▶ Although the toxic shock syndrome caused by *Staphylococcus aureus* was first described in 1978, it can also be caused by streptococci. The authors present 6 patients with TSLS caused by *Streptococcus pyogenes.* All patients required a surgical procedure (usually débridement of a necrotizing soft tissue infection). Surgeons must be aware that the rapid appearance of a TSLS can be caused by streptococci requiring a surgical procedure.—R.J. Howard, M.D., Ph.D.

6 Transplantation

Introduction

The success of transplantation has created problems for the procedure. As the improvement of transplantation has continued, both the number of individuals thought to be candidates for organ transplantation and the types of solid organ transplants performed have grown. However, the number of organ donors has not kept pace with the growth in the recipient pool. A study from Japan (Abstract 140-94-6-1) reports the authors' experience with using living relatives as donors for pediatric liver transplant recipients. This use of related donors was pioneered at the University of Chicago by Broelsch and colleagues. It may be an attractive alternative in countries like Japan that do not have brain death laws. Another way of increasing the donor supply is to use organs from different species. A report by Starzl and colleagues from Pittsburgh (Abstract 140-94-6-2) reports on a xenograft liver transplant to a man who was dying of liver failure caused by active hepatitis B infection but who was not a candidate for a human organ. Although there have only been a small number of reports of xenograft organ transplant in humans, this area of endeavor is receiving widespread attention in the research laboratory, because xenograft organs could go a long way toward solving the problem of donor supply. During this past year, a journal devoted to xenotransplantation has even been established.

One paper (Abstract 140-94-6-3) discusses the costs encountered in organ transplantation, and it also discusses the possibility of using financial incentives to enhance the efficiency of organ procurement efforts. Although financial incentives are currently frowned upon by most transplant surgeons, physicians, and medical ethicists, more discussion is taking place regarding the impact of financial incentives on organ donation.

Several papers deal with the long-term results of organ transplant. One study from Europe (Abstract 140-94-6-4) reports on the results of graft survival as a function of tissue match in more than 100,000 kidney transplant recipients. In these large cooperative trials, there is an effect of tissue typing on graft outcome, something that is difficult to show in a single center. Chronic rejection is an ever-present threat to solid organ transplants. A report of the long-term follow-up of renal allograft recipients from the University of Minnesota (Abstract 140-94-6-13) does not find that tissue typing affects the likelihood of chronic rejection. Another paper from Minnesota (Abstract 140-94-6-5) analyzes the effect on graft loss of death with function. Because transplant center outcome is being increasingly scrutinized as a quality standard, the standard practice of including death with function as a graft loss may be misleading and may give rise to inappropriately low transplant outcome statistics. Another major cause of late graft loss after transplantation is noncompliance (see Abstract 140-94-6-6). A study from the University of Illinois found that as many as 56% of patients are noncompliant in taking medications after transplantation. Others have found noncompliance to be a major source of graft loss. Late graft loss after liver transplantation has also been investigated (see Abstract 140-94-6-7). The common causes of late graft loss are similar to those responsible for graft loss after kidney transplantation. Despite these late graft losses, the recent survival data for patients with liver transplants are remarkable considering the rather low graft survival in the recent past.

An article from the University of Michigan (Abstract 140-94-6-8) investigates survival probabilities for patients receiving dialysis compared with cadaveric renal transplant recipients. This is one of the few valid studies comparing only those patients who are accepted for transplantation and are actually placed on the cadaveric waiting list, rather than all dialysis patients. The authors find that there is no survival advantage to transplantation for the first year after kidney transplantation; however, thereafter, patients who are undergoing transplantation enjoy significant survival compared with patients maintained with dialysis.

Rehabilitation is a major goal of all organ transplantation. The rehabilitation after organ transplantation generally is excellent. Almost one half of patients are employed after heart transplantation (see Abstract 140-94-6-9). A significant proportion (36%) were capable of working but were still unemployed. It is interesting that social factors, such as losing health insurance or disability income, contribute significantly to unemployment after organ transplantation.

Lungs are 1 of the newer solid organs to be transplanted. Just as heart, liver, and kidney transplantation began with rather poor results and achieved superb results with time, so it is with lung transplantation. Lung transplantation graft survival is increasing rapidly. Two papers (Abstracts 140-94-6-10 and 140-94-6-11) document improved results of lung transplant survival.

Richard J. Howard, M.D., Ph.D.

An Appraisal of Pediatric Liver Transplantation From Living Relatives: Initial Clinical Experiences in 20 Pediatric Liver Transplantations From Living Relatives As Donors
Ozawa K, Uemoto S, Tanaka K, Kumada K, Yamaoka Y, Kobayashi N, Inamoto T, Shimahara Y, Mori K, Honda K, Kamiyama Y, Kim HJ, Morimoto T, Tanaka A (Kyoto Univ, Japan)
Ann Surg 216:547–553, 1992   140-94-6-1

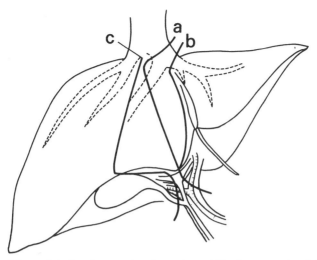

Fig 6–1.—Schema of the lines for parenchymal, vascular, and bile duct transections in living donor graft harvesting. The *a* represents left lobectomy; *b*, lateral segmentectomy; *c*, right lobectomy. (Courtesy of Ozawa K, Uemoto S, Tanaka K, et al: *Ann Surg* 216:547-553, 1992.)

Background.—The graft shortage in pediatric liver transplantation has created a serious medical and social problem. Efforts aimed at resolving this shortage have included, among other therapeutic modalities, the introduction of living related liver transplantation. Although physical benefits for the healthy donor cannot be demonstrated, living donor liver transplantation has definite advantages in terms of graft viability and histocompatibility compared with transplants obtained from cadavers. Initial clinical experience with pediatric patients receiving living related liver transplantations was reported.

Patients and Methods.—Between June 1990 and July 1991, a total of 20 pediatric liver transplantations from living related donors were performed. Fourteen patients had biliary atresia, 2 had Budd-Chiari syndrome, 1 had liver cirrhosis after a hepatitis C viral infection, 1 had progressive intrahepatic cholestasis, 1 had liver cirrhosis, and 1 had protoporphyria. Graft harvesting consisted of 11 left lobectomies, 8 left lateral segmentectomies, and 1 right lobectomy. To maintain optimum viability, the procedures were performed without any vascular control for either the donated graft or the remnant liver. Unnecessary manipulation of the liver was carefully avoided. Figure 6-1 shows the lines for transections in living donor graft harvesting. Donor selection was limited to parents of the recipients. Both FK 506 and steroids were used for immunosuppressive treatment.

Results.—Seventeen of the 20 pediatric recipients have survived, and 15 are well and at home. Two recipients died of postoperative complications after emergency transplantations. Another recipient died of accidental asphyxia at 6 months after operation. Uneventful postoperative courses were noted for all survivors, all of whom were able to resume their normal social lives. In all cases, the arterial ketone body ratio increased to more than 1.0 within 2 days after transplantation. Two patients experienced fairly mild episodes of rejection; both had received ABO-compatible grafts and were successfully treated by FK 506 and steroids.

Conclusion.—It is suggested that living related liver transplantation should not be thought of as merely another option for resolving the pediatric liver transplantation graft shortage. Rather, this procedure should be considered as an independent modality to improve the outcome of liver transplantation.

▶ Because few pediatric liver donors become available, 2 options for pediatric liver recipients are a reduced-size cadaveric organ and partial organs from living relatives. This study from Japan shows that living related liver donation can be done safely with its report on a series of 20 donors. Living related liver donation has 2 advantages: (1) not having significant cold ischemia time, and (2) good tissue-matching between parent and child. Whether these advantages translate into increased long-term graft survival compared to cadaveric transplantation remains to be seen.—R.J. Howard, M.D., Ph.D.

Baboon-to-Human Liver Transplantation
Starzl TE, Fung J, Tzakis A, Todo S, Demetris AJ, Marino IR, Doyle H, Zeevi A, Warty V, Michaels M, Kusne S, Rudert WA, Trucco M (Univ of Pittsburgh, Pa)
Lancet 341:65–71, 1993   140-94-6-2

Introduction.—Previous atempts to transplant baboon kidneys or hearts have failed because of uncontrolled cellular rejection, as well as antibody-mediated endotheliolitis of the graft vessels and parenchymal necrosis. A baboon-to-human liver xenotransplant now is reported, in which both FK 506 and cyclophosphamide were used as immunosuppressants, together with prednisone and prostaglandin, to help mitigate preformed antigraft antibody disorders and cellular rejection.

Case Report.—Man, 35, had had abnormal liver function for 8 years and recurrent bleeding from esophageal varices for 2 years. He had both hepatitis B virus-associated, chronic, active hepatitis and HIV infection. Continuous hospital care had become necessary. At the time of surgery, the patient was jaundiced and had ascites, episodic encephalopathy, and deteriorating liver function. A baboon liver, considered resistant to hepatitis B virus infection, was transplanted using conventional surgical methods. A nonmyelotoxic dose of cyclophosphamide was added to the regimen of FK 506, prednisone, and prostaglandin routinely used in liver allotransplantation.

Stage 3 coma was seen preoperatively, but the patient awoke promptly and was eating and walking within 5 days. The patient lived 70 days after liver transplantation. Biopsy specimens and biochemical monitoring gave little evidence of graft rejection. Several infections developed, the most serious being mixed cytomegalovirus and candidal esophagitis and duodenitis that resulted in recurrent gastrointestinal bleeding. Renal failure also developed and necessitated dialysis; it probably reflected multiple drug toxicity. Several plasmaphereses were done to reduce the serum concentration of bilirubin.

The patient died after cerebral and subarachnoid hemorrhage caused by angioinvasive *Aspergillus* infection. Autopsy demonstrated widespread biliary sludge, primarily representing cellular debris, in the biliary tree, despite an apparently adequate choledochojejunostomy. Multiple bile infarcts were seen throughout the liver. The graft arteries exhibited no evidence of inflammatory or obliterative disease. Baboon DNA was demonstrated in the patient's heart, lung, kidney, and lymph nodes.

Discussion.—This case shows that it is possible to control rejection of a baboon liver xenograft in a human recipient. This patient did not live long enough to answer the question as to whether the transplant can resist hepatitis B virus infection. It is not clear whether HIV-resistant chimeric xenogeneic cells would have a survival advantage over infected autologous cells of the same lineage, or whether this could improve the course of HIV infection.

▶ There have been several previous reports of xenograft kidney or heart transplants into humans. The longest survival of a xenograft transplant into a human involved a chimpanzee kidney, which lasted for approximately 6 months. This report by the Pittsburgh group is another example of a human xenograft, in this case the transplant of a liver from a baboon into a man with liver failure resulting from chronic active hepatitis B. The patient was not a candidate for a human liver transplant because of a high recurrence rate of hepatitis B. This report shows that xenografts can function in humans; however, this and previous reports also emphasize that the xenograft barrier still remains formidable and, as yet, is impossible to overcome. Nevertheless, much research is currently being done on xenotransplantation, and a journal devoted to xenotransplantation has recently been established. Overcoming the xenotransplantation barrier would greatly ease the desperate shortage of cadaveric organs. Nevertheless, the problem will remain formidable for the foreseeable future.—R.J. Howard, M.D., Ph.D.

Organ Procurement Expenditures and the Role of Financial Incentives
Evans RW (Mayo Clinic and Found, Rochester, Minn)
JAMA 269:3113–3118, 1993   140-94-6-3

Background.—Organ procurement expenditures remain a controversial issue. To date, the available information suggests that procurement expenditures, for which the Health Care Financing Administration has been responsible, are extensive. The billed charges for organ procurement were evaluated, and the role of financial incentives to encourage organ donation was examined.

Methods.—A random sample of kidney, heart, liver, heart-lung, and pancreas transplants was used to obtain data on donor organ acquisition charges. The data were based on 28.7% of all United States transplants performed in 1988. Because the range for acquisition charges was considerable, medians, as opposed to means, were used as the measure of central tendency.

Results.—The median charges for donor organ acquisition, using 1988 dollars, were $12,290 for kidney, $12,578 for heart, $16,281 for liver, $12,028 for heart-lung, and $15,400 for pancreas. Since 1983, acquisition charges have increased by 12.9% for kidney, 64.1% for heart, and 61.8% for liver, after adjustment for inflation. Between 9% and 31% of the entire transplant procedure–specific charges were linked with donor organ acquisition.

Discussion.—A broad, unexplained variation in organ procurement charges was noted. Data on actual costs are needed to determine the appropriateness of current charges. Current payment procedures may, in fact, contribute to cost inefficiency. Thus, present billing and payment methods should be reassessed to address issues relative to reimbursement. Finally, financial incentives (generally in the form of a death benefit paid to the deceased's estate or as a single payment to the deceased's family) are increasingly discussed as a means of inducing organ donation. Although such incentives may aid in improving the efficiency of organ procurement, they will add to total transplantation expenditures. Thus, before full-scale implementation, the cost utility of these incentives must be fully established.

▶ Technically, cadaveric organs do not come with a charge and are, thus, "free." However, there are substantial costs for procuring and transporting these organs. This interesting paper discusses the ramifications of the high charges for organ donors and the substantial "profits" to be made from multiple organ donors by organ procurement organizations. The authors also touch on the difficult subject of payment to the families of cadaveric organ donors. This subject has been receiving increasing attention. Some authors have even argued that there should be an open market for live organ donors and that kidneys should be sold to the highest bidder.—R.J. Howard, M.D., Ph.D.

Collaborative Transplant Study: 10-Year Report
Opelz G, for the Collaborative Transplant Study (Univ of Heidelberg, Germany)
Transplant Proc 24:2342–2355, 1992   140-94-6-4

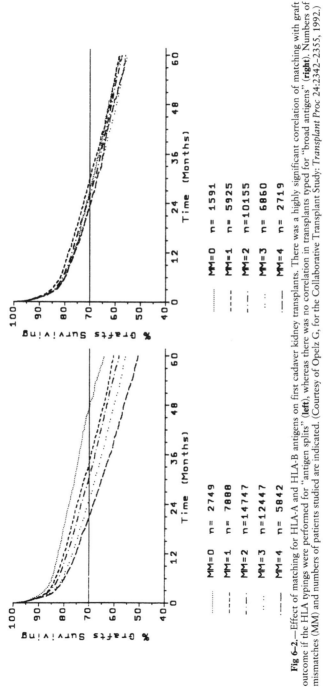

Fig 6-2.—Effect of matching for HLA-A and HLA-B antigens on first cadaver kidney transplants. There was a highly significant correlation of matching with graft outcome if the HLA typings were performed for "antigen splits" (**left**), whereas there was no correlation in transplants typed for "broad antigens" (**right**). Numbers of mismatches (MM) and numbers of patients studied are indicated. (Courtesy of Opelz G, for the Collaborative Transplant Study: *Transplant Proc* 24:2342–2355, 1992.)

The Study.—The Collaborative Transplant Study (CTS) began in 1982 with the goal of combining the experience of many transplant centers to augment knowledge of the factors influencing the outcome of organ transplantation. The CTS is now the largest worldwide effort of its kind. A total of 306 kidney transplant centers in 43 countries are participating actively. As of mid-1992, more than 107,000 kidney transplants had been reported to the CTS, together with 3,000 liver transplants, 1,500 pancreas transplants, 11,000 heart transplants, 500 heart-lung transplants, and 400 lung transplants.

Observations.—The CTS includes a large number of well-matched grafts, making it possible to draw conclusions about the influence of HLA matching on cadaver kidney graft survival (Fig 6–2). The CTS data provide the first convincing evidence of an effect of HLA matching in heart transplantation. There is now unambiguous evidence of the advantage conferred by cyclosporine-based immunosuppression, although cyclosporine has not eliminated the need for histocompatibility matching. The CTS data fail to demonstrate convincing benefit from combination immunosuppression, including the prophylactic use of antithymocyte globulin or monoclonal OKT3.

The Future.—As the CTS enters its second decade, its focus is shifting from early to later post-transplant events that influence the long-term outcome. These include both chronic graft rejection and drug toxicity. In addition, the development of malignancies after organ transplantation is a matter of considerable concern.

▶ The only way that tissue typing can be shown to influence the outcome of cadaveric renal transplantation is through very large cooperative efforts such as the CTS. It is virtually impossible to show that tissue typing affects the transplant outcome when the results of only a single center are examined. Because of an increasing shortage of cadaveric kidneys, there are many transplant centers that ignore tissue typing results. Many centers believe that delayed graft function, which may be increased by kidney sharing, greatly overwhelms the effect of any slight advantage from better matching between donor and recipient.—R.J. Howard, M.D., Ph.D.

Half-Life and Risk Factors for Kidney Transplant Outcome: Importance of Death With Function

Matas AJ, Gillingham KJ, Sutherland DER (Univ of Minnesota, Minneapolis)
Transplantation 55:757–761, 1993   140-94-6-5

Background.—Evaluation of outcomes at transplant centers requires a consistent approach to analyzing data. It has been standard practice to include death with function as graft loss, but this may obscure other significant risk factors and make comparisons between centers problematic.

Objective.—The risk factors for long-term graft survival were examined in 2,230 kidney transplant recipients whose grafts functioned for at least 1 year.

Data Analysis.—Four separate Cox regression analyses were done. The variables for each analysis included whether cyclosporine was used, age at the time of transplantation, donor source, gender, primary transplantation vs. retransplantation, diabetes, and HLA-ABDR mismatches. The first analysis defined graft loss as a return to dialysis, transplant nephrectomy, retransplantation, or patient death. Death with function was censored in the second analysis; the patient was followed until the date of death, but follow-up ceased at the moment before death. The other analyses considered some late deaths to be related to transplantation or immunosuppression. In one, only definitively non–transplant-related deaths were censored, whereas in the other, both these and cardiac deaths were censored.

Results.—When all deaths were censored, age older than 50 years, a cadaver donor source, retransplantation, and diabetes ceased to be risk factors for long-term graft survival. The remaining significant factor was the presence of an antigen mismatch. Patients older than 50 years of age actually had better graft survival when all deaths were censored. Half-life also differed markedly, depending on how death with function was treated. For instance, nondiabetic recipients of living donor kidneys who were younger than 50 years of age had a half-life of 9 years when death with function was considered a graft loss, but they had a half-life of 62 years when death with function was censored.

Conclusion.—Death with function must be taken into account when analyzing the outcome of kidney transplantation. It is suggested that all graft survival data be presented both with and without deaths censored.

▶ Regarding death with graft function as being the same as graft loss may give misleading results when assessing graft survival and risk factors for graft survival. Several risk factors found to be important when death with function is included cease to be risk factors when death with function is excluded from the analysis of the data. Death with function may be even more important in the analysis of late graft loss, because a higher proportion of these patients lose graft function as a result of death with function.—R.J. Howard, M.D., Ph.D.

A Study of Treatment Compliance Following Kidney Transplantation
Kiley DJ, Lam CS, Pollak R (Illinois Inst of Technology, Chicago; Univ of Illinois at Chicago)
Transplantation 55:51–56, 1993   140-94-6–6

Introduction.—Successful transplant surgery requires that the patient comply with an arduous postoperative management program that includes strict dietary regulation, medication schedules, and clinic visits. After rejection and systemic infection, noncompliance reportedly is the major cause of renal allograft failure.

Objective.—The psychological and social variables influencing compliance behaviors were examined in 105 patients followed for at least 18 months after renal allograft transplantation.

Assessment.—In addition to a biographical questionnaire, the patients were evaluated using the Center for Epidemiologic Studies Depression Scale, the Multidimensional Health Locus of Control Scale, and the Social Support Appraisals Questionnaire. In addition, a Health Belief Model Questionnaire, a Patient and Provider Relationship Questionnaire, a Compliance Self-Report Questionnaire, and a Self-Efficacy Questionnaire were specially designed for this study. The signs of compliance included a blood cyclosporine level above 30 ng/mL, less than a 20% gain in body weight, and fewer than 20% missed clinic visits.

Findings.—Twenty-five patients exhibited overall compliance, whereas 29 were noncompliant overall. Twenty-nine patients failed to comply with diet and 27 with medication. None of the patients missed more than one fifth of their scheduled clinic visits. The men were more likely to be noncompliant with medication, and women were more compliant with dietary regulation. Noncompliance was also associated with a larger number of prescribed drugs, depression, unemployment, and the perceived degree of social and family support. Blacks were relatively noncompliant, as were patients with a locus of control ascribed to powerful others. Patients whose grafts failed were more depressed than the others and perceived less benefit from their treatment.

Implications.—Compliance with treatment after renal transplantation is related to how well patients function psychosocially. Three fourths of the study patients failed to comply with either dietary regulation or medication, or both, suggesting a need for clinical interventions that will promote compliance.

▶ This is one of the more thorough studies of patient compliance after kidney transplantation. As many have suspected and as this paper documents, noncompliance with medications can be a major problem after kidney transplantation. The authors found that 56% of their patients were noncompliant with their medications, as determined by a drug cyclosporine level less than 30 ng/mL. It is unfortunate that the authors do not stratify the patients by age, because many of us believe that teenagers have a much higher rate of noncompliance than other transplant recipients.—R.J. Howard, M.D., Ph.D.

Causes of Late Graft Loss After Liver Transplantation
Bäckman L, Gibbs J, Levy M, McMillan R, Holman M, Husberg B, Goldstein

R, Gonwa TA, Klintmalm G (Baylor Univ, Dallas)
Transplantation 55:1078–1082, 1993   140-94-6-7

Background.—Clinical liver transplantation is accepted as routine treatment for end-stage liver diseases. To date, much attention has been given to causes of graft loss early after transplantation. However, there have been no studies focusing on causes of late graft loss after transplantation. The causes of graft loss in liver transplant recipients with grafts functioning for more than 1 year after operation were evaluated.

Patients and Findings.—Between December 21, 1984 and January 14, 1991, 500 consecutive orthotopic liver transplantations were performed in 434 patients at a single center. A total of 362 grafts were functioning for more than 1 year post transplant. After 1 year, 42 grafts (11.6%) were subsequently lost, 33 by death of the patient and 9 by retransplants in 8 patients. Twenty-one of the grafts lost to death were dysfunctioning. In liver transplantation recipients with functioning grafts for more than 1 year, the actuarial 2- and 5-year graft survival rates were 91% and 83%, respectively. During the second year post transplant, the graft loss rate was 3.4 times higher than the loss from 2 to 5 years post transplant. Chronic rejection (26.2%), hepatitis (23.8%), arterial thrombosis/stenosis (11.9%), and recurrent malignancy (9.5%) were the most frequent causes of graft loss. No graft was lost from acute rejection. No differences were noted in the timing of graft loss among the various causes. Pretransplant diagnoses of hepatitis B, chronic rejection, and malignancy were associated with the highest frequency of late graft loss.

Conclusion.—In patients with a functioning graft for more than 1 year post transplant, long-term graft survival was good. The primary causes of graft loss were chronic rejection and recurrent hepatitis. Thus, prevention and treatment of these conditions may further improve the already good results after liver transplantation.

▶ The causes of late graft loss after liver transplantation differ from those responsible for late graft loss after kidney transplantation. Common causes of late graft loss are chronic rejection, arterial thrombosis/stenosis, hepatitis, and recurrent malignancy. Despite these losses, at 1 year, the actuarial survival rate of patients with functioning grafts is excellent.—R.J. Howard, M.D., Ph.D.

Comparison of Survival Probabilities for Dialysis Patients vs Cadaveric Renal Transplant Recipients

Port FK, Wolfe RA, Mauger EA, Berling DP, Jiang K (Univ of Michigan, Ann Arbor)
JAMA 270:1339–1343, 1993   140-94-6-8

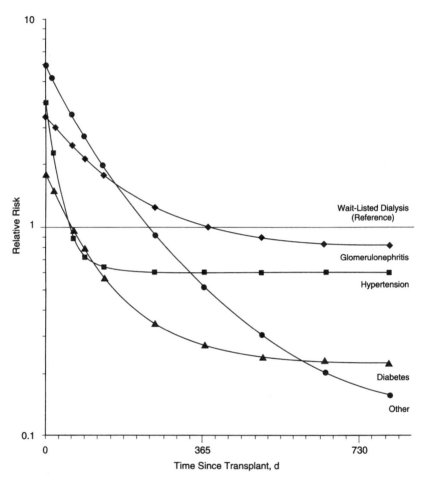

Fig 6-3.—Relative risk of mortality for cadaveric transplant recipients by cause of end-stage renal disease (ESRD) vs. wait-listed patients on dialysis of same cause of ESRD. The reference line is specific for each cause of ESRD. The groups were adjusted (nonproportional Cox model) for the same time since wait-listing and the overall average patient characteristics of age, sex, race, and cause of ESRD. (Courtesy of Port FK, Wolfe RA, Mauger EA, et al: *JAMA* 270:1339-1343, 1993.)

Background.—The number of patients treated for end-stage renal disease (ESRD) with dialysis or transplantation has continued to increase, with more than 160,000 patients undergoing treatment in the United States in 1989. However, the availability of organs for transplants has not increased proportionally. Given these facts and the considerable expense of kidney replacement therapy, it is important to determine accurately the relative death rates for the major forms of therapy—dialysis and transplantation. Previous studies have shown that transplant recipients have much higher survival probabilities than patients receiving dialysis, but many of these studies did not consider patient selection bias or time-to-treatment basis. Therefore, the first study that directly compares adjusted patient survival rates between wait-listed dialysis and transplantation in the cyclosporine era, using the Cox model with a time-dependent covariate in a large population, was undertaken.

Study Design.—In this historical prospective study, enrollment began on the date of wait-listing while a patient with ESRD. From the population-based data of the Michigan Kidney Registry, all patients younger than age 65 years who started ESRD therapy between January 1, 1984 and December 31, 1989 were studied. Patients were followed from ESRD onset ($n = 5,020$) to wait-listing for renal transplant ($n = 1,569$), to receiving a cadaveric first transplant ($n = 799$), and to December 31, 1989. The mortality risk among cadaveric renal transplant recipients was compared with transplant candidates receiving dialysis, using a Cox model with a time-dependent variable based on the waiting time from date of wait-listing to transplantation and adjusted for age, sex, race, and primary cause of ESRD.

Results.—The relative risk of dying was initially higher for transplant patients during the early posttransplant period than for patients receiving dialysis. By day 117, the adjusted death rates were equal between the 2 groups, but transplant recipients surviving beyond that time had a lower relative death rate that appeared to reach a steady state with 68% lower risk than for wait-listed patients receiving dialysis. The cumulative mortality risk was equal for both groups at 325 days after transplantation. The lower long-term risk of dying was most pronounced among patients with diabetes but was not observed among patients with glomerulonephritis as a cause of ESRD (Fig 6–3).

Summary.—The overall mortality risk after renal transplantation is initially increased, and then decreases to a beneficial long-term effect compared with patients receiving dialysis.

▶ The main advantages of transplantation over dialysis that are usually cited have to do with quality-of-life issues, i.e., after transplantation there is no need for patients to go to a dialysis center 3 times per week, nor is there a need for peritoneal dialysis patients to do daily exchanges; there also is a better sense of well being and better rehabilitation. Because of conflicting data, there has been reluctance to say that there is better survival after transplantation. Many of the previous studies comparing transplant recipients with patients undergoing dialysis did not consider selection bias. That is, only the best patients with renal failure were considered for transplantation, whereas all patients receiving dialysis were included in mortality studies. This study does compare "apples with apples" and only considers patients who were accepted for transplantation and placed on a waiting list. It also clearly shows a survival advantage for transplantation after the first year after dialysis.—R.J. Howard, M.D., Ph.D.

Returning to Work After Heart Transplantation

Paris W, Woodbury A, Thompson S, Levick M, Nothegger S, Arbuckle P, Hutkin-Slade L, Cooper DKC (Oklahoma Transplantation Inst, Oklahoma City; Oregon Health Sciences Univ, Portland; Univ of Florida, Gainesville; et al)
J Heart Lung Transplant 12:46–54, 1993   140-94-6-9

Introduction.—Limited economic resources and the failure of many heart transplant recipients to become productive members of society have led to questions about whether heart transplantation is affordable and whether the benefits warrant the cost. Lives have been saved, but the price continues to increase. The factors that influence a transplant recipient's return to work were examined in a series of 250 recipients at 7 regional centers in the United States.

Findings.—Forty-five percent of the patients surveyed were employed, 36% were unemployed, 13% were medically disabled, and 6% were retired. Employed patients typically viewed themselves as physically able to work. Virtually none of them lost health insurance while working, but 42% did lose disability income. Those who were employed were those with the highest education. Disability times were shorter than for unemployed recipients. A large majority of the unemployed believed that they were physically unable to work, a belief inconsistent with the medical findings. One third of this group would lose all health insurance from working, and nearly all would lose disability income. The unemployed tended to be more recent recipients of transplantation and to have a lower level of education and long prior disability times. The 2 centers having definite policies on medical disability certification and employment after transplantation had higher return-to-work rates than did those with more liberal policies (table).

Implications.—Social rehabilitation cannot always be predicted by the medical results of heart transplantation. Employment should be recommended to all heart transplant recipients less than 65 years of age. A policy of being expected to return to work can help motivate younger white-collar workers to resume their work. Blue-collar workers who will not lose health insurance may be referred for job retraining or additional education with vocational rehabilitation.

▶ The goal of organ transplantation is primarily to save lives and secondarily to improve the patient's quality of life and achieve maximal rehabilitation. Although almost half of the patients in this study were employed after heart transplantation, a significant proportion (36%) who were deemed to be capable of working were unemployed. Social factors, such as losing health insurance and losing disability income, may have contributed significantly to their unemployment. Clearly, patients should not be punished for being employed by losing their health insurance.—R.J. Howard, M.D., Ph.D.

Effect of Center Policy on Employment Status After Heart Transplantation

Policy	Definite		Indefinite	
Centers	2		5	
Total number of patients	79		122	
	Total number (%)	White collar† (%)	Total number (%)	White collar† (%)
Employed	48 (61)	34 (71)	64 (52)	44 (69)
Returned to former job	37 (47)	23 (62)	60 (49)	40 (67)
Secured new employment	11 (14)	11 (100)	4 (3)	4 (100)
Unemployed	31 (39)	25 (81)	58 (48)	27 (47)
Made job applications	6 (8)	6 (100)	8 (8)	6 (75)
Plan to seek employment	11 (14)	11 (100)	8 (8)	7 (88)
No plan to seek employment	14 (18)	8 (57)	42 (34)	14 (33)

Note: Data exclude medically disabled and retired patients.
† Includes professionals, students, and homemakers.
(Courtesy of Paris W, Woodbury A, Thompson S, et al: J Heart Lung Transplant 12:46–54, 1993.)

Long-Term Functional Results After Bilateral Lung Transplantation
Dromer C, Velly J-F, Jougon J, Martigne C, Baudet EM, Couraud L, and the Bordeaus Lung and Heart-Lung Transplant Group (Bordeaux Lung and Heart-Lung Transplant Group, Pessac, France)
Ann Thorac Surg 56:68–73, 1993   140-94-6-10

Introduction.—At the study institution, double lung transplantation (DLT) is used for all patients with pulmonary diseases and no severe cardiac dysfunction, and single lung transplantation (SLT) is reserved for patients with pulmonary fibrosis. The long-term functional results of bilateral lung transplantation, both DLT and heart-lung transplantation (HLT), were reviewed and compared with the results published for SLT.

Methods.—Between February 1988 and January 1991, a total of 42 HLTs and 19 DLTs were performed. The HLT group included all 20 patients with primary or secondary pulmonary arterial hypertension and 22 patients with parenchymal disease. The HLT group included patients for whom en bloc DLT performed without vascularization yielded poor results. Forty-two patients who were still alive 6 months after operation were evaluated for short- and long-term pulmonary function.

Results.—The DLT and HLT groups had no significant differences in actuarial survival at 1 year or 3 years after operation (66% vs. 72% and 57% vs. 53%, respectively). One of the 42 survivors required retransplantation, but the others are living almost normal lives. Pulmonary function improved dramatically in all patients within a month after operation; ex-

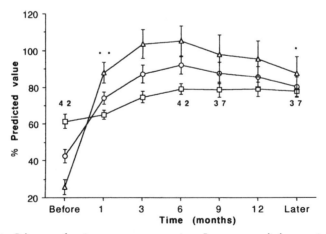

Fig 6–4.—Pulmonary function parameters over time. Parameters studied were vital capacity (*squares*), FEV_1 (*circles*), and $FEFR_{25/75}$ (*triangles*), expressed as percentage of predicted value. Each point represents mean value ± standard error of mean. Values are given before transplantation, at 1 month, every 3 months for 1 year, and "later," which means for 37 patients a mean follow-up of 23.9 months. Figures represent number of patients evaluated at each time. *P < .05 for comparison between later and at 6 months for FEV_1 and $FEFR_{25/75}$. **P < .0001 for comparison between parameters (FEV_1 and $FEFR_{25/75}$) before transplantation and at 1 month afterward. (Courtesy of Dromer C, Velly J-F, Jougon J, et al: *Ann Thorac Surg* 56:68–73, 1993.)

cept for arterial carbon dioxide tension, all parameters showed significant improvement at 6 months. The occurrence of obliterative bronchitis in 6 patients resulted in a slight decrease for the group as a whole in forced expiratory volume in 1 second and forced expiratory flow rate between 25% and 75% of vital capacity. Nevertheless, values remained at more than 75% of predicted (Fig 6–4).

Conclusion.—Previous reports have shown a modest advantage in actuarial survival for SLT over HLT and DLT. In this series of patients, however, both short-term and long-term results of bilateral lung transplantation were excellent. With improvements in surgical procedures and postoperative management, patients undergoing the bilateral procedure achieve greater pulmonary function and have a better chance to recover from complications. It is believed that SLT should be reserved for patients with pulmonary fibrosis and contraindications for bilateral lung transplantation in pulmonary arterial hypertension and chronic obstructive pulmonary disease.

A Decade of Lung Transplantation
Griffith BP, Hardesty RL, Armitage JM, Hattler BG, Pham SM, Keenan RJ, Paradis I (Univ of Pittsburgh, Pa; Children's Hosp, Pittsburgh, Pa)
Ann Surg 218:310–320, 1993   140-94-6-11

Background.—The University of Pittsburgh lung transplantation program began in 1982. Since then, 245 transplantations have been performed. The 10-year experience at that center was reviewed.

Methods and Findings.—The most common transplantation performed was heart-lung (HLT), done in 97 cases. Double-lung transplan-

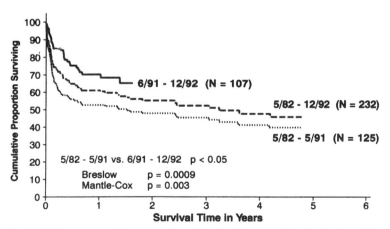

Fig 6–5.—Pulmonary transplantation performed at the University of Pittsburgh. Survival by time interval. (Courtesy of Griffith BP, Hardesty RL, Armitage JM, et al: *Ann Surg* 218:310–320, 1993.)

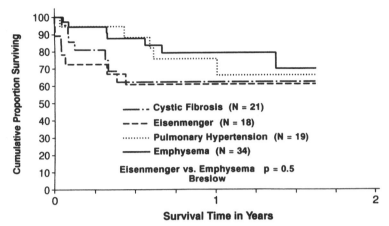

Fig 6–6.—Pulmonary transplant survival by major disease. (Courtesy of Griffith BP, Hardesty RL, Armitage JM, et al: *Ann Surg* 218:310–320, 1993.)

tation (DLT) was done in 80 patients and single-lung (SLT) in 68. The surgery was indicated by primary pulmonary hypertension in 76 patients, obstructive lung disease in 57, Eisenmenger's syndrome in 42, cystic fibrosis in 32, and retransplantation in 13. One hundred fifteen procedures have been performed since May 1991. Heart-lung transplantation has declined from 61% to 15%. Double-lung and SLT have increased from 24% to 43% and from 15% to 42%, respectively. Overall, the 1-, 2-, and 5-year survival rates were 61%, 55%, and 44%, respectively. The 107 patients receiving transplants more recently had a significantly better actuarial survival rate than the 125 early transplant recipients. Those rates at 1 year were 70% and 61%, respectively. The SLT and DLT procedures were more successful overall than HLT. However, HLT has recently been associated with an improved survival rate, from 48% to 72%. One hundred six patients died, 40 of infection, 23 of early allograft dysfunction, 13 of obliterative bronchiolitis, and 10 of operative bleeding (Figs 6–5 and 6–6).

Conclusion.—Lung transplant recipients now have improved long-term outcomes. Further improvements will depend on better treatment for chronic rejection of the airways, histologically defined by obliterative bronchiolitis.

▶ Abstracts 140-94-6–10 and 140-94-6–11 describe the increasing survival rates after lung transplantation. Just as heart, liver, and kidney transplantation began with poor results and the results gradually improved with time, so have the results of lung transplantation improved remarkably in recent years.—R.J. Howard, M.D., Ph.D.

The Significance of a Positive Flow Cytometry Crossmatch Test in Primary Kidney Transplantation

Ogura K, Terasaki PI, Johnson C, Mendez R, Rosenthal JT, Ettenger R, Martin DC, Dainko E, Cohen L, Mackett T, Berne T, Barba L, Lieberman E (Univ of California, Los Angeles; Los Angeles Transplant Society)

Transplantation 56:294–298, 1993   140-94-6-12

Background.—The flow cytometry crossmatch (FCXM) test is more sensitive than the standard microlymphocytotoxicity crossmatch test, and it has the potential of detecting low levels of latent sensitization. There are increasing indications that the FCXM test is useful for evaluating retransplants, but evidence for its validity in assessing first transplants is limited.

Objective.—The efficacy of the T-cell FCXM (T-FCXM) test was examined in 841 primary cadaver donor kidney transplant patients. The group included 468 male and 373 female patients.

Results.—Graft survival rates at 1 year were 82% for patients whose T-FCXM test was negative and 75% for those with positive test results. Graft failures in the first month were 13% more frequent in patients with positive test results, and these patients also had more frequent immunologic failures. A positive T-FCXM test was obtained for 39% of sensitized patients and 8% of those who were not sensitized. Most positive crossmatches were in patients who possessed complement-fixing antibodies.

Recommendations.—Given the scarcity of cadaver kidneys and the many patients awaiting kidney transplantation, it seems appropriate to use available organs in patients who are the most likely to have a successful outcome. The FCXM test should be used prospectively, even though many patients with a positive crossmatch have had successful transplants.

▶ Flow cytometry cross-matching can be used to further refine standard complement-dependent cytotoxicity crossmatch (CDCXM) testing. Patients who had a negative T-FCXM test had a lower primary nonfunction rate and graft failure rate within the first month after transplantation and a higher graft survival at 1 year. Graft survival did not vary among any of the various subgroups of patients, however. Our center is currently willing to transplant patients when negative T-FCXM results are obtained (we still complete the CDCXM, however). With several hundred such cross matches, we have only had 1 test in which the T-FCXM was negative but the CDCXM was positive. The question is whether the differences shown by these authors are enough to justify not performing a kidney transplant when the CDCXM is negative and the FCXM is positive. Our center is currently unwilling to do kidney transplantation in this circumstance when the patient has high panel-reactive antibody (greater than 60%) or for second transplant procedures.—R.J. Howard, M.D., Ph.D.

Risk Factors for Chronic Rejection in Renal Allograft Recipients

Almond PS, Matas A, Gillingham K, Dunn DL, Payne WD, Gores P, Gruessner R, Najarian JS (Univ of Minnesota, Minneapolis)
Transplantation 55:752–757, 1993   140-94-6-13

Introduction.—Chronic rejection is a significant impediment to long-term renal allograft survival. Cyclosporine reduces graft loss caused by acute rejection, but it has had little effect on the occurrence of chronic rejection.

Series.—Risk factors for chronic rejection were sought in 566 patients receiving 587 kidney transplants from 1986 to 1991 who were followed for a year or longer.

Immunosuppression.—Recipients of living related donor kidneys received triple therapy with cyclosporine, prednisone, and azathioprine. Patients given cadaver kidneys received that regimen plus antilymphocyte globulin. Rejection was treated by recycling the prednisone taper. Patients resistant to steroid therapy received further antilymphocyte globulin.

Results.—Chronic rejection was confirmed by graft biopsy in 103 patients, 66 of them cadaver kidney recipients. Chronic rejection reduced the 5-year graft survival rate from 81% to 31%. The risk factors for chronic rejection, determined by logistic regression analysis, included acute rejection, infection, high plasma renin activity, and age over 50 years at the time of transplantation. Only acute rejection and infection were risk factors for patients given living related donor kidneys. The magnitude of these risk factors was evident when comparing times to chronic rejection in patients with and without acute rejection or infection (Fig 6–7).

Conclusion.—Acute rejection is the single most significant risk factor for chronic rejection in renal allograft recipients. These findings suggest the importance of preventing or adequately treating episodes of acute rejection. The role of anticytokine antibody treatment during rejection or infection deserves study.

▶ The authors found several risk factors for chronic rejection. However, there seems to be little that one can do about any of them, except to try to avoid acute rejection and infection (but everyone already does that). Nevertheless, efforts should continue to be directed toward the early events after renal transplantation, because adverse early events have profound long-term consequences. Interestingly, a tissue match between donor and recipient was not a risk factor for chronic rejection.—R.J. Howard, M.D., Ph.D.

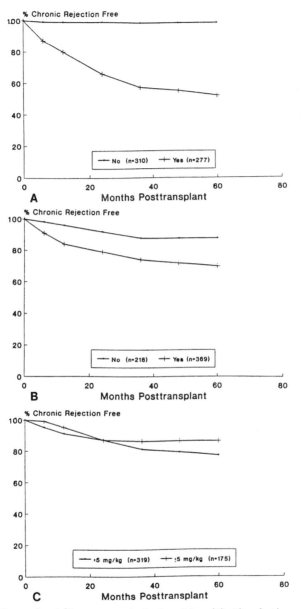

Fig 6–7.—Time to chronic biopsy-proven rejection in recipients (**A**) with and without an acute rejection episode, (**B**) with and without an infection, and (**C**) with a cyclosporine dosage < 5 mg/kg/day at 1 year vs. a larger dosage. (Courtesy of Almond PS, Matas A, Gillingham K, et al: *Transplantation* 55:752–757, 1993.)

A Prospective Randomized Comparison of Quadruple Versus Triple Therapy for First Cadaver Transplants With Immediate Function
Slakey DP, Johnson CP, Callaluce RD, Browne BJ, Zhu Y-r, Roza AM, Adams MB (Med College of Wisconsin, Milwaukee)
Transplantation 56:827–831, 1993   140-94-6-14

Background.—The role of cyclosporin A (CsA) in induction protocols for patients undergoing cadaver renal transplantation is still debated. Many centers currently use induction protocols including antilymphocyte agents such as antilymphocyte globulin (ALG) in the post-transplantation period, withholding CsA until the criteria for satisfactory function have been met. Although this strategy seems to be most beneficial for recipients with delayed graft function, it raises the question of whether prophylactic ALG offers any benefit in first-time adult cadaver renal transplant recipients with immediate graft function.

Methods.—The role of prophylactic ALG in first-time, adult cadaver transplants with immediate graft function was studied in a prospective, randomized comparison of ALG and no ALG. The study subjects were stratified on the basis of diabetes status and age younger or older than 50 years. Sixty-one recipients receiving quadruple therapy received ALG for 7 days in increasing doses. Cyclosporin A, 10 mg/kg/day, was initiated on day 6 in this group. Azathioprine was begun at a dosage of 2.5 mg/kg/day and was adjusted based on white blood cell count. Sixty recipients receiving triple therapy began CsA immediately. Azathioprine was begun at 5 mg/kg/day and was tapered to 2.5 mg/kg/day by day 8.

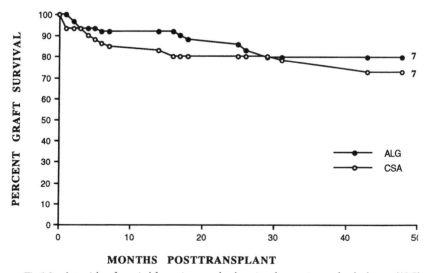

Fig 6–8.—Actuarial graft survival for patients randomly assigned to receive quadruple therapy (ALG) or triple therapy (CsA). There was no significant difference in survival. (Courtesy of Slakey DP, Johnson CP, Callaluce RD, et al: *Transplantation* 56:827–831, 1993.)

Identical dosages of prednisone were given to each group. The patients were followed for 2–4.5 years.

Findings.—Patient survival rates with and without ALG were 93% and 90%, respectively. Actuarial graft survival rates were 79% and 72%, respectively (Fig 6–8). Graft loss from rejection occurred in 6 of the patients given ALG and in 7 not given ALG. Three of 4 high panel-reactive antibody (PRA) recipients in the group immediately given CsA lost their grafts within 30 days, compared with none in the ALG group. Mean time to graft loss was significantly longer in the quadruple therapy group, being 17 and 4 months for the 2 groups, respectively. The total number of rejection episodes and the number of rejection-free were comparable between groups. The use of OKT3 was also similar. There was a higher incidence of cytomegalovirus in the group given quadruple therapy. However, no grafts were lost nor did any patients die as a result. Serum creatinine levels and creatinine clearances were comparable between groups at 1 and 12 months.

Conclusion.—Immediate CsA was not associated with significant nephrotoxicity in these patients. Prophylactic ALG given for 7 days did not reduce the incidence of rejection or lessen OKT3 use in first cadaver transplants. However, it did increase time to graft loss and may protect high-PRA recipients from early graft loss. The groups given the different induction protocols were ultimately similar in patient survival, graft survival, and graft function.

▶ This is one of a small number of prospective, randomized trials investigating the use of ALG as induction therapy for cadaveric renal transplantation. This paper suggests that overall graft survival and function are not affected by induction ALG therapy. Because the course of induction ALG therapy can greatly add to the cost of transplantation, demonstrating equivalent results with cyclosporine alone can reduce the cost of transplantation compared with ALG use. These authors included only first cadaveric recipients who had immediate graft function, and, thus, they excluded one group of patients in whom ALG is claimed to be beneficial: patients who have delayed graft function that may be prolonged by cyclosporine therapy.—R.J. Howard, M.D., Ph.D.

Variation in Expression of Endothelial Adhesion Molecules in Pretransplant and Transplanted Kidneys: Correlation With Intragraft Events
Fuggle SV, Sanderson JB, Gray DWR, Richardson A, Morris PJ (Univ of Oxford, England)
Transplantation 55:117–123, 1993   140-94-6-15

Background.—Acute renal allograft rejection is accompanied by the interstitial infiltration of leukocytes, which is initially mediated by the interaction of endothelial adhesion molecules with their ligands on the

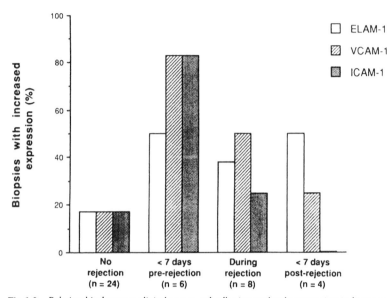

Fig 6–9.—Relationship between clinical status and adhesion molecule expression in biopsy specimens from patients receiving triple-therapy immunosuppression. (Courtesy of Fuggle SV, Sanderson JB, Gray DWR, et al: *Transplantation* 55:117–123, 1993.)

leukocyte cell surface. Inflammatory cytokines can alter the phenotype of the vascular endothelium in ways that promote the adherence of leukocytes to the endothelium. Adhesion molecules also participate in cellular interactions in the effector phase of the response.

Objective and Methods.—Monoclonal antibody staining was used to study the expression of platelet endothelial cell adhesion molecule-1 (PECAM-1, CD31), endothelial leukocyte adhesion molecule-1 (ELAM-1), intercellular adhesion molecule-1 (ICAM-1, CD54), and vascular cell adhesion molecule-1 (VCAM-1) in 20 pretransplant needlecore biopsy specimens and 24 graft biopsy specimens from immunosuppressed patients.

Observations.—In both pretransplant and graft biopsy specimens, PECAM-1 was consistently expressed on endothelia. In contrast, the endothelial expression of ELAM-1 and the proximal tubular expression of ICAM-1 and VCAM-1 varied between pretransplant biopsy specimens. Induced expression of adhesion molecules often was associated with focal leukocyte infiltration before the onset of clinical rejection (Fig 6–9). Greater infiltration of CD45-positive and CD25-positive cells was observed in biopsy specimens exhibiting induced expression of adhesion molecules.

Interpretation.—Induction of the expression of adhesion molecules in renal transplant biopsy specimens is evidence of endothelial activation. This probably facilitates the entry of leukocytes into the graft. Both induced adhesion molecules and HLA class II antigens may render the graft susceptible to damage mediated by allospecific cytotoxic T lymphocytes.

▶ Adhesion molecules may play an important role in allograft rejection. They are induced by inflammatory cytokines and can change endothelial cells in such a way that adherence of leukocytes to vascular endothelium is promoted. These sites to which lymphocytes and macrophages adhere on endothelial cells are called adhesions molecules. This interesting paper demonstrates that these are upregulated in biopsy specimens from rejected kidney transplants.—R.J. Howard, M.D., Ph.D.

Functional and Neurochemical Evidence for Partial Cardiac Sympathetic Reinnervation After Cardiac Transplantation in Humans
Kaye DM, Esler M, Kingwell B, Mcpherson G, Esmore D, Jennings G (Alfred Hosp, Melbourne, Australia)
Circulation 88:1110–1118, 1993   140-94-6–16

Introduction.—There has been considerable debate regarding whether cardiac reinnervation occurs after cardiac transplantation in humans. The issue is relevant for understanding exercise responses after transplantation, the unexplained occurrence of ischemic chest pain, and the heart's responsiveness to adrenergic drugs. Previous studies have used various techniques for evaluating neuronal function, some of them rather indirect. The time course and extent of cardiac reinnervation therefore remain unclear.

Methods.—Both neurochemical and functional tests of neuronal integrity were used to detect sympathetic reinnervation of the transplanted heart in 15 orthotopic cardiac transplant recipients with a mean age of 50 years. Twenty-five healthy volunteers of similar age served as controls. Ten of the transplant patients were classified as "early," having received a transplant less than 18 months previously; 5 were classified as "late," having received their transplant more than 2 years previously. In the neurochemical analysis, the isotope dilution method with coronary sinus venous sampling was used to examine norepinephrine (NE) kinetics at rest and during exercise. The functional assessment included power spectral analysis of heart rate variability and hemodynamic responses to exercise.

Results.—The early transplantation group showed marked attenuation of cardiac NE spillover at rest, a mean of 11 vs. a mean of 105 pmol/min for the late transplantation group and a mean of 103 pmol/min for the controls. Both heart transplant groups had significantly reduced heart rate variability compared with controls, a mean of 59 vs. a mean of 1,673 ms², with signs of a trend toward increasing spectral power in the late group. Cardiac NE spillover during exercise was lower in the early transplantation group than in the controls, a mean of 163 vs. a mean of 1,876 pmol/min. The mean response in the late transplantation group was 1,080 pmol/min. Both transplant groups demonstrated significant depression of the neuronal reuptake process for NE.

Conclusion.—These findings suggest that cardiac sympathetic nerve function is partially restored over time in heart transplant recipients. The reinnervation is at least partly functional, as evidenced by the normalization of the heart rate response to exercise in the late transplant group. However, there are still major abnormalities, including impairment of the uptake process for neuronally released NE and marked attenuation of heart rate variability.

▶ Because of the dictum that neural tissue does not regenerate, it came to be accepted that transplanted organs do not become reinnervated. In the 1993 YEAR BOOK OF SURGERY, a paper presented evidence for reinnervation of renal allografts (1). This more recently abstracted paper provides evidence that cardiac allografts also become reinnervated.—R.J. Howard, M.D., Ph.D.

Reference

1. 1993 YEAR BOOK OF SURGERY, p 141.

7 Endocrine

Introduction

Discussion regarding whether to do preoperative localization studies before parathyroidectomy continues. In general, experienced endocrine surgeons are as good as radiologic studies in identifying the site of large parathyroid glands during the initial operation for hyperparathyroidism. Therefore, many articles suggest that radiologic studies are a waste of money, which may be true for "experienced" endocrine surgeons. However, in the United States, most parathyroid operations probably are not done by these experts; hence, preoperative localization studies may help many surgeons who only occasionally do parathyroidectomies. Even experienced endocrine surgeons obtain localization studies before reoperative surgery. Preoperative localization studies are helpful in approximately 80% (see Abstract 140-94-7–1) of patients who require operation for recurrent or persistent hyperparathyroidism. Preoperative localization studies are even less successful in patients with multiple gland enlargement than they are in patients with single gland enlargement. No doubt this debate about doing preoperative localization studies will continue. Perhaps the development of newer, more reliable tests in the future will prove the worth of preoperative localization studies, even for experienced endocrine surgeons.

The first surgeon to operate on a patient who has hyperparathyroidism has the best opportunity to perform a curative operation and to avoid complications. Complications of recurrent nerve injury and permanent hypocalcemia are greater in patients who have reoperation. Therefore, qualified surgeons should do parathyroid operations and assure themselves they have removed all the diseased tissue. An article from Sweden (Abstract 140-94-7–2) presents a rather high rate of complications after recurrent operation for hyperparathyroidism. Only two thirds of patients who require a second operation will be cured during the second operation, and some patients will require a third, fourth, and even fifth operation. To avoid injuring the recurrent nerves should recurrent hyperparathyroidism develop, many surgeons will autotransplant parathyroid tissue in those who have parathyroidectomy for hyperplasia. Two papers (Abstracts 140-94-7–3 and 140-94-7–4) discuss the long-term function of autotransplanted tissue. Implanted tissue does function, and differential concentrations of parathyroid hormone can be demonstrated between veins of arms that have tissue implants and those that do not. Only a small number of patients who undergo parathyroid autotransplantation for hyperplasia have recurrent hyperparathyroidism. This low number is surprising, because the metabolic drive that led to hyperfunction in the first place (usually renal failure) is still present.

There have been relatively few long-term studies of patients who underwent surgery for hyperparathyroidism. One study reported in this chapter (Abstract 140-94-7–5) follows patients who had been operated on 6 to 32 years previously. Almost 5% of patients had prolonged mild hypocalcemia requiring vitamin D therapy. Whether the results in patients reflect those in patients who underwent surgery performed many years before by inadequately trained surgeons is not discussed. It is to be hoped that patients operated on today would not become hypoparathyroid in the incidence suggested by this paper.

The incidence of parathyroid carcinoma may be changing because of the difference in criteria for diagnosis. Many years ago, the finding of a single mitotic figure on histologic examination was enough to make the diagnosis of parathyroid cancer. Pathologists then decided to make the criteria more stringent, and finding several mitotic figures per high-power field became necessary before they were willing to make the diagnosis of parathyroid cancer. Even more stringent criteria are now required for that diagnosis (see Abstract 140-94-7–6). The authors from Memorial Sloan-Kettering Cancer Center require recurrence, metastases, or frank capillary invasion on histologic examinations before they are willing to make a diagnosis of parathyroid cancer. These different criteria for diagnosis will have to be taken into account in evaluating varying incidences of parathyroid cancer over time.

The surgical treatment of toxic solitary thyroid nodules provides rapid restoration of the euthyroid state compared with treatment with radioactive iodine. However, the long-term rate of hypoparathyroidism does not differ between patients who have radioactive iodine therapy or surgical treatment. Most patients would probably prefer a nonsurgical approach if the complication rates are similar (as they seem to be). Most likely, the great majority of patients are initially treated by nonoperative means, because they are initially seen by endocrinologists who are likely to have a preference for radioactive iodine treatment.

In the 1993 YEAR BOOK OF SURGERY, several articles were presented that discussed the extent of thyroid resection for patients with thyroid cancer. This year Abstract 140-94-7–7 discusses the therapy of papillar microcarcinoma (tumors 1 cm or less in diameter). Despite the increasing tendency toward near total thyroidectomy for these very small tumors, the extent of resection did not seem to affect survival. Medullary carcinoma differs from other thyroid cancers because it has a different cell of origin. Unlike the situation with thyroid cancers of follicular cell origin, total thyroidectomy and dissection of the central lymph node are recommended for patients with medullary carcinoma of the thyroid.

Two papers (Abstracts 140-94-7–8 and 140-94-7–9) discuss adrenocortical cancer. Because currently available chemotherapeutic agents are not effective, an aggressive surgical approach is indicated for these patients, including resection of the adjacent structures if necessary and possible. Aggressive resection may be the only way of preventing or ameliorating the clinical effects of functional tumors.

Computed tomography scanning has eliminated the need for operating on both adrenal glands in patients with unilateral pheochromocytoma. One paper (Abstract 140-94-7–10) advocates removing both adrenal glands in patients with pheochromocytomas when they occur in patients with multiple endocrine neoplasia syndrome. The authors concluded that patients should only have unilateral adrenalectomy because pheochromocytoma did not develop in most patients during follow-up and because 25% of patients having bilateral adrenalectomy had at least 1 episode of acute adrenal insufficiency (1 of these patients died).

Richard J. Howard, M.D., Ph.D.

Parathyroid Re-Exploration
Silver CE, Velez FJ (Albert Einstein College of Medicine, Bronx, NY)
Am J Surg 164:606–609, 1992   140-94-7–1

Introduction.—Patients who require parathyroid reexploration present a challenging surgical problem. The procedure can be difficult and tedious and carries the risk of failure. Researchers reviewed their experience with 27 patients who underwent parathyroid reexploration between 1982 and 1992.

Patients and Methods.—There were 19 cases of primary hyperparathyroidism and 8 of secondary or renal hyperparathyroidism. Twenty of the patients had persistent hyperparathyroidism after the initial surgery, and 7 had recurrent or metachronous disease 2 or more years after an apparently successful initial operation. Patient records were analyzed for the accuracy of preoperative localization tests, factors contributing to failure of the initial surgery, and the relationship of the findings of previous explorations to the current problem. The technical aspects of the reexploration procedure were also reviewed.

Results.—Localization studies, performed in 26 patients, resulted in successful placement in 21 cases. Invasive preoperative localization studies, including arteriography and selective vein catheterization, were successful in 12 of 15 patients. The noninvasive localization procedures performed were thallium-technetium scintigraphy, MRI, CT, and ultrasonography; accurate localization was achieved in 14 of 21 patients. Scintigraphy and MRI were the most useful methods of noninvasive localization. Reexploration was successful, with cure of hyperparathyroidism, in 23 of the 27 patients. The cure rate was 85% for patients with an unsuccessful initial exploration (table) and 85% for those with recurrent disease. All 16 patients with eutopic disease and 7 of 9 patients with ectopic disease were cured. All 4 patients in whom reexploration failed

Results in 20 Patients Who Had an Unsuccessful Initial Exploration

Lesion Location	No. of Patients	Adequate Exploration	Single Gland	Multiple Glands	Super-numerary Gland	Success	Failure
Eutopic	10	0	5	5	0	10	0
Ectopic	8	8	3	5	3	7	1
Unknown location	2	2	0	2	2	0	2
Total	20	10	8	12	5	17	3

(Courtesy of Silver CE, Velez FJ: *Am J Surg* 164:606–609, 1992.)

had multiple gland disease and had abnormal tissue removed at both the first and second operations.

Conclusion.—Previous operative and pathology reports should be carefully reviewed before parathyroid reexploration. In the majority of cases, this analysis together with noninvasive localization studies will lead to successful reexploration. Invasive studies should be needed only when the previous exploration was adequate and noninvasive tests proved inconclusive.

▶ Although preoperative localization studies usually are not helpful when experienced parathyroid surgeons perform the initial operation on patients with hyperparathyroid disease, they can be very helpful before reoperation for persistent or recurrent hyperparathyroidism. As these authors show, such studies successfully located the site of the parathyroid gland in 21 of 26 patients studied. Although reoperation can be extremely frustrating for the surgeon, most glands are found in the normal anatomical location. Only 9 of 27 patients in this series had ectopic parathyroid glands.—R.J. Howard, M.D., Ph.D.

Reoperation for Suspected Primary Hyperparathyroidism
Järhult J, Nordenström J, Perbeck L (Huddinge Univ Hosp, Sweden)
Br J Surg 80:453–456, 1993   140-94-7-2

Objective.—The findings were reviewed in 93 patients having a total of 128 reexplorations for persistent or recurrent hypercalcemia after primary parathyroid surgery. The patients, 72 women and 21 men with a median age of 63 years, were followed for a median of 41 months.

Findings.—Seventy-six patients had persistent and 17 had recurrent hypercalcemia more than 6 months after initial surgery. The median time to relapse was 44 months. About one fourth of patients had a serum calcium level above 3 mmol/L, and the same proportion had symptoms of severe hypercalcemia. Only 23% of venous sampling studies yielded the correct location. Forty-one patients had a single adenoma at reexploration, and 28 had hyperplastic disease. Seven patients were cured even though no abnormal parathyroid was removed at reoperation. The chief causes of failure were undetected adenoma and inadequate resection in patients with multiglandular disease. Two patients had intrathyroidal parathyroid adenomas, and 6 had adenomas in the mediastinum. Nine patients who were not cured were later found to have other disorders. Complications included permanent recurrent nerve paralysis in 9 patients and permanent hypocalcemia in 15.

Conclusion.—Failure to detect an adenoma and failure to remove all involved parathyroid tissue were the chief problems in this series. Reoperation restored normocalcemia in a majority of cases, but this was achieved only with considerable morbidity. Careful risk-benefit analysis should be done in each case before recommending repeated parathyroid surgery.

▶ The first surgeon to operate on a patient for parathyroid disease has the best opportunity to do a curative operation with minimal morbidity. Nine of 93 patients had permanent recurrent nerve paralysis and 15 had permanent hypocalcemia when subjected to reoperation for hyperparathyroidism, numbers which are comparable to those from other series. Inadequate surgery was the reason that most patients required reoperation. Only 14 of 27 patients who required a second reoperation were cured. Curiously, 7 patients were cured even though no abnormal parathyroid tissue was removed at reoperation. The likelihood of cure the first time around is greater in patients who undergo surgery performed by a knowledgeable surgeon.—R.J. Howard, M.D., Ph.D.

Recurrent Hyperparathyroidism Due to Parathyroid Autografts: Incidence, Presentation, and Management
Demeter JG, De Jong SA, Lawrence AM, Paloyan E (Loyola Univ, Maywood, Ill; Edward Hines Jr Hosp, Hines, Ill)
Am Surg 59:178–181, 1993   140-94-7-3

Background.—A small percentage of patients undergoing parathyroidectomy for primary hyperparathyroidism may experience recurrent hyperparathyroidism, primarily because of insufficient excision of hyperfunctioning parathyroid tissue in the neck or a missed ectopic and hyperplastic parathyroid. Although seen less frequently, parathyroid carcinoma and parathyroid autografts may play causative roles. The incidence, clinical characteristics, and outcomes of patients with recurrent hyperparathyroidism resulting from parathyroid autografts were reviewed.

Patients and Findings.—Data on 604 consecutive patients who had surgical treatment for primary hyperparathyroidism between 1965 and 1989 were studied. One hundred patients received parathyroid autografts consisting of portions of 1 or more parathyroid glands. Recurrent hyperparathyroidism developed in 3 patients who had autografts placed in the sternocleidomastoid muscle, for an incidence of 3%. Recurrent disease was diagnosed between 62 and 113 months, with an average of 89 months. A history of neck irradiation was noted for 2 of these patients. In all 3 cases, the autotransplants were from hyperplastic or adenomatous parathyroid tissue. The hyperfunctioning parathyroid tissue was accurately localized via preoperative thallium scans in all 3 patients. At surgery, the hyperfunctioning autografts had grown into a distinct mass with a solitary vascular pedicle and were resected. Histologic evaluation revealed either hyperplastic or adenomatous tissue, corresponding to the histologic type and location of the original tissue transplanted in each patient. Follow-up ranged from 12 to 67 months, with an average of 48 months. All patients remain symptom-free, and none have required oral calcium supplementation.

Conclusion.—Graft-dependent recurrent hyperparathyroidism is caused by autotransplantation of hyperplastic or adenomatous parathyroid tissue. Previous neck irradiation may be a possible risk factor. In instances of recurrent hyperparathyroidism, thallium scanning plays an instrumental role in diagnosis and localization. Excision of the hyperfunctioning autograft is curative, and there is little chance of permanent hypoparathyroidism.

▶ This article also deals with autotransplanted parathyroid tissue and demonstrates that recurrent hyperparathyroidism developed in 3 of 100 patients who underwent parathyroid autotransplantation. It is surprising that hyperplasia does not recur more commonly in individuals receiving autotransplanted tissue, because the drive that led to hyperfunction in the first place (usually renal dysfunction) is still present in most individuals who undergo autotransplantation.—R.J. Howard, M.D., Ph.D.

Determination of the Functioning of Autotransplanted Parathyroid Tissue in Muscle
Karusseit VOL, Falkson CB, Mieny CJ, Ungerer JPJ, Potgieter CD, Van Rensburg BWJ (HF Verwoerd Hosp, Pretoria, South Africa; Univ of Pretoria, South Africa)
S Afr Med J 83:113–114, 1993   140-94-7-4

Introduction.—Subtotal excision of the parathyroid glands has been the traditional surgical treatment for parathyroid hyperplasia. In certain patients, total parathyroidectomy and autotransplantation of some parathyroid tissue in muscle has been advocated. The function of transplanted tissue was assessed in 12 patients who underwent autotransplantation.

Patients and Methods.—During a 6-year period, 20 dialysis and renal transplant patients underwent parathyroid autotransplantation. Parathyroid transplantation was performed in forearm muscle. Twelve of these patients survived for follow-up examination. Blood samples were obtained for determination of parathyroid hormone (PTH) levels.

Results.—Ten of the surviving patients had functional renal transplants, and 2 returned to dialysis. In all 12 cases, there was a difference in levels of PTH between the autografted arm and the nontransplanted arm (Fig 7–1). The intact hormone method was superior to the midmolecule method for demonstrating the functioning of transplanted parathyroid tissue. In 4 patients, midmolecule assays yielded ratios between the transplanted and normal arms of less than 1.5:1; all patients had greater ratios when the intact hormone method was used.

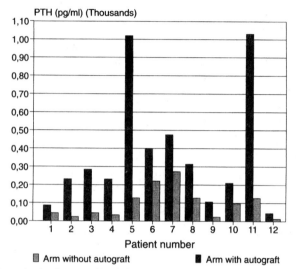

Fig 7–1.—Intact levels of PTH in blood drawn from antecubital veins in transplanted (*filled bars*) and nontransplanted arms (*hatched bars*). All patients have ratio of more than 1.5:1. (Courtesy of Karusseit VOL, Falkson CB, Mieny CJ, et al: *S Afr Med J* 83:113-114, 1993.)

Conclusion.—All these patients undergoing renal transplant and dialysis improved symptomatically after autotransplantation. All but one have intact PTH levels on the transplanted side, and none is clinically hypoparathyroid. Total parathyroidectomy and autotransplantation is indicated in parathyroid hyperplasia and in patients with an ongoing stimulus to hyperplasia.

▶ Autotransplantation has long been used for patients who undergo parathyroidectomy for hyperplasia to obviate the necessity of reentering the neck and risking injury to recurrent laryngeal nerve should hyperparathyroidism recur. This paper demonstrates that these glands function normally when autotransplanted into the muscles of the forearm. It is possible to demonstrate differential venous parathormone levels in the veins of the arms in the autotransplanted individuals.—R.J. Howard, M.D., Ph.D.

Long-Term Effects of Parathyroid Operation on Serum Calcium and Parathyroid Hormone Values in Sporadic Primary Hyperparathyroidism
Lundgren E, Rastad J, Ridefelt P, Juhlin C, Åkerström G, Ljunghall S (Uppsala Univ Hosp, Sweden)
Surgery 112:1123–1129, 1992   140-94-7-5

Objective.—The outcome of parathyroid surgery was examined in 410 patients (median age, 67 years) who underwent surgery for sporadic primary hyperparathyroidism between 1956 and 1984. The mean follow-up was 14 years.

Findings.—After conservative surgery (a mean of 673 mg of abnormal parathyroid tissue being removed), 3.7% of the patients had persistent hypercalcemia and 1.7% had recurrent hypercalcemia. At the same time, 4.7% of the patients had mild hypocalcemia or required vitamin D substitution. Parathyroid hormone (PTH) levels were generally increased in patients with postoperative hyperparathyroidism, normal to increased in those with hypocalcemia or normocalcemia, and low in those requiring vitamin D. Serum creatinine levels correlated closely with the serum PTH. The PTH values in patients who were normocalcemic postoperatively did not differ significantly from those in matched control patients, but the surgical patients had more variable PTH levels.

Conclusion.—Parathyroid surgery is an effective approach to patients having sporadic primary hyperparathyroidism. Nevertheless, secondary hyperparathyroidism may develop during long-term follow-up.

▶ There are relatively few long-term studies of patients who have undergone surgery for hyperparathyroidism. This study investigated a large number of patients who had had operations for primary hyperparathyroidism 6 to 32 years previously. A relatively small fraction had recurrent hypercalcemia, but 3.7% had persistent hypercalcemia, suggesting inadequate initial operation. Significantly, 4.7% of patients had prolonged mild hypocalcemia requiring vitamin D.—R.J. Howard, M.D., Ph.D.

Parathyroid Carcinoma: Diagnosis and Clinical History
Vetto JT, Brennan MF, Woodruf J, Burt M (Mem Sloan-Kettering Cancer Ctr, New York)
Surgery 114:882–892, 1993   140-94-7-6

Background.—Histologic appearance alone often leads to the overdiagnosis of parathyroid carcinoma. One experience was reviewed to assess trends in the treatment and outcome of this unusual disease. To avoid overdiagnosis, cases were identified based on recurrence, metastases, or frank capsular invasion on histologic evaluation.

Methods and Findings.—With this more limited definition, 14 cases of parathyroid carcinoma were identified at the study institution from 1955 to the present. All patients had hypercalcemia. After initial surgery, 2 patients had been free of disease for 31 and 180 months. Six additional patients had a prolonged course and a median survival of more than 80 months. Two of those had reexcision for local recurrence, and 4 had multiple resections for local recurrence or metastases. Reoperations generally resulted in satisfactory but temporary control of hypercalcemia. Six patients died of disease after an aggressive course. Median survival in that group was 47 months. Four of those patients were treated in the

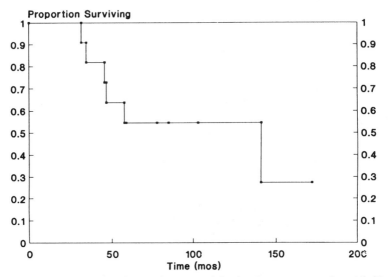

Fig 7–2.—Kaplan-Meier survival curve of patients with local or distant recurrence ($n = 11$). (Courtesy of Vetto JT, Brennan MF, Woodruf J, et al: *Surgery* 114:882–892, 1993.)

1950s, before an aggressive approach to metastatic disease had been adopted. All deaths were the result of hypercalcemia.

Conclusion.—The clinical courses of these patients may reflect the varied biological features of parathyroid carcinoma and the approach to recurrence more than the initial surgery (Fig 7–2). Surgery seems to prolong survival and palliate the symptoms of hypercalcemia in patients with recurrent or distant disease.

▶ Claiming that parathyroid carcinoma is overdiagnosed, these authors have a more stringent diagnosis that includes recurrence, metastases, or frank capillary invasion on histologic examination. Some pathologists claim that finding mitoses in the parathyroid gland establishes the diagnosis of carcinoma. Many cases of parathyroid carcinoma diagnosed in this manner would be excluded from this paper. These different definitions of parathyroid carcinoma lead to variations in the evaluation of the incidence of patients with parathyroid carcinoma.—R.J. Howard, M.D., Ph.D.

Papillary Thyroid Microcarcinoma: A Study of 535 Cases Observed in a 50-Year Period
Hay ID, Grant CS, van Heerden JA, Goellner JR, Ebersold JR, Bergstralh EJ (Mayo Clinic and Found, Rochester, Minn)
Surgery 112:1139–1147, 1992   140-94-7–7

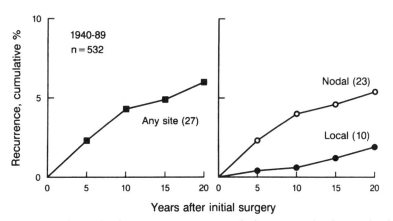

Fig 7-3.—Cumulative risks of tumor recurrence at any site (**left**) or in regional nodes or within thyroid bed (**right**) in PMA of thyroid, based on 532 patients with complete surgical resection (no gross residual tumor) and no distant metastatic lesions on initial examination. *Numbers in parentheses* represent numbers of patients in whom postoperative tumor recurrence occurred. (Courtesy of Hay ID, Grant CS, van Heerden JA, et al: *Surgery* 112:1139-1147, 1992.)

Introduction.—The latest World Health Organization histologic classification has defined papillary microcarcinoma (PMC) as a "papillary carcinoma 1 cm or less in diameter." Data were reviewed on patients who were treated for PMC of the thyroid over 50 years at one institution.

Patients and Methods.—Between 1940 and the end of 1989, a total of 535 patients had thyroid PMC diagnosed and underwent definitive primary surgical therapy of the thyroid at the Mayo Clinic. The mean age at initial diagnosis was 45 years; the mean overall follow-up was 17.5 years. At the conclusion of the study, 400 patients were alive without evidence of thyroid cancer, 2 had died of the disease, and 113 had died of other causes. Disease recurrence and mortality details were obtained from a computerized cancer database.

Results.—In most cases (69%), the initial pathologic diagnosis was made at the time of primary thyroid surgery. Nearly half the diagnoses in the last decade of the study were made by preoperative fine-needle aspiration biopsy, which was introduced in 1980. The median tumor size was 8 mm; 98% of tumors were not locally invasive. Nodal metastases were present in 32% of patients at examination. Bilateral lobe resection was performed in 91% of patients; 10% had radioiodine remnant ablation. The 20-year tumor recurrence rate was 6%, and the death rate from PMC was .4%. Both lethal tumors were DNA aneuploid, and these 2 patients were the only ones in the series who had known distant metastases. Most recurrences were within the first 10 years (Fig 7-3). Node-positive patients and those who had undergone unilateral lobectomy had higher recurrence rates. Total thyroidectomy and radioiodine remnant ablation did not appear to significantly alter recurrence rates.

Conclusion.—Death and locoregional recurrence are both uncommon in patients with PMC. Even the presence of metastases in regional lymph nodes does not signify a life-threatening disease. The recommended treatment for PMC is bilateral lobar resection followed by surveillance of the neck region for up to 5 years. Adjunctive radioiodine ablation is not routinely indicated.

▶ This 50-year review of thyroid PMC (papillary tumors 1 cm or less in diameter) demonstrates that although there was a low incidence of recurrence, essentially nobody dies of PMC and that the life expectancy of these individuals does not differ from that expected in an age-matched population. Significantly, survival was not affected by therapy, although all patients had surgical removal of at least the mass. One might think that with tumors this small they might be incidental findings at operation for another reason. However, only 71 (13%) proved to be incidental findings. Also significant is that over the course of the 50 years of this report, there has been an increasing tendency toward near total thyroidectomy (from 20% to 60% of all patients) for these very small lesions. As reviewed in the 1993 YEAR BOOK OF SURGERY, the extent of thyroid resection for patients with small and large thyroid cancers remains controversial. Surgeons who specialize in endocrine surgery are more likely to perform more extensive resections than are most community surgeons. However, it is difficult to prove that more extensive surgical treatment significantly affects outcome, especially with thyroid PMCs.—R.J. Howard, M.D., Ph.D.

Adrenocortical Carcinoma in Surgically Treated Patients: A Retrospective Study on 156 Cases by the French Association of Endocrine Surgery
Icard P, Chapuis Y, Andreassian B, Bernard A, Proye C (Hôpital Cochin, Paris; Hôpital Beaujon, Paris; Hôpital du Bocage, Dijon, France; et al)
Surgery 112:972–980, 1992   140-94-7–8

Introduction.—Because of the rarity of adrenocortical carcinoma, the prognostic factors, survival rates, and role of adjuvant therapy in patients with this malignant tumor are not well known. Such information regarding a large number of surgically treated adrenocortical carcinomas was collected and reported.

Patients and Methods.—In 1990, members of the French Association of Endocrine Surgery were asked to contribute data on patients with surgically treated adrenocortical carcinomas who were seen since 1978. There were 156 patients at 26 institutions who underwent surgery from January 1978 to March 1991. Ninety-five patients were women and 61 were men. The average age was 47 years. Common symptoms were weight loss, pain, and a palpable abdominal mass. Functional symptoms were found in 52% of patients. Twenty-nine tumors were incidentally discovered. Hormonal studies in 138 patients showed secreting tumors in 62% and nonsecreting tumors in 27%. Nearly half of the patients had locoregional disease or metastases at diagnosis; only 5% had stage I disease. All patients underwent surgery, and complete resection was achieved in 127 cases. The mean tumor weight was 714 g and the mean diameter 12 cm. Mitotane was administered preoperatively in 20 patients and postoperatively in 74 patients.

Results.—Complete follow-up was achieved in all but 3 patients. Five-year actuarial survival rates were 34% overall—42% in the curative group, 53% in the local cancer group, 24% in the regional disease group, and 27% in the reoperative group. Median survival in the palliative group was 6 months. Patients younger than 35 years of age and those with androgen-secreting tumors, precursor-secreting tumors, or nonsecreting tumors had a better prognosis. Only patients with metastases who were treated postoperatively benefitted from mitotane.

Conclusion.—Survival in these patients with adrenocortical carcinoma was influenced by age, extent of disease, radical aspect of the surgical resection, and type of hormonal secretion. Patient sex, tumor size and weight, and tumoral functional status were nonsignificant variables.

An Eleven-Year Experience With Adrenocortical Carcinoma
Pommier RF, Brennan MF (Mem Sloan-Kettering Cancer Ctr, New York)
Surgery 112:963–971, 1992   140-94-7–9

Introduction.—Adrenocortical carcinoma is an aggressive tumor that is rarely encountered in most medical centers. Patients usually arrive with advanced disease, and the prognosis is poor. In a retrospective series of 73 patients, 11 years of experience with this tumor were presented.

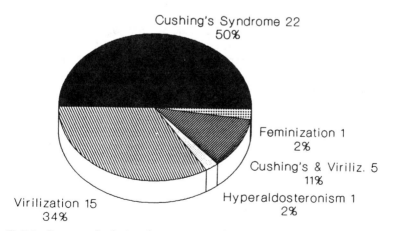

Fig 7–4.—Percentage distribution of 44 patients with functional tumors. (Courtesy of Pommier RF, Brennan MF: *Surgery* 112:963–971, 1992.)

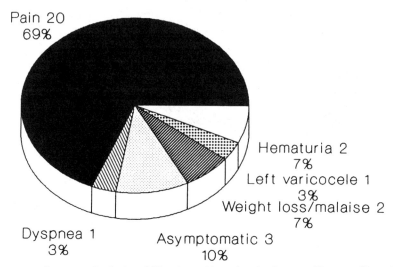

Pain 20
69%

Hematuria 2
7%
Left varicocele 1
3%
Weight loss/malaise 2
7%

Dyspnea 1
3%

Asymptomatic 3
10%

Fig 7-5.—Percentage distribution of 29 patients with nonfunctional tumors. (Courtesy of Pommier RF, Brennan MF: *Surgery* 112:963-971, 1992.)

Patients and Methods.—Follow-up was complete for all patients seen from 1980 through 1991. The study group included 45 women and 28 men. The mean age at diagnosis was 43 years for women and 37 years for men. Signs and symptoms differed according to whether the tumors were functional (Fig 7-4), as in 44 patients, or nonfunctional (Fig 7-5), as in 29 patients. Six patients were judged unresectable at presentation, and 14 were found to be unresectable at exploratory surgery; all 20 of these patients were treated medically. The remaining 53 patients, 4 of whom had distant metastases, underwent complete surgical resections. Ten received postoperative adjuvant therapy, either mitotane (7) or radiation (3).

Results.—Recurrent or metastatic disease developed in 45 of the 53 surgically treated patients, including all 10 who received adjuvant therapy. The mean disease-free interval did not differ significantly for adjuvant vs. no adjuvant therapy groups (2.4 years and 2.5 years, respectively). Recurrent disease in 19 patients was treated with chemotherapy. The mean survival for this group was 19 months. Twenty-six patients with recurrent and metastatic disease underwent 51 reoperations. Their mean survival was 56 months. The overall 5-year survival rate was 35%; patients with complete resection had a 5-year survival rate of 47%.

Conclusion.—Complete resection is the only effective treatment for adrenocortical carcinoma. An aggressive surgical approach is also recommended for recurrent and metastatic disease. No effective chemotherapy is currently available. Mitotane can be quite toxic and without benefit to quality of life or survival.

▶ Abstracts 140-94-7-8 and 140-94-7-9, one a collected experience from France and the other from New York, have similar results. Approximately 40% to 50% of patients have functioning tumors, and the majority of them have advanced disease at presentation. Both papers emphasize an aggressive surgical approach for patients with adrenocortical carcinoma. Currently available chemotherapeutic agents either are not effective or are only partially effective in patients with metastases who received them after operation. An aggressive surgical approach, including reoperation for patients with recurrent disease, appears to be the best approach for these difficult tumors.—R.J. Howard, M.D., Ph.D.

Management of Pheochromocytomas in Patients With Multiple Endocrine Neoplasia Type 2 Syndromes
Lairmore TC, Ball DW, Baylin SB, Wells SA Jr (Washington Univ, St Louis, Mo; Johns Hopkins Univ, Baltimore, Md)
Ann Surg 217:595–603, 1993   140-94-7-10

Introduction.—Pheochromocytomas develop in about 50% of patients with multiple endocrine neoplasia (MEN) type 2A (MEN 2A) and type 2B (MEN 2B). Some clinicians recommend bilateral adrenalectomy in affected patients, even when a pheochromocytoma involves only 1 gland. The optimal surgical management of patients with a pheochromocytoma in a single adrenal gland was investigated.

Patients and Methods.—The records of 58 patients treated between 1956 and 1990 were reviewed. Forty-nine patients had MEN 2A and 9 had MEN 2B. Almost all had clinical signs and symptoms of catecholamine excess (table). Bilateral adrenalectomy was performed when there

Signs and Symptoms of Pheochromocytomas

Signs or Symptoms	MEN 2A or MEN 2B Patients n = 58	Unselected Patients n = 39
Headache	69% (40/58)	72%
Palpitations/tachycardia	62% (36/58)	51%
Hypertension	57% (33/58)	—
Diaphoresis	50% (29/58)	69%
Nausea/vomiting	26% (15/58)	26%
Flushing	21% (12/58)	—
Tremulousness/anxiety	21% (12/58)	26%
Syncope/dizziness	17% (10/58)	3%
None	7% (4/58)	—

(Courtesy of Lairmore TC, Ball DW, Baylin SB, et al: *Ann Surg* 217:595–603, 1993. Modified with permission of Manger WM, Gifford RW Jr: *Pheochromocytoma*. New York, Springer-Verlag, 1977, p 89.)

was radiographic or macroscopic evidence of bilateral pheochromocytoma. Patients underwent a unilateral procedure when there was no evidence of a macroscopic nodule in the contralateral gland. At annual follow-up, recurrence of disease was evaluated by CT scanning and measurement of 24-hour urinary excretion rates of catecholamines and metabolites.

Results.—Thirty-two patients initially underwent bilateral adrenalectomy. Twelve of the 23 patients who had a unilateral procedure subsequently had a pheochromocytoma in the opposite gland. The mean interval from initial operation to recurrence was 11.9 years. During the mean postoperative follow-up of 9.4 years, no patient who underwent unilateral adrenalectomy experienced hypertensive crises or other complications resulting from an undiagnosed pheochromocytoma. Ten patients who had both glands removed, either initially or sequentially, experienced at least 1 episode of acute adrenal insufficiency or addisonian crisis. None of the 102 adrenal glands removed had malignant pheochromocytomas.

Conclusion.—Unilateral adrenalectomy is the treatment of choice for patients with MEN 2A or MEN 2B and pheochromocytoma in a single gland. Recurrence is readily detected, malignant pheochromocytomas are rare, and nearly half the patients will not have a tumor in the opposite adrenal gland for at least 10 years, and some perhaps never will.

▶ This article points out some of the difficulties of surgical decision-making. The authors conclude that patients with MEN 2A or MEN 2B and unilateral pheochromocytoma should only have unilateral adrenalectomy, because in 48% of their patients, pheochromocytomas did not develop during follow-up and because 10 of 43 patients having bilateral adrenalectomy had at least 1 episode of acute adrenal insufficiency and 1 died during a bout of influenza. Other surgeons could look at these same data and come to different conclusions (as, in fact, one did in the discussion). The 11 (48%) patients in whom pheochromocytoma did not develop during follow-up had a mean follow-up of just over 5 years. This follow-up may not have been long enough for a pheochromocytoma to develop. In patients in whom recurrent pheochromocytoma did occur, it did not do so until a mean of just under 12 years. Others might conclude that for younger patients bilateral adrenalectomy is indicated.—R.J. Howard, M.D., Ph.D.

Medullary Carcinoma of the Thyroid: Therapeutic Strategy Derived From Fifteen Years of Experience
Kallinowski F, Buhr HJ, Meybier H, Eberhardt M, Herfarth C (Univ of Heidelberg, Germany)
Surgery 114:491–496, 1993   140-94-7–11

Background.—Medullary thyroid carcinoma (MTC) is locally progressive and metastasizes mainly in the early stages into draining lymph

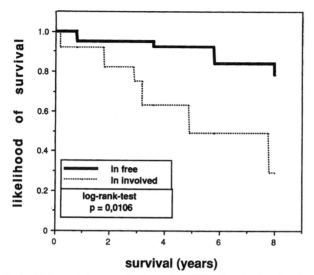

survival (years)

Fig 7–6.—Kaplan-Meier survival curves of patients with MTC with and without lymph node involvement at time of primary operation. (Courtesy of Kallinowski F, Buhr HJ, Meybier H, et al: *Surgery* 114:491-496, 1993.)

nodes. An experience with patients with MTC was reviewed to identify prognostic factors and to develop a stage-related treatment strategy that may improve cure rates.

Methods.—Forty patients were treated for MTC between 1970 and 1985. The mean patient age was 40 years, and the mean length of follow-up was 82 months. Initially, total thyroidectomy was done in 28 patients, subtotal resection in 11, and lobectomy in 1. Initial lymph node dissection consisted of the selective removal of enlarged nodes in most cases. Six patients had unilateral neck dissection. Twenty-six patients had secondary surgery for recurrent disease.

Findings.—At the last follow-up, 10 patients were free of tumor, 12 were scheduled for further therapy, and 6 had persistent but clinically occult disease. Twelve patients had died, with a mean survival of 68 months. The most important prognostic factor was the presence of lymph node involvement at initial surgery (Fig 7-6). All patients with distant disease died within 2 years of receiving their diagnosis. Survival times were increased in women, patients younger than 40 years of age, and patients from familial screening programs.

Conclusion.—Total thyroidectomy and complete dissection of the central lymph node compartment are recommended as primary treatment in patients with MTC. Subsequent treatment by modified radical neck dissection of the lateral compartments is needed in patients with lymph node involvement or increased serum calcitonin concentrations.

▶ Medullary thyroid cancer has a different cell of origin than other forms of thyroid cancer, and its biological behavior differs from that of other thyroid cancers. Most authors recommend total thyroidectomy and central lymph node dissection for patients with MTC. In this series, however, there was no difference in the survival of the patients without positive lymph nodes, regardless of whether subtotal or total thyroidectomy was performed. Lymph node metastasis is the most important predictor of an unfavorable outcome. Because of the high frequency of lymph node metastasis in both symptomatic and asymptomatic patients and because of the poor prognosis for patients with positive lymph nodes, the authors recommend dissection of the central lymph nodes in all patients with MTC.—R.J. Howard, M.D., Ph.D.

Treatment of Toxic Solitary Thyroid Nodules: Surgery Versus Radioactive Iodine
O'Brien T, Gharib H, Suman VJ, van Heerden JA (Mayo Clinic and Found, Rochester, Minn)
Surgery 112:1166–1170, 1992   140-94-7-12

Background.—Continued controversy regarding the correct treatment of toxic solitary thyroid nodules prompted a review of 32 patients with such nodules who were treated between 1970 and 1985.

Patients.—The patients, 24 women and 8 men with a median age of 68 years, all had single toxic nodules and were clinically and/or biochemically hyperthyroid. The median size of the largest nodule diameter was 3.3 cm, and the median radioiodine uptake at 24 hours was 31%. Half the patients were clinically hyperthyroid. Eight of 15 evaluable patients had triiodothyronine toxicosis. The patients were followed for a median of nearly 4 years.

Outcomes.—Nine patients were treated surgically, most often by subtotal unilateral thyroid lobectomy. Two of these patients became hypothyroid within a year after surgery, but there were no surgical complications. None of the surgically treated patients had a recurrent nodule or required retreatment. Twenty-three patients received a median radioiodine dose of 29 mCi. One patient required retreatment, and one had surgery because the nodule persisted. Eight patients (35%) were hypothyroid on follow-up. Nine of 16 patients who were not retreated and who were followed for a year or longer had no evidence of a nodule when last seen.

Conclusion.—Surgical excision is the preferred approach to the solitary toxic thyroid nodule. Radioiodine therapy is a reasonable option when surgery is contraindicated for medical reasons.

▶ The authors favor surgical treatment for toxic solitary thyroid nodules over radioactive iodine therapy because of the rapid restoration of the euthyroid state and the availability of tissue for histologic study. However, patients may favor initial radioactive iodine therapy. Only 1 of 23 patients treated with radioiodine ultimately required operation because of a persistent nodule. The authors do not discuss an alternative strategy of initial treatment with radioactive iodine, reserving surgical therapy for all persistent nodules. This approach would obviate the need for surgery in most patients. The rate of hypothyroidism after radioactive iodine (35%) therapy did not differ significantly from 2 (22%) of 9 patients who became hypothyroid after surgery.—R.J. Howard, M.D., Ph.D.

Normocalcemic Hyperparathyroidism: Biochemical and Symptom Profiles Before and After Surgery
Siperstein AE, Shen W, Chan AK, Duh Q-Y, Clark OH (Univ of California, San Francisco)
Arch Surg 127:1157–1163, 1992   140-94-7-13

Introduction.—Serum calcium has long been the key diagnostic feature and most important predictor of severity of symptoms in patients with primary hyperparathyroidism. In some cases, however, patients are found to be normocalcemic. It is uncertain to what extent patients with normocalcemic hyperparathyroidism benefit from surgery. This question was addressed in a study of surgically treated patients with normocalcemic or minimally hypercalcemic hyperparathyroidism.

Methods.—The patients were divided into 3 study groups: 25 had serum calcium levels below 2.62 mmol/L (normocalcemic), 35 had intermittent hypercalcemia, and 84 had hypercalcemic hyperparathyroidism. Each patient received a questionnaire regarding symptoms and associated conditions before and after parathyroidectomy. All underwent serum chemistry analyses before and after surgery.

Results.—A review of the pathologic reports demonstrated that 104 patients had single adenomas, 27 had hyperplasia, and 11 had multiple adenomas. The 3 groups of patients—normocalcemic, intermediate, and hypercalcemic—were similar in the frequency of their preoperative symptoms and had similar reductions in symptoms postoperatively. Normalization of serum calcium, parathormone, and phosphate levels was also comparable for the 3 groups. Postoperative serum chemistry values showed no statistical differences between normocalcemic, intermediate, and hypercalcemic patients.

Conclusion.—Surgery was effective in reducing symptoms in normocalcemic patients. Findings indicate that factors other than elevated serum calcium levels account for the symptoms of hyperparathyroidism. The cause of normocalcemia despite hyperparathyroidism is complex and multifactorial, and these patients present a diagnostic challenge. Surgery is beneficial, however, both in terms of symptom improvement and correction of metabolic abnormalities.

▶ A small percentage of patients with hyperparathyroidism have elevated parathormone concentrations but are normocalcemic. Patients with normocalcemic hyperparathyroidism have symptoms similar to those of patients with hypercalcemic hyperparathyroidism, and the likelihood of relief with operation is high in both groups. The authors conclude, therefore, that hypercalcemia in and of itself does not cause the symptoms associated with hyperparathyroidism and that surgery should be done in hyperparathyroid patients even if their calcium level is not increased. As one of the authors pointed out in the discussion of the paper by Lundgren (Abstract 140-94-7-5), the likelihood of finding an elevated parathyroid hormone (PTH) level in patients with normocalcemia depends on the assay used. When using a midregion PTH level, 30% to 40% of patients had elevated PTH levels despite having had normocalcemia postoperatively. When they switched to an assay of intact PTH, only 10% of patients had elevated PTH levels. Several different PTH assays were used in this abstracted paper, and we are not told how many were midregion assays and how many were intact assays.—R.J. Howard, M.D., Ph.D.

Hyperparathyroidism in Multiple Endocrine Neoplasia Syndrome

Kraimps JL, Duh Q-Y, Demeure M, Clark OH (Univ of California, San Francisco; Veterans Affairs Med Ctr, San Francisco)
Surgery 112:1080–1088, 1992   140-94-7-14

Background.—Because failed parathyroid operations are more common in patients with primary hyperparathyroidism and multiple endocrine neoplasia (MEN) syndrome, it is important to recognize MEN syndrome in such patients before surgery, so that an appropriate and often more extensive parathyroid operation may be performed. The results of parathyroidectomy in 40 patients with primary hyperparathyroidism and MEN syndrome were analyzed.

Patients and Methods.—Twenty-nine of the 40 patients had initial parathyroidectomy, and 8 of 11 referral patients required reoperation for persistent or recurrent hyperparathyroidism. Subtotal parathyroidectomy was the surgical treatment for patients with hyperplasia.

Results.—Recurrent or persistent hyperparathyroidism developed in 7 of 14 patients with hyperplasia, 3 of 19 with a single adenoma, and in 1 of 7 with double adenomas. Failures in patients with hyperplasia were attributed to missed supernumerary glands in 13% of patients and missed ectopic glands in 33%. Unrecognized hyperplasia contributed to failure in 4 patients with parathyroid tumors (3 patients with solitary tumors and 1 with double tumors). Hypoparathyroidism developed in 1 patient with MEN 2A syndrome and in 3 patients with MEN 1 syndrome.

Conclusion.—There are 2 distinct populations existing among patients who have primary hyperparathyroidism with MEN syndrome and multiple abnormal parathyroid glands. The first population has either single or double adenomas, and these rarely recur. The second population has hyperplasia, and persistence or recurrence of disease is common. Long-term follow-up for these patients is necessary.

▶ Hyperparathyroidism in patients with MEN syndrome seems to differ from hyperparathyroidism in those who do not have this syndrome. The likelihood of recurrence is much greater in the latter patients, especially if they have hyperplasia. They are more likely to have supernumerary glands as well. Some experts recommend that these patients, especially those with MEN 1 syndrome, also have thymectomy and removal of the parathymic fat, because ectopic glands are occasionally found at these sites. Others recommend that patients with MEN syndrome have total parathyroidectomy with autotransplantation because of the likelihood of recurrent hyperparathyroidism.—R.J. Howard, M.D., Ph.D.

Parathyroid Localization Prior to Primary Exploration
Shaha AR, LaRosa CA, Jaffe BM (State Univ of New York, Brooklyn)
Am J Surg 166:289–293, 1993   140-94-7-15

Background.—Controversy exists regarding the use of preoperative parathyroid localization studies before primary exploration. If the preoperative diagnosis of primary hyperparathyroidism is correct, the success of primary surgical exploration exceeds 90% to 95%, precluding the need for preoperative localization. Recent experience suggests that preoperative parathyroid localization studies before primary exploration may be of great value under certain specific conditions.

Patients.—During the past 8 years, 80 parathyroid explorations were performed for primary hyperparathyroidism at 1 institution. In the first 5 years, localization tests included sonography, thallium-technetium scanning, and CT. In the latter 3 years, thallium-technetium scanning was used for specific indications before primary exploration.

Findings.—The enlarged thyroid gland was localized in 24 of 30 patients who underwent thallium-technetium scanning before primary exploration. The specific indications were diagnostic dilemmas, technical problems, and high-risk patient factors. In patients with mild asymptomatic hypercalcemia, preoperative localization confirmed the presence of a parathyroid adenoma and that surgery would be successful. Patient factors included those with high risk because of associated medical problems, including hypertension, congestive heart failure, and other cardiac problems. In those patients, prior localization ensured shorter operative times and less tedious dissections.

Comparison of Various Noninvasive Studies in Parathyroid Localization Before Primary Exploration

	Ultrasound	Thallium-Technetium Scanning	Computed Tomography	Magnetic Resonance Imaging
Sensitivity	55%–88%	59%–96%	68%–95%	57%–82%
Specificity	95%–98%	90%–98%	89%	94%–97%

(Courtesy of Shaha AR, LaRosa CA, Jaffe BM: *Am J Surg* 166:289–293, 1993.)

Discussion. — The use of preoperative parathyroid localization before primary exploration in selected patients helps to achieve the very best results. The 4 currently used noninvasive localization studies—ultrasonography, technetium-thallium subtraction scanning, CT, and MRI, have almost identical success rates (table). Each of these studies has its own advantages and disadvantages, but the technetium-thallium scan is readily available and easy to perform, and it allows easy interpretation as well as localization of ectopic parathyroid glands. The success rates of parathyroid localization using thallium-technetium scanning range from 75% to 80%, with sensitivity and specificity exceeding 90%.

▶ Most experienced parathyroid surgeons are better than localizing studies in identifying the site of abnormal parathyroid glands. However, in certain circumstances, even these experienced parathyroid surgeons may find localizing studies helpful. Most parathyroid surgery in the United States is probably done by surgeons who are not "experts." These are surgeons who do not seek a career as endocrine surgeons and may perform only a small number of parathyroid operations per year. The experts, who tend to be the ones writing the articles, may not need additional studies themselves, but that does not mean that most surgeons performing parathyroid operations would not find preoperative localization studies helpful.—R.J. Howard, M.D., Ph.D.

Parathyroid Localization: Inability to Predict Multiple Gland Involvement
Heller KS, Attie JN, Dubner S (Long Island Jewish Med Ctr, New Hyde Park, NY)
Am J Surg 166:357–359, 1993   140-94-7–16

Background.—About three fourths of solitary parathyroid adenomas can be localized before operation by various imaging techniques. However, because parathyroid exploration without localization is a highly successful procedure, the need for preoperative studies has been questioned. For many patients, the need for bilateral exploration could be avoided if preoperative localization studies were able to distinguish between patients with solitary adenomas and those with multiple gland disease.

Methods.—In a retrospective study, ultrasonography (US), thallium-201/technetium-99m subtraction scintigraphy (TTS), and MRI scans were used to evaluate 16 patients found at surgery to have more than 1 enlarged, hypercellular parathyroid gland. They were drawn from a series of 343 patients who had initial surgery for primary hyperparathyroidism over a 5-year period. Another 4 patients had multiple gland involvement but did not have preoperative localization studies.

Findings.—Magnetic resonance imaging identified 53% of enlarged parathyroid glands compared with just 35% for TTS and 28% for US. Although the addition of MRI or TTS to US improved sensitivity somewhat, the combination still detected only about half the enlarged glands. On their own, none of the 3 techniques was able to predict more than one third of the patients with multiple enlarged glands. In 38% of cases, US did not find any abnormal parathyroid glands, although US plus 1 or both of the other techniques identified at least 1 abnormal gland in 90% of cases.

Conclusion.—None of the imaging techniques investigated can reliably predict multiple parathyroid gland involvement before operation. Although preoperative localization is still justified for quick identification of a solitary adenoma, bilateral surgical exploration is needed for all patients with primary hyperparathyroidism.

▶ Preoperative localization studies are even less successful in patients with multiple gland enlargement than they are in patients with single gland enlargement. This paper demonstrates that justifying preoperative localization studies because they might identify multiple gland enlargement or exclude patients with multiple gland enlargement and avoid the necessity for bilateral neck exploration is not warranted.—R.J. Howard, M.D., Ph.D.

8 Nutrition and Metabolism

Introduction

Twenty-five years have gone by since the use of total parenteral nutrition (TPN) was first introduced into the clinical setting. I consider it to be one of the most important contributions to medicine in the past 50 years. After the initial overenthusiasm, which lasted about 10 years, surgeons began to realize that TPN was associated with specific complications and should only be used in certain patients. In addition, numerous other questions about nutrition and metabolism have been raised. Do current TPN solutions contain appropriate nutrients? Can nutrition modulate organ function in surgical patients? Can the efficacy of nutritional therapy be enhanced by simultaneously providing anabolic agents? How is metabolism controlled in surgical patients sustaining major injury and sepsis?

It is becoming increasingly apparent that nutrition can modulate organ function in hospitalized patients. As a consequence, investigations in this area continue to permeate the literature. In particular, the role of dietary supplements such as omega-3 fatty acids, nucleotides and nucleosides, selected amino acids, and vitamins and minerals continue to be studied in both infants and in adults. Specific sections in this review are devoted to 2 of these nutrients: glutamine and arginine. Newer studies suggest that combinations of nutritional and pharmacologic therapies will play a role in the therapy of critically ill surgical patients. Human growth hormone, which can now be synthesized in large quantities, continues to be the anabolic agent with the most promise.

In recent years, a wealth of information has accumulated concerning the role of cytokines in regulating the body's response to injury, infection, and progressive malignant disease. New knowledge delineating how these key polypeptide molecules control the catabolic response to "stress states" has been generated at a staggering pace. It has become increasingly clear that cytokines work together with classic stress hormones and with other humoral mediators to orchestrate and coordinate the cellular response to critical illnesses. The central role occupied by these polypeptide signals has challenged past teachings and forced us to rethink traditional approaches to treating the host with severe injury and infection. In addition, we are discovering ways of modulating the production of these cytokines using dietary manipulations. The mediators clearly work in conjunction with numerous others, including the glucocorticoids and prostaglandins, to coordinate the stress response. Knowledge of and interest in cytokine biology has led to productive collaborations between clinicians, basic scientists, and industry. Preclinical trials in animals have pointed to both beneficial and detrimental effects of using selective cytokine antagonists to treat experimental sepsis. Moreover, the results appear to be, in part, model-dependent. New studies identifying the function of the CD14 receptor for the LPS/LPS binding protein complex are exciting. Clinical trials designed to determine whether there is a role for cytokine blockade (using monoclonal antibodies and/or receptor antagonists) in critically ill patients are in progress; other studies in patients with cancer are evaluating the potential use of certain cytokines as chemotherapeutic agents. These compounds are expensive and can be associated with significant toxicities. Therefore, it becomes prudent to identify—through carefully designed randomized, prospective trials—specific groups of patients who will benefit from such therapies. Benefits should be measured in terms of a reduction in major complications and improved survival. Other investigations have focused on how cytokine production can be modified; research indicates that the patient's nutritional status and nutrient intake can alter cytokine production.

It is recommended that practicing surgeons become knowledgeable regarding these new treatment options, because it is anticipated that these therapies will become an integral part of the care of critically ill surgical patients in the next several years.

Wiley W. Souba, M.D., Sc.D.

Nutrition and Organ Function

Long-Term Dietary Fish Oil Supplementation Protects Against Ischemia-Reperfusion-Induced Myocardial Dysfunction in Isolated Rat Hearts

Yang BC, Saldeen TGP, Bryant JL, Nichols WW, Mehta JL (Univ of Florida, Gainesville; Univ of Uppsala, Sweden)
Am Heart J 126:1287–1292, 1993   140-94-8-1

Introduction.—Numerous experimental studies have documented the beneficial effects of fish oil on cardiac mortality that were observed in populations consuming large amounts of marine life. Although dietary fish oil has been shown to exert protective effects against arrhythmias and myocardial infarctions after coronary artery occlusion, its effects on ischemia-reperfusion–induced cardiac dysfunction are not known. These effects were examined in rat hearts subjected to global ischemia and reperfusion.

Methods.—Fifteen male Sprague-Dawley rats were fed pellets enriched with fish oil, and 11 received ordinary chow for the 4- to 5-week study period. Three fish oil–fed rats were also fed indomethacin ad libitum for the last 2 days. Isolated hearts from both groups were perfused on a Langendorff apparatus and subjected to 25 minutes of global ischemia and 20 minutes of reperfusion. Measurements of myocardial phospholipid acid content were also obtained.

Results.—At the end of the study, the fish oil–fed rats and control rats were similar in appearance and body weight. In the fish oil–fed group, the myocardial content of long-chain polyunsaturated fatty acid (PUFA) (C20-22) and omega-3 PUFA was increased and that of omega-6 PUFA was decreased. Reduction in the force of cardiac contraction and an increase in cardiac perfusion pressure were noted in both groups after global ischemia and reoxygenation. The reduction in the force of cardiac contraction was less in the hearts of fish oil–fed rats (49%) than in control hearts (63%). Hearts of fish oil–fed rats also had less of an increase in coronary perfusion pressure than control hearts (24% vs. 37%). The cardioprotective effects of fish oil during ischemia and reperfusion were abolished by the administration of indomethacin.

Conclusion.—Four to 5 weeks of fish oil supplementation in rats resulted in a significant change in myocardial phospholipid fatty acid content. The cardioprotective effect of fish oil was modest and was abolished by administration of indomethacin during the last 2 days of the fish oil–rich diet. An indomethacin-sensitive mechanism, probably synthesis of prostacyclin, may be the major contributor to reduced myocardial dysfunction in isolated hearts.

▶ Clinical interest in the interaction between nutrition and organ function has recently been rekindled. More than ever, medical practice must incorporate nutritional considerations, as it is quite clear that nutrition can impact organ function. In this study by Yang and colleagues, dietary fish oil supplementation protected against myocardial dysfunction after ischemia and reperfusion. This may be the result of the ability of these fatty acids to modulate vascular tone, because it has been shown that fish oil can regulate the production of nitric oxide and superoxide anions. The beneficial effects observed by Yang and associates were abolished when a cyclo-oxygenase inhibitor (indomethacin) was administered, indicating an important role for prostaglandins in preserving myocardial function after ischemia. These kinds of studies may lead to specific preoperative nutritional interventions in patients undergoing myocardial revascularization.—W.W. Souba, M.D., Sc.D.

Pretreatment With Glucose Infusion Prevents Fatal Outcome After Hemorrhage in Food Deprived Rats

Alibegovic A, Ljungqvist O (Karolinska Hosp, Stockholm)
Circ Shock 39:1–6, 1993   140-94-8-2

Background.—Patients with poor nutritional status at the time of surgery have an increased incidence of postoperative complications. However, even a 24-hour period of fasting can result in major alterations in body metabolism. The usual period of fasting required before surgery, 16–20 hours, is reported to reduce the hepatic glycogen content in man by 55% to 85%. Such a reduction increased mortality in experimental hemorrhage. Whether the reduced capacity of fluid defense in the fasted animal could be improved by pretreatment with glucose before hemorrhagic stress was determined.

Methods.—Experiments were performed using adult male Sprague-Dawley rats. For 24 hours before the start of the experiments, food was removed but free access to water was allowed. Before 60 minutes of standardized hemorrhage, 20 food-deprived animals were given a 3-hour infusion of either 30% glucose given intravenously or the same volume of .9% NaCl administered at a rate of .3 mL per 100 g of body weight per hour. The animals were closely observed for recovery or death for 7 days. In another 10 rats, 5 in each group, the identical infusion and hemorrhage were performed. The abdomen was opened in these animals, and the liver was examined for liver glycogen content.

Results.—Infusion of glucose resulted in transient hyperglycemia and significantly greater (600%) hepatic glycogen content compared with saline. The glucose-treated rats had substantial hyperglycemia during hemorrhage, whereas glucose levels fell in the saline-treated group. Improved plasma refill was observed in the glucose group. The saline-treated rats had irreversible shock and died within 3 hours of bleeding; in contrast, all glucose-treated rats recovered and survived the 7-day observation period.

Conclusion.—Simple pretreatment with glucose led to hepatic glycogen recovery and was able to prevent death after severe blood loss in the food-deprived rat. Because elective surgery is generally performed after an overnight fast, the findings of this experimental study suggest that glucose infusion during preoperative fasting could improve hepatic glycogen content and enhance the safety of patients.

▶ In this series of rat experiments, Alibegovic and Ljungqvist demonstrated that 24-hour deprivation of food before experimental hemorrhage increased mortality. The investigators showed that administration of glucose to maintain hepatic glycogen reserves is beneficial because it helps support the necessary hyperglycemic response that is essential after severe hemorrhage. The beneficial effects of hyperglycemia are not solely the result of its role as an energy source but, also, its osmotic fluid mobilizing effect. Hyperglycemia and hyperosmolarity have been shown to be associated with improved cardiac function, decreased peripheral vascular resistance, and improved peripheral circulation. The investigators suggest that a preoperative infusion of glucose may be beneficial to patients who have fasted for 6–24 hours before elective surgery.—W.W. Souba, M.D., Sc.D.

Elemental Diet-Induced Bacterial Translocation Can Be Hormonally Modulated

Haskel Y, Xu D, Lu Q, Deitch E (Louisiana State Univ, Shreveport)
Ann Surg 217:634–643, 1993   140-94-8-3

Background.—Previous studies have shown that feeding an elemental diet to mice results in bacterial translocation (BT) that could be prevented by providing dietary fiber. Whether the protective effect of fiber was associated with the stimulation of trophic gut hormones was investigated.

Methods.—The effects of sandostatin and bombesin were assessed in mice given chow or the elemental diet. The ability of bombesin, 10 μg/kg 3 times a day, or sandostatin, 100 μg/kg twice a day, to modulate BT was examined. The mice were killed after 14 days for analysis.

Findings.—The incidence of elemental diet-induced BT was 75%, and it was reduced 9% by fiber and 13% by administration of bombesin (table). Sandostatin did not promote BT in chow-fed mice, but it reversed the protective effect of fiber on BT.

Conclusion.—These findings indicate that elemental diet-induced BT can be hormonally modulated. The beneficial effects of fiber on diet-induced BT also appear to be mediated by hormones.

▶ It has been suggested that the type of enteral diet provided to patients can influence the integrity of the intestinal mucosal barrier. For example, provision of elemental diets to animals can promote BT, and this can be prevented by providing fiber. Hasket et al. showed that the beneficial effects of fiber on BT are hormonally mediated. Administration of the gastrointestinal hormone bombesin prevented diet-induced BT, but it did not prevent bacterial overgrowth in the cecum. Although the mechanisms by which this hormone and others like it may protect the gut mucosal barrier are unclear, it does appear that hormonal modulation of gut permeability is possible. Given the substantial amount of work on growth factors and their ability to enhance cellular proliferation, it is likely that these agents may be used clinically in the future to modulate the nutritional effects on organ function.—W.W. Souba, M.D., Sc.D.

Effect of Bombesin and Sandostatin on Bacterial Translocation in Elemental Diet-Fed Mice

| Group | n | Incidence of BT | | | Magnitude of BT |
		MLN%	Spleen%	Liver%	MLN (CFU g/MLN)
Chow	17	12	0	0	8 ± 6
Elemental diet (ED)	12	75*	8	8	140 ± 43†
ED + fiber	11	9	0	0	27 ± 27
ED + bombesin	16	13	13	13	14 ± 10
ED + sandostatin	12	75*	25	0	153 ± 37†

Note: Data are expressed as mean + standard error of mean.
* $P < .01$ vs. control, ED + fiber and ED + bombesin.
† $P < .05$ vs. control, ED + fiber and ED + bombesin.
(Courtesy of Haskel Y, Xu D, Lu Q, et al: Ann Surg 217:634–643, 1993.)

Early Enteral Feeding Does Not Attenuate Metabolic Response After Blunt Trauma

Eyer SD, Micon LT, Konstantinides FN, Edlund DA, Rooney KA, Luxenberg MG, Cerra FB (Univ of Minnesota, Minneapolis; Methodist Hosp, Indianapolis, Ind; St Paul-Ramsey Med Ctr, St Paul, Minn; et al)
J Trauma 34:639–644, 1993   140-94-8-4

Introduction.—Nutritional support for patients who have critical injuries is typically delayed for at least 24 hours. Enteral feeding soon after trauma, however, may attenuate the stress response and improve patient outcome. This hypothesis was tested in a prospective, randomized clinical trial.

Methods.—Fifty-two patients with blunt trauma who were admitted to a trauma intensive care unit (ICU) entered the study. All had an Injury Severity Score (ISS) of greater than 13 and were likely to require feeding support for at least 7 days. Patients were randomized to receive early enteral feeding (beginning less than 24 hours after ICU admission) or late enteral feeding (beginning more than 72 hours after ICU admission). Feeding was given via nasoduodenal feeding tubes. The primary outcome variable was the degree of metabolic response, as evaluated by urinary excretion of catecholamines and cortisol on study days 5 and 10.

Results.—Fourteen patients, 7 from each feeding group, did not complete the study. The early and late feeding groups were similar in mean age, mean ISS, and male-to-female ratio. The early feeding group had more severe acute lung injuries. The mean time from hospital admission to feeding was 38 hours for the early group and 88 hours for the late group. The target amount of daily nutrient intake was given on 60% of feeding days. Overall, patients in both the early and late feeding groups received 83% of the target amount for the entire study. For the overall study period, the early feeding group received more protein and kilocalories than the late group. Primary outcome variables, as measured by plasma levels of lactate and urinary total nitrogen, catecholamines, and cortisol, did not differ significantly for the 2 groups, nor did individual types of infection. The total number of acquired infections, however, was greater in the early feeding group.

Conclusion.—Early and late enteral feeding groups had similar rates of organ system failure and mortality. The number of ventilator days and ICU days did not differ significantly between groups. Thus, the timing of enteral feeding does not appear to alter the metabolic response to injury or clinical outcome in blunt trauma.

▶ Although it is generally accepted that enteral nutrition is the preferable route of feeding patients and that enteral nutrition is superior to total parenteral nutrition, Eyer and colleagues show that early enteral nutrition (within 24 hours of injury) is not superior to delayed feedings (72 hours). The authors provide data that indicate that early enteral feeding neither attenuated the stress response nor altered patient outcome. These observations are in contrast to those reported by Alexander and by Kudsk, albeit the study design was not comparable. The observations, however, should not detract from my basic recommendation, which is that enteral feeding is superior to parenteral nutrition and that the institution of enteral nutrition in high-risk patients should commence when they have been stabilized hemodynamically. This assumes, of course, that the patient has a usable gastrointestinal tract and that a contraindication to luminal feeding is not present.—W.W. Souba, M.D., Sc.D.

Total Parenteral Nutrition

Role of Parenteral Nutrition in Preventing Malnutrition and Decreasing Bacterial Translocation to Liver in Obstructive Jaundice
Chuang J-H, Shieh C-S, Chang N-K, Chen W-J, Lin J-N (Chang Gung Mem Hosp, Kaohsiung, Taiwan, Republic of China; Chang Gung Mem Hosp, Taipei, Taiwan, Republic of China)
World J Surg 17:580–586, 1993   140-94-8–5

Background.—Patients with obstructive jaundice who require surgery are at risk for significant infectious complications, probably secondary to both impaired immune function and malnutrition. Total parenteral nutrition (TPN) can relieve malnutrition, but at the same time, it may promote bacterial translocation (BT) from the bowel.

Objective and Methods.—Studies were done in dogs undergoing ligation of the common bile duct to learn whether it is possible to prevent malnutrition using TPN without promoting BT. The liver and mesenteric lymph nodes were sampled for quantitative bacterial culture and histologic assessment before and 2 weeks after the interventions.

Results.—Bacterial translocation to the mesenteric nodes was observed in 40% of dogs having common bile duct ligation, whether they were fed conventionally or given TPN. No such translocation was found in control animals, regardless of the method of feeding. Bacterial translocation to the liver was noted in 70% of orally fed animals having common bile duct ligation, significantly more than in any of the other groups (table). These animals lost body weight and had prealbumin values that were consistent with malnutrition. Ligated animals maintained with TPN had a significant increase in alkaline phosphatase levels and histologic findings of cholestasis.

Conclusion.—These findings suggest that TPN can prevent malnutrition and limit BT to the liver in the setting of obstructive jaundice. There is, however, a risk of precipitating cholestasis, which may be prevented by using TPN only in the short term or by performing a drainage procedure.

▶ This study builds on previous investigations that examined the role of malnutrition in endotoxin- or inflammation-induced BT to the liver, bloodstream,

Quantitative Tissue Culture Data

Group	No.	Mesenteric lymph nodes Positive BT *	CFU/g †	Liver Positive BT	CFU/g
I (PO-control)	10	0/10	35 ± 24	0/10	43 ± 24
II (PO-CBDL)	10	4/10*	$4.7 \pm 14.5 \times 10^3$	7/10**	$1.5 \pm 3.2 \times 10^4$
III (TPN-control)	10	0/10	40 ± 27	2/10	69 ± 54
IV (TPN-CBDL)	10	4/10*	$6.7 \pm 19.6 \times 10^3$	2/10	$5.1 \pm 14.1 \times 10^2$

* Positive BT represented a bacterial count of more than 100 CFU/g contained in the respective tissue. All bacteriologic data are expressed as means $\pm$ 1 SD colony-forming units per gram of tissue (CFU/g).

† $P < .05$ vs. group I and III.

** $P < .05$ vs. all other groups.

(Courtesy of Chuang J-H, Shieh C-S, Chang N-K, et al: *World J Surg* 17:580–586, 1993.)

and distant organs. Chuang and associates have demonstrated that malnutrition superimposed on obstructive jaundice will predispose the canine liver to grow a significantly larger number of translocating bacteria. Obstructive jaundice is known to diminish hepatic phagocytosis and impair bacterial clearance, and malnutrition alone may impair intracellular bacterial killing. Previous studies in rodents have documented that obstructive jaundice alone or TPN alone can promote BT from the gut to the mesenteric lymph nodes. In Chuang's study, the discrepancy between the higher rate of translocation to the liver in orally fed dogs with obstructive jaundice (70%) compared to TPN-fed jaundiced animals (20%) is difficult to explain. Despite reduced rates of translocation, those animals in the TPN-obstructed group had a higher degree of cholestasis and a higher alkaline phosphatase level. The authors suggest that TPN may have been responsible for improvements in serum albumin and body weight that resulted in less translocation.—W.W. Souba, M.D., Sc.D.

Effect of Total Parenteral Nutrition Plus Morphine on Bacterial Translocation in Rats
Kueppers PM, Miller TA, Chen C-YK, Smith GS, Rodriguez LF, Moody FG (Univ of Texas, Houston)
Ann Surg 217:286–292, 1993   140-94-8-6

Background.—Both total parenteral nutrition (TPN) and morphine sulfate (MS) are frequently used adjuncts in caring for critically ill patients. Total parenteral nutrition has been shown to produce varying degrees of bacterial translocation (BT), and MS leads to bowel stasis and consequent bacterial overgrowth.

Objective and Methods.—Studies were performed in rats to determine whether the gut stasis produced by parenteral MS leads to increased BT in the setting of TPN. Intestinal transit was estimated from the caudal

Bacterial Translocation to Mesenteric Lymph Nodes

Treatment	Incidence	MLN with >100 CFU	CFU/MLN Mean ± SEM
Control	2/14	0/14	13 ± 9
TPN alone	8/16	1/16	33 ± 14
TPN + MS	15/15*†	15/15*†	2079 ± 811*†
TPN/Gln + MS	6/6*	6/6*†	1009 ± 404

Abbreviations: CFU, colony-forming units; Gln, glutamine.
Note: Numerator in each ratio represents the number of animals in which translocation occurred out of the entire group (denominator).
* P < .05 vs. control.
† P < .05 vs. TPN alone.
(Courtesy of Kueppers PM, Miller TA, Chen C-YK, et al: *Ann Surg* 217:286–292, 1993.)

movement of a fluorescent marker instilled in the proximal duodenum. Quantitative bacterial studies were performed on samples from the various bowel segments as well as the ileocecal mesenteric lymph nodes, spleen, liver, and blood taken by cardiac puncture. The animals were sacrificed after 4 days.

Findings.—By itself, TPN did not alter bowel transit, but transit was prolonged when MS was added to TPN. Morphine sulfate also enhanced bacterial overgrowth and increased BT to the mesenteric nodes (table). Colony-forming units per lymph node increased markedly in animals given both TPN and MS. More than 90% of those animals had bacteria at systemic sites, but this was not observed with TPN alone. The presence of glutamine in TPN fluid did not prevent the effects of combined TPN and MS on BT.

Conclusion.—Bowel stasis caused by chronic MS administration promotes bacterial proliferation in the gut and the translocation of bacteria to mesenteric lymph nodes. Bacteria also migrate to distant organs and enter the systemic circulation.

▶ This study suggests a role for narcotics in promoting BT from the gut when given in conjunction with TPN. Morphine is well known to diminish small intestinal transit, and the authors showed that it also increased the number of viable bacteria in the gut lumen, in particular in the cecum. Simultaneously, the rate of BT to the mesenteric lymph nodes, liver, bloodstream, spleen, and lungs was increased. It was not reported whether morphine alone enhanced translocation, but in conjunction with TPN, the rate of translocation was significantly higher than with TPN alone. Glutamine supplementation of TPN, which has been shown to diminish translocation in other models, was ineffective in reversing the authors' observations.

It would be interesting to study other narcotics to determine whether they have similar effects on translocation. In addition, studies using some of the newer nonsteroidal injectable analgesics, which have been shown to stimulate gut motility, in conjunction with morphine would be important. It is unclear whether the combination of TPN and narcotics plays a role in mediating the presumed intestinal permeability defect that is thought to occur in some critically ill patients, but this rodent study indicates that additional human trials are in order.—W.W. Souba, M.D., Sc.D.

Lateral Hypothalamic Dopaminergic Neural Activity in Response to Total Parenteral Nutrition
Meguid MM, Yang Z-J, Montante A (State Univ of New York, Syracuse)
Surgery 114:400–406, 1993   140-94-8-7

Background.—Clinical observations that total parenteral nutrition (TPN) suppresses food intake prompted a study in rats, which confirmed that TPN lowers food intake in proportion to the amount of cal-

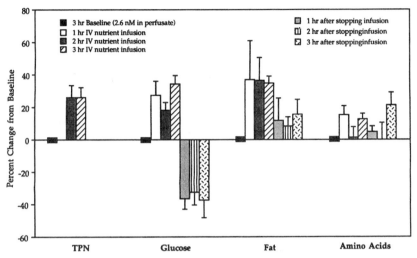

Fig 8–1.—Changes in extracellular dopamine concentration in the lateral hypothalamic area (LHA) during and after stopping different nutrient infusions. The mean of the 3-hour baseline dopamine concentration was 2.6 mmol/L, which represents a 10% extracellular LHA dopamine recovery and is expressed as the baseline. Infusion of TPN-100 raised the dopamine levels above baseline. Infusion of a single macronutrient solution providing 75% of a rat's daily caloric intake raised dopamine levels. Stopping each infusion resulted in either a below-baseline level, a decrease from maximum level, or an unchanged level for the 3-hour measurement period. (Courtesy of Meguid MM Yang Z-J, Montante A: *Surgery* 114:400–406, 1993.)

ories infused. Because the dopaminergic neurons of the lateral hypothalamus modulate food intake, changes in dopamine release from this site were monitored in conjunction with TPN in rats.

Methods.—An intracerebral guide cannula and internal jugular vein catheter were placed and, after 10 days, the rats were fasted and had a 2-mm microdialysis probe placed in the lateral hypothalamus. Dopamine levels were measured by high-performance liquid chromatography before and after 24 hours of infusion of TPN solution, glucose, fat, or amino acid.

Results.—Levels of dopamine in dialysis samples increased significantly during all the nutrient infusions. The increase was most marked with fat infusion, and it was least marked when amino acids were infused (Fig 8–1). The dopamine level decreased to more than one third below baseline after cessation of the infusion of glucose, but it did not change when the fat and amino acid infusions were terminated.

Interpretation.—Infusion of TPN solution or its components has the effect of increasing dopamine levels in the lateral hypothalamus. This may help explain suppressed food intake after the cessation of TPN.

▶ This interesting study by Meguid and colleagues provides insight into the mechanism by which the infusion of hypertonic nutrient solutions suppresses appetite. The authors showed that brain dopaminergic activity, the activity in that portion of the brain that controls appetite, is increased during TPN. This increased activity results in a decrease in the voluntary intake of food, which persists temporarily after stopping the infusion. Although part of this response may be secondary to elevations of nutrient blood concentrations sensed in the brain, more recent studies by this group (unpublished data) also indicate that parenteral nutrition is also sensed in the hepatoportal area, informing the hypothalamus via hepatic afferent nerves to diminish appetite.—W.W. Souba, M.D., Sc.D.

Role of Nucleosides and Nucleotide Mixture in Intestinal Mucosal Growth Under Total Parenteral Nutrition
Tsujinaka T, Iijima S, Kido Y, Homma T, Ebisui C, Kan K, Imamura I, Fukui H, Mori T (Osaka Univ, Japan)
Nutrition 9:532–535, 1993   140-94-8–8

Background.—The intestinal mucosal atrophy associated with total parenteral nutrition (TPN) may be partly a result of deficient intraluminal nutrients and a lack of those nutrients needed for mucosal metabolism. Patients receiving TPN have no dietary source of purines and pyrimidines, and the pool of nucleotides and nucleosides in the intestinal mucosa may be reduced.

Objective and Methods.—The preventive value of a mixture of nucleosides and a nucleotide (OG-VI) was determined in rats given a standard TPN diet for 6 days. The diet provided 250 kcal and 1.78 g of nitrogen per kilogram daily. Study animals also received 2.5 mL/kg of OG-VI daily. A control group was maintained on oral rat chow for the same period.

Results.—Among animals maintained on TPN, jejunal and ileal mucosal weights were significantly greater in those given OG-VI (table). In addition, diamine oxidase activity at both sites was significantly higher when TPN was accompanied by the OG-VI mixture, and a significantly greater bromodeoxyuridine labeling index also was noted.

Conclusion.—To sustain the function of the small intestinal mucosa during TPN, it may be necessary to provide a source of purines and pyrimidines. These nutrients stimulate the proliferation of crypt cells, thereby enhancing the maturity and integrity of the mucosa.

▶ It has been suggested that standard TPN solutions provided to hospitalized patients lack certain key nutrients. In this study, Tsujinaka and associates examined the effects of supplemental nucleotides and nucleosides, which are precursors for DNA biosynthesis, on intestinal mucosal growth in a rat TPN model. The authors reported that addition of OG-VI to TPN stimulated crypt cell proliferation and mucosal growth. Similar clinical trials have yet to be done, but this study suggests that currently used TPN solutions may

Effect of Mixture of OG-VI on Intestinal Mucosal Atrophy Associated With TPN

	TPN + OG-VI Group	TPN Group	Normal Fed Condition
Total wet weight (mg/cm)			
Jejunum	34.3 ± 2.2	33.1 ± 2.7	53.4 ± 8.6
Ileum	31.9 ± 3.8	31.2 ± 3.5	49.9 ± 7.6
Mucosal wet weight (mg/cm)			
Jejunum	22.8 ± 1.8*	20.5 ± 2.0	37.3 ± 8.2
Ileum	19.4 ± 2.2*	16.8 ± 2.3	33.1 ± 8.3
Extractable mucosal protein (mg/cm)			
Jejunum	22.4 ± 2.8*	19.3 ± 2.6	20.3 ± 2.0
Ileum	18.6 ± 4.3	17.2 ± 4.6	17.7 ± 2.3

Note: Values are means ± 1 SD. Extractable mucosal protein was determined in supernatant obtained after centrifugation of mucosal homogenate at 15,000 rpm for 15 minutes at 4°C.
* $P < .05$ vs. TPN group.
(Courtesy of Tsujinaka T, Iijima S, Kido Y, et al: *Nutrition* 9:532–535, 1993.)

lack certain key nutrients that can influence organ function.—W.W. Souba, M.D., Sc.D.

Total Parenteral Nutrition-Associated Cholestasis: Clinical and Histo-pathologic Correlation
Moss RL, Das JB, Raffensperger JG (Children's Mem Hosp, Chicago)
J Pediatr Surg 28:1270–1275, 1993   140-94-8-9

Introduction.—The pathogenesis of cholestatic jaundice, the major complication of total parenteral nutrition (TPN) in infants, is unknown. Although the syndrome has often been defined in terms of serum bilirubin and transaminase levels, these markers do not correlate well with histologic injury to the liver. Histologic changes in the liver were defined in relation to the clinical course of infants receiving TPN, and the effect of enteral feeding on these changes was determined.

Patients and Methods.—Thirty-one infants who underwent surgery for severe gastrointestinal disease or who had biochemical evidence of jaundice were retrospectively identified from records of the study institution during the years 1987–1991. Excluded were infants with defined causes of cholestasis. Necrotizing enterocolitis was the clinical diagnosis in 24 infants. Twenty-one infants were premature and 25 were receiving TPN. At the time of biopsy, 28 of 31 had received some enteral feeding. Results of liver biopsies were available in 23 cases and autopsy specimens in 13.

Results.—There was histologic evidence of cholestasis in 71% of premature infants and 22% of those who were full-term. The infants with cholestasis had received TPN longer (37 days vs. 18 days) and had a shorter period of enteral feeding (17 days vs. 27 days) than infants without cholestasis. Bilirubin levels were elevated in infants with cholestasis, but this marker did not correlate with the extent of histologic damage to the liver. Biliary stasis, the earliest histologic sign of cholestasis, could be seen as early as 5 days after beginning TPN. This change was followed by portal inflammation, bile duct proliferation, and portal fibrosis. Five premature infants who underwent surgery for necrotizing enterocolitis had 2 subsequent biopsies. Despite partial enteral feeding supplemented with TPN, all had progressive liver disease.

Conclusion.—Cholestasis associated with TPN remains a major clinical problem in neonates with diseases of the gastrointestinal tract who require prolonged TPN. Diagnosis of the syndrome must be histologic, because biochemical indices of liver function do not necessarily correlate with liver damage. The TPN solution appears to be directly toxic to the liver, and liver damage is not halted or reversed by partial enteral feeding.

Small Intestinal Mucosa Changes, Including Epithelial Cell Proliferative Activity, of Children Receiving Total Parenteral Nutrition (TPN)
Rossi TM, Lee PC, Young C, Tjota A (Children's Hosp of Buffalo, NY; Med College of Wisconsin, Milwaukee)
Dig Dis Sci 38:1608–1613, 1993   140-94-8-10

Background.—A number of animal studies have indicated a relationship between total parenteral nutrition (TPN) and atrophy of the gut mucosa. A reduction in villus height has been ascribed to the lack of oral nutrient intake. The effect appears to be most marked in the proximal small bowel.

Patients.—Biopsy specimens were taken from the small intestine of 7 children aged 9 months to 5 years who were receiving TPN. Three of the children had inflammatory bowel disease and were maintained with TPN for 1 month. The other 4, who had short-bowel syndrome, required TPN for longer than 9 months. Twenty-two age-matched children with abdominal pain or chronic diarrhea were also studied.

Methods.—Biopsy specimens were maintained in organ culture for the estimation of disaccharidase activities. In addition, DNA was extracted after serial precipitation with perchloric acid, and the incorporation of tritiated thymidine was determined.

Results.—Short-term TPN was associated with slightly reduced activities of lactase, sucrase, and palatinase, but the differences from control values were not significant. Samples from 2 patients receiving long-term TPN exhibited mild focal villus atrophy and reduced disaccharidase activity. The DNA from patients receiving long-term TPN incorporated less thymidine than that from controls, whether on a per-biopsy or per-milligram-of-tissue basis (table).

Conclusion.—As in animals, TPN in children is associated with hypoplastic effects on the small bowel mucosa, but a considerable period of TPN is required for these changes to become evident.

Mucosal Epithelial Cell Proliferative Activity From Small Intestinal Biopsy Specimens of Different Patient Groups

Treatment	Patients (N)	Mucosal weight (mg)	Thymidine incorporation (fmoles)	
			Total	Per milligram tissue
Control (no TPN)	22	4.1 ± 0.5	8.4 ± 1.1	2.7 ± 0.7
IBD (TPN = 1 month)	3	3.1 ± 0.9	5.8 ± 1.7*	2.6 ± 1.1*
SBS (TPN >9 months)	4	3.9 ± 1.6	3.6 ± 1.1*	1.0 ± 0.1*

Note: Values are means ± SEM.
* Significantly different from control group by Student's *t* test (P < .001).
(Courtesy of Rossi TM, Lee PC, Young C, et al: Dig Dis Sci 38:1608–1613, 1993.)

Effect of Total Parenteral Nutrition on Amino Acid and Glucose Transport by the Human Small Intestine
Inoue Y, Espat NJ, Frohnapple DJ, Epstein H, Copeland EM, Souba WW
(Univ of Florida, Gainesville; VA Hosp, Gainesville, Fla)
Ann Surg 217:604–614, 1993   140-94-8-11

Background.—Research indicates that patients given total parenteral nutrition (TPN) have decreased disaccharidase enzyme activity. However, morphologic changes are minimal, with only slight reductions in villous height occurring. The effect of TPN on small intestinal amino acid and glucose transport activity was determined.

Methods.—By random assignment, 6 patients received TPN and 7 received a regular oral diet for 1 week before abdominal surgery. Ileum and jejunum were obtained during surgery. Brush-border membrane vesicles (BBMV) were prepared by means of magnesium aggregation/differential centrifugation. Using a rapid mixing/filtration method, transport of L-MeAIB, a selective system A substrate; L-glutamine; L-alanine; L-arginine; L-leucine; and D-glucose was assayed with and without sodium.

Findings.—Vesicles had approximately 18-fold enrichments of enzyme markers, classic overshoots, transport into an osmotically active space, and similar 1-hour equilibrium values. Total parenteral nutrition reduced the carrier-mediated transport velocity of all substrates but glutamine across ileal BBMVs by 26%–44%. A generalized reduction in nutrient transport was also observed in the jejunum of 1 patient receiving TPN, although glutamine was least affected. Kinetic assessment of the system A transporter showed that the uptake reduction was caused by a decrease in carrier maximal velocity of transport, consistent with a decreased number of functional carriers in the brush-border membrane.

Conclusion.—Total parenteral nutrition reduces brush-border amino acid and glucose transport activity. The finding that glutamine transport is not downregulated within 1 week of bowel rest may further underscore the importance of glutamine's metabolic role as a gut fuel and in the body's response to catabolic stresses.

▶ Abstracts 140-94-8-9 through 140-94-8-11 suggest that TPN is associated with certain specific morphologic and biochemical alterations in the gut and may cause complications. As in studies in rodents, it has been found that TPN does result in mucosal atrophy in humans, but a considerable period is required for these changes to become apparent. These histologic changes are accompanied by a decrease in the activities of several brush-border amino acid transporters, the exception being glutamine, which suggests that the transport of glutamine is a high priority for the gut. Cholestatic jaundice can occur in some patients, and the diagnosis is definitively made histologically and not on the basis of abnormal liver function tests. In a more recent unpublished study that was presented at the American Surgical Association in April 1994, major complications in patients randomized postoperatively to receive TPN or 5% dextrose solutions after pancreaticoduodenectomy were significantly higher in the TPN group. These reports not only point out that TPN should be used only when it is indicated, but they emphasize that additional clinical trials should (1) define the absolute indications for TPN; (2) examine the role of specific nutrient supplements (e.g., nucleotides, glutamine) in reversing morphometric and biochemical alterations, and in maintaining mucosal function; and (3) continue to investigate the mechanism by which TPN solutions become toxic.—W.W. Souba, M.D., Sc.D.

Glutamine

Glutamine and the Preservation of Gut Integrity
van der Hulst RRWJ, van Kreel BK, von Meyenfeldt MF, Brummer R-JM, Arends J-W, Deutz NEP, Soeters PB (Academisch Ziekenhuis, Maastricht, The Netherlands)
Lancet 341:1363–1365, 1993   140-94-8-12

Background.—The addition of glutamine to total parenteral nutrition (TPN) improves nitrogen balance and enhances protein synthesis. In ani-

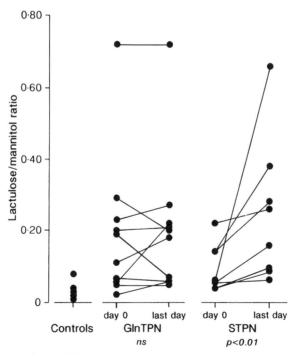

Fig 8–2.—Intestinal permeability in controls (*n* = 12) and patients (glutamine-enriched TPN, *n* = 10; standard TPN, *n* = 8). Lactulose/mannitol ratio before and after 2 weeks of TPN; *P* < .01 day 0 vs. last day in STPN; *P* < .001 controls vs. STPN and Gln TPN day 0 and last day. (Courtesy of van der Hulst RRWJ, van Kreel BK, von Meyenfeldt MF, et al: *Lancet* 341:1363-1365, 1993.)

mals, glutamine preserves gut structure and function. It is not known whether the same is true for humans. In a randomized, prospective study, the effects of glutamine-peptide–enriched TPN on mucosal structure and intestinal permeability were investigated.

Methods.—Twenty patients with inflammatory bowel disease or neoplastic disease received either glutamine-dipeptide–enriched TPN or standard TPN for 10–14 days. Blood tests, duodenoscopy with biopsies, and an intestinal permeability test were performed at baseline and on the last day of TPN. Intestinal permeability was measured as the ratio between urine lactulose and mannitol concentrations after enteral administration. Ten patients with dyspepsia who had normal histologic findings were controls for mucosal structure. Twelve healthy volunteers served as controls for urine tests.

Results.—Intestinal permeability did not change in the glutamine TPN group, but it increased significantly in the standard TPN group (Fig 8–2). The enhanced permeability could not be clearly attributed to altered excretion of lactulose or mannitol. The lactulose/mannitol ratio was significantly higher in all patients than in controls. Intestinal villus height was unchanged in the glutamine TPN group but decreased slightly in the standard TPN group. Crypt depth did not differ significantly between groups and was unchanged by TPN. However, villus height was lower in the glutamine group before and after parenteral nutrition and decreased only after 2 weeks of parenteral nutrition in the standard TPN group.

Conclusion.—The excretion ratio of lactulose and mannitol is a reliable measure of intestinal permeability. Adding glutamine dipeptide to total parenteral nutrition preserves gut permeability and mucosal structure.

Glutamine is Essential for Epidermal Growth Factor-Stimulated Intestinal Cell Proliferation
Ko TC, Beauchamp RD, Townsend CM Jr, Thompson JC (Univ of Texas, Galveston; Shriners Burn Inst, Galveston, Tex)
Surgery 114:147–154, 1993   140-94-8–13

Background.—Through an unknown mechanism, glutamine stimulates the growth of intestinal mucosa in vitro. The role of glutamine in enterocyte proliferation stimulated by epidermal growth factor (EGF) was investigated, and specific EGF mitogenic actions that required glutamine were identified.

Methods.—A nontransformed rat intestinal mucosal cell line, IEC-6, was stimulated with EGF, 20 ng/mL, with and without glutamine, 0.1 to 10 mmol/L. Protein synthesis, DNA, and RNA were measured by determining incorporation of tritiated thymidine, tritiated uridine, and ^{14}C-leucine. Cell numbers and messenger RNA levels of early growth response genes *zif268*, *jun-B*, and *c-myc*, were also determined.

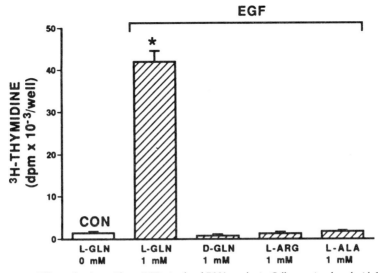

Fig 8–3.—Effects of amino acids on EGF-stimulated DNA synthesis. Cells were incubated with EGF (20 ng/mL) and 1 mmol/L of either L-glutamine (*L-GLN*), D-glutamine (*D-GLN*), L-arginine (*L-ARG*), or L-alanine (*L-ALA*). Tritiated (^{3}H)-thymidine incorporation was determined after 24 hours. Control (*CON*) received no EGF or L-glutamine. $P < .05$ vs. CON. (Courtesy of Ko TC, Beauchamp RD, Townsend CM Jr, et al: *Surgery* 114:147–154, 1993.)

Results.—Glutamine was required for EGF stimulation of DNA, RNA, and protein synthesis and cell replication. Among L-glutamine, D-glutamine, L-arginine, and L-alanine, only the addition of L-glutamine to EGF stimulated DNA synthesis (Fig 8–3). The addition of glutamine, 1 or 10 mmol/L, to EGF significantly increased cell number after 3 days (Fig 8–4). The EGF-activated expression of *zif268, jun-B,* and *c-myc* occurred without glutamine.

Conclusion.—The EGF-stimulated proliferation of intestinal mucosal cells requires glutamine. The mitogenic effects of EGF can be divided into glutamine-independent and glutamine-dependent pathways. Glutamine-independent activity includes the signal transduction that triggers expression of early growth response genes. The glutamine-dependent activity includes DNA, RNA, and protein synthesis.

▶ Glutamine is a classified and a nonessential amino acid, and it is currently absent from TPN solutions because of its relatively short shelf life. The studies by van der Hulst and associates (Abstract 140-94-8–12) and by Ko and colleagues (Abstract 140-94-8–13) further attest to the importance glutamine occupies in intestinal mucosal growth and function. When TPN is supplemented with glutamine, the mucosal atrophy and permeability defect that develop with standard glutamine-free solutions are no longer observed. Furthermore, glutamine is essential for mucosal growth in vitro. It is possible that mucosal glutamine requirements are increased in "stressed" patients

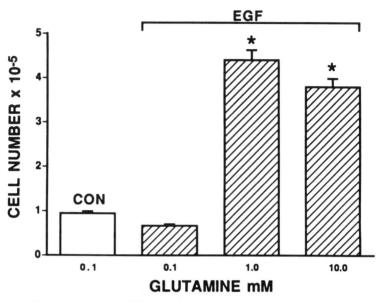

Fig 8–4.—Effects of glutamine on EGF-stimulated IEC-6 cell growth. Cells were treated with EGF (20 ng/mL) plus glutamine (.1, 1, or 10 mmol/L), and cell numbers were counted after 72 hours. Control (CON) cells received only .1 mmol of glutamine per L. $P < .05$ vs. CON. (Courtesy of Ko TC, Beauchamp RD, Townsend CM JR, et al: *Surgery* 114:147–154, 1993.)

and that the availability of glutamine is rate-limiting. Provision of exogenous glutamine may provide the "extra" needs and result in an improvement in gut function.—W.W. Souba, M.D., Sc.D.

Glutamine and Cancer

Souba WW (Harvard Med School, Boston)
Ann Surg 218:715–728, 1993   140-94-8-14

Background.—Glutamine, the most abundant amino acid in blood and tissues, is essential for tumor growth. Marked changes in organ glutamine metabolism are typical in hosts with cancer. The role of glutamine in tumor growth was reviewed, with consideration of the alterations in interorgan glutamine metabolism associated with tumor development and the potential benefits of glutamine nutrition in patients with cancer.

Methods.—Data from investigations of glutamine metabolism and nutrition of the cancer host were compiled and summarized.

Results.—In vivo and in vitro studies of glutamine metabolism in cancer have demonstrated that many tumors are avid glutamine consumers. Host glutamine depletion is a hallmark of progressive tumor growth (Fig 8-5). Glutamine depletion occurs partly because the tumor acts as a

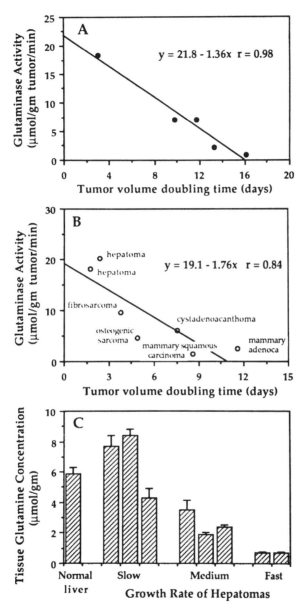

Fig 8–5.—Correlation between tumor growth and the rate of intracellular glutamine metabolism. **A,** relationship between phosphate-dependent glutaminase activity and tumor doubling time in 5 different hepatomas; data modified from Linder-Horowitz et al. **B,** positive correlation between phosphate-dependent glutaminase activity and tumor doubling time in seven solid malignancies of different tissue origin; data modified from Knox et al. **C,** negative correlation between tumor glutamine concentration and cell proliferation (growth rate) in hepatomas; data modified from Sebolt et al. (Courtesy of Souba WW: *Ann Surg* 218:715–728, 1993.)

Is Glutamine a Conditionally Essential Amino Acid in the Host With Cancer?

Definition: A conditionally essential amino acid is one that is nonessential during health but is required in the diet in certain pathophysiologic states because tissue utilization exceeds the capacity for endogenous biosynthesis. Provision of the nutrient (glutamine) in the diet during the disease state (cancer) improves tissue metabolism, structure, and function.

Hypothesis: In the host with cancer, glutamine is a conditionally essential amino acid. Its provision counteracts the glutamine depletion that develops with progressive tumor growth and it also attenuates host tissue injury associated with tumor growth and antineoplastic therapy.

Evidence that glutamine may be conditionally essential in the tumor-bearing host

Required Effect/Criteria	Evidence/Examples
Decrease in blood and tissue glutamine concentrations	Tumor-bearing animals develop glutamine depletion in blood[5,28,29] and skeletal muscle.[5,26]
Atrophy or dysfunction of a specific tissue(s)	Tumor-bearing rats exhibit impaired intestinal glutamine metabolism,[35] villous atrophy,[29] and bacterial translocation.[36,37] Rats treated with radiation therapy or chemotherapy develop bacteremia,[58,63] mucosal atrophy,[59,60] or mucosal damage[61,63,64] when no glutamine is provided in the diet.
Effects of conditionally essential nutrient (glutamine) repletion	

"glutamine trap," nearly doubling the normal rate of glutamine extraction. Another mechanism of glutamine depletion is cytokine-mediated changes in glutamine metabolism in host tissues. Studies in animals as well as in humans suggest that hosts with cancer may benefit from pharmacologic doses of dietary glutamine (table).

Required Effect/Criteria	Evidence/Examples
Correct tissue glutamine depletion	Glutamine-enriched diets restore muscle glutamine in tumor-bearing rats.[54,55]
Enhance cellular utilization	Feeding glutamine-enriched diets to rats receiving whole abdominal radiation increases gut uptake of circulating glutamine.[63]
Improvement in tissue morphology and function	Glutamine-enriched diets increase intestinal villous height in the tumor-bearing rat (M. Torosian, University of Pennsylvania, personal communication). Glutamine-enriched TPN increases gut mucosal glutathione levels in the tumor-bearing rat.[55] Glutamine-enriched enteral diets improve recovery and enhance mucosal healing after chemotherapy or radiation therapy.[58,61,63,64] Glutamine-enriched enteral diets increase carcass weight in tumor-bearing rats.[54]
Improvement in protein economy	Glutamine nutrition improves nitrogen balance in bone marrow transplant patients.[74]
Improvement in outcome	Glutamine nutrition decreases infections and shortens hospital stay in bone marrow transplant patients.[74]

(Courtesy of Souba WW: *Ann Surg* 218:715–728, 1993.)

Conclusion.—Knowledge of glutamine metabolism regulation in the tumor-bearing host will lead to improved nutritional support regimens for patients with cancer.

▶ Glutamine is a primary fuel for rapidly proliferating malignant cells. Marked derangements in interorgan glutamine metabolism occur in the host with cancer. These impairments lead to glutamine depletion, which can be attenuated with glutamine-enriched diets. The growing tumor consumes enormous amounts of glutamine to support cellular biosynthetic and energy requirements. Recent studies in hepatomas (1) demonstrate that glutamine transport rates are accelerated by 10- to 30-fold in hepatomas compared to normal human hepatocytes. The transport of glutamine into the cytoplasm of hepatomas is mediated by a carrier protein that is distinctly different from that which is operating in normal hepatocytes. The Km (affinity) of this "new" carrier is quite low (approximately 100 μM), indicating that tumor cells adapt so that they can extract glutamine efficiently, even at low ambient concentrations. This may explain the several studies that show that supplemental glutamine in vivo does not appear to stimulate tumor growth. Methods of selectively blocking glutamine uptake by malignant cells may prove to be a useful treatment strategy.—W.W. Souba, M.D., Sc.D.

Reference

1. Bode BP, Souba WW: Modulation of cellular proliferation alters glutamine transport and metabolism in human hepatomas. *Ann Surg* In press.

Arginine

Arginine-Supplemented Diets Improve Survival in Gut-Derived Sepsis and Peritonitis by Modulating Bacterial Clearance: The Role of Nitric Oxide

Gianotti L, Alexander JW, Pyles T, Fukushima R (Univ of Cincinnati, Ohio; Shriners Burn Inst, Cincinnati, Ohio)
Ann Surg 217:644–654, 1993   140-94-8-15

Background.—Dietary arginine enhances resistance to infection. However, its role in transfusion-induced immunosuppression and gut-derived sepsis has not been defined. The effect of arginine on survival rates and host defense mechanisms was investigated in a murine model of transfusion-induced immunosuppression.

Methods.—Balb/c mice were fed one of the following: laboratory chow; an unsupplemented AIN-76A diet; or an AIN-76 diet supplemented with 2% arginine, 2% arginine plus Nω-nitro-L-arginine (NNA), or 4% glycine. After 10 days, the mice were transfused with allogeneic blood. Cecal ligation and puncture (CLP) or gavage with 10^{10} *Escherichia coli* and a 20% burn injury were performed 5 days later. Four hours after the burn injury, mesenteric lymph nodes, liver, and spleen were harvested.

Results.—Post-CLP survival was significantly higher among arginine-supplemented mice (56%) compared with AIN-76A-fed mice (28%) and chow-fed mice (20%). All arginine-supplemented mice survived the gavage and burn, whereas survival was only 50% in both the glycine-supple-

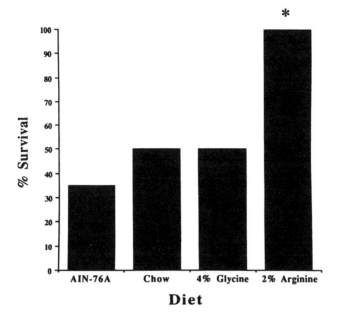

*

Diet

Fig 8–6.—Survival rates of animals fed with either laboratory chow, AIN-76A semipurified diet, 4% glycine-supplemented diet, or 2% arginine-supplemented diet undergoing blood transfusions, bacterial gavage (10^{10}), and a 20% burn injury. * P < .01 vs. all other diets. (Courtesy of Gianotti L, Alexander JW, Pyles T, et al: *Ann Surg* 217:644-654, 1993.)

mented and chow-fed mice and 35% in the AIN-76A group (Fig 8-6). Again, the difference was significant. Among arginine-supplemented mice, treatment with NNA significantly decreased survival from 95% to 30.5%. Radionuclide counts revealed greater translocation to the mesenteric lymph nodes among AIN-76A mice; however, no diet-related difference in translocation to liver or spleen was observed. Based on quantitative colony counts and the calculated percentage of viable bacteria

Number of *Escherichia coli* as Measured by CFU/G of Tissue

Diet	Mesenteric Lymph Nodes	Liver	Spleen
Arginine	0*	483 ± 137†	162 ± 108*
Glycine	4,240 ± 2,649	3,913 ± 1,362	2,338 ± 1,591
Chow	1,434 ± 251	2,622 ± 776	1,625 ± 435
AIN-76A	15,216 ± 10,899	5,762 ± 1,186	13,857 ± 10,468

Note: Values are means ± SEM.
* P < .05 vs. all other diets.
† P < .05 vs. glycine and AIN-76A.
(Courtesy of Gianotti L, Alexander JW, Pyles T, et al: *Ann Surg* 217:644-654, 1993.)

remaining, immune defense against translocated organisms was significantly enhanced by arginine (table); these benefits were reversed by NNA.

Conclusion.—Arginine supplementation affects infection-related mortality. Apparently, this benefit is mediated by enhanced bactericidal mechanisms via the arginine–nitric oxide pathway.

Arginine Stimulates Wound Healing and Immune Function in Elderly Human Beings

Kirk SJ, Hurson M, Regan MC, Holt DR, Wasserkrug HL, Barbul A (Sinai Hosp of Baltimore, Md; Johns Hopkins Med Insts, Baltimore, Md)

Surgery 114:155–160, 1993   140-94-8-16

Background.—Physiologic immune function and tissue repair processes of the extremities may be suboptimal in the elderly. Arginine enhances immune function and may promote wound healing. The effect of oral arginine supplementation on wound healing and T-cell function in elderly humans was investigated in a randomized double-blind study.

Methods.—For 2 weeks, 30 healthy elderly adults received daily supplements of 30 gm of arginine aspartate containing 17 g of free arginine; 15 volunteers received placebo syrup. A polytetrafluoroethylene catheter was inserted subcutaneously into the right deltoid region to assess fibroplastic wound responses. Catheters were analyzed for α-amino nitrogen, an indicator of protein accumulation; hydroxyproline, an index of repar-

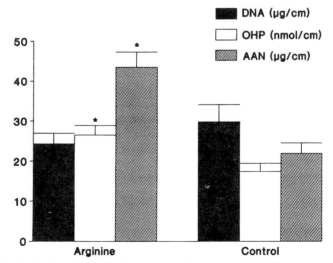

Fig 8–7.—Biochemical analysis of polytetrafluoroethylene catheters in arginine and control groups. *Abbreviations:* OHP, hydroxyproline; AAN, α-amino nitrogen. (Courtesy of Kirk SJ, Hurson M, Regan MC, et al: *Surgery* 114:155–160, 1993.)

ative collagen synthesis; and DNA accumulation, an index of cellular infiltration. A 2- × 2-cm split-thickness wound was created to examine epithelialization. Assessment of the mitogenic response of peripheral blood lymphocytes to concanavalin A, phytohemagglutinin, pokeweed mitogen, and allogeneic stimuli was performed at the beginning and end of supplementation.

Results.—Arginine significantly enhanced collagen deposition, reflected by higher wound-catheter accumulation of hydroxyproline, which was a mean 26.49 nmol/cm in the arginine-treated group and 17.41 nmol/cm in controls (Fig 8–7). Total protein content also significantly increased with arginine supplementation: accumulated α-amino nitrogen was a mean 43.47 μg/cm with arginine supplementation compared with only 21.95 μg/cm with placebo. Neither the DNA content of the catheters nor the rate of wound epithelialization was influenced by arginine. Greater peripheral blood lymphocyte responses to mitogenic and allogeneic stimuli occurred with arginine supplementation, and serum levels of insulin-like growth factor-1 significantly increased.

Conclusion.—Arginine supplementation may improve wound healing and immune response in the elderly.

Arginine Transport in Human Liver: Characterization and Effects of Nitric Oxide Synthase Inhibitors
Inoue Y, Bode BP, Beck DJ, Bland KI, Souba WW (Univ of Florida, Gainesville; Monsanto Co, St Louis, Mo; Harvard Med School, Boston)
Ann Surg 218:350–363, 1993   140-94-8-17

Background.—Hepatocyte intracellular availability and the subsequent biosynthesis of nitric oxide may be regulated by plasma arginine. Little is known about arginine transport across the human hepatocyte plasma membrane.

Methods.—Plasma membrane transport of ³H-L-arginine was characterized in hepatic plasma membrane vesicles (HPMVs) and in hepatocytes isolated and cultured from human liver biopsy specimens. The effects of nitric oxide synthase inhibitors ω-nitro-L-arginine methyl ester (L-NAME) and N-methylarginine (NMA) on arginine transport were examined in HMPVs and in cultured cells.

Results.—Arginine transport was saturable, Na⁺-independent, and sensitive to temperature and pH (Fig 8–8). Lysine, homoarginine, and ornithine inhibited arginine transport. Significant attenuation by nitric oxide synthase inhibitors suggests that the nitric oxide synthase enzyme may share a structurally similar arginine-binding site. On the basis of Dixon plot analysis, blockade occurred by competitive inhibition. In vivo lipopolysaccharide treatment of rats doubled the stimulation of saturable hepatic arginine transport. The lipopolysaccharide-induced arginine transport was inhibited by L-NAME, suggesting that arginine transport

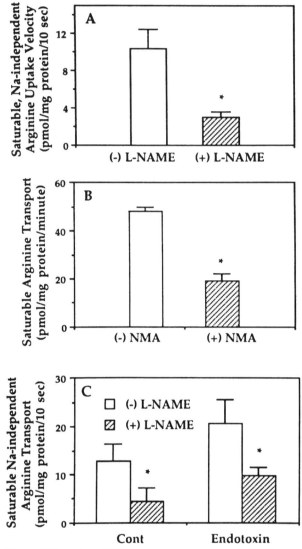

Fig 8–8.—Effects of NO synthase inhibitors on arginine transport. **A,** the 10-second transport of [³H] arginine by human HPMVs was assayed in the presence of 10 mM of L-NAME. **B,** the 60-second transport of [³H] arginine by human female hepatocytes was measured in the presence of 5 mM of NMA. **C,** the 10-second transport of [³H] arginine by rat HPMVs from control and LPS-treated rats was assayed in the presence of 10 mM of L-NAME. (Courtesy of Inoue Y, Bode BP, Beck DJ, et al: *Ann Surg* 218:350–363, 1993.)

by human hepatocytes is mediated primarily by the Na⁺-independent transport system y⁺.

Conclusion.—The ability of arginine derivatives to block nitric oxide production may derive from their inhibition of the nitric oxide synthase enzyme as well as from their ability to competitively inhibit arginine transport across the hepatocyte plasma membrane. The use of selective arginine derivatives that compete with arginine at the plasma membrane level may modulate septic response.

Endotoxin Stimulates Arginine Transport in Pulmonary Artery Endothelial Cells

Lind DS, Copeland EM III, Souba WW (Univ of Florida, Gainesville)
Surgery 114:199–205, 1993   140-94-8-18

Background.—The pulmonary endothelium has a key role in metabolizing arginine, the exclusive precursor molecule for nitric oxide. The endothelial production of nitric oxide is increased during endotoxemia, even though the circulating arginine level is reduced. It is possible that

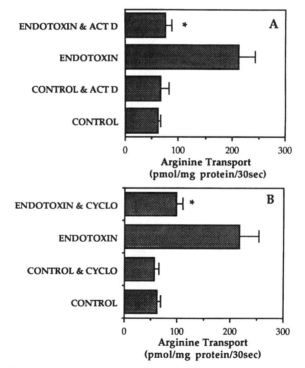

Fig 8–9.—Effect of actinomycin D and cycloheximide on endotoxinstimulated arginine transport. Cells were incubated with saline solution (control) or endotoxin (10 μg/mL) for 12 hours in presence (**A**) or absence (**B**) of actinomycin D (*Act D*, 4 μmol/L, also for 12 hours) or cycloheximide (*Cyclo*, 10 μmol/L for 8 hours). Thirty-second Na⁺-independent transport of [³H] L-arginine was measured. Data represent mean ± SEM of at least 3 separate determinations done in duplicate. *P <.01 vs. control. (Courtesy of Lind DS, Copeland EM III, Souba WW: Surgery 14:199–205, 1993.)

endotoxin stimulates carrier-mediated arginine transport in the pulmonary endothelium.

Methods.—The uptake of tritiated L-arginine by endothelial cells of the porcine pulmonary artery was estimated in the presence and absence of sodium ion. Cell monolayers were incubated with varying concentrations of *Escherichia coli* endotoxin, and arginine transport was monitored. Transport affinity and the peak rate of arginine metabolism were measured over a range of arginine concentrations. Uptake was also estimated after exposing cells to actinomycin D, a transcriptional inhibitor, and cycloheximide, which inhibits protein synthesis.

Findings.—Three fourths of total arginine transport by the endothelial cells was mediated by a high-affinity, sodium-independent transport system. Endotoxin stimulated this form of transport twofold to fivefold in a time- and dose-dependent manner. Accelerated arginine transport was noted within 2 hours of exposure to endotoxin and peaked at 12 hours. Peak transport velocity increased 68% in endotoxin-exposed cells, with no change in transport affinity. The endotoxin-related increase in arginine uptake was prevented by both actinomycin D and cycloheximide (Fig 8-9).

Conclusion.—Endotoxin stimulates arginine transport by pulmonary artery endothelial cells through a process that requires de novo RNA and protein synthesis. This response may serve to support arginine-dependent biosynthetic pathways in the lung in the presence of sepsis. Further studies are needed before rational treatment will be possible. The nonspecific inhibition of the arginine–nitric oxide pathway might have adverse effects.

▶ Arginine is another so-called "designer" nutrient that may be required in increased amounts by the body during stress states. Arginine possesses a strong ability to stimulate pituitary growth hormone secretion, which may, in part, explain its effects on wound repair. Supplemental dietary arginine has been shown to stimulate wound healing in both animals and in man. Arginine-supplemented diets also improve survival in gut-origin sepsis by improving bacteria clearance, an effect that appears to involve the nitric oxide pathway.

Arginine is the exclusive precursor for the biosynthesis of nitric oxide, an important bioregulatory molecule that has numerous functions. Although initially described for its role in regulating vascular tone, nitric oxide also plays a key role in modulating immune function. Arginine transport into cells from the blood occurs predominantly via the system y^+ transport protein, the activity of which is enhanced significantly in endothelial cells incubated with endotoxin. Treatment of animals with endotoxin also enhances hepatic arginine uptake. Compounds that block nitric oxide synthase also block arginine transport, suggesting the potential for novel dietary methods of controlling arginine availability and possibly of nitric oxide production.—W.W. Souba, M.D., Sc.D.

Growth Hormone

Growth Hormone Treatment After Abdominal Surgery Decreased Carbohydrate Oxidation and Increased Fat Oxidation in Patients With Total Parenteral Nutrition
Mjaaland M, Unneberg K, Bjøro T, Revhaug A (Tromsø Univ Hosp, Norway; Univ of Oslo, Norway)
Metabolism 42:185–190, 1993   140-94-8-19

Introduction.—Nutritional support alone does not readily correct net protein loss after surgical trauma, but growth hormone (GH) can improve nitrogen balance in this setting, as well as after injury. The effect is followed by increased fat mobilization and oxidation. It may be especially useful to conserve protein through fat oxidation after stress.

Objective.—The effects of GH on fat and carbohydrate metabolism were examined in 20 patients having elective gastrointestinal surgery, half of whom received recombinant human GH.

Methods.—Treated patients received 24 IU of GH subcutaneously each morning after surgery. Parenteral nutrition was given; it supplied 125% of the basal metabolic rate with a nitrogen content of 5.7 g/m². Equal parts of glucose and Intralipid were delivered via a central venous catheter.

Results.—Patients given GH had a significant increase in resting energy expenditure compared with placebo recipients. A decrease in respiratory quotient resulted from both increased fat oxidation and reduced oxidation of carbohydrate (table). Venous levels of free fatty acids and both venous and arterial glycerol levels were higher in GH-treated patients, but there were no significant differences in plasma levels of glucose, lactate, or pyruvate. Forearm flux studies showed an increase in free fatty acid efflux in the GH-treated patients and higher glycerol efflux than in the placebo group. The GH recipients had higher plasma levels of insulin and glucagon than did the placebo patients. Levels of insulin-like growth factor also were increased.

Discussion.—Administration of GH in conjunction with nutritional support promotes lipolysis both generally and in forearm tissues. Fat oxidation and energy expenditure both increase, whereas carbohydrate oxidation lessens. Fat is a preferred source of energy in patients receiving parenteral nutrition after abdominal surgery.

Afternoon Restins Energy Expenditure (REE), Respiratory Quotient (RQ), and Fat and Carbohydrate Oxidation

Group	Day −1	Day 1	Day 2	Day 3	Day 4	Day 5	ANOVA
REE (%BMR)							
GH	104 ± 5	127 ± 4†	124 ± 3†	134 ± 4‡	126 ± 5*	128 ± 7	†
PL	98 ± 2	111 ± 2	109 ± 3	107 ± 4	112 ± 1	112 ± 3	
RQ							
GH	.80 ± .03	.78 ± .02	.79 ± .02	.82 ± .02	.80 ± .02*	.77 ± .01*	†
PL	.82 ± .01	.85 ± .03	.84 ± .01	.92 ± .05	.88 ± .03	.91 ± .06	
Carbohydrate oxidation (g/m²/24 h)							
GH	72 ± 20	55 ± 12	59 ± 12	80 ± 13	68 ± 15	43 ± 8†	*
PL	65 ± 9	92 ± 21	79 ± 4	98 ± 14	110 ± 16	91 ± 4	
Fat oxidation (g/m²/24 h)							
GH	47 ± 8	71 ± 9	62 ± 6*	60 ± 8*	60 ± 7*	73 ± 4†	†
PL	45 ± 3	43 ± 9	41 ± 4	31 ± 5	31 ± 7	46 ± 8	

Note: Measurements were taken at 4:00 PM preoperatively and on the first 5 postoperative days (8 hours after GH or placebo injection) in patients treated with GH and placebo (PL). The results are means ± standard error of the mean.
* $P < .05$.
† $P < .01$.
‡ $P < .001$; between-group differences.
(Courtesy of Mjaaland M, Unneberg K, Bjøro T, et al: *Metabolism* 42:185–190, 1993.)

Anabolic Therapy With Growth Hormone Accelerates Protein Gain in Surgical Patients Requiring Nutritional Rehabilitation

Byrne TA, Morrissey TB, Gatzen C, Benfell K, Nattakom TV, Scheltinga MR, LeBoff MS, Ziegler TR, Wilmore DW (Harvard Med School, Boston)
Ann Surg 218:400–418, 1993   140-94-8-20

Background.—The impact of adjunctive exogenous growth hormone (GH) on protein accumulation and the composition of weight gain were investigated in a group of stable, nutritionally compromised postoperative patients receiving standard hypercaloric nutritional therapy.

Methods.—Fourteen patients with severe gastrointestinal dysfunction participated in the study. After 7 days of following a standard nutritional regimen that provided approximately 50 kcal/kg/day and protein, 2 g/kg/day, 4 patients continued receiving the standard nutritional therapy and 10 received GH, .14 mg/kg/day. Body fat, mineral content, lean mass, total body water, extracellular water, and body protein were determined on day 7 of standard therapy and after 3 weeks of GH treatment.

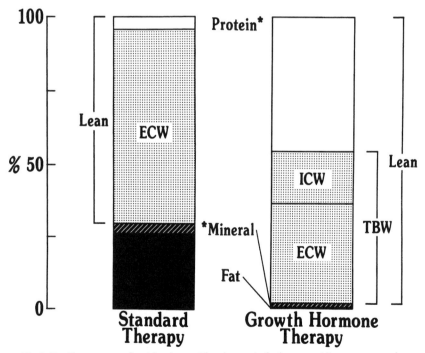

Fig 8–10.—Components of weight change. The changes in body composition are expressed as a percentage of the change in body weight. The percentage of weight change as protein was significantly greater in the GH-treated patients (P < .02) than in those receiving standard nutritional therapy. Patients receiving STD gained significantly more mineral content (P < .02) and tended to deposit a greater proportion of body weight as fat and extracellular water. (Courtesy of Byrne TA, Morrissey TB, Gatzen C, et al: *Ann Surg* 218:400-418, 1993.)

Results.—Patients who received GH gained minimal body fat but significantly more lean mass (mean, 4.311 kg) compared with patients receiving standard nutritional therapy (mean, 1.988 kg) (Fig 8–10). Similarly, GH-treated patients gained significantly more protein, (mean, 1.417 kg) compared with those on standard nutritional therapy (mean, .086). The increase in lean mass in GH-treated patients was not accompanied by an inappropriate expansion of extracellular water. In contrast, patients receiving standard therapy stored a greater proportion of body weight as extracellular water and significantly more fat compared with GH-treated patients. Growth hormone significantly increased substrate oxidation and the use of available energy, which significantly increased the efficiency of protein deposition by 66%.

Conclusion.—In stable adult patients receiving aggressive nutritional therapy, adjunctive GH accelerates protein gain without increasing body fat or expanding extracellular water. Because GH therapy facilitates nutritional repletion, it may shorten the postsurgical convalescence of malnourished patients after major procedures.

Growth Hormone Treatment Improves Serum Lipids and Lipoproteins in Adults With Growth Hormone Deficiency

Cuneo RC, Salomon F, Watts GF, Hesp R, Sönksen PH (St Thomas' Hosp, London; Northwick Park Hosp, Harrow, England)
Metabolism 42:1519–1523, 1993   140-94-8–21

Background.—Hypercholesterolemia and hypertriglyceridemia are prevalent among growth hormone (GH)–deficient children and adults.

Demographic Characteristics and Serum Lipid, Lipoprotein, and Apolipoprotein Levels for Adults With GH Deficiency and Control Subjects

	GH-Deficient	Normal	P
Sex (M:F)	16:8	15:8	—
Age (yr)	38 ± 2	37 ± 2	.74
Height (cm)	169.5 ± 2.0	175.2 ± 2.1	.06
Weight (kg)	80.9 ± 3.8	77.5 ± 3.9	.54
Total cholesterol (mmol · L^{-1})	5.85 ± 0.22	4.89 ± 0.17	.002
Triglycerides (mmol · L^{-1})	2.18 ± 0.36	1.24 ± 0.09	.017
HDL cholesterol (mmol · L^{-1})	0.83 ± 0.06	1.26 ± 0.06	<.001
LDL cholesterol (mmol · L^{-1})	4.10 ± 0.20	3.06 ± 0.16	<.001
Apo A-1 (g · L^{-1})	1.36 ± 0.04	1.44 ± 0.04	.16
Apo B (g · L^{-1})	1.01 ± 0.05	0.84 ± 0.04	.011

Note: Data are presented as means ± standard error of the mean.
(Courtesy of Cuneo RC, Salomon F, Watts GF, et al: *Metabolism* 42:1519–1523, 1993.)

These dyslipidemias are well-recognized risk factors for cardiovascular and coronary artery disease. Six-month treatment with GH decreased serum cholesterol levels in adults with severe GH deficiency. More detailed information about the dyslipidemias and effects of long-term GH treatment in that adult population was provided.

Methods.—Twenty-four adults with a 12-month history of GH deficiency received either recombinant human GH (rhGH), administered for 6 months as subcutaneous injection of .07 U/kg of body weight, or placebo. Twenty-three age-, weight-, and gender-matched normal volunteers served as controls. Fasting venous blood samples were obtained before treatment and after 1, 3, and 6 months.

Results.—At baseline, patients had significantly higher serum concentrations of cholesterol, low-density-lipoprotein (LDL) cholesterol, apolipoprotein B (apo B), and triglycerides, and lower concentrations of high-density-lipoprotein (HDL) cholesterol compared with controls (table). The serum HDL cholesterol concentration was diminished in 75% of patients. Serum cholesterol was elevated in 39% of patients; triglycerides in 26%; LDL cholesterol in 39%; and apo B in 25%. After 6 months' treatment with rhGH, mean total serum cholesterol, mean LDL cholesterol, mean HDL:LDL ratio, mean apo B level, and mean apo B:A-1 ratio all decreased significantly; HDL cholesterol and apo A-1 levels did not change.

Conclusion.—Hyperlipidemia may increase the risk for cardiovascular disease in adults with GH deficiency. Long-term treatment with rhGH improves lipid and lipoprotein profiles in these patients. However, the impact of long-term rhGH treatment on cardiovascular mortality remains to be assessed.

▶ Human recombinant growth hormone can now be synthesized because of advances in genetic engineering and the use of "smart" bacteria. Although currently expensive, it is anticipated that, in the future, substantial quantities of this naturally occurring pituitary compound will be produced inexpensively. Aside from the use of GH in pituitary dwarfism, specific indications for the use of GH in catabolic surgical patients have not yet been formulated. Nonetheless, it appears that GH is safe and will promote positive nitrogen balance, increase muscle mass and strength, and improve serum lipid profiles in patients at risk for coronary artery disease. Growth hormone has been shown to increase the uptake of amino acid from the gut lumen. I think this peptide will be used in combination with nutritional therapy in the future and is likely to be an important component of metabolic therapy in some chronically catabolic patients.—W.W. Souba, M.D., Sc.D.

Miscellaneous

Tumor Necrosis Factor-α Mediates Changes in Tissue Protein Turnover in a Rat Cancer Cachexia Model

Costelli P, Carbó N, Tessitore L, Bagby GJ, Lopez-Soriano FJ, Argilés JM, Baccino FM (Università di Torino, Italy; Universidad de Barcelona; Louisiana State Univ, New Orleans; et al)

J Clin Invest 92:2783–2789, 1993   140-94-8-22

Background.—Rats bearing the ascites hepatoma Yoshida AH-130 provide a suitable model for studying the mechanisms underlying cancer-related cachexia. Previous studies suggest that tumor growth can rapidly cause weight loss that is associated with the hypercatabolism of tissue protein. Tumor necrosis factor (TNF) is found in the plasma shortly after tumor implantation.

Objective.—The role of TNF in mediating changes in muscle protein turnover was examined in rats bearing AH-130 tumor, using a goat polyclonal antibody against murine TNF IgG.

Observations.—Fractional rates of protein degradation were increased in the gastrocnemius muscle, heart, and liver of tumor-bearing rats, but fractional synthesis rates were similar to those in control animals. Tumor necrosis factor appeared in the circulation in the hypercatabolic animals, and there were hormonal changes including a fall in plasma insulin level and a rise in corticosterone. Daily treatment with anti-TNF IgG decreased rates of protein degradation at all sites in the tumor-bearing animals, compared with those given a nonimmune IgG preparation (table). The active antibody also lessened the changes in plasma insulin and corticosterone associated with tumor growth.

Conclusion.—These findings implicate TNF in the altered protein metabolism associated with tumor growth in this model, but protection was far from complete.

▶ Tumor necrosis factor-α(cachectin) plays an important role in mediating cancer cachexia as well as in mediating the metabolic response to infection. In this study, treatment of rats with the Yoshida hepatoma with an anti-TNF antibody decreased the tumor-induced increases in protein synthetic rates but did prevent weight loss. Tumor necrosis factor appears to be necessary to augment hepatic amino acid uptake to support the synthesis of key hepatic defense proteins in some animal tumor models. It is of interest that TNF has been used as a tumor cytotoxic agent as well. Collectively, studies such as this indicate that additional work is necessary to sort out the role of TNF and selective cytokine blockade in patients with advanced malignant disease.—W.W. Souba, M.D., Sc.D.

Tissue Weight and Protein in AH-130 Tumor-Bearing Rats

Tissue	Day 4 Tumor bearers				Day 7 Tumor bearers			
	Controls	None	IgG	Anti-TNF	Controls	None	IgG	Anti-TNF
Muscle	631±9 (3)	509±12 **(7)	516±22 **(3)	558±9 **(4)‡	660±17 (3)	476±22 **(6)	483±21 **(3)	567±26 *(5)‡
Protein	59.4±0.9 (3)	47.4±2.5 *(7)	51.3±1.5 **(4)	52.8±1.1 **(3)	64.5±0.7 (3)	39.2±3.1 **(6)	40.3±1.4 **(3)	53.2±2.3 (4)‡***§
Heart	395±18 (3)	324±11 **(7)	305±10 **(3)	303±8 **(4)	391±9 (3)	255±7 **(6)	249±13 **(3)	248±14 **(5)
Protein	47.3±3.7 (3)	37.6±3.0 **(5)	45.7±1.7 (4)‡‡	50.0±2.6 (4)‡‡	50.4±3.0 (3)	32.6±3.2 **(6)	42.9±1.3 (3)	41.7±0.9 *(4)‡
Liver	5,532±94 (3)	4,898±157 *(7)	4,910±123 *(3)	4,773±235 *(3)	6,711±11 (3)	4,411±100 **(6)	4,776±174 **(3)	5,234±252 **(5)‡‡
Protein	1,132±12 (3)	898±27 **(5)	942±43 *(4)	894±27 **(4)	1,432±43 (3)	865±19 **(6)	932±14 **(3)	988±73 **(5)
Kidney	1,008±47 (3)	880±13 **(7)	841±18 *(3)	820±40 *(4)	1,124±36 (3)	742±12 **(6)	811±23 **(3)‡	793±34 **(5)
Protein	246±18 (3)	198±8 **(7)	199±7 **(3)	191±10 **(4)	277±21 (3)	170±11 **(6)	173±13 **(3)	178±14 **(5)

Note: Data are means ± SEM for the number of animals indicated in parentheses. Tissue net weight and total protein expressed as milligrams per 100 g of initial body weight. Statistical significance of the differences: *tumor bearers vs. controls (untreated nontumor bearers); ‡nonimmune IgG- or anti-TNF-treated vs. untreated tumor bearers; §nonimmune IgG vs. anti-TNF treatment. *‡P < .05; **‡‡§P < .01.
(Courtesy of Costelli P, Carbó N, Tessitore L, et al: J Clin Invest 92:2783–2789, 1993.)

The Effect of Dietary Protein Depletion on Hepatic 5-Fluorouracil Metabolism

Davis LE, Lenkinski RE, Shinkwin MA, Kressel HY, Daly JM (Philadelphia College of Pharmacy and Science; Univ of Pennsylvania, Philadelphia)
Cancer 72:3715–3722, 1993   140-94-8-23

Background.—Tumor-bearing hosts frequently have protein calorie malnutrition and, as a result, are susceptible to toxicity from 5-fluorouracil (5-FU). The mechanism underlying this susceptibility is not understood.

Objective and Methods.—The effects of protein depletion on the in vivo hepatic metabolism of 5-FU in rats were examined by using ^{19}F-nuclear magnetic resonance (NMR) spectroscopy. Animals received either a normal 21.5% protein diet or a low 2.5% protein diet for 25 days before 5-FU was injected intraperitoneally. Serum 5-FU pharmacokinetics were studied at the same time by high-performance liquid chromatography. Hepatic dihydropyrimidine dehydrogenase (DPD) activity was assayed spectrophotometrically.

Findings.—In animals given the low-protein diet, the time to initial detection of fluoro-β-alanine in the liver was significantly prolonged, as was the duration of the 5-FU signal. Both the clearance of 5-FU and hepatic DPD activity were significantly lower in the low-protein group. These animals had more 5-FU toxicity, as evidenced by diarrhea, weight loss, and leukopenia (table). Mortality was 85% in the low-protein group, compared with 12% in animals given a normal-protein diet.

Conclusion.—Protein depletion augments the toxic effects of 5-FU in the rat. As a noninvasive test ^{19}F-NMR spectroscopy may prove useful in determining how to adjust chemotherapy to minimize toxicity.

Effect of Protein-Depleted Diet on 5-FU Toxicity

	RD (n = 10) (mean ± SD)	LPD (n = 9) (mean ± SD)	P value
Weight loss, day 5 after 5-FU (g)	16 ± 14	36 ± 17	<0.05*
Lymphocyte count Day 5 after 5-FU (mm³)	5775 ± 2239 (n = 6)	1767 ± 993 (n = 3)	<0.05* ---
Diarrhea	Mild, 3/10	Severe, 9/9	<0.01†
Survival, day 7 after 5-FU	9/10	1/9	<0.01†

Abbreviations: RD, regular diet; LPD, low-protein diet; SD, standard deviation.
* Independent *t* test.
† Chi-square analysis.
(Courtesy of Davis LE, Lenkinski RE, Shinkwin MA, et al: Cancer 72:3715–3722,1993.)

▶ This study provides insight into one possible mechanism by which toxicity develops from aggressive chemotherapeutic regimens in the malnourished patient with cancer. It appears that the nutritional status of the patient with cancer is one factor that affects the disposition and toxicity of antineoplastic drugs that undergo extensive hepatic metabolism. Animal studies have demonstrated that protein-calorie malnutrition can increase the morbidity and mortality associated with administration of 5-FU. Most dosage regimens are based on body surface area and do not take host malnutrition into account.—W.W. Souba, M.D., Sc.D.

The Two-Edged Sword of Large-Dose Steroids for Spinal Cord Trauma

Galandiuk S, Raque G, Appel S, Polk HC Jr (Univ of Louisville, Ky)
Ann Surg 218:419–427, 1993   140-94-8-24

Background.—Spinal cord injury remains the most consequential form of nonfatal trauma, in terms of both quality of life and costs. High-dose steroid treatment has been reported to lessen the extent of neurologic damage, and the publicity gained by this study led to wide acceptance of steroid use. The immunosuppressive actions of steroids, however, raise the possibility that treated patients may be at increased risk of severe pneumonia.

Objective.—The effects of steroid treatment were studied in 32 patients having cervical or upper thoracic spinal injuries. Eighteen neurologically intact patients were reviewed, and 14 patients with high-dose steroids were evaluated prospectively. Treated patients received 30 mg of methylprednisolone per kg intravenously, followed by a dose of 5.4 mg/kg/hr for 23 hours.

Results.—Steroid-treated patients were hospitalized longer than the others. Pneumonia developed in 79% of the steroid-treated group and in half the patients not given steroid treatment. The number of episodes per patient did not differ significantly. The expression of monocyte class II antigens was reduced in steroid-treated patients, as was the ratio of T-helper to T-suppressor cells. Some host defenses were elevated for a short time in the steroid group, but later responses were blunted and delayed. Patients with infection had reduced monocyte antigen expression and relatively low helper/suppressor cell ratios regardless of whether they received steroids.

Discussion.—Steroid treatment of cord-injured patients may preserve neurologic function, but it also increases the risk of pneumonia and significantly prolongs hospital time. It is to be hoped that the adjunctive use of cytokines or immunostimulants will eliminate some of the adverse side effects of steroid treatment while maintaining its neuroprotective action.

▶ This study strongly suggests that length of hospital stay is significantly greater in spinal cord injuries treated with steroids. This may be associated with the immunosuppressive effects of steroid therapy, and it translates into an increase in hospitalization costs of more than $50,000 per patient. It remains unclear to what extent these disadvantages offset the putative benefits of high-dose steroid therapy in this group of patients.—W.W. Souba, M.D., Sc.D.

Effect of Ibuprofen on the Inflammatory Response to Surgical Wounds
Dong Y-L, Fleming RYD, Yan TZ, Herndon DN, Waymack JP (Shriners Burns Inst, Galveston, Tex; Univ of Texas, Galveston)
J Trauma 35:340–343, 1993   140-94-8-25

Introduction.—Severely injured patients often become immunosuppressed and, as a result, may be at an increased risk of infection. It is possible that immune suppression in this setting is a result of excessive prostaglandin synthesis and that cyclooxygenase suppression could prevent it.

Study Design.—The effects of the cyclooxygenase inhibitor ibuprofen on the inflammatory response were examined in rats subjected to a 30% total-body-surface area burn. Ibuprofen was given intraperitoneally in a

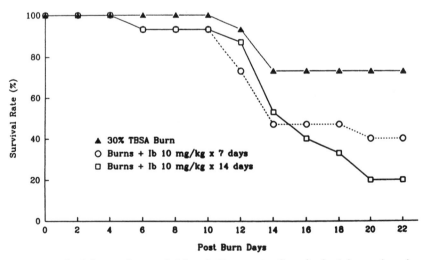

Fig 8–11—Survival curves for rats administered either a carrier, ibuprofen for 7 days, or ibuprofen for 14 days after burn injury. The animals were subjected to cecal ligation and puncture on postburn day 10. (Courtesy of Dong Y-L, Fleming RYD, Yan TZ, et al: *J Trauma* 35:340–343, 1993).

dose of 5 mg/kg twice daily for either 1 or 2 weeks. The cecum was ligated and punctured 10 days after burn injury.

Results.—Ibuprofen administration led to a decrease in neutrophil chemiluminescence, reduced lymphocyte blastogenesis, and infiltration of a sponge matrix by helper/inducer T lymphocytes. Survival after cecal ligation and puncture was reduced by ibuprofen treatment (Fig 8–11).

Conclusion.—These findings suggest that the cyclooxygenase system produces metabolites that promote the survival of severely injured rats.

▶ Ibuprofen is a cyclooxygenase inhibitor that blocks the endogenous synthesis of prostaglandins. In previous studies (1), administration of ibuprofen before administration of endotoxin to healthy volunteers has been shown to reduce fever, heart rate, and subjective discomfort. In this study, ibuprofen diminished the immune response and increased mortality in burned rats subjected to intraperitoneal sepsis. It appears that prostaglandins are important mediators of the inflammatory response that enhance survival under certain circumstances. Whether inflammatory responses should be blocked in critically ill patients may be dependent on the severity of the illness.—W.W. Souba, M.D., Sc.D.

Reference

1. Revhaug A, et al: *Arch Surg* 123:162, 1988.

9 Growth Factors and Wound Healing

Introduction

The first growth factor discovered was nerve growth factor, which was identified some 40 years ago. Since then, a number of additional growth factors have been identified and purified. This field has stimulated great interest because of the numerous clinically relevant problems that potentially involve peptide growth factors. Growth factors occupy a central role in wound healing, inflammatory responses, and cellular differentiation. In general, growth factors regulate cell proliferation, but they also possess multiple biological activities that appear to be independent of growth. They are likely to play a role in controlling cellular metabolic activity. Despite major advances in our understanding of how growth factors work, significant gaps in our knowledge of their mechanism of action remain.

Growth factors regulate the cellular machinery that controls biosynthesis of nucleic acid and subsequent mitosis. Growth factors act on target cells by binding to specific cell surface protein receptors that subsequently "transduce" this signal to the nucleus of the cell. The signal, once received, initiates a number of events, which may include (1) expression of certain genes that also control proliferation and differentiation; (2) enhancement of amino acid uptake by the cell to support protein biosynthesis; and (3) stimulation of angiogenesis.

A number of articles published during this past year have continued to demonstrate the ability of growth factors to enhance wound repair. Most of these studies have not been clinical in nature; thus, the specific use of growth factors in patients with defects in wound healing requires additional research. It is known that the topical application of epidermal growth factor can accelerate the healing of donor sites used for skin grafting. It has been shown in animal studies that basic fibroblast growth factor can stimulate healing of gastric ulcerations. Certain growth factors enhance amino acid transport, presumably to provide the necessary substrate for de novo protein biosynthesis. Because there appears to be inadequate production of growth factor by chronic nonhealing wounds, it is likely that this impairment is important in the failure to heal. Similarly, excessive production of growth factors or altered expression of their receptors may be involved in the formation of hypertrophic scarring.

In the future, growth factors will be used in clinical medicine to enhance healing or to promote differentiation. It should be pointed out that there is compelling evidence to indicate that these proteins are also involved in the process of carcinogenesis and in the growth of established tumors. Transfection of normal cells with certain growth factor expression vectors can lead to transformation. Thus, the use of such therapies will require a better understanding of these events as well.

Wiley W. Souba, M.D., Sc.D.

Biology of Wound Healing

Inhibition of Cell Proliferation by Chronic Wound Fluid
Bucalo B, Eaglstein WH, Falanga V (Univ of Miami, Fla)
Wound Rep Reg 1:181–186, 1993   140-94-9-1

Background.—Occlusive wound dressings may improve chronic wound repair through the stimulatory action of fluid accumulating underneath the dressings. The in vitro proliferative effects of chronic wound fluid obtained from under a polyurethane membrane applied to venous ulcers for 24 hours were investigated.

Methods.—The proliferative effects of this fluid on human dermal fibroblasts, endothelial cells, and keratinocytes were determined by measuring cell counts and DNA synthesis. The fluid was obtained from 6 patients, 63 years of age or older, who had venous ulcers treated with occlusive dressings. The ulcers had been present for at least 6 months with no signs of reepithelialization.

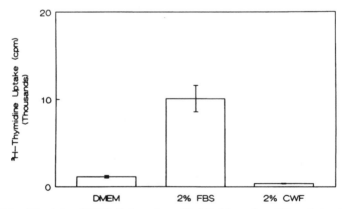

Fig 9–1.—Abbreviation: DDEM, Dulbecco's modified Eagle's medium. Effect of chronic wound fluid on incorporation of tritiated thymidine by cultures of human dermal fibroblasts. Cultures in which 2% chronic wound fluid was added also contained 2% fetal bovine serum (*FBS*). Results represent mean ± standard deviation of measurements from quadruplicate wells. (Courtesy of Bucalo B, Eaglstein WH, Falanga V: *Wound Rep Reg* 1:181–186, 1993.)

Findings.—Chronic wound fluid inhibited the proliferation of human dermal fibroblasts and did not stimulate the proliferation of microvascular endothelial cells or keratinocytes. As measured by tritiated thymidine uptake, DNA synthesis by human dermal fibroblasts showed a 30-fold mean inhibition after the addition of chronic wound fluid to 2% fetal bovine serum (Fig 9-1). After the fluid was heated to 100°C, the inhibitory activity of the fluid on fibroblast proliferation was blocked and was mainly limited to a fraction of chronic wound fluid enriched in components less than 30 kd in molecular weight. However, this did not occur at 56°C. Chronic wound fluid reduced the viability of fibroblasts at concentrations ranging from 1% to 4% and in the presence of serum, as shown by the reduced ability of the cells to exclude trypan blue. The viability of endothelial cells, as evidenced by an increased release of tritiated adenine, was also reduced under these conditions.

Conclusions.—Fluid from chronic wounds is either not stimulatory or is detrimental to cell proliferation in vitro. Wound occlusion is a complex phenomenon that is not limited to the retention of wound fluid. It affects the physical features of ulcers as well as the inflammatory cells recruited into the wound site. Nevertheless, attempts should be made to more effectively remove some components of the chronic wound exudate, a step that may result in better outcomes.

▶ Wounds fluids contain substantial quantities of growth factors that serve to stimulate cellular growth, which results in wound healing. The concentration of these growth factors changes over time as the wound heals. Fluid derived from acute, normally healing wounds stimulates the proliferation of endothelial cells and fibroblasts. In contrast, this study by Bucallo and colleagues demonstrates that fluid from chronic wounds inhibits the proliferation of human fibroblasts and fails to stimulate the proliferation of microvascular endothelium. This observation suggest that chronic wound fluids may contain lower concentrations of growth factors than does fluid from normally healing wounds. It also suggests that nonhealing wounds may not produce growth factors. The cause for this inadequate production of growth factor is unclear, but it may be the result of ischemia or the presence of some toxic factor that may be produced.—W.W. Souba, M.D., Sc.D.

Collagen Synthesis in Intact Skin Is Suppressed During Wound Healing

Ihlberg L, Haukipuro K, Risteli L, Oikarinen A, Kairaluoma MI, Risteli J (Univ of Oulu, Finland)

Ann Surg 217:397–403, 1993   140-94-9–2

Background.—Surgical injury stimulates the synthesis of acute-phase proteins while, at the same time, it inhibits the production of albumin. Net catabolism of skeletal muscle proteins also takes place. Total collagen synthesis appears to be transiently inhibited after surgery. It seems

Concentrations of PICP and PIIINP in Blister 1-Fluid at Different Times Before and After Operation

Day	PICP (µg/L) Median	(Range)	p Value*	PIIINP (µg/L) Median	(Range)	p Value*
-1	228	(137 to 601)	—	140	(35 to 356)	—
+1	145	(47 to 233)	0.01	68	(21 to 172)	0.17
+2	102	(53 to 249)	0.02	76	(24 to 132)	0.04
+4	159	(76 to 244)	0.03	66	(44 to 84)	0.06
+7	152	(84 to 207)	0.06	56	(32 to 72)	0.03

* Postoperative medians were compared with preoperative medians by using Wilcoxon signed-rank sum test.
(Courtesy of Ihlberg L, Haukipuro K, Risteli L, et al: *Ann Surg* 217:397–403, 1993.)

possible that wound healing takes priority over the synthesis of structural and peripheral collagen after surgical wounding.

Objective.—Concentrations of the carboxyterminal propeptide of type I procollagen (PICP) and the aminoterminal propeptide of type III procollagen (PIIINP) were compared in wound fluids from 10 surgical patients and in fluid from suction blisters of intact skin. Serum levels of PICP and PIIINP also were measured by specific radioimmunoassays.

Results.—The absolute concentrations of PICP and PIIINP in blister 1-fluid are presented in the table. Levels of both PICP and PIIINP in blister fluid decreased after operation. At the same time, concentrations in wound fluid increased. The median increase in PICP was nearly 50-fold 4 days after operation, whereas PIIINP increased 11-fold. Increases of more than 400-fold were apparent 7 days after operation for both PICP and PIIINP. Serum levels of both propeptides increased at most postoperative intervals. The median concentration of albumin decreased from 33 g/L before operation to 22 g/L on the fourth postoperative day.

Conclusion.—Collagen synthesis may be suppressed peripherally in the first postoperative week, at the same time that synthesis is increasing rapidly in the wound tissue. It may be possible to limit the loss of structural collagen that tends to occur after major surgery and trauma in high-risk patients.

▶ Ihlberg and colleagues noted that concentrations of the propeptides of type I and type III collagen were diminished in skin suction blisters during the first week after major abdominal surgery. In contrast, peptide concentrations were increased in fluids from the midline wound. The authors suggest that wound healing takes priority over the synthesis of peripheral collagen after surgical stress. In vitro studies indicate that inflammatory mediators (cytokines) and glucocorticoids diminish the growth of fibroblasts, the main source of collagen. Growth factors preferentially elaborated in the surgical wound may account for the increase in synthesis noted in these wounds. Suction blister injury is limited to the epidermis, which is a different injury than a full-thickness abdominal wall incision.—W.W. Souba, M.D., Sc.D.

Regulation of Extracellular Matrix Proteins and Integrin Cell Substratum Adhesion Receptors on Epithelium During Cutaneous Human Wound Healing In Vivo
Juhasz I, Murphy GF, Yan H-C, Herlyn M, Albelda SM (Wistar Inst of Anatomy and Biology, Philadelphia; Univ of Pennsylvania, Philadelphia)
Am J Pathol 143:1458–1469, 1993   140-94-9-3

Introduction.—A key component in the process of cutaneous wound healing is the migration of keratinocytes over the injured dermis to form a new epidermal layer. The migrating epidermal keratinocytes are exposed during the wound healing process to a provisional wound bed containing extracellular matrix (ECM) material that includes fibrin, fibrinogen, fibronectin, tenascin, and vitronectin. Little is known, however, about the regulation of the ECM adhesion receptors (integrins) that are ultimately responsible for cell migration. This process was studied in a human in vivo model.

Methods.—Full-thickness human skin grafts were transplanted onto inbred mice aged 6-8 weeks with severe combined immunodeficiency. The donor skin consisted of human neonatal foreskin. Four to 6 weeks after engraftment, deep excisional wounds involving both the epidermal and dermal layers were made. The wounded skin grafts with the surrounding murine skin were subsequently removed for analysis by immunohistochemistry. The studies centered on the changes in the expression of cell matrix proteins and epithelial integrins.

Results.—The changes in the ECM proteins associated with wounding included loss of laminin and type IV collagen in the region of the wound and expression of tenascin and fibronectin. Alterations were also observed in the integrins on the migrating keratinocytes. During the stage of active migration 1 to 3 days after wounding, there was marked upregulation of the α_v subunit and de novo expression of the fibronectin receptor (α_5 β_1). After epithelial integrity had been established in the later stages of wound healing, redistribution of the α_2, α_3, α_6, and β_4 collagen–lamimin-binding integrin subunits to suprabasal epidermal layers was observed.

Conclusion.—During human cutaneous wound healing, changes in the type and distribution of ECM components are accompanied by changes in the expression of integrins on the migrating keratinocytes. Keratinocytes were found to upregulate fibronectin–fibrinogen-binding integrins and redistribute collagen–laminin-binding integrins. The human skin/severe combined immunodeficient chimera is a useful model for studying the process of human wound repair.

▶ Juhasz and associates have demonstrated that during wound healing, changes in the type and distribution of ECM components are accompanied by changes in the expression of integrins on the migrating keratinocytes. These changes in keratinocytes are accompanied by upregulation of plasminogen activators, synthesis of keratins, and the expression of growth factors. All these factors appear to work together in the control of normal wound healing. Derangements in some or all of these mechanisms are likely to explain the abnormal wound healing that is observed in patients with chronic nonhealing wounds and in patients in whom hypertrophic scarring develops. As our knowledge of the regulation of wound healing is enhanced, we should be able to modulate some of these alterations to improve or accelerate wound healing in our patients.—W.W. Souba, M.D., Sc.D.

Growth Factors

▶↓ I have chosen to comment on all of the following abstracts collectively, because they all focus on the role of specific growth factors in regulating cellular repair or growth. Proliferative and antiproliferative growth factors are found in fluids from virtually all wounds, and they help control the healing process. It is of interest that some chronic wound fluids do not appear to contain measurable levels of certain proliferative wound fluids. During wound repair, there appears to be an elaboration of these factors and their receptors, which are variably expressed as a function of time and the course of the wound. Growth factors have been shown to influence fibroblasts in wounded tissues differently than in nonwounded tissue. Also of interest is that the various cells that make up the healing wounds (e.g., endothelial cells, fibroblasts, inflammatory cells, and keratinocytes) work together in the control of wound healing. One cell type may secrete a specific growth factor that serves to "turn on" another cell. An important part of this response is the fibronectins, proteins that comprise a portion of the extracellular matrix and promote cell migration. Growth factors are not only produced in wounded tissues but, in general, are constantly secreted by cells in normal tissues. Their production helps regulate normal cellular growth and metabolism. They are also secreted into the gut lumen, where they act to modulate mucosal growth and turnover.

A variety of different growth factors have now been identified, and the genes encoding either for their biosynthesis or for the synthesis of their receptors have been cloned. Now that these substances have been purified, numerous in vivo and in vitro studies have been done, providing insight into how they work. Despite the large amount of recent research on growth factors, it is apparent that our understanding of the control of wound healing still has major gaps. As these gaps are filled in, specific roles for growth factors in modulating cellular growth and proliferation in the clinical setting will be better understood.—W.W. Souba, M.D., Sc.D.

Identification of Multiple Proliferative Growth Factors in Breast Cyst Fluid
Ness JC, Sedghinasab M, Moe RE, Tapper D (Children's Hosp and Med Ctr, Seattle; Univ of Washington, Seattle)
Am J Surg 166:237–243, 1993   140-94-9-4

Background.—Gross cystic disease of the breast, a common benign disorder that is associated with an increased risk of breast cancer, and cancer itself are both hormonally induced states characterized by abnormal proliferative responses. In vitro studies of breast cancer cell lines suggest that the autocrine or paracrine secretion of peptide growth factors may have a role in progressive breast cancer by stimulating the proliferation of epithelial cells. A preliminary study of breast cyst fluids demonstrated increased mitogenic activity in samples from women at the highest risk.

Objective and Methods.—Samples of breast cyst fluid were obtained from 226 women and analyzed in a blinded manner. Mitogenic activity was estimated using an in vitro cell proliferation assay that measures the incorporation of tritiated thymidine into embryonic mouse fibroblasts. In addition, levels of epidermal growth factor (EGF), transforming growth factors (TGFs) α and β, insulin-like growth factors (IGFs) I and II, and platelet-derived growth factor (PDGF) were determined by radio-immunoassay.

Findings.—Fluid samples from all subtypes of cysts contained significant amounts of proliferative growth factors. For the first time, breast cyst fluid was shown to contain IGF-II, PDGF, and TGF-β. Concentrations of PDGF, TGF-β, and EGF in breast cyst fluid were several-fold greater than those reported for serum, whereas levels of IGF-I and IGF-II were substantially lower in cyst fluid. No TGF-α was found in the first 100 samples tested. Concentrations of EGF and IGF-II correlated with apocrine type 1 cysts.

Implications.—Fluid samples from a wide range of benign breast cysts contain growth factors that are associated with normal and transformed epithelial cell proliferation. The profile of growth factors in breast cyst fluid might provide an indication of the relative amount of such factors expressed by the breast tissue in a given case, as well as the degree of responsiveness of the breast tissue to the prevailing hormonal milieu.

Epidermal Growth Factor Receptor Distribution in Burn Wounds: Implications for Growth Factor-Mediated Repair
Wenczak BA, Lynch JB, Nanney LB (Vanderbilt Univ, Nashville, Tenn)
J Clin Invest 90:2392–2401, 1992   140-94-9-5

Introduction.—Numerous peptide growth factors, including epidermal growth factor (EGF) and platelet-derived growth factor, have been shown in vivo and in vitro to stimulate various aspects of wound healing. The EGF receptor (EGF-R) has been associated with key events connected with wound repair. To help define endogenous mechanisms of growth factor-mediated repair, the presence of the EGF-R was evaluated in healing wound tissues removed from burn patients.

Methods.—Skin specimens were collected from 32 patients with either partial thickness or full-thickness burns during routine burn incision and autografting procedures. The patients ranged in age from 8 months to 77 years and had burns involving 2% to 88% of total body surface area. In the early postburn period (days 2–4), the epithelial margins surrounding the burns were examined for the presence of the EGF-R. Immunohistochemical studies were performed on postburn days 5, 7–10,

12, and 16. Other areas examined were closely associated sweat ducts, sebaceous glands, and hair follicles.

Results.—In the early postburn period, prominent staining for the EGF-R was observed in undifferentiated, marginal keratinocytes and adjacent proliferating, hypertrophic epithelium, as well as in both marginal and nonmarginal hair follicles, sweat ducts, and sebaceous glands. Although the EGF-R was depleted along leading epithelial margins during the late postburn period, the immunoreactive EGF-R remained intensely positive in the hypertrophic epithelium and all skin appendages. There was a positive correlation between increased detection of the immunoreactive EGF-R and the presence of [^{125}I] EGF binding in the hypertrophic epithelium and proliferating cell nuclear antigen distributions.

Conclusions.—The findings indicate that immunoreactive EGF-Rs can be detected as early as 2 days after a burn injury. The intense localization of the EGF-R suggests that the requisite receptors for EGF and its related ligands are expressed at this time in the proliferative cell population. During the later phases of wound repair, the dynamic equilibrium of EGF-Rs appears to shift toward downregulation. The presence of the EGF-R is a common denominator in the burn wound healing process and appears to have a multifunctional role in epithelial repair.

Effect of Epidermal Growth Factor on Cell Proliferation in Normal and Wounded Connective Tissue
Malcherek P, Schultz G, Wingren U, Franzén L (Univ of Linköping, Sweden; Univ of Florida, Gainesville; Sahlgrenska Hosp, Gothenburg, Sweden)
Wound Rep Reg 1:63–68, 1993   140-94-9–6

Introduction.—There is evidence that epidermal growth factor (EGF) plays a central role in tissue repair, including stimulation of connective tissue repair in the perforated rat mesentery. The mechanism of accelerated wound closure is unclear, but it may involve stimulation of mitosis, contraction, migration, or angiogenesis by EGF. The effect of EGF on connective tissue cell was examined during the initial phase of repair in perforated and unwounded mesentery.

Methods.—Laparotomies were performed in Sprague-Dawley rats, including standardized scalpel perforations in the center of the mesenteric "windows." Half the windows were left as internal controls. Starting on the day of laparotomy, the rats were treated with intraperitoneal injections of EGF, 10 μg dissolved in phosphate-buffered saline solution, or the saline solution alone. Treatments were applied twice a day for 4 consecutive days. The results were assessed in terms of cell proliferation, as reflected by the mitotic index of fibroblasts and mesothelial cells or the DNA content of individual fibroblast cell nuclei.

Results.—Proliferation during the early postoperative period was enhanced by laparotomy alone, with increased numbers of S+ G2 fibroblasts and a higher mitotic index. By the third day of treatment, the mitotic index in perforated windows was increased by EGF treatment, compared with that of controls treated with phosphate-buffered saline only. However, unwounded tissues showed no significant increase in either S+ G2 fibroblasts or mitotic index. Wounded tissue also showed a significantly higher proliferative response after EGF treatment.

Conclusions.—These experimental results demonstrate a proliferation of connective tissue cells by EGF in wounded, but not in unwounded, tissue. Enhanced fibroblast proliferation may be important to the EGF-induced enhancements in connective tissue repair. Further studies will be needed to determine the extent to which EGF affects other mechanisms of repair.

Human Keratinocytes Are a Major Source of Cutaneous Platelet-Derived Growth Factor

Ansel JC, Tiesman JP, Olerud JE, Krueger JG, Krane JF, Tara DC, Shipley GD, Gilbertson D, Usui ML, Hart CE (Oregon Health Sciences Univ, Portland; Rockefeller Univ, New York; Univ of Washington, Seattle; et al)
J Clin Invest 92:671–678, 1993   140-94-9-7

Purpose.—One of the main mitogenic factors involved in cutaneous wound healing appears to be platelet-derived growth factor (PDGF). In human dermal wounds, PDGF appears to be derived from both platelets and monocytes. No reports have addressed the production of PDGF by human keratinocytes. The production of PDGF by human keratinocytes in culture was reported.

Observations.—Cultured human keratinocytes demonstrated both A and B chain PDGF mRNA at Northern blot analysis. Keratinocyte-conditioned culture media contained significant levels of only PDGF-AA polypeptide (Fig 9–2). However, the AB and BB isoforms were also present in detergent-solubilized cell extracts. The PDGF receptors were not expressed in cultured keratinocytes at analysis for either mRNA levels or polypeptide expression. Immunostaining of cryosections of human cutaneous wounds revealed constitutive expression of both the PDGF A and B chains by normal and newly reconstituted wound epidermis. Immunostaining showed no evidence of PDGF receptor polypeptide expression in the epidermis.

Conclusions.—These results suggest that keratinocytes are an important source of PDGF for cutaneous wound healing. The absence of PDGF receptor expression suggests this growth factor plays no autocrine role in keratinocyte growth. This and other recent studies suggest that keratinocytes are a major source of cytokines with a direct influence on adjacent dermal constituents.

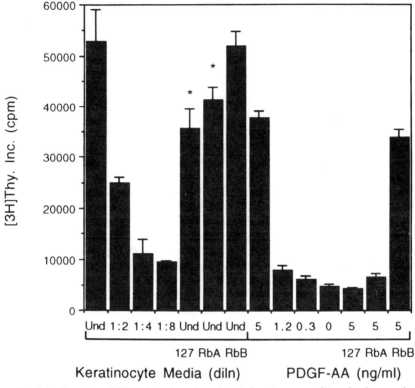

Fig 9–2.—Detection of PDGF-AA mitogenic activity in keratinocyte-conditioned culture media. Increasing amounts of purified PDGF-AA and dilutions of concentrated keratinocyte-conditioned culture media were analyzed for mitogenic activity by ability to stimulate [^{3}H]-thymidine incorporation into murine 3T3 cells. Anti-PDGF antibodies 127:122 (*127*), rabbit anti-PDGF A chain IgG (*RbA*), or rabbit anti-PDGF B chain IgG (*RbB*) were added to purified AA, 5 ng/mL, and to undiluted keratinocyte concentrate (*Und*). Both anti-PDGF-AA antibodies were able to significantly inhibit mitogenic activity in conditioned media sample, demonstrating presence of PDGF-AA, whereas no inhibitory activity was observed with anti-PDGF B chain antibody. Results are expressed as cpm of [^{3}H]-thymidine incorporation ± standard deviation for triplicate determinations. *P < .05. (Courtesy of Ansel JC, Tiesman JP, Olerud JE, et al: *J Clin Invest* 92:671–678, 1993).

Macrophages and Fibroblasts Express Embryonic Fibronectins During Cutaneous Wound Healing

Brown LF, Dubin D, Lavigne L, Logan B, Dvorak HF, Van De Water L (Harvard Med School, Boston; Beth Israel Hosp, Boston)
Am J Pathol 142:793–801, 1993   140-94-9–8

Background.—The fibronectins (FNs) are a group of adhesive glycoproteins that participate in wound healing. The proteins form through alternative splicing of a single gene transcript at 3 sites (EIIIA, EIIIB, and V). The matrix that forms shortly after tissue injury consists of fibrin and extravasated plasma FN lacking the EIIIA and EIIIB domains. A local increase in messenger RNA (mRNA) for FN is found within 2 days of skin excision in the rat, and wounds of this age express so-called "embryonic" FN containing the EIIIA and EIIIB domains.

Objective and Methods.—In situ hybridization studies were done using probes for the different FN mRNAs to identify the cells that synthesize the various isoforms of FN. Probes for collagen and lysozyme served to distinguish between fibroblasts and macrophages. Partial-thickness punch biopsy wounds were made on the flanks of adult rats.

Results.—Macrophages were the major cells expressing FN mRNA 2 days after wounding. Many of them expressed mRNAs for embryonic FN. After 7–10 days, when the wound was maturing, fibroblasts were the major source of embryonic FN.

Conclusion.—In addition to phagocytosing wound debris and providing degradative enzymes and cytokines, wound macrophages appear to synthesize embryonic FNs that contribute to the extracellular matrix needed for wound repair. The FNs may act through promoting cell migration. Alternative splicing of FNs by both macrophages and fibroblasts may prove to be a point in the wound-healing process at which therapeutic intervention is feasible.

PDGF and FGF Reverse the Healing Impairment in Protein-Malnourished Diabetic Mice
Albertson S, Hummel RP III, Breeden M, Greenhalgh DG (Shriners Burn Inst, Cincinnati, Ohio; Univ of Cincinnati, Ohio)
Surgery 114:368–372, 1993   140-94-9-9

Objective.—Chronic malnutrition has serious negative effects on tissue repair, and even brief alterations in nutritional intake have been shown to have adverse effects. Growth factors have been shown to improve healing in impaired models, but not after malnutrition. The effects of growth factors on altered tissue repair caused by malnutrition were investigated.

Methods.—Adult female C57BL/KsJ-db mice, including genetically diabetic animals and their nondiabetic littermates, were used in the tests. The animals were fed either regular rat chow or a 1% protein diet for 1 or 2 weeks before receiving a full-thickness skin wound to the back. These wounds were then treated topically for 5 days with vehicle, platelet-derived growth factor (PDGF), 10 μg, or basic fibroblast growth factor (bFGF), 1 μg.

Results.—Wound analysis demonstrated significant impairment of wound closure in the malnourished animals. Wound closure was not enhanced by growth factors in the nondiabetic mice, regardless of whether they ate a normal or restricted diet. However, tissue repair was significantly enhanced by growth factors in the diabetic mice (table). The de-

Percent of Wound Closure in Diabetic Animals Fed Regular Chow (*Reg chow*) or 1% Protein Diet (PD) Ad Libitum Starting 1 Week Before Wounding and Continuing Until Death on Day 21

Treatment	Day 15	Day 18	Day 21	% Wt Δ*	Histologic score†
Reg chow (n = 7)	37.4 ± 10.1	54.1 ± 7.8	62.2 ± 8.4‡	−6.7 ± 5.1	8.2 ± 0.4
PD (n = 6)	42.6 ± 6.1	51.6 ± 3.5	41.2 ± 3.2	−27.0 ± 2.6	5.0 ± 1.0§
PD + bFGF (n = 5)	73.4 ± 4.0‖	82.8 ± 3.3‖	75.6 ± 4.8‡	−27.0 ± 1.2	8.4 ± 1.1
PD + PDGF (n = 9)	61.5 ± 4.9	80.0 ± 3.6‖	86.7 ± 2.7‖	−29.0 ± 1.2	6.6 ± 0.7

Notes: Values are expressed as mean ± standard error of mean. Wounds were treated topically with vehicle, bFGF (1 μg), or PDGF (10 μg) per day for 5 days, starting at wounding.
* Percentage of change in body weight from day of wounding until death.
† From wounds harvested at day 21.
‡ P < .05 vs. PD by RM-ANOVA and Tukey's test.
§ P < .05 vs. Reg chow or PD + bFGF by Kruskal-Wallis test.
‖ P < .05 vs. Reg chow or PD.
(Courtesy of Albertson S, Hummel RP III, Breeden M, et al: *Surgery* 114:368–372, 1993.)

creased cellularity and granulation tissue of the protein-depleted diabetic wounds were reversed by treatment with growth factors.

Conclusions.—In this study, growth factors enhanced healing in diabetic mice that ate a protein-restricted diet. No such effect was noted in their nondiabetic counterparts. The difference may be related to the different healing mechanisms of the 2 groups: contraction in the nondiabetic animals vs. formation of granulation tissue and reepithelialization in diabetic animals. Studies of this type may one day lead to strategies for optimizing healing in patients at risk for failed healing.

Application of Basic Fibroblast Growth Factor May Reverse Diabetic Wound Healing Impairment
Phillips LG, Abdullah KM, Geldner PD, Dobbins S, Ko F, Linares HA, Broemeling LD, Robson MC (Univ of Texas, Galveston)
Ann Plast Surg 31:331–334, 1993   140-94-9-10

Introduction.—Fibroblasts cultured from diabetic wounds are prematurely senescent with abnormal insulin receptors. Manipulation of the diabetic fibroblast may improve or reverse impairments in wound healing characteristic of patients with diabetes. The effect of the application of basic fibroblast growth factor (bFGF) in an animal model of diabetic-impaired wound healing was examined.

Methods.—The experiment used male Sprague-Dawley rats that were divided into 2 groups: normal (NL) and strepto-zotocin-induced diabetic (SD). With the animals under general anesthesia, a 6-cm dorsal incision was made through the skin and panniculus carnosus. Both NL and SD wounds were injected with 0.1 mL of 1 of 3 solutions: saline, growth factor vehicle, and 10 μg of bFGF. The wounds were then closed with interrupted, full-thickness sutures of 4-0 nylon. The animals were euthanized at 7, 10, 14, or 21 days after wounding. Breaking strength of the wound was assessed with the Instron Tensiometer 4201.

Results.—All NL wounds were stronger than all SD wounds at 7 and 10 days. By day 14, there were no differences between the NL and SD wounds treated with bFGF. The SD wounds treated with bFGF were statistically significantly stronger than both SD wounds injected with saline or vehicle, an advantage that persisted at least 21 days. Light microscopy examination of 21-day wound clefts revealed the bFGF-treated SD wound specimen to be narrow, mature, well-organized, and indistinguishable from an NL wound. These characteristics were not apparent in SD vehicle-treated wounds at 21 days.

Conclusion.—Because of the defect inherent to the diabetic fibroblast, bFGF is a logical choice for manipulation of diabetic wounds. Application of a 10-μg dose of bFGF might aid in the healing of these wounds.

Autocrine Control of Wound Repair by Insulin-Like Growth Factor I In Cultured Endothelial Cells
Taylor WR, Alexander RW (Emory Univ, Atlanta, Ga; Atlanta Veterans Affairs Med Ctr, Decatur, Ga)
Am J Physiol 265:801C–805C, 1993   140-94-9-11

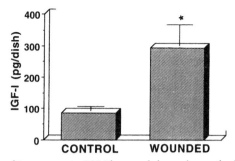

Fig 9–3.—Release of immunoreactive IGF-I by wounded monolayers of cultured endothelial cells. Confluent monolayers of endothelial cells were wounded and placed in medium supplemented with 10% fetal calf serum for 24 hours. The cells were then washed 3 times and placed in serum-free medium for 3 hours. Radioimmunoassay was used to measure IGF-I in conditioned medium. Results are from 5 experiments performed in triplicate. *P < .001. (Courtesy of Taylor WR, Alexander RW: *Am J Physiol* 265:801C–805C, 1993.)

Introduction.—During percutaneous transluminal coronary angioplasty, the endothelial surface of the artery is denuded and the underlying vessel is mechanically injured. In response to this injury, the vessel wall components proliferate. The regeneration process is regulated by both blood borne and endogenous growth factors. To increase understanding of the autocrine growth factors involved in endothelial cell wound repair, a tissue culture model of endothelial wounding was studied.

Methods.—Cultured porcine aortic endothelial monolayers were mechanically wounded by passing a sterile 7-mm glass rod over the culture surface. Autoradiography with labeled thymidine was used to quantify proliferation at the wound edge.

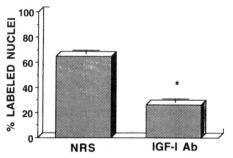

Fig 9–4.—Inhibition of autocrine growth by IGF-I antibody. Monolayers were wounded and processed. Cultures were treated with either nonimmune serum (NRS) or IGF-I antibody (IGF-I Ab) at 1:1,000 dilution. Control cultures were incubated with [³H]-thymidine in serum-free medium for 24 hours and wounded immediately before fixing. Autoradiography was performed, and proliferation was quantified by dividing the number of labeled cells by the total number of cells per high-power field. Results are from total of 3 experiments performed in duplicate. *P < .001. (Courtesy of Taylor WR, Alexander RW: *Am J Physiol* 265:801C–805C, 1993.)

Results.—In wounded cultures incubated in media supplemented with 10% fetal calf serum, a mean of 81% of the nuclei at the wound edge were labeled. In serum-free media, a mean of 65% nuclei at the wound edge were still labeled, indicating a significant autocrine component to wound repair. The potential role of insulin-like growth factor I (IGF-I) in the wound repair process was evaluated using a radioimmunoassay. There was nearly a 200% increase in production of IGF-I in wounded cultures compared to that in nonwounded cultures (Fig 9-3). When wounded cultures were incubated with inactivating concentrations of anti-IGF-I, only 26% of the wound edge nuclei were labeled (Fig 9-4).

Conclusions.—These results indicate there is a significant autocrine contribution to the control of the proliferative response of cultured endothelial monolayers to mechanical injury. The secretion of IGF-I is significantly increased in these wounded monolayers and appears to contribute to these autocrine mechanisms.

Exogenous Transforming Growth Factor-β_2 Enhances Connective Tissue Formation in Transforming Growth Factor-β_1-Deficient, Healing-Impaired Dermal Wounds in Mice
Ksander GA, Gerhardt CO, Olsen DR (Celtrix Pharmaceuticals, Inc, Santa Clara, Calif)
Wound Rep Reg 1:137–148, 1993   140-94-9-12

Introduction.—The transforming growth factor-β (TGF-β) appears to have a critical role in the regulation of development and tissue repair. In clinical reports, local topical treatment with exogenous TGF-β_2 has been beneficial in macular hole disease. The level of endogenous TGF-β_1 was compared in dressing-impaired wounds and air-exposed wounds in mice, and the response to treatment with exogenous TGF-β_1 and TGF-β_2 was characterized.

Methods.—Wounds were created in the mid-dorsum of adult female Swiss Webster mice. In a previous study, it was reported that connective tissue formation in full-thickness dermal wounds in mice and guinea pigs is severely impaired when the wounds are covered with synthetic, adherent, moisture vapor-permeable membrane (SAM). This dressing-induced impairment was reversed with exogenous TGF-β_1 or TGF-β_2. In this study, wounds were treated with a single application of TGF-β immediately after wounding and before application of SAM. At various periods, the wounds were excised and prepared for histologic, immunohistochemical, and histomorphometric investigation.

Results.—As reported previously, there was significantly less connective tissue in SAM-covered sites than in air-exposed wounds treated with 1.2 μg of TGF-β_1. Treatment at this dose significantly increased the amount of connective tissue in SAM-covered sites, but it had no effect on the amount of connective tissue in air-exposed wounds. This finding, confirmed by immunolocalization studies with an anti-TGF-β_1 antibody, indicated that the quantity of endogenous TGF-β_1 in SAM-covered wounds was less than that in air-exposed wounds. Histologic analysis confirmed that exogenous TGF-β_2 stimulates enhanced cellularity and connective tissue formation.

Conclusion.—Through a variety of mechanisms, TGF-β_2 stimulates repair in healing-impaired wounds that are also deficient in endogenous TGF-β_1. A single application of exogenous TGF-β_2 substitutes for the endogenous TGF-β_1 that is deficient in the SAM-covered wounds and can directly stimulate connective tissue formation.

Transforming Growth Factor-β Enhances Connective Tissue Repair in Perforated Rat Mesentery But Not Peritoneal Macrophage Chemotaxis
Franzén LE, Schultz GS (Univ Hosp, Linköping, Sweden; Univ of Florida, Gainesville)
Wound Rep Reg 1:149–155, 1993   140-94-9-13

Purpose.—The perforated rat mesentery model was used to examine the effect of transforming growth factor (TGF)-β on connective tissue

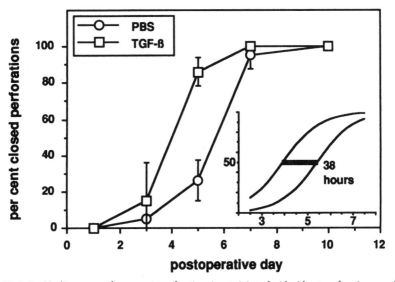

Fig 9–5.—Healing curves of mesenteric perforations in rats injected with either transforming growth factor-β (TGF-β) or phosphate-buffered saline solution for 4 days, beginning at the day of operation. The *inset* shows the curves after a logistic transformation of the values from days 3, 5, and 7. The estimated improvement in the time to reach 50% healing for the TGF-β group is 38 hours, as illustrated by the *horizontal line*. Each point represents the mean ± SEM. (Courtesy of Franzén LE, Schultz GS: *Wound Rep Reg* 1:149-155, 1993.)

repair. The influx of macrophages into the peritoneal cavity and their mitogenic activity were also assessed.

Methods.—Male rats were laparotomized, and mesenteric wounds were created with a scalpel. Intraperitoneal injection of .5 μg of TGF-β occurred daily for 2 or 4 days. After 1-10 days, the animals were injected with tritiated thymidine and then decapitated. Macrophages were collected by peritoneal washing, and the number of closed perforations were counted to assess connective tissue repair. Autoradiography was used to quantitate labeled cells.

Results.—Administration of TGF-β for either 2 or 4 days accelerated perforation closure on days 3–7 post injury (Fig 9-5). Laparotomy significantly increased leukocyte influx and macrophage-labeling index. However, administration of TGF-β did not significantly influence leukocyte influx or macrophage-labeling index.

Conclusions.—Transforming growth factor-β stimulated connective tissue repair in the perforated rat mesentery. This effect was not exerted through an increase in macrophage number, but the actual mechanism of this effect remains unknown.

Epidermal Growth Factor Promotes Wound Repair of Human Respiratory Epithelium
Zahm J-M, Pierrot D, Puchelle E (INSERM U314, Université de Reims, France)
Wound Rep Reg 1:175–180, 1993   140-94-9–14

Introduction.—Reepithelialization of the airway mucosa is essential for the repair of airway epithelial wounds. Epidermal growth factor (EGF) is a peptide that stimulates cell proliferation and is found in the lung. The effect of growth factors (e.g., EGF) on the wound repair process of respiratory epithelium has not been studied. Therefore, an in vitro human surface respiratory epithelium wound repair model was used to study the effect of EGF on wound repair.

Methods.—Human surface epithelial cells were cultured from nasal polyp explants on a type I collagen gel in defined serum-free media. After mechanical injury, image analysis techniques were used to measure outgrowth area, ciliated surface, ciliary beating frequency, and rate of wound repair in the presence of 0, 5, 10 and 20 ng of EGF per mL.

Results.—There was a significant dose-dependent increase in the outgrowth area (Fig 9-6), the percentage of surface covered by ciliated cells, and the ciliary beating frequency. At 10 ng of EGF per mL, the wound repair rate was increased by 29%.

Conclusions.—Epidermal growth factor may play an important role in the regeneration of respiratory epithelium after injury. Epidermal growth factor may prove to be an effective treatment for respiratory epithelial wounds, after its in vivo efficacy is assessed in animal trials.

Outgrowth area (mm²)

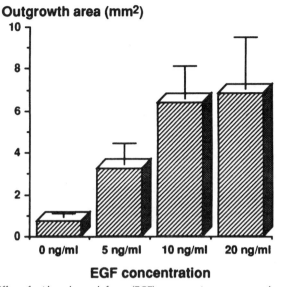

EGF concentration

Fig 9–6.—Effect of epidermal growth factor (EGF) concentrations on outgrowth area obtained from human nasal polyp explants. *Bars* represent mean of 10 measurements. An increase in EGF concentration induced a significant increase ($P < .05$) in the outgrowth area. (Courtesy of Zahm J-M, Pierrot D, Puchelle E: *Wound Rep Reg* 1:175–180, 1993.)

Regulation of Collagen Synthesis and Messenger RNA Levels in Normal and Hypertrophic Scar Fibroblasts In Vitro by Interferon Alfa-2b

Tredget EE, Shen YJ, Liu G, Forsyth N, Smith C, Harrop AR, Scott PG, Ghahary A (Univ of Alberta, Edmonton, Canada)
Wound Rep Reg 1:156–165, 1993   140-94-9-15

Introduction.—Hypertrophic scars (HTS) and keloids, dermal forms of fibroproliferative disorders, commonly occur after thermal and traumatic injury of the skin. In these conditions, components of the inflammatory process appear to activate dormant fibroblasts leading to cellular proliferation and excessive matrix synthesis. The effect of interferon on collagen metabolism has been examined in normal tissues and other fibroproliferative disorders, but no previous study has investigated the potential benefits of interferon (IFN) α-2b in HTS fibroblasts after burn injury.

Methods.—Four patients who were burned with HTS agreed to have dermal biopsy specimens taken for analysis. With the biopsy area under local anesthesia, 6-mm punch biopsy specimens were obtained from HTS that were hyperemic, raised, thickened, and pruritic. Biopsy specimens of uninjured normal skin were also taken from each patient at an anatomical site matched to the burn site. Fibroblast cultures were prepared and exposed to IFN α-2b.

Results.—In both HTS and normal fibroblasts, IFN α-2b reduced collagen protein synthesis and type I messenger RNA levels. These changes were not apparent, however, until after approximately 72 hours. Four pairs of normal and HTS fibroblasts showed significant reductions in collagen synthesis, accompanied by significant reductions in type I but not type III procollagen messenger RNA. In contrast to normal skin fibroblasts, HTS fibroblasts recovered completely from the effects of IFN α-2b on procollagen type I messenger RNA within 48 hours after treatment was discontinued; the reduction in type I procollagen messenger RNA persisted beyond 72 hours in normal skin fibroblasts treated with IFN α-2b.

Conclusion.—Collagen synthesis is reduced in both normal and hypertrophic fibroblasts by IFN α-2b, although the hypertrophic fibroblast may remain less sensitive to the growth factor. Findings have implications for the dosage and duration of IFN α-2b therapy in patients with burn-related HTS.

Clinical Aspects of Wound Healing

Clinical and Experimental Studies of Cigarette Smoking in Microvascular Tissue Transfers

Gu Y-D, Zhang G-M, Zhang L-Y, Li G-F, Jiang J-F (Shanghai Med Univ, People's Republic of China)
Microsurgery 14:391–397, 1993   140-94-9-16

Background.—The harmful effects of cigarette smoking on the circulatory system are well documented. Recently, the harmful effect of smoking on the microcirculation of replanted toes has been reported. Three patients who underwent free tissue transfer and had postoperative circulatory crisis caused by cigarette smoke were studied. Animal experiments that demonstrate the harmful effects of smoking on the healing of endothelia at the anastomotic vessel site were described.

Complete Coverage Rate of Sutures at Different Postoperative Times

	24 hr		48 hr		120 hr		240 hr	
Group †	No.	Percent‡	No.	Percent	No.	Percent	No.	Percent
Con	9	28	10	31	20	64	28	87
Before	6	19	7	22	7	22	12	37
After	5	16	6	18	7	22	9	28

Note: χ2 test: At 24 and 48 hours between Con, Before, and After, $P > .05$. At 120 and 240 hours, Con vs. Before and After, $P < .01$. Before vs. After, $P > .05$.
† Con, control group; *Before,* preoperative smoking group; *After,* the postoperative smoking group.
‡ No. means the number of sutures that were completely covered by various components. Percent represents the number of sutures being completely covered/32—the number of sutures of 4 anastomotic sites of 2 rats—× 100%.
(Courtesy of Gu Y-D, Zhang G-M, Zhang L-Y, et al: *Microsurgery* 14:391–397, 1993.)

Case Report.—Patient, 36, who was a 1-pack/day smoker, had a crushed left thumb. The patient stopped smoking for 1 week before reconstruction of the thumb with a second toe transfer. Vessel condition was good, and dissection and anastomosis were satisfactory. The patient's condition was excellent until 50 hours post surgery, when the patient smoked 1 cigarette. One hour later, the skin temperature decreased, the skin color became pale, swelling appeared, and capillary back flow decreased. Spasm of the anastomotic site and distal artery were discovered, and thrombosis was suspected. Reanastomosis was performed, but necrosis developed.

Methods.—Fifty-eight male Wistar rats were randomly divided into 3 groups: preoperative smoking group, postoperative smoking group, and control group. All rats underwent carotid artery anastomosis.

Results.—The complete suture covering rate was significantly higher in the control group than in either of the smoking groups (table). After 5 days, the endothelium filling rate in the needle holes was 75% in the control group, but it was only 16% in the preoperative smoking group and 19% in the postoperative smoking group.

Conclusions.—Circulatory crisis caused by smoking is a significant cause of failure in patients with microvascular tissue transfer. Patients must be educated on the harmful effect of active and passive smoking, and all smoking must be prohibited around these patients.

▶ You cannot overemphasize to your patients the importance of smoking cessation before and after surgery. With regards to microvascular surgery, nicotine has been shown to cause vasoconstriction of the cutaneous blood vessels, impaired endothelialization of the vascular anastamosis, and promotion of platelet deposition at vascular anastamotic sites. Even passive smoke can lead to circulatory crisis in a microvascular tissue transplant.—W.W. Souba, M.D., Sc.D.

Organization and Development of a University Multidisciplinary Wound Care Clinic
Steed DL, Edington H, Moosa HH, Webster MW (Univ of Pittsburgh, Pa)
Surgery 114:775–779, 1993   140-94-9–17

Introduction.—Leg ulcers are a major public health problem in the United States. The cost of treating these wounds is estimated to exceed 1 billion dollars annually. Researchers describe the establishment of a multidisciplinary wound care clinic and its benefits to patients and to physicians in training.

Methods.—The Wound Healing/Limb Preservation Clinic at the University of Pittsburgh was organized as an outpatient facility staffed by the departments of surgery, vascular surgery, and dermatology. The clinic's operations are coordinated by a full-time research nurse clinician. Patients also have access to other members of the wound care team, including a plastic surgeon, an orthopedist, a podiatrist, a pedorthist, and specialists in hyperbaric medicine and in the fitting of compression stockings and pumps. The clinic was established in response to a number of perceived needs: an underserved patient population, continuity of care, training of personnel interested in wound care, evaluation of therapies, and basic science research in the area.

Results.—During the clinic's first 4 years and 3 months of operation, 683 patients with nonhealing wounds of the lower extremities were evaluated. Duration of the ulcer before the visit to the clinic ranged from 1 month to 62 years. The primary causes of ulcers were venous stasis (41%), diabetic neuropathy (27%), and arterial insufficiency (17%). Patients underwent 179 operations, including 86 operating room débridements, 48 amputations, 23 arterial bypasses, and 14 skin grafts. Twelve patients received hyperbaric oxygen therapy, and 56 were admitted to the hospital for intravenous antibiotic treatment of cellulitis. The overall rate of wound healing for the 261 patients with complete follow-up was 54%. To date, 132 patients have been entered into randomized, prospective trials of topical growth factors.

Conclusion.—The Wound Healing/Limb Preservation Clinic offers a multidisciplinary approach that has benefited patients with chronic leg ulcers. Patient compliance has improved; residents and nurses have gained valuable experience; and new information on the pathogenesis and management of problem leg ulcers has been generated.

▶ Multidisciplinary clinics offer benefits to both the patients and the physicians involved in the effort. They foster the development of clinical trials and provide a mechanism by which data from all patients can be maintained in a centralized fashion. Invariably, they tend to provide better care from the standpoint that multiple disciplines are involved in diagnosis, treatment strategies, and follow-up. A cooperative, multidisciplinary-care, patient-focused approach will have several advantages in a capitation health care model.—W.W. Souba, M.D., Sc.D.

Suture Length to Wound Length Ratio and Healing of Midline Laparotomy Incisions
Israelsson LA, Jonsson T (Univ of Lund, Sweden)
Br J Surg 80:1284–1286, 1993   140-94-9-18

Introduction.—Continuous suture techniques for the closure of midline laparotomy incisions are both rapid and safe. Although several studies have examined the question of suture length, an optimal ratio of suture length to wound length has not been established. In a prospective study, researchers sought to determine how this ratio affects healing of midline laparotomy wounds.

Patients and Methods.—Subjects were 454 patients who underwent abdominal procedures through a midline incision from August 1989 to March 1991. The length of the incision was measured after closure of the fascia, and the length of suture remnants was determined to calculate the ratio of suture length to wound length. Wound infections were classified as major or minor. At 12 months after surgery, surviving patients were examined for the presence of incisional hernia.

Results.—The mean length of the incision was 27 cm, and the mean ratio of suture length to wound length was 3.6. The incidence of minor and major wound infection was 4% and was not affected by the suture length to wound length ratio. Follow-up was possible in 363 patients. The overall incidence of incisional hernia 1 year after surgery was 18.7%. When the ratio of suture length to wound length was less than 4, hernia occurred in 23.7% of the patients. In contrast, the incidence of hernia was only 9% when the ratio was greater than or equal to 4. These 2 groups of patients with hernia were similar in other recorded variables including age, degree of contamination, suture material used, and mean length of incision. Multivariate analysis identified suture length to wound length ratio, age, and major wound infection as independent risk factors for the development of hernia.

Conclusion.—Continuous suturing gives the best results when the ratio of suture length to wound length is 4:1. A ratio greater than or equal to 4 results in a lower incidence of hernia in patients with midline laparotomy incisions.

▶ This paper suggests that the likelihood of a midline incisional hernia developing can be reduced by suturing the fascia of the wound with a ratio greater than or equal to 4. In other words, the length of suture material used in closing the fascia should be greater than 4 times the length of the wound. The study suggests that the incidence of incisional hernia is 2.5 times greater when the ratio was less than 4. Presumably, such lower ratios result in enough fascial ischemia to lead to necrosis and, apparently, development of a hernia in the fascia.

The amount of suture one uses when closing a midline wound in a running fashion depends on the size of the fascial bites, as well as on the spacing of the sutures and the extent to which the running stitch is "tightened up" during the suturing. A more carefully designed study would sort out these different factors, because each of them could independently influence the development of a hernia.

Excluding the suture length used for tying the knots at either end of the incision and assuming that (1) facial sutures are placed exactly 1 cm from the edge; (2) fascial sutures are placed exactly 1 cm apart; and (3) the fascia is exactly 2 mm thick, one can calculate that the ratio of suture length to wound length needed for a closure that opposes the fascia without any tension is 4.68. It would also be important to define a ratio that was too large, because wounds that are closed too loosely can also result in an incisional hernia.—W.W. Souba, M.D., Sc.D.

Hyaluronate Metabolism Undergoes an Ontogenic Transition During Fetal Development: Implications for Scar-Free Wound Healing

Estes JM, Adzick NS, Harrison MR, Longaker MT, Stern R (Univ of California, San Francisco)
J Pediatr Surg 28:1227–1231, 1993   140-94-9-19

Background.—In contrast to the scar formation that characterizes healing in the adult, fetal cutaneous wounds heal through a regenerative process that totally restores the normal architecture of the skin. Hyaluronic acid (HA) is a prominent component of the fetal extracellular matrix, and it may have a key role in regeneration.

Methods.—Fluid samples from wounds were aspirated from subcutaneous cylinders placed in fetal and adult sheep 3, 7, and 14 days after implantation. The fluids were analyzed by using sensitive assays for both HA and HA-stimulating activity (HASA).

Findings.—The levels of both HA and HASA were higher in fetal than in adult wound fluids. The difference was most marked when fluids were sampled at 75 and 100 days' gestation (Fig 9–7). These samples contained elevated amounts of HA and HASA for up to 2 weeks after wounding. The levels of HA were significantly lower in wound fluid taken at 120 days' gestation, and they also were more transient. The level

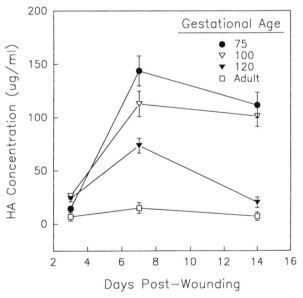

Fig 9–7.—Levels of HA in fetal and adult wound fluid in micrograms per milliliter. Fluid obtained from Hunt-Schilling wound chambers in fetal and adult sheep was assayed for HA at 3, 7, and 14 days post wounding. Samples were taken and averaged from 3 to 4 wound cylinders in each of 2 animals and are expressed as mean and standard deviation. (Courtesy of Estes JM, Adzick NS, Harrison MR, et al: *J Pediatr Surg* 28:1227–1231, 1993.)

of HASA as related to the interval after wound production correlated with the level of HA. Wounds healed without scarring before 120 days' gestation, but there was scarring after this time.

Interpretation.—High levels of HA and HASA in wound fluid correlate with the scar-free fetal wound healing in this ovine model. The findings support a mechanistic function for HA and the factors that regulate its deposition during tissue repair.

Fetal Wound Healing: The Ontogeny of Scar Formation in the Non-Human Primate
Lorenz HP, Whitby DJ, Longaker MT, Adzick NS (Univ of California, San Francisco)
Ann Surg 217:391–396, 1993   140-94-9-20

Introduction.—Because the fetus has unique healing characteristics, there has been interest in the repair of human facial defects in utero when scarring and fibrosis do not occur. Before such procedures can be attempted, however, several questions about the biology of fetal repair must be considered. A model of fetal wound healing was developed by using the rhesus monkey to determine how scar formation develops.

Methods.—Full-thickness wounds were created in fetal rhesus monkey lips from 75 through 114 days' gestation. Control adult incisional wounds were made on the maternal thorax. The fetal lip wounds were harvested at 14 days post wounding and prepared for histologic and immunohistochemical studies. Sections for histology were stained with either hematoxylin-a eosin or Masson's trichrome; an indirect immunohistochemical technique was used to stain for human type I or type III collagen.

Results.—All wounds had completely healed in 14 days, with restoration of epidermal and dermal continuity. In the fetus of 75 days' gestation, lip wounds healed with complete restoration of normal tissue architecture. However, in the fetuses of 85 to 100 days' gestation, the wounds healed with an absence of hair follicles and sebaceous glands. The dermal collagen pattern in these fetuses remained reticular and similar to that in unwounded dermis. At 107 days, a thin scar was observed in the wound, indicating a transition to scar formation between 100 and 107 days gestation in the nonhuman primate. With term at 165 days, this transition occurs early in the third trimester. All adult wounds healed with scar formation.

Conclusion.—A transition from scarless repair characteristic of fetal wound healing to adult-type repair with scar formation occurs early in the third trimester in the nonhuman primate. The process of transition is gradual, spanning several weeks in the primate fetus. The transition wound, not previously described, has a pattern that is neither regeneration nor classic scar. If these findings could be extrapolated to the human fetus, it would mean that in utero repair during the third trimester would be associated with classic scar formation and contracture.

▶ The absence of scarring in fetal wounds has been correlated with a sparse inflammatory response (reduced infiltration macrophages and monocytes), reduced angiogenesis, and the absence of certain growth factors, including transforming growth factor-β and basic fibroblast growth factor. Fibrosis and angiogenesis are 2 features of adult wound repair that are not evident in scarless fetal healing. With time, in utero, there is a sequential loss of regenerative capabilities in nonhuman primate fetal skin. Hyaluronic acid is a mucopolysaccharide that appears to play a central role in wound healing with regards to the organization and structure of the extracellular matrix. It also facilitates cellular proliferation and motility, and promotes the maintenance of the undifferentiated state during the early stages of embryonic organ development. The observation that fetal wound fluids contain significantly higher quantities of HA than do fluids from adult wounds suggests an important mechanistic function for this mucopolysaccharide in promoting scarless repair in utero. However, last in gestation, this capacity is lost and a transition from scarless repair to adult-type repair occurs early in the third trimester. As human fetal surgery becomes more established, the possibility of intervention becomes more feasible, and it appears that the timing of repair to ensure scarless healing will be quite important.—W.W. Souba, M.D., Sc.D.

10 Gastrointestinal

Esophagus

INTRODUCTION

It has long been recognized that Barrett's esophagus is related in some way to excessive gastroesophageal reflux. Recent studies have attempted to define and quantitate those abnormalities that characterize patients with reflux who have Barrett's esophagus compared with those who do not have the disease. Several have been identified: increased exposure to both acid and alkaline refluxate, a significantly lowered lower esophageal sphincter pressure, a significantly shorter lower esophageal sphincter length, more nonpropulsive contractions in the distal esophagus, and a greater degree of duodenogastric reflux. It is generally thought that in these patients, even the most successful antireflux procedure does not reverse the underlying pathology or protect against the development of adenocarcinoma. A recent study (Abstract 140-94-10-2) suggests, however, that repeated episodes of photoablation associated with potent suppression of gastric acid secretion can accomplish the former goal and may, therefore, interdict the latter result.

There is continuing interest regarding the use of adjuvant and neoadjuvant therapy in patients with potentially resectable carcinoma of the esophagus. Esophageal endosonography may be an important methodology for selecting and stratifying patients, especially for neoadjuvant therapy It is highly sensitive and specific with respect to defining the depth of esophageal involvement and predicting the presence of lymph node metastases. Unfortunately, the technique appears to be unreliable in detecting tumor infiltration into mediastinal organs such as the trachea. More important, it cannot be accomplished in up to one third of patients preoperatively because of luminal narrowing. Neoadjuvant radiation therapy has recently been tested in a large Scandinavian study (Abstract 140-94-10-4). The data suggest that there is a small but real benefit to this approach. On the other hand, a large phase III trial (Abstract 140-94-10-5) evaluating cisplatin-based neoadjuvant chemotherapy produced extremely disappointing results, including greater morbidity, increased postoperative mortality, and no survival benefit. Similarly, a well-designed prospective trial of adjuvant radiotherapy for this disease was equally disappointing (Abstract 140-94-10-6). It demonstrated increased morbidity and mortality associated with early appearance of metastatic disease and reduced overall survival.

It is always wise to obtain objective information in patients seen with esophageal symptoms suggestive of gastroesophageal reflux disease. In almost half, some other cause or no cause whatsoever may be discovered. Whether to add an antireflux procedure to the repair of paraesophageal hiatus hernias remains controversial. One experienced group believes that this should be accomplished only selectively. In their hands, the outcome is excellent. Only 2 of the 100 patients who underwent anatomical repair without an associated antireflux procedure had reflux postoperatively. In a similar vein, it has recently been suggested that it is unnecessary to add a "completion" myotomy to the surgical repair of esophageal perforations secondary to pneumatic dilation for achalasia because, in many patients, dysphagia is completely relieved in the long term by this approach (Abstracts 140-94-10-8 and 140-94-10-9). The addition of fundoplication to elective myotomy in patients with achalasia continues to excite debate. A recent 2- to 6-year evaluation of patients undergoing total (360-degree) gastric wrap showed that the vast majority of patients will experience progressive dysphagia after this procedure. Furthermore, as many as 30% may require reoperation. Whether a similar untoward result accompanies less-than-total fundoplication remains to be determined.

Wallace P. Ritchie, Jr., M.D., Ph.D.

Functional Foregut Abnormalities in Barrett's Esophagus
Stein HJ, Hoeft S, DeMeester TR (Univ of Southern California, Los Angeles)
J Thorac Cardiovasc Surg 105:107–111, 1993   140-94-10-1

Background.—Patients with gastroesophageal reflux disease are predisposed to the development of Barrett's esophagus. The factors underlying this predisposition are not well understood.

Methods and Findings.—In 15 patients with Barrett's esophagus, 24 with esophagitis, and 22 healthy persons, the symptoms, esophageal acid and alkaline exposure, lower esophageal sphincter resistance, esophageal clearance function, gastric secretory state, gastric emptying, and duodenogastric reflux were assessed. Compared with patients with esophagitis, patients with Barrett's esophagus had less heartburn and regurgitation but a greater frequency and duration of reflux episodes and percent of time that pH was less than 2, 3, and 4 and greater than 7 on ambulatory 24-hour esophageal pH monitoring (Fig 10–1). Patients with Barrett's esophagus also had a reduced lower esophageal sphincter resistance and contraction amplitude in the distal region of the esophagus. An increased frequency of nonperistaltic contractions and contractions less than 30 mm Hg on 24-hour ambulatory esophageal motility monitoring, increased basal and stimulated gastric acid secretion, and a greater prevalence of excessive duodenogastric reflux were also noted in patients with Barrett's esophagus.

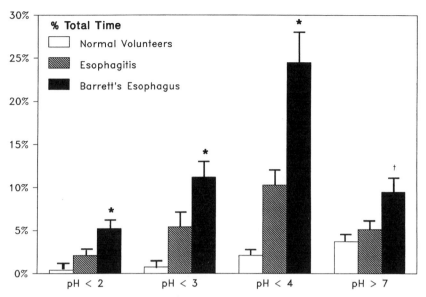

Fig 10–1.—Mean esophageal acid and alkaline exposure on ambulatory 24-hour esophageal pH monitoring in normal volunteers, patients with esophagitis, and patients with Barret's esophagus. *P < .01 vs. esophagitis and normal volunteers; †P < .05 vs. esophagitis and normal volunteers. (Courtesy of Stein HJ, Hoeft S, DeMeester TR: *J Thorac Cardiovasc Surg* 105:107–111, 1993.)

Conclusion.—Although patients with Barrett's esophagus have fewer symptoms than those with esophagitis, the former group has a substantially greater esophageal acid and alkaline exposure. This appears to result from persistent reflux of highly concentrated gastric acid and duodenal contents across a mechanically defective lower esophageal sphincter in combination with inefficient esophageal clearance function.

▶ For many years, this productive group has been in the forefront of defining and quantitating those abnormalities of gastroesophageal function that predispose to Barrett's esophagus in some patients with gastroesophageal reflux but not in others. Using very sophisticated methodologies, these authors indicate that there is a plethora of differences. In addition to the previously described increased exposure to both acid and alkaline refluxate when compared with patients with esophagitis only and with healthy individuals, patients with Barrett's esophagus have significantly lowered resting pressures, a significantly shorter lower esophageal sphincter length, significantly more nonpropulsive contractions (which are also weaker) in the distal esophagus, a greater gastric acid output, and more duodenogastric reflux on gastric pH monitoring. All of this points, in my opinion, to virulent and end-stage gastroesophageal reflux disease. Of interest is the authors' recommendation that in view of the compromised contractility of the distal esophagus, the best approach is a Colles gastroplasty associated with a Belsey repair. Many surgeons would demur, believing that a floppy Nissen performed in the abdomen is quite efficacious, even if the esophagus is modestly foreshortened.—W.P. Ritchie, Jr., M.D., Ph.D.

Restoration of Squamous Mucosa After Ablation of Barrett's Esophageal Epithelium

Berenson MM, Johnson TD, Markowitz NR, Buchi KN, Samowitz WS (Salt Lake City VA Med Ctr, Utah; Univ of Utah, Salt Lake City)
Gastroenterology 104:1686–1691, 1993   140-94-10-2

Background.—The source of the tissue in Barrett's esophagus is most likely metaplastic, and metaplastic epithelium has the theoretical potential to revert to normal. It was hypothesized that squamous epithelium could be restored in patients with Barrett's esophagus if the columnar tissue characteristic of the condition was ablated while gastric acid secretion was suppressed.

Patients and Methods.—Ten men ranging in age from 27 to 72 years were studied. All had symptomatic gastroesophageal reflux disease of 5 to 25 years' duration and esophageal columnar tissue repeatedly documented for periods of 1 to 11 years. During treatment with 40 mg of omeprazole daily, the patients underwent videotaped endoscopies at 2- to 5-week periods to argon laser photoablate the columnar tissue, obtain biopsy specimens, and assess results. Areas of ablation were specified as islands, tongues, extensions, or patches. Patients remained in the study for periods ranging from 6 weeks to 38 weeks.

Results.—Most ablated areas were retreated 1 to 6 times. After a single treatment, nearly all areas showed endoscopic evidence of partial or complete re-epithelialization with squamous tissue. Biopsy specimens confirmed endoscopic assessments in all but 1 instance. A biopsy specimen showed squamous regrowth over a bed of granulation tissue. Another biopsy specimen revealed glandular mucosa persisting beneath stratified squamous tissue. The only complication reported was mild retrosternal pain for 2–3 days after laser treatment.

Conclusion.—Esophageal columnar epithelium is known to be premalignant. Regression of the columnar epithelium and restoration of squamous esophageal mucosa was accomplished in these patients with Barrett's esophagus by a combination of omeprazole and argon laser ablation. It was speculated that suppression of acid reflux allowed the multipotential precursor cell to differentiate normally. Long-term follow-up in larger patient groups is needed before photoablation can be accepted as a therapy for Barrett's epithelium.

▶ This study is interesting, although it is unlikely to have much clinical applicability, at least in the near future. It is widely accepted that even the most stringent program of nonoperative therapy and the most carefully performed and eminently successful antireflux procedures do not interdict the small but real probability of the development of adenocarcinoma in Barrett's esophagus. Furthermore, there is little evidence that either approach causes regression of the disease. In this study, however, the authors demonstrate that, for a relatively short period at least, repeated episodes of photoablation therapy associated with potent suppression of gastric acid secretion can accomplish this last goal in some patients. True clinical efficacy, however, will rest on the demonstration that similar results can be achieved long term and that all areas of Barrett's epithelium can be ablated using these techniques.—W.P. Ritchie, Jr., M.D., Ph.D.

Endosonography in Patient Selection for Surgical Treatment of Esophageal Carcinoma
Fok M, Cheng SWK, Wong J (Univ of Hong Kong)
World J Surg 16:1098–1103, 1992   140-94-10-3

Objective.—In patients with esophageal cancer, the findings at endosonography (ES) have been found to correlate well with the surgical findings. Still to be determined, however, is whether the information provided by ES results in any change in treatment. The usefulness of ES in the preoperative staging of patients with esophageal carcinoma, how

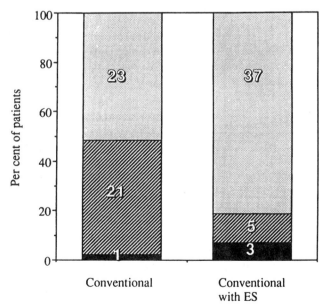

Fig 10–2.—Proportions of correct staging, understaging, and overstaging made by conventional methods of preoperative assessment and with endosonography (ES). The accuracy of conventional staging is 51%, and the accuracy of ES is 82%. *Numbers* in the bar charts indicate number of patients. *Open squares,* correct stage; *striped squares,* understaged; *filled squares,* overstaged. (Courtesy of Fok M, Cheng SWK, Wong J: *World J Surg* 16:1098–1103, 1992).

it affects the decision to resect, and whether it predicts the type of resection were analyzed in a prospective study.

Methods.—The study sample comprised 89 consecutive, unselected patients with esophageal cancer. In each, disease was staged by both the conventional preoperative methods and the new American Joint Commission of Cancer operative staging classification. Sixty-two patients underwent resection, 22 had a bypass operation, and 5 had no operation. Endosonography was attempted in all patients, but the examination was unsuccessful in 19 cases because of total or near-total obliteration of the esophageal lumen, and it was incomplete in 13 cases because of distal tumor obstruction. The analysis was focused on the 45 patients who had a satisfactory ES examination and a transthoracic resection.

Results.—Endosonography had a sensitivity of 89% in defining the depth of esophageal involvement and a specificity of 96%. The sensitivity and specificity for lymph node metastasis were 85% and 86%, respectively. However, ES was not able to detect tumor infiltration to mediastinal organs and the extent of intra-abdominal spread. Preoperative staging with ES had an accuracy of 82%, compared with just 51% for conventional staging (Fig 10-2). In 31% of patients, ES correctly identified a more advanced stage of disease than conventional staging. However, ES made no difference in the evaluation of resectability or in the prediction of whether resection was curative or palliative.

Conclusion.—Endosonography is an accurate method for staging the depth of esophageal involvement and lymph node metastases in patients with esophageal carcinomas. However, for patients in whom surgery is the preferred method of treatment, even if it is to be only palliative, ES has not helped in guiding the decision to operate or what type of resection to perform.

▶ This study indicates that in patients with esophageal carcinoma in whom it can be performed successfully, ES is highly sensitive and specific with respect to defining the depth of esophageal involvement and predicting the presence of lymph node metastases. As such, it should prove useful in stratifying patients for studies of neoadjuvant therapy in this otherwise dismal disease. There are 3 caveats, however. First, an accurate ES evaluation may not be possible in up to one third of patients because of luminal narrowing. Second, ES is unreliable in detecting tumor infiltration into mediastinal organs (e.g., the trachea) and in identifying intra-abdominal disease. Finally, in this series at least, the results of ES evaluation did not affect the decision of whether to operate (or the type of operation to be performed) in patients in whom surgery was judged to be the appropriate method of treatment based on conventional staging technologies. All this aside, the bottom line is well stated in an accompanying editorial, which can be paraphrased as follows: For the information to be useful, it must be used.—W.P. Ritchie, Jr., M.D., Ph.D.

Pre-Operative Radiotherapy Prolongs Survival in Operable Esophageal Carcinoma: A Randomized, Multicenter Study of Pre-Operative Radiotherapy and Chemotherapy: The Second Scandinavian Trial in Esophageal Cancer

Nygaard K, Hagen S, Hansen HS, Hatlevoll R, Hultborn R, Jakobsen A, Mäntyla M, Modig H, Munck-Wikland E, Rosengren B, Tausjφ J, Elgen K (Ullevaal Hosp, Oslo, Norway; Norwegian Radium Hosp, Oslo, Norway; Rikshospitalet, Oslo, Norway; et al)

World J Surg 16:1104–1110, 1992   140-94-10-4

Background.—Surgery is generally recommended for patients with squamous cell carcinoma of the esophagus who are judged operable. However, because the prognosis after surgical resection is poor, adjuvant therapy has been used in a number of trials. The nature of these studies

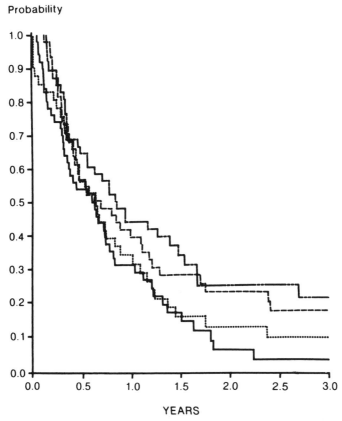

Probability

YEARS

Fig 10–3.—Actuarial survival curves for 4 treatment groups. Group 1, *dotted line;* group 2, *solid line;* group 3, *long and short dashed line;* and group 4, *dashed line.* (Courtesy of Nygaard K, Hagen S, Hansen HS, et al: *World J Surg* 16:1104–1110, 1992.)

Probability of Being Alive After Start of Treatment in Each of 4 Groups

Group	Time after treatment		
	12 months	24 months	36 months
1	0.34	0.13	0.09
2	0.31	0.06	0.03
3	0.44	0.25	0.21
4	0.39	0.23	0.17
1 + 2	0.32	0.09	0.06
3 + 4	0.42	0.24	0.19

(Courtesy of Nygaard K, Hagen S, Hansen HE, et al: *World J Surg* 16:1104–1110, 1992.)

has made it difficult to draw definite conclusions as to the value of such therapy. The effects of combined treatment in esophageal carcinoma were examined in a multicenter trial.

Methods.—Eligibility criteria for patients with histologically verified squamous cell carcinoma of the esophagus included age younger than 75 years, Karnofsky performance state 50; no other diseases contraindicating surgery; and tumor stage T1 or T2, NX, MO, located at least 21 cm from the incisor teeth or below the fifth thoracic vertebra. The 186 eligible patients were randomized to receive surgery alone (group 1); preoperative chemotherapy and surgery (group 2); preoperative irradiation and surgery (group 3); or preoperative chemotherapy, radiation therapy, and surgery (group 4). Chemotherapy consisted of 2 cycles of cisplatin and bleomycin. Radiation therapy, at a total of 35 Gy, was given in 20 fractions over 4 weeks. A standard combined laparotomy and right-sided thoracotomy was the surgical approach.

Results.—Chemotherapy caused nausea and vomiting in most patients, and 8 did not complete the regimen. All patients completed radiation therapy. The incidence of postoperative complications and the number of leakages in anastomoses were similar for the 4 groups. Overall, the postoperative mortality rate (death within 1 month after operation) was 15%; the rate was 13% in group 1, 15% in group 2, 11% in group 3, and 24% in group 4. Actuarial survival curves for the 4 treatment groups for up to 3 years are shown in Figure 10–3. Esophageal resection was classified as being curative in 82 patients, and these patients had a significantly better survival than those having a palliative resection. Three-year survival was significantly higher in pooled groups receiving radiation therapy, compared with the pooled groups not receiving such treatment. Preoperative chemotherapy did not improve survival, and there was no interaction between radiation therapy and chemotherapy. Women had a significantly better survival rate than men. The probabilities of being alive at various time intervals are shown in the table.

Conclusion.—Preoperative irradiation significantly improved intermediate-term survival in patients with esophageal carcinoma. The chemotherapy regimen used, however, yielded no benefit and may have contributed to morbidity and mortality.

▶ The need for effective adjuvant or neoadjuvant therapy in patients with squamous cell carcinoma of the esophagus is obvious. This large Scandinavian study of preoperative chemotherapy and radiotherapy has a number of virtues: (1) An appropriate control group (surgery alone) was included; (2) relatively large numbers of patients were enrolled; (3) standard regimens were evaluated; and (4) statistical analysis was rigorous. Although, like any human enterprise, it can be criticized on a number of grounds (and Dr. T.R. DeMeester does so with vigor in an accompanying editorial), none of its faults are fatal, in my view. The data suggest that, in this disease, there is a small but real benefit to preoperative radiotherapy but not to preoperative chemotherapy, even in combination with radiotherapy. As the accompanying figures indicate, however, the overall prognosis is still miserable. How to improve it further is still a very cogent question.—W.P. Ritchie, Jr., M.D., Ph.D.

Randomized Trial of Preoperative Chemotherapy for Squamous Cell Cancer of the Esophagus
Schlag PM, for the Chirurgische Arbeitsgemeinschaft fuer Onkologie der Deutschen Gesellschaft fuer Chirurgie Study Group (Univ of Heidelberg, Germany)
Arch Surg 127:1446–1450, 1992   140-94-10–5

Objective.—Seventy-seven patients with histologically proved squamous cell cancer of the esophagus, who were considered to be potentially curable by surgery alone, participated in a phase III trial of preoperative chemotherapy. The patients were younger than 68 years of age and had a Karnofsky performance status greater than 70%. None had evidence of distant metastasis.

Treatment.—Only 46 patients agreed to randomization. Twenty-four patients were randomized to undergo immediate surgery alone. Tumors confined to the esophagogastric junction were treated by abdominothoracic esophagectomy. The others underwent surgery via a thoracoabdominocervical approach. The celiac, paraesophageal, and paratracheal nodes were resected and continuity was restored by interposing stomach tissue. The remaining 22 randomized patients received fluorouracil and cisplatin preoperatively. Fluorouracil was given by infusion in a dose of 1 g per m² daily for 5 days. Cisplatin was infused in a dose of 20 mg per m² on days 1-5. Treatment was repeated twice at 3-week intervals if there was at least a minor response to initial treatment. Thirteen patients who did not agree to randomization chose to receive chemotherapy before surgery, whereas 18 chose surgery alone. In all, 34 of the patients received chemotherapy.

Results.—Two patients died preoperatively of treatment-related myelotoxicity. Two others had severe myelotoxicity, and 1 had marked nephrotoxicity. Two patients were proved to have a complete remission, and 11 had a major response. Four others had a minor response to chemotherapy. Chemotherapy did not improve the resectability of disease. Severe pulmonary disorders developed in 48% of patients given chemotherapy and 31% of those having surgery only. Postoperative mortality was increased by chemotherapy, and there was no apparent survival benefit. Both groups had a median survival of 10 months.

Conclusion.—Despite a high response rate to preoperative chemotherapy, these patients experienced significant drug-related morbidity and mortality, and the overall prognosis was not improved. For these reasons, entry of patients into the trial ceased.

▶ This study makes the important point that, in terms of neoadjuvant therapies, the results derived from phase II (nonrandomized) trials, no matter how encouraging, cannot begin to define the real benefit of a therapeutic strategy. In this particular case, the cisplatin-based regimen used appeared to improve the resectability rate and prolonged survival in carefully performed phase II studies of squamous cell carcinoma of the esophagus. The randomized effort reported here clearly shows that this is not the case. A substantially greater morbidity, primarily pulmonary, an increase in postoperative mortality, and no survival benefit were associated with this very intense regimen. Neoadjuvant strategies are clearly needed in this dismal disease. However, this is not one of them.—W.P. Ritchie, Jr., M.D., Ph.D.

Postoperative Radiotherapy for Carcinoma of the Esophagus: A Prospective, Randomized Controlled Study
Fok M, Sham JST, Choy D, Cheng SWK, Wong J (Univ of Hong Kong; Queen Mary Hosp, Hong Kong)
Surgery 113:138–147, 1993   140-94-10–6

Introduction.—Most patients who undergo resection of esophageal carcinoma will have locoregional recurrence or distant metastasis as a result of residual disease or systemic micrometastases. Accordingly, there is great interest in possible multimodal approaches to improving control of local and systemic disease. The use of postoperative radiotherapy in patients with esophageal carcinoma was investigated.

Methods.—The study sample comprised 130 patients with esophageal carcinoma. After stratification for curative resection (CR) or palliative resection (PR), the patients were randomized to receive either postoperative radiotherapy or no additional treatment. The resection was curative in 60 cases and palliative in 70; half of each group was assigned to receive radiotherapy. The radiation dose was 4.900 cGy, with a 350 cGy fraction after CR and 5.250 cGy at the same dose rate after PR.

Results.—No complications were observed during radiation therapy. At follow-up, 37% of the radiotherapy group had complications in the

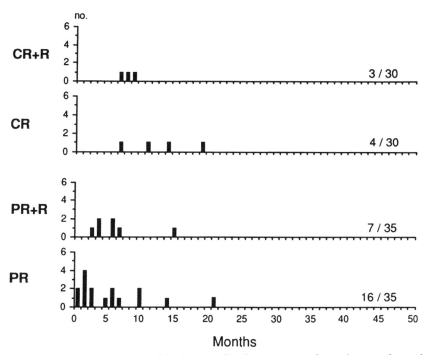

no.

CR+R   3 / 30

CR   4 / 30

PR+R   7 / 35

PR   16 / 35

Months

Fig 10–4.—Incidence and time of development of local recurrence in radiation therapy and control groups. After palliative resection, significantly more patients in control group had local recurrence. *Abbreviations:* CR+R, curative resection plus radiation therapy; PR+R, palliative resection plus radiation therapy. (Courtesy of Fok M, Sharm JST, Choy D, et al: *Surgery* 113:138-147, 1993.)

intrathoracic stomach, compared with only 6% of the control group. Gastric ulcers developed in 17 of 24 patients in the radiotherapy group, and 5 died as a result of bleeding. Local recurrence was significantly less common for PR patients who received radiotherapy (20% vs. 46%), but there was no difference in the CR groups (10% vs. 13%) (Fig 10-4). Patients who received radiotherapy were less likely to have intrathoracic recurrence.

Among patients with residual mediastinal tumor, tracheobronchial obstruction resulted in death in 33% of the control patients vs. 7% of the radiotherapy patients. There was no difference in local extrathoracic or anastomotic recurrence. However, the rate of distant metastasis was 40% for CR plus radiation therapy, 30% for CR only, 69% for PR plus radiotherapy, and 51% for PR only (Fig 10-5). Metastases developed in 5 months in PR patients who received radiation therapy vs. 8.5 months for the PR only group. The time to onset was 10 to 11 months in both CR groups. The median postoperative survival was 9 months in the radiotherapy groups vs. 15 months in the control groups (Fig 10-6).

Conclusion.—The shorter survival in patients with esophageal carcinoma who received postoperative radiotherapy was the result of irradia-

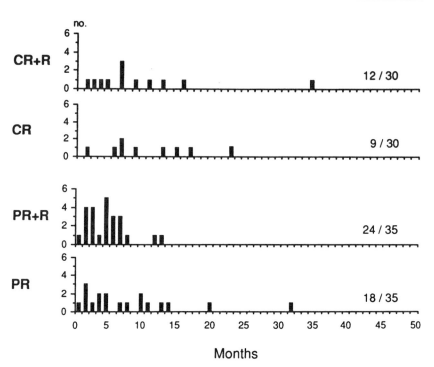

Fig 10–5.—Incidence and time of development of metastasis in radiation therapy and control groups. After palliative resection, significantly more patients in radiation therapy group had metastasis in early postoperative period. *Abbreviations:* CR +R, curative resection plus radiation therapy; PR +R, palliative resection plus radiation therapy. (Courtesy of Fok M, Sham JST, Choy D, et al: *Surgery* 113:138–147, 1993.)

tion-related deaths and early metastasis. Such combination therapy appears useful only for patients who have residual mediastinal tumor after operation, in whom it can reduce the incidence of local recurrence in the tracheobronchial tree.

▶ This skilled and energetic group has designed and brought to fruition a prospective, randomized, and controlled trial of the use of adjuvant radiotherapy for carcinoma of the esophagus. The results seem totally clear-cut. Those patients who were receiving adjuvant radiotherapy experienced increased morbidity and mortality because of extremely difficult to treat radiation injury to the intrathoracic stomach used as an esophageal substitute. Early appearance of metastatic disease and reduced overall survival were also noted in this group compared with the control patients. These data clearly mitigate against the use of radiotherapy, at least as delivered in this study, in the adjuvant setting for this disease.—W.P. Ritchie, Jr., M.D., Ph.D.

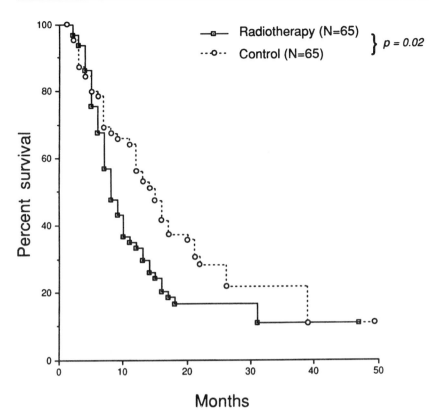

Months

Fig 10–6.—Kaplan-Meier cumulative survival curve of radiation therapy and control groups, combining both curative and palliative resection. Survival was significantly worse for patients who underwent postoperative radiation therapy. (Courtesy of Fok M, Sham JST, Choy D, et al: *Surgery* 113:138–147, 1993.)

Value of Physiologic Assessment of Foregut Symptoms in a Surgical Practice
Costantini M, Crookes PF, Bremner RM, Hoeft SF, Ehsan A, Peters JH, Bremner CG, DeMeester TR (Univ of Southern California, Los Angeles)
Surgery 114:780–787, 1993   140-94-10-7

Background.—Esophageal symptoms are generally nonspecific. With physiologic testing techniques such as esophageal manometry and 24-hour pH monitoring of the distal esophagus, more precise diagnoses can be made. The reliability of symptoms in the diagnosis of gastroesophageal reflux disease was examined, and esophageal motility disorders were assessed by functional tests.

Methods.—Three hundred sixty-five patients who were referred for suspected esophageal functional disease were studied. The symptomatic

Relationship Between Proved Esophageal Function Abnormalities and Abnormalities
Suspected on Symptomatic Basis

		Detected Abnormality		
Suspected Abnormality	N =	GERD	Motility Disorder	No Esophageal Disease
GERD	161	105 (65.2%)	11 (6.8%)	45 (28%)
Motility Disorder	95	31 (32.6%)	35 (36.8%)	29 (31%)
Non-Cardiac Chest Pain	34	9 (26%)	17 (50%)	8 (24%)
Aspiration	30	12 (40%)	5 (17%)	13 (43%)
Abdominal Pathology	45	14 (31%)	12 (27%)	19 (42%)
T O T A L	365	171	80	114

(Courtesy of Costantini M, Crookes PF, Bremner RM, et al: *Surgery* 114:780–787, 1993.)

evaluation was compared with the findings on esophageal manometry and ambulatory 24-hour pH monitoring of the distal esophagus.

Findings.—The symptomatic diagnosis, based on the patients' main complaint, was gastroesophageal reflux in 44%, esophageal motor disorder in 26%, chest pain of esophageal origin in 9%, reflux and aspiration in 8%, and abdominal abnormalities in 12%. The symptomatic diagnosis was considerably affected by findings on the esophageal function tests. Gastroesophageal reflux and motility disorders were detected in all symptomatic groups. A large number of patients in each group tested normal (table).

Conclusion.—Symptomatic complaints are not reliable for diagnosing esophageal abnormality. Objective assessment is needed in these patients to avoid inappropriate medical or surgical treatment.

▶ If one makes the assumption that ambulatory 24-hour pH monitoring and standard (but carefully performed) esophageal manometry are highly specific and sensitive for detecting, respectively, gastroesophageal reflux disease and esophageal motility disorders (and there is absolutely no reason to doubt this assumption), then this paper has a very important message for the practicing surgeon. Although it is often possible to suspect one or the other by careful history, objective evidence of these disorders is absolutely essential in their management if surgery is contemplated. As the authors emphasize, a careful history points to the appropriate functional assessment to be made; the results of that assessment indicate whether (and which) surgical intervention should be undertaken.—W.P. Ritchie, Jr., M.D., Ph.D.

Surgical Repair of Esophageal Perforation Due to Pneumatic Dilation for Achalasia: Is Myotomy Really Necessary?

Pricolo VE, Park CS, Thompson WR (Rhode Island Hosp, Providence; Brown Univ, Providence, RI)
Arch Surg 128:540–544, 1993   140-94-10–8

Background.—Perforation of the esophagus is a rare complication of pneumatic dilation of achalasia. Most recommendations have been for esophageal repair combined with esophagocardiomyotomy, but the need for the latter procedure has not been established.

Patients.—The results of repair were reviewed in 6 patients with achalasia who had an esophageal perforation secondary to pneumatic dilation. Myotomy was not part of the reconstructive procedure. The patients were 4 men and 2 women aged 53 to 87 years, all of whom had undergone dilation for the relief of dysphagia and who had symptoms of perforation within 1 hour of the procedure.

Technique.—Under broad-spectrum antibiotic coverage, the distal esophageal tear is approached through a left posterolateral thoracotomy. A cervical incision is made in one patient with a high esophageal perforation. The edges are débrided of nonviable tissue and reapproximated with interrupted nonabsorbable sutures. Where feasible, the repair is supported with a patch of gastric fundus. A draining gastrostomy and feeding jejunostomy are left in place.

Results.—Four patients had an uncomplicated recovery and were discharged 10–15 days after surgery. One patient required reoperation for bleeding secondary to a duodenal ulcer, and 1 patient had a suture line leak repaired after a mediastinal abscess developed. The latter patient also had acalculous cholecystitis develop and died of multiple organ system failure secondary to sepsis. None of the 5 surviving patients had recurrent dysphagia when followed for 1–12 years. Two patients had occasional symptoms of gastroesophageal reflux that responded to postural change and medical treatment.

Conclusion.—When repairing a distal esophageal perforation resulting from pneumatic dilation of achalasia, it is not necessary to add a myotomy.

▶ One of the discussants of this paper paraphrased a vastly overused adage about fixing things that aren't broken by asking: "If it's already broke, why break it some more?" Although the numbers of patients included in this series are far too small to provide a definitive answer, we, too, have been impressed that patients with small, contained, well-draining perforations after pneumatic dilation for achalasia have a very good long-term result after being treated nonoperatively. This suggests they may have undergone all the myotomy that they will ever need.—W.P. Ritchie, Jr., M.D., Ph.D.

Long-Term Effect of Total Fundoplication on the Myotomized Esophagus

Topart P, Deschamps C, Taillefer R, Duranceau A (Université de Montréal)
Ann Thorac Surg 54:1046–1052, 1992   140-94-10-9

Introduction.—Esophageal myotomy is an effective palliative procedure for patients having achalasia or diffuse esophageal spasm, but the value of adding an antireflux procedure at the distal end of the myotomized esophagus remains uncertain. In a total of 17 patients undergoing esophagocardiomyotomy from 1978 to 1983, the long-term effects of a 360-degree short fundic wrap were evaluated.

Patients.—Thirteen patients with achalasia and 4 with diffuse esophageal spasm underwent surgery. The 9 men and 8 women were aged 19 to 68 years. All the patients initially had typical symptoms of their motor disorders.

Clinical Results.—Dysphagia and regurgitation lessened substantially immediately after surgery but, after 2 years, 5 patients (29%) were symptomatic. Only 3 of 12 patients followed for 6 years or longer remained totally asymptomatic. Five patients required further surgery because of esophageal emptying problems and related symptoms.

Objective Findings.—The distal transverse esophageal diameter increased progressively after surgery and exceeded 6 cm at 10 years. Esophageal stasis increased from 32% to 75% in this interval. Resting esophageal pressures decreased significantly after surgery, and peak contraction pressures also decreased. The resting pressure gradient in the area of the lower esophageal sphincter decreased from 25.5 to 7.4 mm Hg after surgery and remained stable thereafter. No significant exposure to acid was found in the 8 patients monitored. Endoscopy disclosed esophageal dilatation and retention but no evident damage from reflux esophagitis.

Discussion.—If an antireflux procedure is to be added to esophageal myotomy, the best type of repair remains controversial. Total fundoplication appears inappropriate when added to the freshly myotomized esophagus because progressive esophageal dilatation and retention ensue, leading to poor emptying. A 29% rate of reoperation is unacceptable.

▶ This paper is certain to add fuel to the fire surrounding the burning question of whether one should add an antireflux procedure to standard myotomy in patients undergoing operation for either achalasia or, less commonly, diffuse esophageal spasm. Only 3 of 12 patients who were initially subjected to "Heller" myotomy with a 360-degree gastric wrap remained asymptomatic after 6 years. In addition, almost 30% of patients ultimately required further surgery because of dysphagia. All of this was a consequence of progressive decreases in resting intra-esophageal pressure and in peak esophageal contraction pressures over time. It is of interest that despite a marked reduction in lower esophageal sphincter pressure (occurring even in the face of the wrap), no abnormalities in 24-hour esophageal pH recordings were observed, suggesting that the wrap may have been unnecessary in the first place. This round goes to the antifundoplicationists, or at least to those who advocate something less than a 360-degree wrap.—W.P. Ritchie, Jr., M.D., Ph.D.

Stomach and Duodenum

INTRODUCTION

The potential for curing gastrinoma or for rendering patients engastrinemic, at least, has increased dramatically during the past decade because of the identification of the "gastrinoma triangle" and the realization that many tumors in that triangle will be found in the duodenum. Although intraoperative ultrasound is often helpful in identifying these lesions, recent studies clearly indicate that duodenotomy followed by careful palpation of the entire duodenum is the best method of localizing and extirpating them (Abstracts 140-94-10–10 and 140-94-10–11). Gastric outlet obstruction secondary to non–Zollinger-Ellison-related duodenal ulcer is an uncommon complication, but it almost always requires surgical therapy when it occurs. A recent prospective trial (Abstract 140-94-10–12) indicates that, compared with highly selective vagotomy with Jaboulay gastroduodenostomy and with selective vagotomy and antrectomy with B-II gastrojejunostomy, highly selective vagotomy with posterior-dependent gastrojejunostomy is associated with superior outcomes in the long term.

A more common problem is the perforated gastric or duodenal ulcer (Abstract 140-94-10–13). A number of recent reports clearly indicate that perforated gastric ulcers are more lethal than perforated duodenal ulcers. In both diseases, operative mortality is a function of the duration of the perforation as well as the presence of significant concurrent medical illness in afflicted patients. Regardless of whether the ulcer is considered to be "acute" or "chronic," simple closure of the perforation is associated with a very high risk of ulcer recurrence, particularly in gastric ulcer. The Roux stasis syndrome (postprandial bloating and nausea associated with a Roux-en-Y gastrojejunostomy) continues to be a perplexing clinical problem (Abstract 140-94-10–14). Although the etiology is not totally clear, current evidence suggests that delayed gastric emptying and Roux limb dysmotility are important factors. The best treatment, in all probability, is to not perform the Roux in the first place.

Finally, as is the case with other organ systems, the laparoscope can be used to treat potentially lethal upper abdominal diseases in poor-risk patients (Abstract 140-94-10–15). In one instance, for example, an acute gastric volvulus caused by a large paraesophageal hiatus hernia was reduced and fixed to the anterior abdominal wall laparoscopically with a good long-term result.

Wallace P. Ritchie, Jr., M.D., Ph.D.

A Prospective Study of Intraoperative Methods to Diagnose and Resect Duodenal Gastrinomas

Sugg SL, Norton JA, Fraker DL, Metz DC, Pisegna JR, Fishbeyn V, Benya RV, Shawker TH, Doppman JL, Jensen RT (NIH, Bethesda, Md)

Ann Surg 218:138–144, 1993   140-94-10–10

Background.—Duodenal gastrinomas are an increasingly common finding in patients with Zollinger-Ellison syndrome. Some have advocated intraoperative endoscopy with transillumination (IOE) at surgery to detect these tumors, and others have recommended routine duodenotomy (DX).

Methods.—Whether DX should be routinely done in those with Zollinger-Ellison syndrome was investigated in a prospective study of 35 patients. The ability of DX to detect gastrinomas was compared with that of palpation, intraoperative ultrasound (IOUS), and IOE.

Findings.—Thirty-three patients (94%) had tumors detected and excised. Twenty-seven (77%) had duodenal gastrinomas excised. The average duodenal tumor size was .8 cm, which was significantly smaller than the pancreatic and lymph node tumors found in this series. Standard palpation after a Kocher maneuver identified 19 of the 31 (61%) duodenal tumors, and IOUS showed only 8 tumors (26%) and no new lesions. With IOE, 20 duodenal gastrinomas (164%) and 6 new lesions were identified. Duodenectomy identified 100% of the duodenal tumors and 5 additional lesions. The morbidity rate was 17%. One patient had a duodenal fistula after surgery and later recovered. None of the patients died.

Conclusion.—The duodenum is the most common location for gastrinomas (77%) in patients with Zollinger-Ellison syndrome. Duodenectomy should be performed routinely in patients with this syndrome to detect and remove duodenal gastrinomas.

Duodenal Gastrinomas, Duodenotomy, and Duodenal Exploration in the Surgical Management of Zollinger-Ellison Syndrome

Thompson NW, Pasieka J, Fukuuchi A (Univ of Michigan, Ann Arbor)

World J Surg 17:455–462, 1993   140-94-10–11

Background.—The duodenum is a more common site of primary gastrinoma than has been thought, but these tumors are often missed at conventional exploration. As many as 40% of patients with a biochemical diagnosis of Zollinger-Ellison syndrome (ZES) have had negative findings on laparotomy in the past decade. Detection of gastrinomas requires duodenotomy and careful palpation of the everted mucosa.

Recent Experience.—Seven patients with duodenal gastrinomas were encountered in the past 2 years at 1 institution. Four of them had sporadic ZES, whereas 3 had the multiple endocrine neoplasia type I

(MEN-I) syndrome. All 7 patients had malignant gastrinomas in the duodenum as evidenced by metastatic lymph nodes and, in 1 instance, liver metastasis as well. The 4 patients with sporadic ZES became eugastrinemic after local tumor excision, removal of involved nodes, and lobectomy in the 1 patient with hepatic metastasis. Two of the 3 patients with MEN-I also became eugastrinemic after surgery, which in these cases included distal pancreatectomy.

Conclusion.—Duodenotomy should be performed in patients with sporadic ZES in whom no pancreatic tumor is found and in all patients with ZES associated with MEN-I, regardless of whether a pancreatic tumor is seen. If a duodenal tumor is found, the regional lymph nodes should be removed.

▶ Abstracts 140-94-10–10 and 140-94-10–11 illustrate that exciting new information is emerging concerning the location and potential curability of gastrinomas in patients with ZES. It is now apparent that, in sporadic cases at least, many—if not most—gastrinomas are located in the duodenum. They are almost always small, may be multiple, and are frequently associated with lymph node metastasis. Although intraoperative ultrasound is an important adjunct, the Bethesda group has shown clearly that duodenotomy followed by careful palpation of the entire duodenum is the best method of localizing and extirpating these tumors. The Ann Arbor group agrees and reminds us of the importance of resecting all suspicious lymph nodes in the area. Furthermore, they suggest that patients with MEN-I, who were hitherto thought to be incurable, may also benefit from this approach.—W.P. Ritchie, Jr., M.D., Ph.D.

Prospective Randomized Study Comparing Three Surgical Techniques for the Treatment of Gastric Outlet Obstruction Secondary to Duodenal Ulcer
Csendes A, Maluenda F, Braghetto I, Schutte H, Burdiles P, Diaz JC (Univ of Chile, Santiago)
Am J Surg 166:45–49, 1993   140-94-10–12

Objective.—Early and late results of 3 different procedures used to treat patients with gastric outlet obstruction secondary to duodenal ulcer were compared. This serious complication occurs in approximately 6% to 8% of patients with duodenal ulcers.

Patients and Methods.—Seventy-two men and 18 women took part in the prospective clinical trial. The mean age of the group was 47 years, and the mean duration of chronic duodenal ulcer was 88 months. All had gastric outlet obstruction as diagnosed by clinical history, endoscopic examination, and the saline load test. After laparotomy, the patients were randomized to receive highly selective vagotomy (HSV) plus gastrojejunostomy, HSV plus Jaboulay gastroduodenostomy, or selective

Late Follow-up of Patients Who Underwent Surgery for Gastric Outlet Obstruction

	HSV + GJ (n = 28)	HSV + J (n = 27)	SV + A (n = 28)
Mean follow-up (m)	91 (36-132)	116 (72-156)	91 (30-120)
Endoscopy	12 (40%)	13 (45%)	12 (43%)
Visick I	24 (80%)	19 (70%)*	21 (75%)
Visick II-III	3 (11%)	5 (19%)	4 (14%)
Visick IV	---	3 (11%)	3 (11%)

Abbreviations: GJ, gastrojejunostomy; J, Jaboulay; A, antrectomy.
* P < .01.
(Courtesy of Csendes A, Maluenda F, Braghetto I, et al: *Am J Surg* 166:45–49, 1993.)

vagotomy (SV) plus antrectomy. The mean duration of follow-up was 98 months.

Results.—Six patients were lost to follow-up, and 1 died of acute pancreatitis in the early postoperative period after HSV plus Jaboulay anastomosis. The postoperative courses of the 3 groups were similar. With long-term follow-up, there was a significantly better outcome after HSV plus gastrojejunostomy than after HSV plus Jaboulay anastomosis, but not after SV plus antrectomy (table). Gastric acid output, measured late after surgery in 24 patients, was similar for the 3 groups. Recurrent ulcers were found only in patients treated with HSV plus Jaboulay anastomosis. Three patients in the SV plus antrectomy group had severe alkaline gastritis.

Conclusion.—Highly selective vagotomy plus gastrojejunostomy is recommended as the treatment of choice for patients with duodenal ulcer and gastric outlet obstruction. Patient selection is highly important to the success of this procedure. Excluded from this series were patients with a severe deformity of the duodenal bulb but without evidence of gastric retention and with normal results on the saline test.

▶ Cicatricial gastric outlet obstruction is an uncommon complication of chronic duodenal ulcer disease in the United States, and it is likely to become even more so as the use of triple-therapy directed against *Helicobacter pylori* becomes more widespread. Until now, however, this may not have been the case in Chile, where the authors were able to randomize a total of 90 patients with reasonably well-documented gastric outlet obstruction in the short space of 4 years. The data suggest that HSV complemented by posterior-dependent gastrojejunostomy is probably associated with superior outcomes compared with HSV with Jaboulay gastroduodenostomy and with SV and antrectomy with a Billroth II gastrojejunostomy. This is almost entirely because of either more patients in the last 2 groups having been classified as Visick grade IV because of recurrent ulcer (HSV + Jaboulay) or the development of alkaline reflux gastritis (SV + antrectomy). It is of interest that dumping occurred in only 1 patient subjected to the resective procedure. One of the major advertised advantages for using HSV is that it maintains the innervation of the antrum intact. For this reason, gastric emptying of solids and semisolids is maintained near normal in nonobstructed patients with duodenal ulcer disease requiring operation; therefore, dumping is almost a nonexistent problem. The question arises: Why go to the trouble of performing an HSV if one is to bypass the pylorus anyway? Why not perform truncal vagotomy, which is technically simpler and is accomplished more rapidly? The authors' argument is new (to me) and interesting: Gastric stasis, frequently encountered early after truncal vagotomy and gastrojejunostomy, is not a problem after HSV and gastrojejunostomy, because the antropyloric pump is maintained intact. This is an intriguing thought.—W.P. Ritchie, Jr., M.D., Ph.D.

Perforated Gastric and Duodenal Ulcer: An Analysis of Prognostic Factors
Hamby LS, Zweng TN, Strodel WE (Univ of Kentucky, Lexington)
Am Surg 59:319–324, 1993   140-94-10–13

Background.—The surgical management of perforated ulcers continues to be a subject of discussion, because it is still unclear whether patients benefit from simple ulcer closure rather than definitive operation. The risk factors associated with operative morbidity and mortality were examined, and the long-term outcomes of definitive operation and simple ulcer closure were compared.

Method.—The records of 84 patients who underwent operation for perforated ulcer were reviewed. Demographic data were collected, along with information regarding antecedent ulcer history, concomitant medical illness, medications, ulcer location, degree of peritoneal contamination, complications, and outcome. Operative mortality was defined as death during hospitalization or within 30 days of operation. A complication was seen as an event prolonging hospitalization or contributing to death. Follow-up was done by telephone interviews, and recurrent ulcers were documented radiographically, endoscopically, or surgically.

Results.—Surgery was done in 84 patients with perforated ulcer. The majority were perforations in the duodenum. Sixty-one percent of patients had a definitive operation, and the rest had simple ulcer closure. Thirty-seven percent of the patients had 40 complications. These patients were significantly older and were more likely to have a preexisting illness and be hospitalized at the time of perforation. Eighteen percent of the patients died in hospital. Factors contributing to death included advanced age, pulmonary disease, perforation lasting longer than 24 hours, and use of steroids. Patients with gastric ulcers had a higher mortality rate than patients with gastroduodenal ulcers. Follow-up over a mean of 48 months for discharged patients showed that those who received definitive operation had a significantly lower recurrent ulcer rate than those treated with simple closure.

Conclusion.—Categorical data modeling showed that age (greater than 42 years), hospitalization at the time of perforation, and the presence of one or more significant medical conditions are directly related to a stepwise increase in complications and death after operative treatment of perforated ulcer. Patient outcome from surgery appears to be independent of the procedure performed, although the definitive procedure offers a lower rate of ulcer recurrence and is, therefore, to be recommended.

▶ Despite the virtual disappearance of elective surgery for peptic ulcer disease, surgeons are still called upon with some regularity to treat its complications, including perforations. This paper was selected because it tends to reinforce lessons about this condition that are deserving of emphasis. First, perforated gastric ulcers are a more lethal entity than are perforated duodenal ulcers, probably because afflicted patients are older, are more hemodynamically unstable on admission, and experience greater delay between perforation and definitive therapy (1). Second, as noted by others, operative mortality is a function of the duration of perforation, the presence of significant concurrent medical illness, and advanced patient age (this last point is probably a reflection of the second). Additional risk factors include steroid use and in-hospital perforation, which has also been noted by others. Missing from the list—but still important—is the presence of perioperative shock (or a systolic blood pressure less than 90 mm Hg). Third, simple closure of the perforation is associated with a higher risk of recurrence of ulcers than is a definitive ulcer operation, irrespective of ulcer acuity or chronicity. That no differences in operative mortality were noted between these 2 options in the study from the University of Kentucky is interesting, but its significance is unclear because the series was not performed in a prospective and randomized way.

For me, the bottom line is this: In the absence of significant risk factors, patients with perforated peptic ulcers are all best served by a definitive ulcer operation—and parietal cell vagotomy is a very good one.—W.P. Ritchie, Jr., M.D., Ph.D.

Reference

1. *Ann Surg* 209:693, 1989.

Manometric and Scintigraphic Studies of the Relation Between Motility Disturbances in the Roux Limb and the Roux-En-Y Syndrome
van der Mijle HCJ, Kleibeuker JH, Limburg AJ, Bleichrodt RP, Beekhuis H, van Schilfgaarde R (Univ Hosp, Groningen, The Netherlands)
Am J Surg 166:11–17, 1993   140-94-10–14

Background.—Patients frequently complain of abdominal pain, fullness, nausea, and vomiting after a Roux-en-Y gastrojejunostomy. This syndrome is thought to be caused by slow gastric emptying, and/or Roux-limb stasis, or both. Whether slow gastric emptying and Roux-limb stasis can be attributed to motility disorders in the Roux limb was investigated.

Method.—Thirty-seven patients who had undergone Roux-en-Y gastrojejunostomy were studied. Twenty-six had symptoms of Roux-en-Y syndrome, and 11 were asymptomatic. Radionuclide studies were used to assess gastrojejunal transit, and manometry was used to investigate the motility of the Roux limb.

Results.—Slow gastric emptying, Roux-limb stasis, or a combination of both was found in 20 of the 26 symptomatic patients, compared with only 4 of the 11 asymptomatic patients. The basic motor patterns, the interdigestive motor cycle, and the fed state were found in most patients. Motility disturbances were present in 34 of the 37 patients, but they were significantly more frequent in the symptomatic group and in patients with Roux-limb stasis. However, there appeared to be no relationship between motility disorders and slow gastric emptying. The principal finding was a pause in the fed state, which was exclusive to patients with very slow gastric emptying. Aberrant propagation of the migrating motor complex and the absence of a fed state were not seen in patients with normal gastrojejunal transit.

Conclusion.—The frequency of motility disorders found in symptomatic patients with Roux-limb stasis indicates a causative relationship between motility disorders and the Roux-en-Y syndrome. However, because no correlation was seen between motility disorders in the Roux limb and slow gastric emptying, it is unlikely that Roux-limb stasis is responsible for slow gastric emptying.

▶ It is becoming increasingly apparent that the etiology of the very troublesome Roux stasis syndrome (postprandial bloating, nausea, and vomiting after creation of a Roux-en-Y gastrojejunostomy) is much more complex than originally thought. The results of this study, taken in association with a second study performed by the same group (1), suggests that at least 2 possibly independent factors may be responsible: slowed gastric emptying and Roux-limb stasis.

A considerable body of experimental evidence supports these assertions, especially the second. The authors suggest that vagotomy may be the major reason for the former, whereas interruption of proximal duodenal pacesetter potentials may be responsible for the latter. Under any circumstance, the syndrome is extremely difficult to treat. The clinical lesson is that, for some patients, the Roux may be as much a disease as a cure and should never be undertaken unless the indications are absolutely clear. In particular, creating a Roux in a patient with already delayed gastric emptying is a prescription for disaster.—W.P. Ritchie, Jr., M.D., Ph.D.

Reference

1. *Br J Surg* 80:60, 1993.

Laparoscopic Reduction of Acute Gastric Volvulus
Koger KE, Stone JM (Stanford Univ, Calif)
Am Surg 59:325–328, 1993   140-94-10-15

Background.—The various types of gastric volvulus are classified by anatomical configuration, with torsion about the longitudinal axis of the stomach—organoaxial volvulus—occurring in about two thirds of cases. This type of volvulus, commonly associated with paraesophageal hernia, is referred to as an "upside-down" stomach, reflecting the rotation of the stomach into the thoracic cavity. A new surgical technique for correction of organoaxial gastric volvulus with associated paraesophageal hernia was reported.

Case Report.—Woman, 75, was seen with acute onset of upper abdominal pain, first with vomiting and then with nonproductive retching. She had a known paraesophageal hernia but was considered a poor surgical risk because of obesity and cardiopulmonary disease. After intravenous hydration was started and a nasogastric tube was placed, upper gastrointestinal barium radiography was per-

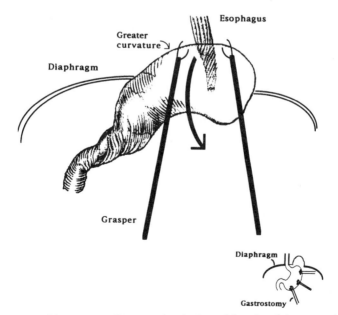

Fig 10–7.—Schematic view of laparoscopic reduction and detorsion of the organoaxial gastric volvulus. **Inset,** percutaneous endoscopic gastrostomy tubes arrayed along the greater curvature of the stomach. (Courtesy of Koger KE, Stone JM: *Am Surg* 59:325–328, 1993.)

formed, disclosing an intrathoracic gastric volvulus with gastric outlet obstruction.

The volvulus was managed by laparoscopic reduction and detorsion of the stomach (Fig 10-7). Three pull-type percutaneous endoscopic gastrostomy tubes were then placed on the greater curvature of the stomach—the fundus, body, and antrum—to produce a broad and secure area of fixation. The paraesophageal hernia was left unrepaired. The gastrostomy tubes were removed after 2 months. Gastric detorsion and fixation were confirmed by postoperative barium radiography. The patient was following a regular diet with normal bowel function at 1-year follow-up.

Discussion.—A technique of laparoscopic detorsion and percutaneous endoscopic gastropexy was reported in a patient at poor surgical risk who had acute gastric volvulus. The relatively simple procedure avoids the morbidity of laparotomy and provides for rapid recovery of gastric function.

▶ Here is another inventive—even ingenious—use of the laparoscope to treat a potentially lethal disease in a poor-risk patient. It is interesting that the patient has done well for at least 1 year, even though the paraesophageal hernia sac was not excised and no attempt was made to close the diaphragmatic defect, both of which are considered important in the open technique.—W.P. Ritchie, Jr., M.D., Ph.D.

Biliary Tract

INTRODUCTION

Open cholecystectomy has much in common with the steam locomotive: it is infrequently used and remembered with fondness by many. A recent report of open cholecystectomy in almost 43,000 patients (Abstract 140-94-10–16) reminds us that it is an extremely safe and effective operation. The overall mortality rate approximates that of anesthesia, even in poor-risk patients. The morbidity is very acceptable, including an extraordinarily low incidence of common bile duct injury. The report represents the gold standard, perhaps in perpetuity, against which laparoscopic cholecystectomy must ultimately be measured.

The widespread use of laparoscopic cholecystectomy has produced 1 very surprising result (Abstract 140-94-10–17): Despite a 25% reduction in unit cost for the operation, overall expenditures have increased by almost 12%, which is entirely caused by the rate of cholecystectomy having increased by almost 60%. The precise reasons for greater utilization are not clear, but they could relate, at least in part, to the extension of the procedure to those previously considered too "unfit" for open cholecystectomy. In view of the demonstration that postoperative pulmonary function is substantially better after laparoscopic cholecystectomy than after open cholecystectomy, such as extension may be very appropriate in some circumstances.

Whether to add operative cholangiography routinely to laparoscopic cholecystectomy remains a matter of some debate. An experienced Canadian group (Abstract 140-94-10-19) suggests that selected preoperative endoscopic retrograde cholangiopancreatography, with stone extraction if applicable, is a reasonable current approach until greater facility is obtained in performing laparoscopic cholangiography and common bile duct exploration. One likely casualty of the increased use of laparoscopic cholecystectomy may be incidental appendectomy. This is good. At least when performed in conjunction with open cholecystectomy in patients aged 65 or older, incidental appendectomy is of no benefit whatsoever (Abstract 140-94-10-20). Finally, advances in the treatment of established gallstone diseases continue to be matched by advances in our understanding of their pathogenesis. A key step is the nucleation of cholesterol crystals followed by crystal growth. A recent study (Abstract 140-94-10-21) indicates that gallbladder mucin may be responsible for accelerating that growth once nucleation has occurred.

Wallace P. Ritchie, Jr., M.D., Ph.D.

Open Cholecystectomy: A Contemporary Analysis of 42,474 Patients

Roslyn JJ, Binns GS, Hughes EFX, Saunders-Kirkwood K, Zinner MJ, Cates JA (Med College of Pennsylvania, Philadelphia; Univ of California, Los Angeles; Northwestern Univ, Evanston, Ill; et al)
Ann Surg 218:129–137, 1993   140-94-10–16

Background.—The recent introduction of several modalities for the treatment of cholelithiasis has challenged the more traditional cholecystectomy, which has long been considered the gold standard of treatment. The lack of contemporary data on open cholecystectomy, how-

TABLE 1.—Effect of Age on Outcome

	Age (yr)	
	< 65	> 65
No.	30,059	12,415
% of group	70.8	29.2
Morbidity rate (%)	10.2	25.7*
No. of deaths	9	62
Mortality rate (%)	0.03	0.50*
Length of stay (days)	4.7	7.3*
Charges ($)	5,980	9,728*

*P < .0001 vs. age < 65 years.
(Courtesy of Roslyn JJ, Binns GS, Hughes EFX, et al: *Ann Surg* 218:129–137, 1993.)

TABLE 2.—Impact of Disease Status on Outcome

Disease Status

	Chronic	Acute	Complicated
No.	27,892	13,246	1,336
% of group	65.7	31.2	3.1
Morbidity rate (%)	11.9	19.4*	25.2*
No. of deaths	29	34	8
Mortality rate (%)	0.10	0.26*	0.60*
Length of stay (days)	4.8	6.6*	8.6*
Charges ($)	5,881	9,043*	12,510*

* P < .0001 vs. chronic cholecystitis.
(Courtesy of Roslyn JJ, Binns GS, Hughes EFX, et al: *Ann Surg* 218:129–137, 1993.)

ever, has impeded efforts to define the role of these alternative treatments; a study was, therefore, undertaken to evaluate the outcome of open cholecystectomy as it is currently practiced.

Methods.—All open cholecystectomies performed by surgeons in California and Maryland during a recent 12-month interval were evaluated in this population-based study. A total of 42,474 patients were assessed, representing nearly 8% of all patients in the United States undergoing cholecystectomy during any recent 12-month interval. The patients were grouped according to diagnosis-related information (DRG-197 and DRG-198) and were then categorized by principal diagnosis and divided into 3 clinically homogeneous subgroups, including acute, chronic, and complicated cholecystitis. The data consisted of information collected from January 1, 1989 to December 31, 1989, by using computerized analysis of Uniformed Billing (UB-82) discharge analysis information from all non-Veterans Administration acute care hospitals in the 2 states. This information was supplemented with a 5% random sample of Medicare UB-82 data from patients discharged between October 1, 1988 and September 30, 1989 in other states.

Results.—The mean length of stay was no more than 6 days, and in-hospital–based charges were $7,076. The overall morbidity was 14.7%, which included all complications, regardless of severity. Complication rates were significantly increased in elderly patients, at 25.7%, vs. 10.1% in those younger than 65 years. The overall mortality rate was .17%. A 17-fold increase in the death rate for elderly patients was noted, compared to that in younger patients (Table 1). In those with acute and complicated cholecystitis, death rates were .26% and .60%, respectively. These rates were 2.5 and 6 times greater, respectively, than those in patients with chronic disease (Table 2). Increased mortality rates were associated with acute and complicated disease, emergency admission, and age greater than 64 years. With chi-square analysis, the presence of complicated disease and age greater than 65 years were found to be critical factors, with age greater than 65 years representing the single most important determinant of a fatal outcome. Hypertension, congestive heart failure, and diabetes had an independent impact on mortality. Factors not associated with mortality included obesity, asthma, previous coronary artery bypass, and hypothyroidism.

Conclusion.—Open cholecystectomy is a safe, effective treatment for cholelithiasis, with an almost zero mortality rate. The ultimate role of alternative treatment should be assessed in relation to current data on open cholecystectomy.

▶ The rapidity with which laparoscopic cholecystectomy has come to dominate the entire treatment of a specific disease entity has no parallel in modern medical history. That being the case, however, this report has 2 major virtues (among many). First, it provides a very thorough snapshot (taken just before the procedure became an endangered operative species) of the outcomes associated with open cholecystectomy, based on an analysis of 8% of all individuals undergoing the operation in one year's time in the United States. Second, it provides an important gold standard against which the results of laparoscopic cholecystectomy can be judged in the future. This is of some importance because it is totally unrealistic to think that a true randomized comparison of the two methods will ever be made in this country or elsewhere; the public (and, in all probability, the profession) won't accept it.

The report indicates that, in a heterogeneous group of patients undergoing surgery done by an equally heterogeneous group of surgeons, open cholecystectomy is an extraordinarily safe and effective operation. The overall mortality rate is extremely low (much lower than results from previous studies done a decade or so ago would suggest), even in the face of advanced years and acute or complicated disease. The overall morbidity rate seems high (14.7%), but the vast majority of these complications were of no consequence. Of special interest are the data relative to bile duct injuries. In some series of laparoscopic cholecystectomy, these have been reported in up to 1% of patients. Because this entity was not recorded as a separate modifier in the large databases used, the authors decided to consider all complications identified as "accidental operative lacerations" or "postoperative fistula" to be bile duct injuries. By this definition (which, if anything, overestimates the true incidence of the problem), bile duct injury occurred in 91 of the almost 43,000 patients who had surgery (.21%). The authors are quick to point out that these data should not be interpreted as indicating a bias on their part for open cholecystectomy. Rather, they have sought to provide us with a benchmark against which laparoscopic cholecystectomy can be measured once it is a "mature" procedure. They have succeeded admirably.—W.P. Ritchie, Jr., M.D., Ph.D.

Increased Cholecystectomy Rate After the Introduction of Laparoscopic Cholecystectomy

Legorreta AP, Silber JH, Costantino GN, Kobylinski RW, Zatz SL (US Quality Algorithms and US Healthcare, Blue Bell, Pa; Univ of Pennsylvania, Philadelphia)
JAMA 270:1429–1432, 1993   140-94-10–17

Background.—Laparoscopic, or "closed," cholecystectomy has been rapidly replacing "open" cholecystectomy. The closed procedure substantially reduces length of hospital stay, resulting in reduced costs. However, the overall costs may be higher because the procedure may be done more often and the readmission rate may be increased.

Methods and Findings.—Inpatient and outpatient expenditures, incidence rates, and length of hospitalization for 6,909 enrollees in a health maintenance organization (HMO) with gallbladder complaints from 1988 through 1992 were analyzed. The incidence of cholecystectomy and total HMO expenditures on gallbladder disease have risen since closed cholecystectomy was introduced. The rate of cholecystectomy procedures per 1,000 enrollees rose from 1.35 in 1988 to 2.15 in 1992. Total yearly expenditures for gallbladder disease per 1,000 HMO enrollees (in 1992 dollars) increased by 11.4%, despite a 25.1% decrease in unit cost (physician and hospital cost) for cholecystectomy procedures. There were no significant changes in the rate of appendectomies or inguinal hernia repairs or total expenditures for them in that period (Figs 10-8 and 10-9).

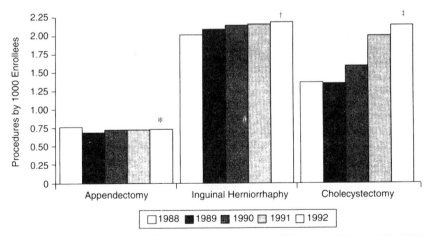

Fig 10–8.—Rates per 1,000 enrollees for selected procedures. *1992 through 1988, $P > .677$; †1992 through 1988, $P > .317$; and ‡1992 through 1988, $P < .001$. (Courtesy of Legorreta AP, Silber JH, Costantino GN, et al: *JAMA* 270:1429–1432, 1993.)

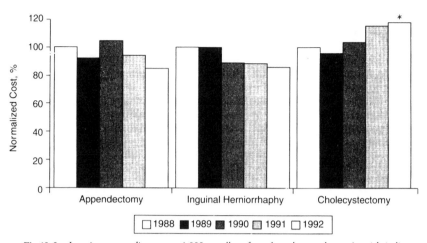

Fig 10–9.—Inpatient expenditures per 1,000 enrollees for selected procedures. *Asterisk* indicates 1992 vs. 1990, 1992 vs. 1989, and 1992 vs. 1988; *P* < .001. (Courtesy of Legorreta AP, Silber JH, Costantino GN, et al: *JAMA* 270:1429–1432, 1993.)

Conclusion.—The introduction of laparoscopic gallbladder procedures has increased cholecystectomy rates and the resultant costs in this HMO population. The use of this new technology, touted as reducing health-care costs, may actually increase costs because of changes in the indications for gallbladder surgery.

▶ This fascinating paper, which deserves to be read in its entirety, demonstrates how the Law of Unintended Consequences can become operative when a new technology confronts an old disease. Despite a 25% reduction in unit cost for cholecystectomy during the period studied (the laparoscopic era), overall expenditures rose by almost 12%, which was entirely caused by the rate of cholecystectomy increasing by nearly 60% during the same period. The rates of appendectomy, which is nondiscretionary, and of herniorrhaphy, which has the same discretionary attributes as cholecystectomy, remained the same.

An accompanying editorial suggests that laparoscopic cholecystectomy may be "too much of a good thing," because its undoubted patient-friendly character may have led physicians to liberalize the indications for gallbladder extirpation. It would certainly be unfortunate if cholecystectomy is now being recommended for patients who are "dyspeptic," "gaseous," have "sluggish" gallbladder emptying or, God forbid, have truly asymptomatic stones. All of these, in my opinion, are totally inappropriate indications for operation. On the other hand, the increased rate may reflect treatment of a backlog of "procrastinators," those who have tolerated their typical symptoms of biliary colic because of fear of the open approach. It might also reflect extension of the procedure to those considered too "unfit" for open cholecystectomy. All would agree, I believe, that laparoscopic cholecystectomy is appropriate under these circumstances.

Only time will tell which of these explanations is correct. If the former is true, the rate of cholecystectomy is likely to remain at the new and higher set point; if the latter is true, however, cholecystectomy rates should, in time, return toward previous levels. One final note: In the future, in calculating cost:benefit ratios, the equally important but more difficult to quantitate costs associated with days missed from work because of biliary colic or days saved for work because of decreased postoperative morbidity must also be considered.—W.P. Ritchie, Jr., M.D., Ph.D.

Pulmonary Function After Laparoscopic Cholecystectomy
Schauer PR, Luna J, Ghiatas AA, Glen ME, Warren JM, Sirinek KR (Univ of Texas Health Sciences Ctr, San Antonio)
Surgery 114:389–399, 1993   140-94-10-18

Purpose.—In patients undergoing abdominal surgery, pulmonary complications are a major cause of morbidity and mortality. These complications could potentially be reduced by the use of laparoscopic procedures, which minimize disruption of the abdominal skin and musculature. The effects of laparoscopic cholecystectomy and open cholecystectomy on postoperative pulmonary function were compared.

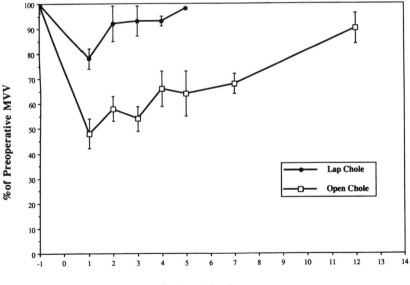

Postoperative day

Fig 10–10.—Postoperative maximum voluntary ventilation (MVV.). *Abbreviations: Lap*, laparoscopic; *Chole*, cholecystectomy. (Courtesy of Schauer PR, Luna J, Ghiatas AA, et al: *Surgery* 114:389–399, 1993.)

Methods.—Forty consecutive patients undergoing elective cholecystectomy were randomized to different surgical units, which used either laparoscopic or open cholecystectomy. Pulmonary risk factors were equal in the 2 groups. Before operation, both groups underwent pulmonary function studies, oxygen saturation measurements, and chest radiography; these studies were repeated after surgery until levels returned to baseline. The narcotic requirements and the occurrence of pulmonary complications in the 2 groups were also compared.

Results.—Postoperative pulmonary impairment was reduced by 30% to 38% by laparoscopic cholecystectomy in all areas studied, including forced vital capacity, forced expiratory volume in 1 second, forced expiratory flow, midexpiratory phase, maximum forced expiratory flow, maximum voluntary ventilation, total lung capacity, and oxygen saturation. Patients in the laparoscopic cholecystectomy group returned to baseline pulmonary function 4 to 10 days sooner than those in the open cholecystectomy group (Fig 10–10). All pulmonary complications, including atelectasis, hypoxia, and pneumonia, were more common in the open cholecystectomy group. Atelectasis was also more severe in the open cholecystectomy group. Patients in that group needed 8 times more postoperative pain medication than those in the laparoscopic cholecystectomy group.

Conclusion.—Laparoscopic cholecystectomy reduces the postoperative pulmonary complication rate compared with open cholecystectomy. This advantage results from significant reductions in both pulmonary compromise and narcotic requirements. Laparoscopic cholecystectomy is the procedure of choice for patients undergoing elective cholecystectomy; the benefits of laparoscopy should be transferrable to other major abdominal operations as well.

▶ This well-done study is representative of a number of sophisticated efforts that compare alterations in a variety of physiologic functions (e.g., "stress" hormone release, hemodynamic alterations, etc.) after laparoscopic, as opposed to open, cholecystectomy. In this instance, the results are clear (and probably can be translated to other upper abdominal procedures, such as fundoplication and myotomy for achalasia): Postoperative pulmonary function is substantially better after laparoscopic cholecystectomy than after open cholecystectomy. Whether these differences can be completely explained on the basis of the size of the incision needed to access the abdominal cavity is not certain. Whatever the explanation, however, data such as these provide a powerful argument for extending laparoscopic cholecystectomy to patients deemed too "unfit" for open cholecystectomy based on compromised pulmonary function (vide supra).—W.P. Ritchie, Jr., M.D., Ph.D.

Cholecystectomy Without Operative Cholangiography: Implications for Common Bile Duct Injury and Retained Common Bile Duct Stones
Barkun JS, Fried GM, Barkun AN, Sigman HH, Hinchey EJ, Garzon J, Wexler

MJ, Meakins JL (Mcgill Univ, Montreal)
Ann Surg 218:371–379, 1993   140-94-10-19

Introduction.—The advent of laparoscopic cholecystectomy has had many clinical benefits, but it has also necessitated much reassessment of traditional practices, including the need for routine operative cholangiography.

Study Plan.—Data were collected prospectively on the first 1,300 patients who underwent laparoscopic cholecystectomy on an elective or urgent basis at 4 McGill University teaching hospitals. More than two thirds of the patients were women; the mean patient age was 49 years. Endoscopic retrograde cholangiopancreatography (ERCP) was done preoperatively in 106 patients who were considered to be at risk for a common bile duct stone, most often because of abnormal liver function, jaundice, a dilated common duct, or pancreatitis.

Results.—Open cholecystectomy proved necessary in 6.2% of patients. There was one postoperative death (.08%), and 4.8% of the patients had postoperative complications. Fifty patients (3.8%) were found to have common duct stones at preoperative ERCP (table). Of 49 patients having ERCP postoperatively, 17 were found to have retained common duct stones. The overall incidence of choledocholithiasis during a median follow-up of 22 months was 5.2%. The rate of complications associated with ERCP was 9%; pancreatitis was most frequent. Five common bile duct injuries (.4%) were recognized. Eight patients underwent open exploration of the common bile duct.

Conclusion.—It is possible to perform laparoscopic cholecystectomy safely, without routine intraoperative cholangiography, through relying on preoperative ERCP in patients at risk for common duct stones.

▶ At some time in the future, it seems likely that most general surgeons who perform laparoscopic cholecystectomy will also be capable of carrying out simultaneous intraoperative cholangiography and common bile duct explora-

Management of Common Bile Duct Stones

Prevalence of CBD Stones (1300 Patients)

Detection	No.	%	Treatment
Preoperative	45	3.5	ERCP sphincterotomy
Operative	6	0.5	Open CBDE
Postoperative	17	1.3	ERCP sphincterotomy
Total	68	5.2	

(Courtesy of Barkun JS, Fried GM, Barkun AN, et al: *Ann Surg* 218:371-379, 1993.)

tion efficiently, safely, and to good effect. This is not the case at present, however. Until that era arrives, the approach advocated by the authors (the use of ERCP, when applicable, in selected patients with stone extraction) seems quite reasonable for the vast majority of patients having surgery in other than a teaching setting. There is one point of interest: The argument that intraoperative cholangiography prevents common bile duct injury in the laparoscopic setting does not impress the McGill group. The rate of bile leak in their series was low (.9%) and comparable to that reported in other series, in which intraoperative cholangiography was used more routinely.—W.P. Ritchie, Jr., M.D., Ph.D.

Appendectomy Incidental to Cholecystectomy Among Elderly Medicare Beneficiaries
Warren JL, Penberthy LT, Addiss DG, Mcbean AM (Health Care Financing Administration, Baltimore, Md; US Dept of Health and Human Services, Atlanta, Ga)
Surg Gynecol Obstet 177:288–294, 1993   140-94-10-20

Background.—The benefit of performing incidental appendectomy in elderly individuals is a controversial subject. The operation is commonly performed to eliminate the risk of future appendicitis. However, in most elderly patients, the probability of acute appendicitis developing is extremely low, and performing an incidental appendectomy prolongs operative time, increases the duration of anesthesia, and raises costs. Moreover, it may lead to increased infection. The characteristics and outcomes of Medicare patients who received appendectomy incidental to cholecystectomy were compared with those of patients who received only cholecystectomy.

Method.—A total of 8,936 patients undergoing cholecystectomy with incidental appendectomy were compared with a group of 44,461 patients undergoing cholecystectomy without incidental appendectomy. The study controlled for age, race, gender, and comorbidity status. The adverse outcomes of incidental appendectomy—including wound infections, other infections, extensive complications, and death within 30 days of admission were examined.

Results.—During the 6-year study, 3.78 incidental appendectomies were performed for every 100 cholecystectomies. White patients were more likely to have incidental appendectomies than were black patients, and men were more likely to undergo the procedure than were women. The likelihood of having the incidental operation decreased significantly with age. The group that underwent incidental appendectomy experienced an 83% higher rate of infection than the group that did not. The former group also experienced a higher risk of other infections, extensive postoperative complications, and mortality at 30 days. The preventive effect of incidental appendectomy on morbidity and mortality from future instances of appendicitis was found to be negligible. For patients aged 65–69 years, 115 incidental appendectomies would be required to prevent one future instance of appendicitis, and 4,472 incidental operations would have to be performed to prevent a single future death from acute appendicitis.

Conclusion.—Appendectomy cholecystectomy increases the risk for wound infection in elderly patients. Although the procedure is often done to prevent morbidity and mortality from future instances of appendicitis, the risk of acute appendicitis in elderly individuals is small. With these results in mind, the surgeon should carefully weigh the risks and benefits of incidental appendectomy for elderly patients.

▶ Outcome analysis is here to stay. The gurus of managed care need it, the Health Care Financing Administration is doing it, and it is a clearly defined goal of the Clinton Health Care Plan. All physicians, including surgeons, should welcome it, with the proviso that the methodologies involved be valid and meaningful. In some instances, this proviso has, in all probability, been ignored (e.g., in studies on the outcomes of coronary bypass performed by individual hospitals and individual surgeons in New York State and Pennsylvania; garbage in and garbage out, in my opinion). In this study, however, the results deserve respect because the number of patients is large (more than 53,000), because the statistical analysis is appropriate and because the outcomes are clear. The message is also clear: The performance of incidental appendectomy coincident with open cholecystectomy in patients aged 65 or older is not appropriate. Indeed, it is probably not appropriate in patients who are much younger than this. The temptation to do such surgery will surely be less as open cholecystectomy becomes increasingly rare.—W.P. Ritchie, Jr., M.D., Ph.D.

Bovine Gallbladder Mucin Accelerates Cholesterol Monohydrate Crystal Growth in Model Bile
Afdhal NH, Niu N, Gantz D, Small DM, Smith BF (Boston City Hosp; Boston Univ)
Gastroenterology 104:1515–1523, 1993   140-94-10–21

Objective.—Gallbladder mucin accelerates the nucleation of cholesterol crystals, which is an early phase of gallstone formation, but the process whereby the crystals mature into macroscopic stones is poorly understood. For this reason, a novel model system was developed to learn how mucin influences the growth of cholesterol monohydrate crystals.

Methods.—Cholesterol crystals of uniform size were incubated in model bile preparations having varying cholesterol saturation indices at 37°C. Crystal size was estimated by measuring the length and width of individual crystals by polarizing light microscopy and calculating the average crystal area. In this system, it is possible to study the growth of preformed crystals independently of significant de novo crystal nucleation.

Observations.—The degree of crystal growth depended on the extent to which cholesterol was supersaturated in the bile. Adding bovine gallbladder mucin in concentrations of .5 to 8 mg of accelerated crystal growth per mL in supersaturated bile in a manner that depended on both concentration and time, compared with control incubations with bovine serum albumin or model bile only. Crystal growth was associated with a progressive decrease in cholesterol saturation and with an increase in the total mass of cholesterol crystals. The total number of crystals declined, suggesting a net transfer of cholesterol to larger crystals.

Clinical Implication.—These findings indicate that gallbladder mucin may, through accelerating the growth of cholesterol crystals, contribute to the postnucleation maturation of cholesterol gallstones.

▶ Cholesterol gallstone formation is a complex process involving the secretion of cholesterol supersaturated bile by the liver, the nucleation of cholesterol crystals in the gallbladder, and, finally, growth of those crystals into macroscopic gallstones. The prevention of any of these events has the potential for prophylaxis (if not treatment) of gallstone disease in susceptible patient populations that, admittedly, are difficult to identify. This study demonstrates that, under extremely carefully controlled conditions, bovine gallbladder mucin accelerates cholesterol crystal growth once nucleation has occurred. In the stomach at least, a wide variety of agents (e.g., the nonsteroidal anti-inflammatory drugs) inhibit mucin secretion. Might the same not be true in the gallbladder?—W.P. Ritchie, Jr., M.D., Ph.D.

Pancreas

INTRODUCTION

The virtue of using early endoscopic retrograde cholangiopancreatography with endoscopic papillotomy in patients with acute biliary pancreatitis has been explored in a prospective trial (Abstract 140-94-10-22). The data indicate that this approach results in a reduction in biliary sepsis in patients predicted to have either mild or severe pancreatitis. On the other hand, the procedure does not appear to alter the course of the pancreatitis per se.

Acute pancreatitis in elderly patients (Abstract 140-94-10-23) is a serious condition, particularly if no obvious underlying etiology is found. In these patients, multiple organ system failure develops early, and substantial morbidity and mortality occurs. An important underlying factor may be hypoperfusion of the pancreas resulting from concomitant congestive heart failure. Pancreatic pseudocysts frequently develop in proximity to major splanchnic vessels and, on occasion, the patients are seen with life-threatening hemorrhage. A recent review of 13 such patients (Abstract 140-94-10-24) indicates that angiographic identification and embolization of the involved artery is the appropriate initial treatment. Pseudocyst drainage should rapidly follow to prevent recurrent hemorrhage.

An important communication has provided new information concerning the advantages of decompressing a dilated pancreatic duct in patients with mild-to-moderate chronic pancreatitis (Abstract 140-94-10-25). Those advantages include almost immediate relief of pain and, equally important, prevention of progression of the disease to major exocrine and endocrine insufficiency. In patients with near end-stage pancreatitis, ductal decompression also results in prompt pain relief; however, it does not prevent further deterioration of pancreatic function.

In patients with chronic pancreatitis confined to the head of the gland, classic pancreaticoduodenectomy with pylorus preservation produces excellent long-term results (Abstract 140-94-10-26). However, the short-term cost is great because the procedure is difficult and the perioperative course is often stormy. In the hands of expert and experienced surgeons, pancreaticoduodenectomy can be performed with a mortality rate less than that associated with jaywalking on a busy street (Abstract 140-94-10-27). This attests to the virtue of concentrating expertise in the hands of a few surgeons who perform the procedure over and over again.

The latest addition to the list of potential islet cell tumor markers is labelled somatostatin analogue (Abstract 140-94-10-28). However, its sensitivity and specificity, compared with more standard localizing techniques (including intraoperative ultrasound), are not as yet defined.

Wallace P. Ritchie, Jr., M.D., Ph.D.

Early Treatment of Acute Biliary Pancreatitis by Endoscopic Papillotomy
Fan S-T, Lai ECS, Mok FPT, Lo C-M, Zheng S-S, Wong J (Univ of Hong Kong)
N Engl J Med 328:228–232, 1993   140-94-10-22

Background.—Conservative management of acute biliary pancreatitis is successful in most patients, but biliary sepsis and other complications develop in other patients, with associated mortality rates ranging from 13% to 50%. Endoscopic papillotomy within 24 hours of hospital admission may reduce the incidence of complications in these patients.

Treatment.—In a prospective, randomized trial, 195 patients with acute biliary pancreatitis were assigned to 1 of 2 treatment groups. Within 24 hours of admission, 97 patients underwent emergency endoscopic retrograde cholangiopancreatography (ERCP), which was followed by endoscopic papillotomy for ampullary and common bile-duct stones. The remaining 98 patients received initial conservative treatment and selective ERCP with or without endoscopic papillotomy only when their condition deteriorated.

Results.—There were 127 patients with biliary stones. Overall, the incidence of local and systemic complications was similar in the 2 treatment

Complications of ERCP and Endoscopic Papillotomy in 195 Patients With
Acute Pancreatitis, According to the Predicted Severity of Disease and the
Location of the Stone

VARIABLE	NO. OF PATIENTS	POST-ERCP SERUM AMYLASE	ABDOMINAL PAIN	POST-PAPIL-LOTOMY BLEEDING
		IU/liter	*no. of patients*	
Emergency ERCP (n = 97)				
Mild				
No stone	22	990 (57–4785)	0	0
Gallbladder stone only	14	1345 (100–8090)	1	0
Common-bile-duct stone	20	549 (22–6385)	0	2
Severe				
No stone	11	364 (64–2900)	0	0
Gallbladder stone only	11	948 (151–3003)	0	0
Common-bile-duct stone	19	1162 (131–9080)	1	2
Conservative treatment (n = 98)				
Mild				
No stone	23	284 (65–3310)	1	0
Gallbladder stone only	15	274 (35–2190)	1	0
Common-bile-duct stone	20	320 (86–9500)	0	0
Severe				
No stone	12	197 (75–1270)	0	0
Gallbladder stone only	12	174 (80–7710)	0	0
Common-bile-duct stone	16	404 (80–2168)	1	4

Note: Median values are given for serum amylase, with ranges shown in parentheses. The
severity of disease was predicted on the basis of urea and glucose levels at admission.
(From Fan S-T, Lai ECS, Mok FPT, et al: N Engl J Med 328:228–232, 1993. Courtesy of Fan
S-T, Choi TK, Lai ECS, et al: Gut 30:1591–1595, 1989.)

groups, but the incidence of biliary sepsis was significantly lower in patients who underwent emergency ERCP with or without endoscopic
papillotomy, particularly among patients with severe pancreatitis. All patients with biliary sepsis had persistent ampullary or common–bile-duct
stones. If only patients with biliary stones were analyzed, the morbidity
rate in patients who underwent emergency ERCP was not significantly
lower than that in patients in the conservative-treatment group. The hospital mortality rate was slightly lower in patients who underwent emergency ERCP. The incidence of exacerbation of abdominal pain after
ERCP with or without endoscopic papillotomy and the incidence of

bleeding after endoscopic papillotomy were the same irrespective of the timing of the procedure (table).

Conclusion.—The combination of emergency ERCP and endoscopic papillotomy within 24 hours after admission is indicated in the management of acute pancreatitis, regardless of the predicted severity and suspected cause.

▶ This well-designed and carefully conducted study sought to test the hypothesis that early ERCP with endoscopic papillotomy could reduce the incidence of complications in patients with suspected gallstone pancreatitis. It was accomplished by randomizing patients to receive "universal" ERCP or to "conservative" treatment with selective ERCP. For the two thirds of patients in each group who had associated pancreatitis and lithic disease of the biliary tract, the hypothesis appears to be correct. There was a substantial reduction in morbidity in the treated vs. the nontreated group (16% vs. 33%). A trend toward decreased mortality was also apparent. However, the authors have made a more global conclusion than this. They recommend early ERCP and papillotomy on a routine basis, "irrespective of the predicted severity and suspected cause."

That recommendation is based on there having been no episodes of biliary sepsis (cholangitis, cholecystitis) in the entire treated group, including patients without gallstones, compared with 13 episodes in the entire observed group, also including patients without gallstones. That translates into one having had to perform ERCP in 98 patients to obviate 13 episodes of biliary sepsis. This might be cost effective in Hong Kong, where gallstones and gallstone pancreatitis are very common, but it probably would not be so in the Western world, where alcohol-related pancreatitis is the clear front-runner. Furthermore, the paper clearly demonstrates that early and routine ERCP do not obviate the progression of pancreatitis to either local complications or to the more lethal systemic ones. This having been said, there is a clear and important message in this paper: Irrespective of the cause of pancreatitis, early ERCP with attempted endoscopic papillotomy is a safe procedure.—W.P. Ritchie, Jr., M.D., Ph.D.

Acute Pancreatitis of Unknown Etiology in the Elderly
Browder W, Patterson MD, Thompson JL, Walters DN (East Tennessee State Univ, Johnson City)
Ann Surg 217:469–475, 1993   140-94-10-23

Background.—The incidence of acute pancreatitis is increasing among elderly patients, and in a significant number of these patients, a cause for this condition cannot be explicitly defined. An experience with acute pancreatitis in patients older than 60 years was reviewed, and patients without a clearly defined cause for pancreatitis and those with a well-documented cause were compared with respect to morbidity and mortality.

TABLE 1.—Clinical Outcome of Acute Pancreatitis in
Elderly Patients

	Unknown Etiology	Known Etiology
Morbidity*	48%	22%
Mortality	24%	8.3%
Hospital stay (Mean)	14.8 ± 3.5 days	12.9 ± 1.4 days
SICU stay †	4.4 ± 1.3 days	1.6 ± .44 days

Abbreviation: SICU, stay in intensive care unit.
* P < .05. The most common causes of morbidity were pulmonary failure and congestive heart failure.
† Mean ± standard error of the mean; significant at P < .05.
(Courtesy of Browder W, Patterson MD, Thompson JL, et al: Ann Surg 217:469-475, 1993.)

TABLE 2.—Organ System Failure Scoring in Acute Pancreatitis

Organ System	Criteria for Scoring *
1. Cardiovascular	Mean arterial pressure < 50 mm Hg
	Pulse < 50
	Ventricular tachycardia/fibrillation
	Cardiac arrest
	Acute MI
2. Pulmonary	Ventilatory rate < 5 or > 50
	FIO_2 > 0.4
	PEEP > 5 mm Hg
3. Renal dialysis	Serum creatinine ≥ 3.5 mg %
4. Neurologic	Glasgow coma scale ≤ 6
5. Hematologic	Hematocrit < 20%
	Leukocyte count < 3,000
	Platelets < 50,000
	DIC
6. Hepatic	Bilirubin > 3 mg %
	SGPT > 100
7. Gastrointestinal	Stress ulcer
	Acalculous cholecystitis
	Necrotizing enterocolitis
	Bowel perforation

Abbreviations: DIC, disseminated intravascular coagulation; FIO_2, forced inspiratory oxygen; MI, myocardial infarction; PEEP, positive end-expiratory pressure; SGPT, serum glutamic pyruvic transaminase.
* Presence of any one of the criteria resulted in 1 point for that organ system. Scoring ranges from 0 to 7.
(From Browder W, Patterson MD, Thompson JL, et al: Ann Surg 217:469-475, 1993. Courtesy of Tran DD, Cuesta MA: Am J Gastroenterol 87:604-608, 1992.)

Patients and Methods.—A total of 93 patients with acute pancreatitis diagnosed between 1987 and 1991 were studied. Diagnoses were confirmed by elevated serum amylase concentration and the presence of inflammatory changes in the pancreas, which was determined with CT and/or ultrasound or surgical intervention. When the history and laboratory findings excluded any known etiologic factor and a normal biliary tract was revealed during ultrasound, the patients were classified as having pancreatitis of unknown cause.

Results.—Seventy-two patients had a well-documented cause for their pancreatitis. The remaining 21 were classified as having an unknown cause. The length of hospital stay, time in the surgical intensive care unit, and morbidity and mortality were higher in patients without established causes (Table 1). Three of the deaths in the unknown-cause group were from multiple organ failure. At autopsy, 2 of the 3 cadavers had pancreatic necrosis. Two other deaths were caused by early cardiorespiratory failure and were not associated with pancreatic necrosis. Two patients in the unknown-cause group underwent surgical intervention, which consisted of pancreatic debridement and drainage for pancreatic necrosis. At hospital admission, an organ failure score was obtained (Table 2). In patients who subsequently died, the mean organ failure score was significantly higher. Patients in the unknown-cause group had a significantly higher organ failure score compared with those with established causes. Hypotension at admission, length of symptoms before admission, and number of Ranson's criteria were not found to be predictive of subsequent mortality, although the functional status of the various organ systems was.

Conclusion.—Elderly patients with acute pancreatitis of unknown cause experience a more severe disease, with higher mortality. These patients also have a greater compromise of organ function. Aggressive support of such organ systems may be useful in treating such patients.

▶ As many as 40% of patients aged 60 years or older with documented acute pancreatitis will have no obvious underlying etiologic risk factor, such as gallstones, alcoholism, etc., for their disease. Many do have underlying congestive heart failure, however, which suggests that hypoperfusion and relative ischemia of the pancreas may be responsible. This is entirely speculative. The sobering fact of the matter is that, in this group, when the etiology is unclear, multiple organ system failure is a very common sequela, surgical ICU stays are long, and the morbidity and mortality are substantial. Furthermore, bad outcomes occur rapidly and appear to be a consequence of systemic collapse rather than the severity of the underlying pancreatitis. How does one interdict this course? Here are 3 suggestions: First, perform ERCP early in such patients in an attempt to define and treat a cause, if present. Second, monitor all elderly patients with acute pancreatitis, especially those with an obscure etiology, in the setting of the intensive care unit and treat accordingly. Third, frequently assess the pancreas with dynamic CT scanning. Should infected fluid collections appear, drain them; if pancreatic necrosis is apparent, débride it and do so repeatedly.—W.P. Ritchie, Jr., M.D., Ph.D.

Arterial Hemorrhage Complicating Pancreatic Pseudocysts: Role of Angiography
Adams DB, Zellner JL, Anderson MC (Med Univ of South Carolina, Charleston)
J Surg Res 54:150–156, 1993   140-94-10-24

Background.—Pancreatic pseudocysts often develop in direct proximity to the major splanchnic arteries and their branches, and they present a life-threatening risk of major arterial hemorrhage. The initial symptoms and outcomes of patients with pancreatic pseudocysts were reviewed, and the role of angiography in the diagnosis and management of this complication were assessed.

Patients.—A record review identified 180 patients with pancreatic pseudocysts who were managed surgically. Thirteen of the patients had arterial hemorrhage. Demographic data, the location and site of pseudocysts, involved vessels, clinical presentation, diagnostic studies, types of management employed, number of units of blood transfused, the length of hospital stay, morbidity, and mortality findings were analyzed for the patients with arterial complications.

Findings.—In the 13 patients with arterial complications of pancreatic pseudocysts, the underlying cause was chronic pancreatitis secondary to alcohol abuse in 10 patients and trauma in 3 patients. The clinical manifestation of pseudocyst bleeding was variable but most often included a sudden onset of abdominal pain and clinical findings suggesting hypovolemia. The bleeding site was identified with selective visceral angiography in 9 patients. Contrast-enhanced CT scans demonstrated evidence of bleeding in 5 of 7 patients. Hemorrhage was controlled by angiographic embolization in 6 patients and by surgery in 7 patients. The patients treated with angiographic embolization had less average blood loss than patients treated operatively, but the length of the hospital stay was similar for the 2 groups.

Conclusion.—As demonstrated in other research, the most common cause of pancreatic pseudocysts in this group of 180 patients was chronic pancreatitis secondary to long-term alcohol abuse. The 13 patients with arterial complications were commonly seen with acute pain in the region of the cyst, evidence of gastrointestinal or intra-abdominal bleeding, and findings suggesting acute hypovolemia. The patients managed angiographically required less transfused blood and had no mortality or procedure-related morbidity. Diagnostic dynamic CT scans and angiography and management of bleeding with angiographic embolization have substantially improved outcome in patients with arterial hemorrhage complicating pancreatic pseudocysts.

▶ Bleeding from eroded splanchnic vessels is an uncommon but dreaded complication of pancreatic pseudocysts. This paper reminds us that, in 1994, angiographic identification and embolization of the involved artery is the initial treatment of choice and is far better than ill-advised attempts at operative control. Subsequent pseudocyst drainage should be done early, however, to avoid recurrent hemorrhage.—W.P. Ritchie, Jr., M.D., Ph.D.

Progressive Loss of Pancreatic Function in Chronic Pancreatitis Is Delayed by Main Pancreatic Duct Decompression: A Longitudinal Prospective Analysis of the Modified Puestow Procedure
Nealon WH, Thompson JC (Univ of Texas, Galveston)
Ann Surg 217:458–468, 1993   140-94-10-25

Background.—Chronic pancreatitis may be associated with abdominal pain and/or exocrine and endocrine insufficiency. Functional deficits may result in pancreatic malabsorption, steatorrhea, diabetes mellitus, or unrelenting abdominal pain. The reason for operative drainage in these patients is relief of abdominal pain through a resectional or decompressive procedure. Previously, a significant delay in functional impairment in patients who underwent surgery was reported. The effect of operative drainage of the main pancreatic duct on the functional derangements associated with chronic pancreatitis was evaluated using a prospective, randomized approach.

Patients.—A total of 143 patients with chronic pancreatitis underwent endoscopic retrograde cholangiopancreatography, the Bentiromide-para-aminobenzoic acid test, a 72-hour fecal fat test, the oral glucose tolerance test, and fat meal–stimulated pancreatic polypeptide release. These tests were used to classify chronic pancreatitis as mild/moderate (M/M) or severe (Table 1). Eighty-three patients had an M/M grade at

---

TABLE 1.—5-Point System to Grade the Severity of Chronic Pancreatitis

Test	Threshold	Points Assigned
ERCP	Cambridge "severe"	1
OGTT/insulin	Abnormal hyperglycemia	1
Lipomul PP	Flat response	1
72-hour fecal fat	More than 7 g/24°	1
Benteromide/PABA	Less than 50% absorption	1
		Total 5 points

Note: The system for grading the severity of chronic pancreatitis is based on 5 measures: 0, 1, or 2 points = mild/moderate grade; 3–5 points = severe grade. Each of 5 tests—fat-stimulated pancreatic pancreatic polypeptide (PP), oral glucose tolerance test (OGTT), Bentiromide PABA, 72-hour fecal fat, and endoscopic retrograde cholangiopancreatography (ERCP)—are performed. Abnormal results in each test are assessed 1 point.
(Courtesy of Nealon WH, Thompson JC: *Ann Surg* 217:458–468, 1993.)

TABLE 2.—Chronic Pancreatitis
Follow-Up
Mild/Moderate (n = 83)

	Initial Evaluation	Follow-Up	Progressed To Severe
Operated	47/47	41/47 (87%)	6/47 (13%)
Non-operated	38/36	8/36 (22%)	28/36 (78%)

Note: Eighty-three patients were initially graded as mild/moderate chronic pancreatitis. The changes in severity grade from initial evaluation to follow-up for mild/moderate stage in patients who underwent operation and those who did not are shown.
(Courtesy of Nealon WH, Thompson JC: Ann Surg 217:458–468, 1993.)

initial evaluation; 47 of these patients underwent an operative drainage procedure and 36 did not. Patients were examined at 16-month intervals for a mean follow-up of 47.3 months.

Results.—Of the 47 patients with M/M disease who were operated upon, 87% preserved their functional grade during follow-up. Only 22% of the 36 patients who were not operated upon preserved their grade (Table 2). In a separate prospective study, 17 patients with chronic pancreatitis classified as M/M disease and nondisabling abdominal pain were randomized to operative or nonoperative treatment. Nine patients underwent surgery and eight did not. At follow-up, 7 of the 9 patients who had surgery and 2 of 8 nonsurgical patients preserved their functional grade.

Conclusion.—In patients with chronic pancreatitis, high intraductal pressure may contribute to the ongoing loss of function and an ongoing level of subacute inflammation. Surgical patients with chronic pancreatitis maintained their functional grade during follow-up more frequently than nonsurgical patients. These data support early operative drainage of the main pancreatic duct before significant and irreversible loss of function.

▶ For years, gastroenterologists have disparaged the modified Peustow procedure as ineffective and unnecessary. They argue that decompression of the main pancreatic duct does not prevent progressive loss of pancreatic exocrine and endocrine function; furthermore, even without operation, pain ultimately disappears as a consequence of pancreatic "burnout." This excellent paper clearly demonstrates that this viewpoint is specious. In patients defined as having M/M disease, 87% preserved their functional grade on extended follow-up after operation compared with only 22% of those who did not undergo surgery. Furthermore, relief of pain was achieved in 85% of the former group compared with only 1.3% of the latter group. This was true even though many patients continued to abuse alcohol. In contrast, in patients classified as having severe pancreatitis, operative decompression relieved pain but did not prevent deterioration of pancreatic function. The essence of the message is that in the patient with chronic pancreatitis with suitable ductal anatomy, rather than wait until complete functional decompensation has occurred, a policy of early operation is clearly appropriate.—W.P. Ritchie, Jr., M.D., Ph.D.

The Whipple Procedure for Severe Complications of Chronic Pancreatitis
Traverso LW, Kozarek RA (Virginia Mason Med Ctr, Seattle)
Arch Surg 128:1047–1053, 1993   140-94-10–26

Introduction.—Surgical removal of the head of the pancreas may be necessary in patients with chronic pancreatitis who experience certain types of complications. One preferred method for removing the pancreatic head is the pylorus-preserving Whipple (PPW) procedure. The indications for removal of the head of the pancreas in patients with severe complications of chronic pancreatitis were reviewed, and the short- and long-term results of PPW were assessed.

Patients and Methods.—Of 28 patients treated between 1986 and 1993, 3 who had previously undergone a vagotomy and antrectomy were not candidates for PPW. These patients underwent standard pancreaticoduodenectomy, and the remaining 25 had PPW. Preoperative

---

Reasons for Resection of the Pancreatic Head in 28 Patients

Expanding pseudocyst(s) in head--pain (n = 7)
Pancreatic duct blowout (n = 5)
Biliary obstruction (n = 5)
Arteriovenous fistula bleeding into cyst (n = 3)
Pleural fistula (n = 1)
Multiple pseudocysts in head--pain (n = 8)
Pancreatic and bile duct obstruction (n = 5)
Pancreatic duct blowout (n = 4)
"Pseudotumor" 8 and 12 cm (n = 2)
Biliary and pancreatic duct obstruction--pain (n = 9)
Diffuse calcified and enlarged head (n = 5)
Pancreatic duct blowout and cutaneous fistula (2 patients) (n = 3)
Duodenal obstruction (n = 2)
Pancreatic duct obstruction--pain (n = 4)
Diffuse calcified and enlarged head (n = 4)
Pancreatic duct blowout (n = 1)

Note: *n* equals the total number of patients within each subheading.
(Courtesy of Traverso LW, Kozarek RA: *Arch Surg* 128:1047–1053, 1993.)

endoscopic retrograde cholangiopancreatography and CT revealed expanding pseudocysts, pancreatic duct disruption, arteriovenous fistula, or calcified obstructive fibrosis of the bile duct, pancreatic duct, and/or duodenum (table). The goal of PPW is to preserve a functioning pylorus, the entire stomach, and the first part of the duodenum.

Results.—No deaths were associated with the procedure. Ten of the 28 patients experienced postoperative complications. Four had gastric outlet dysfunction secondary to retrogastric amylase-rich fluid collections and 3 had adult respiratory distress syndrome related to a prolonged (14 to 19 hours) operation time. There was one wound infection. Two patients died during the first year after surgery; one died of lung cancer, and the other committed suicide. At an average follow-up of 27.2 months, all patients reported relief of pain and all but one had returned to full physical activity and work or school. All but one patient had gained or maintained weight. The incidence of diabetes increased from 44% to 56% during follow-up. Although none had recurrent pancreas problems, 28% had resumed drinking alcohol.

Conclusion.—Patients with chronic pancreatitis who require PPW have difficult and urgent clinical problems. These operations were performed as a last option, and the procedures were quite lengthy. Nevertheless, results were successful and all patients enjoyed symptomatic relief. Key elements to a good outcome are preoperative endoscopic and radiologic assessment, drainage, and stenting procedures.

▶ There is a growing conviction among knowledgeable pancreatic surgeons that there exists a subset of patients with chronic pancreatitis (cohort size unknown) in whom the disease is confined to the head of the gland only. Conventional bypass or drainage procedures performed in this group are likely to fail, it is thought, because this portion of the gland is left in place and can act as a continuous "pacemaker" for smoldering inflammation. Based on this premise, a number of operative strategies have evolved designed specifically to treat this group. They include the Begar procedure (excision of only the pancreatic head with preservation of the duodenum and common duct [1]); the Frey procedure (resection of the ventral pancreatic head only [2]); and some variation of classical pancreaticoduodenectomy.

In this report, a skilled group of pancreatic surgeons detail their results with the last approach, usually accomplished using the pylorus preservation technique. The relatively long-term outcomes (27 months on average) are very commendable: 88% of patients were totally pain-free, 96% had maintained or gained weight, and 96% had returned to normal activity. This is not an operation for the faint-hearted; the procedure is bloody, tedious, and time-consuming because of the intense inflammation encountered. Undoubtedly as a consequence, perioperative morbidity is relatively high. The authors rightly stress the great value of obtaining preoperative visceral angiography with evaluation of the portal venous phase. In the first place, it may prompt an alteration in the planned operation (e.g., early splenectomy in the face of splenic venous thrombosis). In the second place, it may alert the surgeon to the presence of an anomalous right hepatic artery which, if inadvertently sacrificed during the procedure, will result in an ischemic common bile duct. There is one ethical question: Is it worth expending this much effort (7 to 19 hours in the operating room per case) and this many resources (20 units of blood in some instances and a hospital stay ranging from 8 to 68 days) on a group of patients, 82% of whom are alcoholic to begin with and almost 30% of whom resumed drinking in the early postoperative period?—W.P. Ritchie, Jr., M.D., Ph.D.

References

1. *Surgery* 97:467, 1985.
2. *Pancreas* 2:701, 1987.

One Hundred and Forty-Five Consecutive Pancreaticoduodenectomies Without Mortality
Cameron JL, Pitt HA, Yeo CJ, Lillemoe KD, Kaufman HS, Coleman J (Johns Hopkins Med Insts, Baltimore, Md)
Ann Surg 217:430–438, 1993   140-94-10-27

Background.—In past years, pancreaticoduodenectomy has carried high hospital morbidity and mortality rates, and in the 1970s, many thought that the procedure should be abandoned. More recent findings, however, suggest marked reductions in both morbidity and mortality.

Series.—The outcome of pancreaticoduodenectomy was examined in 145 consecutive patients (mean age, 59 years) who underwent surgery from 1988 to 1991. Thirty-seven patients were aged 70 years or older, and 4 were older than 80 years of age. The most common indication was

TABLE 1.—Preoperative Risk Factors

	≤69 Years (n = 108)	≥70 Years (n = 37)	P
Prior MI	5%	14%	NS
Hypertension	19%	32%	NS
Diabetes	18%	19%	NS
Chronic obstructive pulmonary disease	1%	3%	NS
Peripheral vascular disease	2%	8%	NS
Etoh abuse	26%	22%	NS
Smoking	38%	16%	.02
Prior biliary surgery	36%	38%	NS

(Courtesy of Cameron JL, Pitt HA, Yeo CJ, et al: *Ann Surg* 217:430–438, 1993.)

TABLE 2.—Pancreaticoduodenectomy in 145 Patients

Postoperative Complications	≤69 Years (%) (N = 108)	≥70 Years (%) (N = 37)	P
Delayed gastric emptying	32	46	NS
Pancreatic fistula	19	22	NS
Intraabdominal abscess	10	5	NS
Wound infection	6	11	NS
Pancreatitis	7	3	NS
Bile leak	6	3	NS
Cholangitis	5	5	NS
Small bowel obstruction	1	0	NS
Pneumonia	1	0	NS
Dehiscence	1	0	NS
None	52	38	NS

(Courtesy of Cameron JL, Pitt HA, Yeo CJ, et al: *Ann Surg* 217:430–438, 1993.)

pancreatic adenocarcinoma. Preoperative risk factors are found in Table 1.

Surgery.—The mean operating time exceeded 7 hours, and blood loss averaged 970 mL. Patients received a mean of 1.4 units of blood replacement. Only 9 patients had total pancreatectomy. The pylorus was preserved in 81% of cases. Eight patients underwent partial resection of the portal or superior mesenteric vein with reanastomosis. The mean postoperative hospital stay was 19 days.

Outcome.—Fifty-two percent of the patients had postoperative complications, most frequently delayed gastric emptying or pancreatic fistula formation (Table 2). There were no life-threatening complications. Two patients required reoperation during the initial hospitalization. No patient died within a month of surgery. Complications were no more frequent in the older patients.

Conclusion.—Given proper patient selection, pancreaticoduodenectomy may be done in patients of any age, with benign or malignant disease, with a minimal risk of death in hospital.

▶ This is an extremely impressive report. In the 11 years between 1969 and 1980, approximately 50 Whipple procedures were performed at the Johns Hopkins Hospital. The hospital mortality rate approached 25%. Between 1980 and 1992, however, the number of pancreaticoduodenectomies had increased almost sixfold, and the hospital mortality rate had decreased almost 10-fold. What made the difference? Improved anesthetic techniques, better methods of patient support in the intensive care unit, and a heightened capacity to treat complications effectively (the complication rate is still high at 52%). All these factors must have played a role. However, it seems clear that the ability to concentrate great expertise and experience in the hands of a few surgeons who perform the procedure over and over again must be a major factor. In this instance, specialization is a hero and not the villain that some health care policy makers would like to make it out to be.—W.P. Ritchie, Jr., M.D., Ph.D.

Use of Isotope-Labeled Somatostatin Analogs for Visualization of Islet Cell Tumors
van Eyck CHJ, Bruining HA, Reubi J-C, Bakker WH, Oei HY, Krenning EP, Lamberts SWJ (Erasmus Univ, Rotterdam, The Netherlands)
World J Surg 17:444–447, 1993   140-94-10-28

Objective.—In vitro autoradiographic studies demonstrate that most endocrine tumors show a high concentration of somatostatin receptors, in contrast to the virtual absence of binding sites in surrounding normal tissue. These findings agree with the clinical observation that tumor hormone secretion is suppressed after octreotide administration. The feasibility of in vivo detection of somatostatin receptor-positive tumors after administration of a radioactive iodine-labeled analogue was examined.

Methods.—Two isotope-labeled somatostatin analogues were injected intravenously in 25 patients with suspected somatostatin receptor-positive islet cell tumors. The analogues used were ^{123}I-Tyr-^{3}-octreotide and ^{111}In-Octreotide. A gamma camera was used to make planar or emission CT images.

Results.—These imaging studies demonstrated the primary tumor—as well as distant metastases, previously unrecognized in some cases—in 20 of 25 patients (table). Somatostatin receptors were also detected in vitro

Incidence of Somatostatin Receptors on Endocrine Pancreatic Tumors In Vitro (Seen by Autoradiography) and In Vivo (Seen by Scintigraphy)

Tumor	Incidence of somatostatin (analog) receptors	
	In vitro	In vivo
VIPomas	7/8 (87%)	1/1
Gastrinomas	5/5 (100%)	10/11 (91%)
Glucagonomas	3/3 (100%)	1/1
Insulinomas	8/11 (72%)	5/8 (63%)
GRF-omas	4/4 (100%)	—
"Nonfunctioning" islet cell tumors	4/4 (100%)	2/2
Somatostatinomas		1/2

Note: Eight of these tumors have been investigated both in vitro and in vivo. In all cases the results of the in vitro and in vivo investigations were parallel.
(Courtesy of van Eyck CHJ, Bruining HA, Reubi J-C, et al: World J Surg 17:444–447, 1993.)

in these tumors, suggesting that the in vivo ligand binding to the tumor in fact reflected binding to specific somatostatin receptors. In tumors with somatostatin receptors detected in vivo, octreotide had a good suppressive effect on hormonal hypersecretion.

Discussion.—This study describes somatostatin receptor scintigraphy as a simple, painless, noninvasive technique for the diagnosis of islet cell tumors and carcinoids. It may be of considerable value in localizing primary tumors and metastases. Prospective studies are needed to compare this new method with other techniques and to establish its sensitivity and specificity.

▶ Most functioning islet cell tumors are suppressible with somatostatin. This suggested to Dr. Lamberts and his clever colleagues that these tumors must contain somatostatin receptors. They further reasoned that if this was the case, the primary tumor and its metastases, if present, could be visualized scintigraphically by injecting radiolabelled somatostatin analogues. As this paper indicates, they reasoned correctly. The potential clinical use of this technique obviously remains to be determined. A not-so-educated guess is that it may possibly be helpful in making the diagnosis, but it may not be so helpful in terms of precise localization.—W.P. Ritchie, Jr., M.D., Ph.D.

Small Intestine and Appendix

INTRODUCTION

Multivariant analysis has been applied to the outcomes experienced in a large number of patients undergoing operation for intestinal Crohn's disease in an attempt to identify those who are prone to early symptomatic recurrence. In one study (Abstract 140-94-10-29), the number of anastomoses performed was found to be the most important prognostic factor, followed by inflammation at the resection margins. Patients requiring an ileostomy had a lower early recurrence rate than those who did not. It is of importance that marginal inflammation was a predictor for early recurrence only in those patients with multiple anastomoses. Whether the margins of resection should be extended in this group is unclear.

Small-bowel obstructions at trochar sites after laparoscopic surgery are being noted with increasing frequency. One recent report (Abstract 140-94-10-30) advises fascial closure of all such sites that are 10 mm or more in extent, even if it means enlarging the incision. It seems almost gratuitous to add that if the bowel obstruction is itself managed laparoscopically, it is best to gain access using new ports of entry.

The long-term recurrence rate in patients with successfully treated small-bowel obstruction has also recently been reassessed (Abstract 140-94-10-31). Overall, approximately 35% to 40% of such patients will experience a reobstruction within 4 to 10 years. The greatest risk appears to be in those who have had several previous bouts of obstruction; conversely, the least risk is encountered in those whose obstruction was on the basis of hernia. Fortunately, reoperation is required to relieve recurrent obstruction in only 10% to 20% of patients.

A disturbing report from a large children's hospital (Abstract 140-94-10-32) indicates that, compared with a decade ago, patients with acute appendicitis are more frequently first seen in emergency departments, the initial diagnosis is more likely to be inaccurate, definitive therapy is more likely to be delayed, and patients experience greater morbidity and even mortality. The reasons for this deteriorating pattern of treatment is unclear, but most possibilities have considerable societal ramifications. Comparisons of laparoscopic with open appendectomy continue to appear.

A recent report from Hong Kong (Abstract 140-94-10-33) suggests that, in the Hong Kong patient population at least, the laparoscopic approach offers little in the way of advantage when the diagnosis seems secure. Costs were not analyzed in this study, however. A related study (Abstract 140-94-10-34) attempts to define the role of preoperative ultrasonography in diagnosing acute appendicitis. The results were interpreted as indicating that this modality has a higher positive and negative predictive value than does the surgeon's clinical impression at the time of admission. However, it seems certain that those cases about which the surgeon was initially unsure might well have declared themselves in a short period. Furthermore, the surgeon correctly disregarded the ultrasonic impression of a normal appendix in a number of instances and found surgical pathology (not always appendiceal) in every case. Finally, a case report is included (Abstract 140-94-10-35) that reemphasizes how ill-advised it is to perform a barium enema in patients with suspected perforations of the lower gastrointestinal tract, the opinion of our radiologist colleagues notwithstanding.

Wallace P. Ritchie, Jr., M.D., Ph.D.

Prediction of Early Symptomatic Recurrence After Intestinal Resection in Crohn's Disease

Heimann TM, Greenstein AJ, Lewis B, Kaufman D, Heimann DM, Aufses AH Jr (Mount Sinai School of Medicine, New York)
Ann Surg 218:294–299, 1993   140-94-10-29

Background.—Most patients with Crohn's disease will have endoscopic signs of perianastomotic recurrence within one year of intestinal resection. Most of these recurrences are initially asymptomatic; however, some patients have aggressive disease, with rapid progression to linear ulcerations and stenosis and early symptomatic recurrence. Clinical criteria that would predict which patients are at high risk of early symptomatic recurrence after intestinal resection for Crohn's disease were sought in a prospective study.

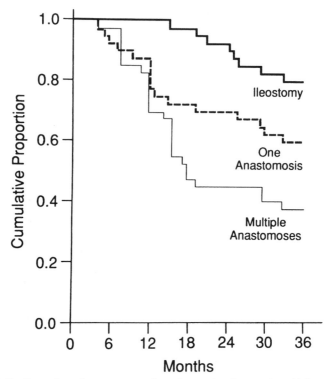

Fig 10–11.—Comparison of recurrence rates for patients undergoing resection with ileostomy with 1 anastomosis and multiple anastomoses. (Courtesy of Heimann TM, Greenstein AJ, Lewis B, et al: *Ann Surg* 218:294-299, 1993.)

Methods.—The study sample comprised 164 patients with a mean age of 36 years at surgery who underwent nonemergent intestinal resection for Crohn's disease over 13 years. Fifty-six percent of patients had involvement of both the large and small intestine; 31% had involvement of the small intestine only, and 13% had involvement of the large intestine only. Twenty-one percent had skip areas. A mean of 54 cm of bowel was resected. Abscess or fistula was the indication for surgery in 51% of patients and obstruction was the indication in 41%. The analysis sought associations between preoperative, intraoperative, and follow-up data and the outcome of early recurrence, defined as symptomatic recurrent disease within 36 months of surgery.

Findings.—Forty percent of patients had early symptomatic recurrence. On multivariate analysis, the number of anastomoses was found to be the most important predictor of early recurrence (Fig 10–11), followed by inflammation of the resection margins (Fig 10–12). The early recurrence rate was significantly lower in patients requiring an ileostomy than in those with single or multiple anastomoses. Inflammation at the margins was unrelated to early recurrence in patients requiring ileostomy

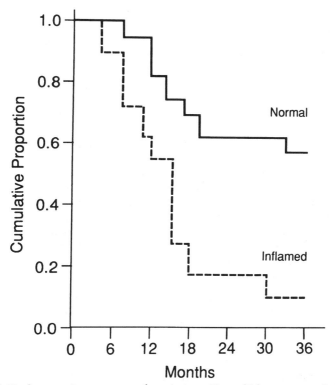

Fig 10–12.—Symptomatic recurrence rate for patients requiring multiple anastomoses. Patients with microscopic inflammation at the margins had significantly higher symptomatic recurrence rates than those with normal margins (P <.01). (Courtesy of Heimann TM, Greenstein AJ, Lewis B, et al: *Ann Surg* 218:294-299, 1993.)

or a single anastomosis. In contrast, 91% of patients with multiple anastomoses who had inflammation at either margin had early recurrence. Patients with multiple anastomoses and normal margins had the same recurrence rate as patients with a single anastomosis (42%).

Conclusion.—For patients undergoing intestinal resection for Crohn's disease, the risk of early symptomatic recurrence is high when extensive disease requires multiple resections and anastomoses, especially when the margins are inflamed. Ileostomy, when compared to anastomosis, appears to lower the risk of early recurrence. More study is needed to determine whether the postresection course of the disease can be altered by avoiding multiple anastomoses and using adjuvant medical therapy.

▶ Of 164 patients undergoing nonemergent intestinal resection for Crohn's disease at the Mount Sinai Hospital in New York between 1976 and 1989, symptomatic recurrence developed in 40% within the short space of 3 years. Interestingly, multivariant analysis suggested that the probability of early recurrence was less in patients who required an ileostomy as part of their therapy and also in the subset of patients requiring multiple anastomoses who had no histologic evidence of inflammation at the margins of resection. This last observation challenges what has, for years, been conventionally thought and conventionally taught, namely, remove gross disease and pay no attention to the microscopic marginal appearance (1, 2). This approach, along with the introduction of stricturoplasty, has undoubtedly saved some patients from the ravages of the short-bowel syndrome. The issue is whether it has also predisposed them to early recurrence. From a practical point of view, should surgeons now revert to trying to achieve histologically negative margins? The answer is no; not as a general rule. Recall that negative margins were of benefit only in those patients (28) requiring multiple anastomoses, a patient group with undoubtedly more severe disease than average. What of the protective effect of ileostomy? This could reflect a patient population with primarily colonic Crohn's without small-bowel involvement in the first place. One thing seems certain: Crohn's disease is complex and fascinating; as physicians and surgeons, we are a long way from understanding all of its nuances.—W.P. Ritchie, Jr., M.D., Ph.D.

References

1. *Ann Surg* 192:311, 1980.
2. *Dis Colon Rectum* 34:909, 1991.

Postoperative Bowel Obstruction Following Laparoscopic Surgery
Patterson M, Walters D, Browder W (East Tennessee State Univ, Johnson City)
Am Surg 59:656–657, 1993   140-94-10-30

Introduction.—Laparoscopic surgery is an increasingly frequently used approach to treating symptomatic cholelithiasis, and it also is increasingly being applied to such conditions as appendicitis and inguinal hernia. Laparoscopy also is finding more applications in gynecologic surgery. Herniation of a viscus into the abdominal trocar entry site has occasionally been mentioned, but infrequently reported.

Patients.—Three patients had bowel obstruction secondary to visceral herniation into a trocar entry site after laparoscopic surgery. One patient had undergone laparoscopic cholecystectomy, another had had a bilateral inguinal herniorrhaphy, and the third had undergone removal of an ectopic pregnancy. The patient who had herniorrhaphy had his incarcerated bowel reduced laparoscopically, but the other 2 patients had open surgery.

Implications.—Bowel obstruction may not be clinically obvious in these patients. It appears wise to provide fascial closure of all trocar sites that are 10 mm or more in extent, either directly or under laparoscopic visualization. It may be necessary to enlarge the incision, especially in an

Chapter 10-Gastrointestinal / **293**

obese patient. If bowel obstruction is itself managed laparoscopically, it is best to make a new incision.

▶ My consulting on 4 personal cases similar to those described here (all occurring after gynecologic laparoscopy) prompted inclusion of this paper. Although it may seem like preaching to those already in church, there is one point of the sermon: Close all fascial defects.—W.P. Ritchie, Jr., M.D., Ph.D.

Long-Term Outcome After Hospitalization for Small-Bowel Obstruction
Landercasper J, Cogbill TH, Merry WH, Stolee RT, Strutt PJ (Gundersen/Lutheran Med Ctr, La Crosse, Wis)
Arch Surg 128:765–771, 1993   140-94-10–31

Introduction.—Small-bowel obstruction, which accounts for nearly 20% of all surgical admissions for acute abdominal conditions, is known to have a high rate of recurrence. There are few studies, however, on the long-term outcome after hospital discharge. In a review of 309 consecutive hospitalizations for small-bowel obstruction over a 5-year period, the recurrence rate of small-bowel obstruction and its relationship to the cause of obstruction and method of treatment were investigated.

Patients and Methods.—The patient group had a mean age of 61 years; 59% were women and 41% were men. Ninety-two percent had undergone laparotomy. Patients were managed with nasogastric intubation, intravenous fluid, and close observation on admission. Most patients with classic signs of infarction or admission roentgenograms indicating complete obstruction underwent celiotomy; those whose condition did not improve within 72 hours generally also underwent laparotomy. The duration of hospital stay averaged 20 days for patients undergoing surgery and 8 days for those treated without operation. Follow-up averaged 53 months and extended up to 129 months.

Results.—Recurrent obstruction developed in 34% of all patients by 4 years and in 42% by 10 years. The rate of recurrence was 29% for patients who underwent surgery and 53% for those treated without operation. Patients with prior multiple obstructions had a higher recurrence rate (50%) than those without this factor (40%). None of the patients with hernia who were treated surgically had a recurrence; in contrast, the recurrence rate after surgery for patients with malignant neoplasms was 56%. Eleven of the 142 patients who died during follow-up had small-bowel obstruction listed as a contributing cause of death.

Conclusion.—Most cases of small-bowel obstruction result from adhesions, and no uniformly effective means of preventing this problem has been found. Although surgery lessens the risk of recurrent small-bowel obstruction, it does not eliminate it. Most recurrences occur within 4 years. Many factors need to be considered in deciding upon a course of treatment. The lower recurrence rate associated with surgery must be weighed against the costs and potential risks of operation.

▶ It is always refreshing to find new information about old and very common diseases. This paper is one of the few of which I am aware that traces the long-term (average follow-up, more than 4 years) outcome of a large number of patients initially hospitalized with mechanical small-bowel obstruction. It indicates that they are exposed to a 34% and 42% chance, respectively, of experiencing a recurrent small-bowel obstruction within 4 and 10 years. Patients at particular risk are those who were initially successfully treated nonoperatively, those with multiple prior episodes of obstruction, and those in whom obstruction developed in the setting of associated malignancy. This reobstruction rate is higher than many might anticipate. There is good news, however. The data also indicate that recurrent small-bowel obstruction in this setting necessitates operation only 10% to 20% of the time.—W.P. Ritchie, Jr., M.D., Ph.D.

Does the Current Health Care Environment Contribute to Increased Morbidity and Mortality of Acute Appendicitis in Children?
Linz DN, Hrabovsky EE, Franceschi D, Gauderer MWL (Case Western Reserve Univ, Cleveland, Ohio)
J Pediatr Surg 28:321–328, 1993   140-94-10–32

Background.—Early diagnosis and treatment are the most reasonable way to improve outcomes in patients with acute appendicitis. Changes in health care delivery that encourage primary physicians to act as "gatekeepers," however, may be resulting in delayed surgical referrals. Whether current gatekeeper controls on health care lead to increased treatment delays and morbidity in children with acute appendicitis was investigated.

Methods.—Experience with acute appendicitis at a large children's hospital over 2 periods 10 years apart was reviewed. One hundred seven consecutive children who underwent surgery for acute appendicitis from July 1988 through June 1990 were compared with 119 children treated between July 1978 through June 1980.

Findings.—The groups were similar in age, sex ratio, race, antecedent diseases, and negative appendectomy rate. More patients in the more recent group were seen initially in an emergency department or urgent care setting. The initial diagnosis was significantly less accurate in the more recent group. Although the length of time that elapsed before seeing a physician was comparable between groups, the length of time before seeing a surgeon was significantly different, being 41.2 hours in the earlier group and 56.4 hours in the later group. There was no significant between-group difference in time from seeing the surgeon to operation. The more recent group had a higher morbidity rate, although the difference was nonsignificant. Morbidity was more complex in the more recent group; 6 patients had 2 or more complications and 2 children died. In the earlier group, only 1 patient had multiple complications, and no one died. In a multiple logistic regression analysis, variables affecting the presence of complications included time to physician, time to surgeon, and pathology. The length of hospital stay did not differ between groups.

Conclusion.—At the children's hospital studied, it now takes more time for children with acute appendicitis to reach the pediatric surgeon, with a subsequent trend toward more frequent and complex morbidity. These findings may be attributed to changes in the initial physician-contact setting, greater misdiagnosis, and delayed surgical referral.

▶ The data provided in this paper are indisputable. At this particular children's hospital in Cleveland, compared with statistics from 10 years ago, patients with acute appendicitis were more likely to be seen in emergency departments; the initial diagnosis was more likely to be inaccurate; definitive surgical intervention was more likely to be delayed; and, as a consequence, patients experienced greater morbidity and (sadly) mortality. The answer to the question posed by the title is unequivocally "yes." The difficulty comes when one attempts to decide which part of the "current health care environment" is responsible. Is it a problem of parental indifference? Is it a problem of the gatekeepers obstructing access? Is it a problem of poorly trained emergency room physicians? Is it a problem of a changing natural history of disease? Is it a combination of all of these? Gatekeeper-bashing is popular and may even be appropriate under some circumstances. However, this particular paper tells us only that something is badly amiss; what it is and how to correct it are far from clear.—W.P. Ritchie, Jr., M.D., Ph.D.

Laparoscopic Versus Open Appendicectomy: Prospective Randomised Trial
Tate JJT, Dawson JW, Chung SCS, Lau WY, Li AKC (Chinese Univ of Hong Kong)
Lancet 342:633–637, 1993   140-94-10–33

Introduction.—It has proved difficult to randomly evaluate new laparoscopic surgical methods, because surgeons need to become experienced with the new methods and subsequently tend to favor one approach or the other. Nevertheless, whether there are differences in outcome in patients randomly assigned to undergo either open appendicectomy (OA) or laparoscopic appendicectomy (LA) was determined.

Study Design.—Three surgical teams admitted to the study 140 patients who had a clinical diagnosis of acute appendicitis for which a gridiron incision in the right iliac fossa would be appropriate, and who also were suitable for laparoscopy. The 70 patients assigned to the OA group and the 70 in the LA group were similar in age, gender, and the duration of symptoms. Acute appendicitis was histologically confirmed in 80% of the patients in both groups, and perforation occurred in 17% in both groups.

Outcome.—The mean time required for LA was 70.3 minutes, compared with 46.5 minutes in the OA group. No major intraoperative complications occurred in either group. Fourteen patients in the LA group (20%) required conversion to an open operation. Pain scores and analgesic needs were comparable in the 2 groups, as were times to the resumption of diet and discharge from the hospital. About three fourths of the patients in each group had returned to work 3 weeks postoperatively. Wound problems after discharge were somewhat less frequent after LA, but not significantly so.

Conclusion.—There are no substantial differences in the postoperative course after OA and LA.

▶ This study differs from one reviewed last year in these pages (1) in that it was unable to identify significant differences between laparoscopic and traditional appendectomy in terms of complications, postoperative pain and analgesic requirement, time to reintroduction of diet, and hospital stay. Furthermore, at the time of the initial postoperative follow-up, equivalent numbers of patients had returned to work (74% to 79%). Keeping in mind that a type 2 statistical error is common in studies such as these, the results, if true, suggest that very little benefit may accrue from use of the laparoscopic approach in patients in whom the diagnosis is reasonably certain. Perhaps the greatest boon to be gained from this technique will be for those who were previously admitted to the hospital to "rule out" appendicitis. In such instances, a reasonable strategy is to perform diagnostic laparoscopy early (within 6 hours of admission) and to discharge the patient posthaste if no surgical problem is found.—W.P. Ritchie, Jr., M.D., Ph.D.

Reference

1. 1993 YEAR BOOK OF SURGERY, pp 254.

Accuracy of Ultrasound in the Diagnosis of Acute Appendicitis Compared With the Surgeon's Clinical Impression
Wade DS, Morrow SE, Balsara ZN, Burkhard TK, Goff WB (US Naval Hosp, San Diego, Calif)
Arch Surg 128:1039–1046, 1993   140-94-10–34

Rationale.—The clinical diagnosis of acute appendicitis has been reported to be accurate in 50% to 80% of cases. It is especially difficult to make this diagnosis clinically in the very young, elderly persons, and women of reproductive age.

Objective.—The accuracy of clinical diagnosis, as made by the surgeon, was compared with that of abdominal ultrasound examination in a prospective series of 107 patients admitted with suspected appendicitis. The series included 71 male patients and 28 female patients whose mean ages were 26 and 21 years, respectively, and 8 children with a mean age of 10.6 years. Eighty-one patients were operated on.

Ultrasound Criteria.—The ultrasonographic diagnosis of appendicitis included a noncompressible, immobile, blind-ended structure having the appearance of a target. The visualized structure must have exceeded 6 mm in greatest diameter.

Findings.—An ultrasonographic diagnosis of appendicitis was 85.5% sensitive and 84% specific, and it had positive and negative predictive values of 88% and 80%, respectively. Its overall accuracy was 85%. In contrast, the surgeon's clinical impression at the time of admission was 71% accurate overall. A clinical diagnosis of appendicitis was 63% sensitive and 82% specific and had positive and negative predictive values of 83% and 62%, respectively.

Conclusion.—Abdominal ultrasonography is a more accurate means of diagnosing acute appendicitis than clinical assessment by the surgeon. However, 24% of patients with normal ultrasound findings were ultimately found to have appendicitis at operation. Therefore, ultrasonography cannot be relied upon to the exclusion of the surgeon's careful and repeated examination. Ultrasonography may be most helpful when the surgeon is unwilling to operate immediately.

▶ Ultrasound may be a useful tool by which to complement clinical judgment; however, the perceptive surgeon will easily recognize that papers like this do not support the proposition that ultrasound should supplant a carefully performed history and physical examination as the gold standard in the diagnosis of acute appendicitis. Even though 18 patients with appendicitis at operation were initially selected for observation by the surgeon but then underwent surgery after the ultrasound image was obtained, it seems certain that many (if not all) of these would have declared themselves clinically during a period of observation and would then have been safely managed operatively. It is manifestly unfair, in my view, to include these patients as clinical false negatives. More importantly, the surgeon overrode the ultrasonic declaration of appendiceal normality in 5 cases and found appendicitis in all 5. Furthermore, 2 other patients did not have ultrasound results that were positive for appendicitis, but they underwent surgery anyway and were found to have other conditions mandating exploration: a tubo-ovarian abscess and a perforated duodenal ulcer. Ultrasound should complement clinical evaluation, not the reverse. Parenthetically, the increasingly widespread use of early diagnostic laparoscopy in patients previously admitted as "rule out appendicitis" may make studies like this moot.—W.P. Ritchie, Jr., M.D., Ph.D.

Perforation Associated With Barium Enema in Acute Appendicitis
Shust N, Blane CE, Oldham KT (Univ of Michigan Hosps, Ann Arbor)
Pediatr Radiol 23:289–290, 1993   140-94-10–35

Introduction.—A child suspected of having atypical acute appendicitis had a barium enema examination that led to appendiceal perforation and extravasation of contrast medium. Emergency appendectomy was followed by life-threatening septic complications. This care prompted a review of the literature to better define contraindications to barium enema examination.

Impressions.—The barium enema has long been used to assess children who might have appendicitis as well as those whose appendix has been perforated. No complications were reported in 4 studies totaling more than 1,000 barium enema examinations. Barium spill into the peritoneum appears to be very rare, whether or not the appendix has ruptured. A diligent literature search yielded a single report of leakage. It may be that obstruction of the proximal appendix, which precedes distal suppurative changes, prevents filling of the more distal, friable part of the appendix, the part that is at risk of perforating.

▶ In those antedeluvian times when I was growing up in the field of surgery, performing a barium enema in patients with suspected perforations, particularly of the lower gastrointestinal tract, was a sure invitation to leave the residency program. As this case illustrates, barium mixed with enteric content is a potent—and often lethal—adjuvant to infectious peritonitis. Despite the assertions of the authors to the contrary in relation to safety, such studies should never be performed on patients who might have a hole in the gastrointestinal tract, especially the lower tract.—W.P. Ritchie, Jr., M.D., Ph.D.

Colon and Rectum

INTRODUCTION

A comparatively early but relatively large experience with laparoscopic colectomy, primarily sigmoid colectomy and right hemicolectomy, has been reported (Abstract 140-94-10-36). Forty-one percent of patients required conversion to celiotomy. There were no deaths, but almost one quarter of the patients had major complications. If the procedure was successfully completed laparoscopically, the hospital stay was significantly shorter than that associated with traditional approaches. However, the cost of open right hemicolectomy was less than when conversion was necessary. The yield of lymph nodes in patients who had surgery for malignant disease was comparable and adequate.

Same-admission colostomy closure was evaluated on a busy trauma service (Abstract 140-94-10-37). The approach seemed safe, provided strict guidelines were adhered to, and it probably saved 1 to 3 days of hospitalization. An examination of data from several large tumor registries suggests that total colectomy with ileorectal anastomosis is a very viable alternative to restorative proctocolectomy in patients with familial adenomatous polyposis (Abstract 140-94-10-38). The authors of the report think that the procedure is eminently justifiable as a primary treatment for most patients, because the risk of invasive adenocarcinoma developing in the retained rectal stump (and the risk of dying of that carcinoma) is extremely low if strict surveillance methodologies are used.

When patients undergoing restorative proctocolectomy for mucosal ulcerative colitis are matched in all respects except underlying disease to patients undergoing the same procedure for familial adenomatous polyposis, the long-term functional outcomes are comparable and very acceptable (Abstract 140-94-10-39). This is true despite a somewhat higher incidence of pouch-related complications and inflammation in the colitis group. Although these results are in contrast to those obtained in other series, it seems clear that restorative proctocolectomy is an extremely valuable approach to both groups of patients.

The results of an anorectal advancement flap repair of rectovaginal and other complicated anorectal fistulas have been reported and appear to be strikingly good: Diverting colostomies are avoided, sphincter function is preserved, and 94% of fistulas are successfully closed (Abstract 140-94-10-40). Notable exceptions include those patients whose fistulas are related to radiation-induced injury and those which are associated with fulminant Crohn's disease.

A randomized comparison of three nonsurgical treatments of first- and second-degree hemorrhoids has been completed (Abstract 140-94-10-41). The results suggest that infrared coagulation may be the best nonoperative treatment modality available for this disease. However, given that only approximately one third of patients treated in this manner ultimately become totally asymptomatic, one wonders if there might not still be room for surgical hemorrhoidectomy in some patients. Finally, an experience with low anterior resection as definitive treatment for complete rectal prolapse (Abstract 140-94-10-42) indicates that this operation is still an excellent alternative to rectal suspension operations.

Wallace P. Ritchie, Jr., M.D., Ph.D.

Laparoscopic Colectomy: A Critical Appraisal
Falk PM, Beart RW Jr, Wexner SD, Thorson AG, Jagelman DG, Lavery IC, Johansen OB, Fitzgibbons RJ Jr (Creighton Univ, Omaha, Neb; Univ of Southern California, Los Angeles; Cleveland Clinic Florida, Fort Lauderdale; et al)
Dis Colon Rectum 36:28–34, 1993   140-94-10–36

Objective.—The advent of successful laparoscopic biliary surgery has led to the application of laparoscopic methods for many thoracic and abdominal operations. The outcome of laparoscopic colorectal surgery in 66 patients was examined.

Patients and Operations.—The series included 28 men with a mean age of 63 years and 38 women with a mean age of 58 years. The most frequent procedures were sigmoid colectomy and right hemicolectomy. Fewer patients underwent low anterior resection, colectomy with an ileal pouch-anal anastomosis, and abdominoperineal resection. Forty-one percent of the patients were converted from laparoscopic colectomy to celiotomy. Data on the results of conventional sigmoid colectomy and right hemicolectomy were acquired from the same centers.

Findings.—There were no deaths, but 24% of the patients had major complications. The mean postoperative hospital stay was significantly shorter when surgery was laparoscopically completed than when conversion was necessary or traditional surgery was performed. The cost of right hemicolectomy was less for conventionally managed patients than when conversion was necessary, but no such difference was found for sigmoid resection. The yield of lymph nodes in patients operated on for malignant disease was comparable in all groups.

Conclusion.—Colorectal surgery may be done laparoscopically with acceptable morbidity as long as the surgeon is properly trained. Although the hospital stay is shortened, it remains to be established that total hospital costs will decline.

▶ This multicenter, retrospective study describes an early but large experience with laparoscopically performed colon resection, primarily right hemicolectomy and sigmoid resection. It contains a number of interesting observations, including an analysis of in-hospital costs. Although the length of stay for both procedures was significantly less using the laparoscopic approach, the overall hospital costs were not different relative to those associated with open colectomy. This was so because of the larger operating room costs associated with laparoscopy—a function, no doubt, of our love affair with disposables (and of an increased operating time). In my view, this infatuation should end.

In this same connection, the high conversion rate (41%) is of some concern because, in these instances, the costs of the traditional procedure are additive to those of the laparoscopic one. Parenthetically, one of the reasons (admittedly infrequent) for conversion was that the lesion was not found in the resected specimen. This serves as a reminder that, no matter how good laparoscopic procedures become, the tactile sense will always be denied us.—W.P. Ritchie, Jr., M.D., Ph.D.

Same Admission Colostomy Closure (SACC): A New Approach to Rectal Wounds: A Prospective Study
Renz BM, Feliciano DV, Sherman R (Emory Univ, Atlanta, Ga)
Ann Surg 218:279–293, 1993   140-94-10–37

Objective.—The safety of a policy of same admission colostomy closure (SACC) was examined in 30 consecutive patients with traumatic rectal wounds at or below the pelvic peritoneal reflection of the rectum. Gunshot injuries were responsible for 27 cases. All but 5 of the patients had associated injuries.

Criteria.—A rectal wound was diagnosed when a hole or blood was evident on digital anorectal examination, when proctoscopy or laparotomy revealed a hole or blood, or when a transpelvic missile trajectory was combined with blood on digital examination or proctoscopy and there was no other explanation.

Management.—Wounds near the peritoneal reflection were repaired at laparotomy. All patients had fecal diversion, most often via sigmoid loop colostomy. The presacral space was drained through the perineum. Healing was assessed by a peranal contrast enema 5–10 days after injury. If the patient was doing well clinically at this time, had a normal contrast enema, was without infection, and had normal anal continence, SACC was offered.

Results.—Twenty-three of the 30 patients had an unrepaired extraperitoneal rectal wound. Only 2 patients had distal colorectal washout. Eight patients had evidence of leakage on contrast enema examination. Six of them had unrepaired wounds, for a leakage rate of 26% in this group. Sixteen patients underwent SACC a mean of 12 days after injury. Three patients had complications other than fever, none of them related to the healed rectal wound. The mean hospital stay after SACC was 5.4 days. Two patients (12.5%) had a fistula develop after SACC. They were among the first 7 patients operated on, who had a simple single- or double-layer colostomy closure using absorbable sutures. The 9 subsequent patients had resection of a loop or an end stoma, followed by a hand-sewn 1- or 2-layer end-to-end anastomsis. None of these patients had complications.

Conclusion.—Contrast enema testing is a reliable means of confirming healing of a traumatic rectal wound. Once a wound is shown to be sealed, the colostomy may be safely closed. At the cost of a minor emotional setback, SACC saves 1–3 days of hospital time.

▶ This paper shows that (1) the current approach to penetrating rectal injury, including proximal diversion and presacral drainage, is appropriate; (2) even without rectal washout, the majority of rectal wounds heal rapidly (within 7 to 10 days); and (3) colostomy closure can be accomplished safely if no leakage from a rectal wound is apparent at that time on contrast enema, the patient is doing well clinically, and there is no evidence of sphincter incompetence. On the downside, the process is very labor-intensive and some patients are not emotionally prepared for 2 operations within the same hospitalization.—W.P. Ritchie, Jr., M.D., Ph.D.

Rectal Cancer Risk in Patients Treated for Familial Adenomatous Polyposis

De Cosse JJ, Bülow S, Neale K, Järvinen H, Alm T, Hultcrantz R, Moesgaard F, Costello C, and the Leeds Castle Polyposis Group (New York Hosp/Cornell Med Ctr, New York; Hvidovre Hosp, Copenhagen; St Mark's Hosp, London; et al)

Br J Surg 79:1372–1375, 1992   140-94-10–38

Objective.—Because total colectomy with ileorectal anastomosis (IRA) leaves patients with familial adenomatous polyposis (FAP) at risk of having rectal cancer, 2 studies were done to determine the extent of this risk.

Scandinavian Study.—The incidence of rectal cancer was estimated in 297 unselected patients from national registers in Denmark, Finland, and Sweden who underwent total colectomy and IRA for FAP and were followed for at least one year. The median age at the time of surgery was 27 years. Thirty-five patients (12%) had colonic cancer within a year of IRA, and 3 (1%) had rectal cancer. Thirteen patients (4.4%) subsequently had rectal cancer. The cumulative risk of rectal cancer developing after IRA was 3.1% at 5 years, 4.5% at 10 years, 9.4% at 20 years, and 13.1% at 25 years.

Registry Study.—Data on 50 patients having FAP and invasive rectal cancer were obtained from 11 polyposis registries. The patients represented 3.7% of all those registered who were at risk after IRA when surgery was done before mid-1986. Eleven of the 50 patients had invasive colonic cancer at the time of surgery. The median interval from IRA to the detection of invasive cancer was 11 years. Forty-five evaluable patients had a 5-year survival rate of 71%, and 29 patients had a 10-year survival rate of 55%.

Conclusion.—Combining the results of both series, patients with FAP had a 2% risk of dying of rectal cancer within 15 years after IRA. This procedure is warranted as primary treatment for most patients with FAP. These patients must be followed all their lives.

▶ This paper tells us that total colectomy with IRA 10 cm to 15 cm from the anal verge may still be a very appropriate operation for patients with FAP. Careful analysis of data from several well-kept registries suggests that such patients have only a 13% chance of rectal cancer developing at 25 years after operation and only a 2% chance of dying of that cancer at 15 years. Patient selection is key, however. Surveillance proctoscopy must be performed religiously every 6 months, something the noncompliant individual may have difficulty dealing with over a 40- to 50-year period.—W.P. Ritchie, Jr., M.D., Ph.D.

Similar Functional Results After Restorative Proctocolectomy in Patients With Familial Adenomatous Polyposis and Mucosal Ulcerative Colitis

Tjandra JJ, Fazio VW, Church JM, Oakley JR, Milsom JW, Lavery IC (Cleveland Clinic Found, Ohio)
Am J Surg 165:322–325, 1993   140-94-10-39

Background.—Restorative proctocolectomy with an ileoanal reservoir has been a significant advance in the treatment of familial adenomatous polyposis (FAP) and mucosal ulcerative colitis (MUC). Patients with polyposis tended to be in better health than those with colitis, and restorative proctocolectomy has generally been thought to yield better results in the former group.

Study Population.—The clinical and functional results of restorative proctocolectomy were compared in 39 pairs of patients with FAP and MUC who were individually matched for surgeon, the type of ileal pouch created, and the technique of ileal pouch–anal anastomosis. Nineteen S-pouches and 20 J-pouches were created. Twenty-one anastomoses were stapled and 18 were hand-sewn with mucosectomy. The 2 groups were also matched for age (median, 30 years) and gender. The median follow-up after operation was 32 months.

Results.—The operating time and average hospital stay were similar in the 2 groups, as was the volume of blood lost (about 650 mL). Complications, including pouch-related septic problems, were more frequent in the MUC group. The functional outcome, in terms of daytime and nighttime stool frequencies and the ability to defer defecation, were similar in the MUC and FAP groups. In each group, 87% of patients were continent during the day and 49% were continent at night. Patient ratings of the quality of their lives and health and the degree of satisfaction with the outcome of surgery were identical in the 2 groups.

Conclusion.—Restorative proctocolectomy provided a comparable functional outcome in closely matched patients having diagnoses of FAP and MUC. Pouchitis was more often a problem in patients with colitis.

▶ Patients with FAP are considered to be ideal candidates for restorative proctocolectomy, and rightly so. The importance of this paper is the demonstration that, when patients with this condition are matched with those having MUC in every respect except the underlying disease, the functional outcome after approximately 3 years is exactly the same and is very good, despite a somewhat higher incidence of pouch-related complications and inflammation in the latter group. This operation is a major step forward in the treatment of both diseases.—W.P. Ritchie, Jr., M.D., Ph.D.

Endorectal Advancement Flap Repair of Rectovaginal and Other Complicated Anorectal Fistulas

Kodner IJ, Mazor A, Shemesh EI, Fry RD, Fleshman JW, Birnbaum EH (Washington Univ, St Louis, Mo; Jewish Hosp, St. Louis, Mo)

Surgery 114:682–690, 1993   140-94-10-40

Introduction.—In the past, the surgical repair of rectovaginal and complicated anal-perineal fistulas has frequently been followed by complications and failure of the repair. A series including 107 patients who had an endorectal advancement flap repair within the past 10 years was reviewed.

Patients.—The patients included 98 women and 9 men with a mean age of 38 years. Seventy-one patients had a low rectovaginal fistula, 28 had an anterior anal-perineal fistula, and 8 had a posterior anal-perineal fistula. The most common cause of fistula formation was obstetric injury, followed by cryptoglandular abscess or fistula and Crohn's disease.

Technique.—The operative technique used preserves the sphincter muscle and covers the internal opening of the fistulous tract with healthy rectal wall. A broad-based, inverted U-shaped flap is elevated starting just distal to the mucocutaneous junction. The flap consists of mucosa, submucosa, and part of the thickness of the internal sphincter; its base is twice as wide as its apex. The fistulous tract is curetted, and counter drainage is provided with either a self-contained suction drain or a mushroom-tip catheter. The flap is sewn in place using interrupted 2-0 chromic gut sutures. The mucocutaneous junction is repaired with 3-0 chromic gut sutures.

Results.—There were no deaths, but 17 patients (16%) had a persistent or recurrent fistula. Nine of these patients successfully underwent a second operation. Recurrence of the fistula did not destroy sphincteric function in patients who had reconstruction simultaneously. Continence was unchanged in 80% of the patients and improved in 18%. Two patients, who still had intestinal flow diversion, were not evaluable.

Conclusion.—The endorectal advancement flap operation is a safe and effective means of repairing low rectovaginal and anal-perineal fistulas. It improves sphincter function and avoids the need for fecal diversion.

▶ For many surgeons, placement of a seton has been the procedure of choice in the treatment of rectovaginal or other complex anal-perineal fistulas, particularly when they are located in an anterior position and where a high probability of sphincter involvement exists. Unfortunately, this approach produces a high incidence of both incontinence and recurrences. The treatment strategy advocated by this group of skilled colorectal surgeons clearly warrants attention. Diverting colostomies are avoided, sphincter function is preserved, and, eventually, 94% of fistulas are successfully closed. According to the authors, the approach is suitable for any fistula that can be visualized (and probed) with the important exceptions of those that are a consequence of radiation injury to the rectum and those that are associated with fulminant and uncontrolled Crohn's disease. Even in this last group, however, if nonoperative treatment renders the tissue mobile and supple, an advancement flap can often be performed with reasonable results.—W.P. Ritchie, Jr., M.D., Ph.D.

Optimal Nonsurgical Treatment of Hemorrhoids: A Comparative Analysis of Infrared Coagulation, Rubber Band Ligation, and Injection Sclerotherapy
Johanson JF, Rimm A (Univ of Illinois, Rockford; Med College of Wisconsin, Milwaukee)
Am J Gastroenterol 87:1601–1606, 1992   140-94-10-41

Background.—Although numerous nonoperative treatments for the management of hemorrhoids have been suggested, none has been reported as being consistently more efficacious than the others. Data from multiple randomized, controlled clinical trials were compared to assess the efficacy of infrared photocoagulation (IRC), injection sclerotherapy, and rubber band ligation, and to determine the optimal nonoperative hemorrhoid treatment.

Methods.—The meta-analysis was limited to those approaches that have been compared in randomized, controlled clinical trials. Patients were classified as responders if symptoms were resolved after treatment. Five clinical trials involving 863 patients were analyzed. Of these, 2 compared IRC with rubber band ligation, 2 compared sclerotherapy with rubber band ligation, and 1 compared all 3 procedures.

TABLE 1.—Pooled Response Rates 12 Months After IRC or
Rubber Band Ligation (RBL)

Outcome	No. of Events/ No. of Patients		Pooled Rate Difference	p Value
	IRC	RBL		
Treatment response				
Asymptomatic	85/204	79/185	0.049	0.23
No improvement	59/204	47/185	0.026	0.24
Additional therapy	29/184	8/150	0.106	0.0002
Complications				
Pain	11/307	45/226	0.233	0.02
Bleeding	24/307	12/226	0.010	0.24

(Courtesy of Johanson JF, Rimm A: *Am J Gastroenterol* 87:1601–1606, 1992.)

TABLE 2.—Pooled Response Rates 12 Months After Injection
Sclerotherapy or Rubber Band Ligation (RBL)

Outcome	No. of events/ No. of patients		Pooled Rate Difference	p Value
	Sclero	RBL		
Treatment response				
Asymptomatic	44/175	60/163	0.104	0.07
No improvement	61/175	40/163	0.069	0.19
Additional therapy	39/171	14/163	0.128	0.009
Complications				
Pain	43/81	30/62	0.011	0.46
Bleeding	6/162	7/146	0.010	0.13

(Courtesy of Johanson JF, Rimm A: *Am J Gastroenterol* 87:1601–1606, 1992.)

Results.—No significant differences in treatment response were noted between IRC and rubber band ligation at a 12-month follow-up, although 3 times as many patients initially treated with IRC underwent additional treatments for symptom recurrence. Each technique was comparable with respect to effective treatment of first- and second-degree hemorrhoids. However, a fivefold difference in development of pain was noted in patients treated with rubber band ligation (Table 1). The symptomatic response rate at 12 months was better in those treated with rubber band ligation compared to those who underwent sclerotherapy, although this difference was not statistically significant (Table 2). Nearly 3 times more patients initially treated with sclerotherapy needed additional treatment. Although stratification by hemorrhoid severity revealed comparable response rates for first-degree hemorrhoids, rubber band ligation was significantly better than sclerotherapy in the treatment of second-degree hemorrhoids. The complication rates of these 2 methods were similar.

Conclusion.—In this meta-analysis, statistically significant differences between various nonoperative approaches for hemorrhoid treatment were revealed. Rubber band ligation had a better long-term effect but was associated with a significantly higher incidence of post-treatment pain. However, fewer and less severe complications were noted in patients treated with IRC. When all factors are considered, IRC may represent the optimal nonoperative hemorrhoid treatment.

▶ In this report, a new and powerful statistical methodology (meta-analysis) is applied to the treatment of an ancient and uncomfortable surgical disease: first- and second-degree hemorrhoids. Of the 3 nonoperative treatments evaluated, IRC and rubber band ligation were equally efficacious in the long term and better than injection sclerotherapy. However, more treatments were required in the IRC group to achieve this end than in the rubber-banded group.

On the other hand, rubber banding was associated with a significantly higher incidence of post-treatment pain. When the infrequent but lethal problem of pelvic sepsis after rubber band ligation is also taken into account, the conclusion of the authors seems reasonable: Infrared coagulation may be the best nonoperative treatment modality available for this disease. It should be pointed out, however, that only 79 of 185 patients in the rubber band group and 85 of 204 in the infrared group ultimately became totally asymptomatic. Might not some of the remaining patients be candidates for treatment the old-fashioned way?—W.P. Ritchie, Jr., M.D., Ph.D.

Anterior Resection for the Treatment of Rectal Prolapse: A 20-Year Experience
Cirocco WC, Brown AC (Saint Vincent Health Ctr and Hamot Med Ctr, Erie, Pa)
Am Surg 59:265–269, 1993   140-94-10–42

Introduction.—For definitive treatment of the difficult problem of complete rectal prolapse, anterior resection compares well with the widely used rectal suspension operations. Rectal suspension procedures are associated with inherent risks of hemorrhage and infection, and all procedures carry the risk of recurrent rectal prolapse. Twenty years of experience with anterior resection for rectal prolapse were reviewed.

Patients.—The study comprised 35 women and 6 men with an average age of 56 years, all of whom were undergoing their first attempt at surgical correction for rectal prolapse. Fifty-one percent had some anal incontinence, and 41% were seen with constipation. The operation consisted of anterior resection and presacral drainage, with complete mobilization of the rectum to the level of the coccyx and levator ani muscles, followed by resection and anastomosis. The anastomosis was hand-sewn in all but 2 cases, in which it was stapled. Patients were followed up for an average of 6 years.

Outcomes.—There were 3 recurrences at 2–5.5 years postoperatively. After surgery, 90% of patients seen with anal incontinence had either no change or improved continence. Three fourths of patients seen with constipation were either improved or unchanged in this area. The morbidity rate was 15%, including 3 incisional hernias, 2 cases of small bowel obstruction, and 1 of stroke.

Conclusion.—In properly selected patients, anterior resection is the procedure of choice for patients with complete rectal prolapse. Most surgeons are familiar with the procedure, which offers a cure while limiting the risks of rectal suspension procedures. Long-term recurrence and complication rates are low.

▶ This report reemphasizes that low anterior resection used as therapy for complete rectal prolapse remains an excellent alternative to rectal suspension operations. Not only does it avoid the complications associated with placement of prosthetic material, but it is also a standard skill in the armamentarium of the well-trained general surgeon.—W.P. Ritchie, Jr., M.D., Ph.D.

Spleen

INTRODUCTION

Splenectomy remains the mainstay of treatment for patients with idiopathic thrombocytopenic purpura (ITP). It seems intuitively obvious that the site of platelet sequestration is predictive of the outcome of the procedure. Until recently, however, that assertion has not been proved. To address this issue, autologous labelled platelets were administered to 51 patients with persistent drug-resistant ITP (Abstract 140-94-10-43). All patients subsequently underwent splenectomy. Eighty-one percent of the patients had a splenic sequestration site. In these, platelet counts had normalized in 87% by 3 years postoperatively. In contrast, those patients with mixed or hepatic sites of sequestration had a minimal response. This technique may help in better selecting patients for the procedure.

Two studies (Abstracts 140-94-10-44 and 140-94-10-45) remind us that splenectomy for hematologic disease can be associated with the unusual, but potentially lethal, problem of portal vein thrombosis. The diagnosis is difficult to make, and therapy is often delayed at the expense of enteric viability. The issue of prophylaxis using platelet inhibitors in the pediatric patient undergoing this operation is unsettled but potentially important.

Wallace P. Ritchie, Jr., M.D., Ph.D.

Splenectomy in Idiopathic Thrombocytopenic Purpura: Its Correlation With the Sequestration of Autologous Indium-111-Labeled Platelets
Lamy T, Moisan A, Dauriac C, Ghandour C, Morice P, Le Prise PY (Hopital Pontchaillou, Rennes, France; Centre Eugène Marguis, Rennes, France; Hosp of St-Brieuc, France)
J Nucl Med 33:182–186, 1993   140-94-10-43

Introduction.—Splenectomy can increase the chances of definitive remission in patients with idiopathic thrombocytopenic purpura (ITP), with an overall effectiveness of 72% at a minimum 6-month follow-up. There is ongoing debate about whether the platelet sequestration site is related to the outcome of the operation. The results of ^{111}In-labeled autologous platelet sequestration studies in 111 patients with ITP were analyzed.

Methods.—All patients with a clinical diagnosis of ITP over a 6½-year period underwent ^{111}In-labeled platelet sequestration study. Fifty-one patients with persistent, drug-resistant ITP went on to undergo surgery, in-

Outcome 3 Months After Splenectomy (51 Patients)

Sequestration site	Number	Complete remission	Partial remission	Failures
Splenic	38	33	1	4
Mixed	9	2	0	7
Hepatic	4	0	0	4
Platelet counts 10⁹/liter*		322 (110)	85	32 (9)

* Mean–1 standard deviation.
(Courtesy of Lamy T, Moisan A, Dauriac C, et al: *J Nucl Med* 33:182–186, 1993.)

dependent of the results of these studies. The analysis focused on whether the isotopic results could accurately predict a beneficial response to surgery.

Results.—Eighty-one percent of the patients had a splenic sequestration site, 12% had a mixed site, and 7% had a hepatic site. Surgery was done more than 6 months after diagnosis in 33 patients and earlier in 18 patients at high risk of bleeding. The outcome for all 51 patients at 3 months after splenectomy is shown in the table. At a median follow-up of 3 years, platelet count had normalized in 87% of patients with splenic sequestration, compared with just 15% of those with mixed or hepatic sequestration.

Conclusion.—Sequestration studies using autologous ¹¹¹In-labeled platelets appear to be useful in patients with ITP. These studies demonstrate that thrombocytopenias meeting the accepted clinical and biological criteria for ITP do not necessarily result from excessive destruction. In addition, because splenectomy is much more likely to be successful in patients with splenic sequestration, these studies can help the clinician decide whether splenectomy should be performed.

▶ More often than not, successful surgical therapy is a function of successful patient selection. Not surprisingly, this paper suggests that, in addition to the response to steroids and IgG, the site of platelet sequestration (splenic vs. mixed or hepatic) is an important predictor of outcome in patients with ITP. Surgeons would do well to consider this before subjecting patients to splenectomy for this indication.—W.P. Ritchie, Jr., M.D., Ph.D.

Portal Vein Thrombosis After Elective Splenectomy: An Underappreciated, Potentially Lethal Syndrome

Rattner DW, Ellman L, Warshaw AL (Harvard Med School, Boston)
Arch Surg 128:565–570, 1993   140-94-10-44

Introduction.—Portal vein thrombosis (PVT) is widely recognized in patients with cirrhosis and liver tumors. However, it may be more com-

Characteristics of Patients With Portal Vein Thrombosis After Splenectomy

Patient No.	Age, y/ Sex	Diagnosis	Spleen Weight, g
1	67/M	Myeloid metaplasia	707
2	73/M	Lymphosarcoma cell leukemia	5530
3	52/F	Autoimmune hemolytic anemia	280
4	58/F	Lymphoma	1280
5	52/M	Chronic lymphocytic leukemia	5200
6	76/M	Gastric carcinoma	160
7	46/M	Sarcoidosis	775

(Courtesy of Rattner DW, Ellman L, Warshaw AL: *Arch Surg* 128:565–570, 1993.)

mon than is appreciated in patients who have had splenectomy. Seven patients with thrombosis of the portal and splenic vein after elective splenectomy were studied.

Patients.—The patients were seen during a 12-year period at a hospital where more than 1,000 splenectomies were performed. Six had portal or superior mesenteric vein thrombosis after splenectomy, and one had acute postoperative splenic vein thrombosis producing a similar syndrome. Myeloproliferative disorders were the most common underlying illnesses (table). Symptoms, including abdominal pain, diarrhea, and nausea, developed during the initial hospitalization in 3 patients, shortly after discharge in 2, and up to 18 months postoperatively in the remaining 2. None were initially suspected of having PVT. The final diagnosis was made by ultrasound plus color Doppler in 3 patients, contrast-enhanced CT in 2, and laparotomy and autopsy in one each.

Outcomes.—There were 2 deaths, both in patients with a long interval from the onset of PVT to correct diagnosis and therapy. The other 5 patients were given a diagnosis earlier and survived. Treatment included intravenously administered heparin sodium for 1–2 weeks, followed by warfarin sodium after discharge. In one patient, streptokinase was given before heparinization, resulting in complete thrombolysis. All patients received broad-spectrum antibiotics during their initial treatment. Serial ultrasound documented recanalization of the portal vein in 2 patients.

Discussion.—The authors report a series of patients with PVT after splenectomy. At least 2 pathogenetic factors appear to be operable: a hypercoagulable state and stasis in the splenic vein stump. Portal vein thrombosis should be suspected in postsplenectomy patients who have fever and abdominal complaints. Urgent thrombolytic treatment and long-term anticoagulation therapy may preserve the patient's life and bowel integrity.

Thrombosis of the Portal Venous System After Splenectomy for Pediatric Hematologic Disease
Skarsgard E, Doski J, Jaksic T, Wesson D, Shandling B, Ein S, Babyn P, Heiss K, Hu X (Hosp for Sick Children, Toronto)
J Pediatr Surg 28:1109–1112, 1993   140-94-10–45

Purpose.—Splenic, portal, and mesenteric vein thrombosis have been reported as rare and potentially fatal complications of splenectomy for hematologic diseases in adults. Two pediatric cases and 1 in a woman aged 18 years represent the first reports of postsplenectomy splanchnic venous thrombosis in such patients.

Patients.—The patients were a boy aged 13 years with hereditary elliptocytosis (HE), a boy aged 13 years with thalassemia intermedia (TI), and a woman aged 18 years with idiopathic thrombocytopenic purpura

Patients With and Without Venous Thrombosis After Splenectomy

	Patients Without Thrombosis (n = 15)	Patients With Thrombosis (n = 4*)
Median age (yr)	6	13
Sex	10 M, 5 F	2 M, 2 F
Diagnosis		
ITP	6	1
HS	5	2
TM	1	1
SS	2	0
ALL	1	0
Preoperative steroids	6 YES, 9 NO	1 YES, 3 NO
Median preoperative hemoglobin (g/L)	108	92
Median preoperative platelets (x 10^9/L)	215	307
Median operating time (min)	80	85
Median estimated blood loss (mL)	30	30
Median resuscitation volume (mL)	500	675
Medium postoperative hemoglobin (g/L)	125	113
Medium postoperative platelets (x 10^9/L)	575	631
Splenic mass (g)	235	549

Abbreviations: HS, hereditary spherocytosis: *TM,* thalassemia minor; *SS,* sickle cell disease; *ALL,* acute lymphoblastic leukemia.
* Three patients were symptomatic and 1 was asymptomatic.
(Courtesy of Skarsgard E, Doski J, Jaksic T, et al: *J Pediatr Surg* 28:1109–1112,1993.)

(ITP). The patients underwent splenectomy over a 10-year period and presented 4–13 days after splenectomy with abdominal pain and nausea, with or without fever. Imaging findings, including abdominal Doppler ultrasound or CT, or both, showed the following: in the patient with HE, an intraluminal filling defect with partial obstruction to flow in the right branch of the portal vein; in the patient with TI, splenic vein thrombosis with complete occlusion of the main portal and proximal superior mesenteric veins; and in the patient with ITP, complete thrombosis of the splenic vein, proximal superior mesenteric vein, and portal vein with retrogastric collateralization. The patient with HE had complete resolution of his vascular obstruction without treatment, but the other 2 patients had portal venous cavernomatous transformation with hepatofugal flow after 6 months of systemic anticoagulation therapy. All patients were asymptomatic at most recent follow-up.

Surveillance Program.—This experience prompted a program of routine postoperative ultrasound study in splenectomized pediatric patients. Sixteen consecutive asymptomatic postsplenectomy patients were studied at a median of 51 days postoperatively. This program identified 1 case of asymptomatic left portal venous thrombosis, which recanalized without treatment. The only significant predictors of thrombosis in these patients were older age and larger splenic mass (table).

Conclusion.—Thrombosis of the portal venous system is a potentially serious complication of splenectomy in children with hematologic disease. It should be considered in all children with abdominal pain after splenectomy. A routine postoperative surveillance program, such as the 1 described in this study, may also be considered. Aspirin prophylaxis may be warranted for patients with high-risk characteristics: massive spleen enlargement, older age, and possibly a high postoperative platelet count.

▶ Taken together, Abstracts 140-94-10–44 and 140-94-10–45 remind us that there are 2 diseases we will never diagnose: the disease we have never heard of and the disease we don't think about. Portal or superior mesenteric venous thrombosis after elective splenectomy, an uncommonly encountered but potentially devastating complication, falls into the second category. Obviously, it is no respecter of age, although it may be more lethal in adults. The principal common denominator of afflicted patients in these studies is the presence of underlying hematologic disease which may produce a hypercoagulable state, either in and of itself or after treatment. As the Harvard Medical School group (Abstract 140-94-10–44) also emphasizes, factors such as stasis in the splenic venous stump may also be important. Presenting signs and symptoms are usually vague, and the diagnosis can be very difficult to make. For these reasons, appropriate therapy may be delayed at the expense of enteric viability. Treatment with thrombolytic agents is an intriguing suggestion but only appropriate early in the course of the disease before the bowel becomes compromised.

The Toronto group (Abstract 140-94-10–45) raises the interesting question of whether long-term platelet inhibition with acetylsalicyclic acid might not be appropriate in the pediatric patient undergoing splenectomy for hematologic indications. To adopt that suggestion would require a much better definition of the risk-benefit ratio of this approach than is currently available. However, if the problem in the pediatric age group is more common than appreciated, might we not be dealing in the future with patients requiring complex operations for cavernous transformation, including hepatic transplantation? If so, some sort of prophylaxis would clearly be in order.—W.P. Ritchie, Jr., M.D., Ph.D.

Hernia

INTRODUCTION

An early but carefully performed and analyzed series of patients undergoing a standard preperitoneal hernia repair laparoscopically has been reported (Abstract 140-94-10-46). In contrast to laparoscopic cholecystectomy, the advantages of an endoscopic approach to hernia repair relative to traditional approaches is much less clear. There are probably 3 principal issues: cost, early return to gainful activity, and durability. Only a prospective trial will provide a scientifically acceptable perspective on each of these issues. Obturator hernias are rare but potentially lethal. A report of 13 patients seen in a 5-year period (Abstract 140-94-10-47) indicates that patients are overwhelmingly female, overwhelmingly old, and overwhelmingly emaciated. Classic signs of small-bowel obstruction may be present, but this is not invariable because many patients have a Richter-type hernia. The classic finding of numbness along the inner thigh is frequently absent. As with any mechanical small-bowel obstruction in the elderly, aggressive fluid resuscitation and early operation should be the rule.

Wallace P. Ritchie, Jr., M.D., Ph.D.

Laparoscopic Herniorrhaphy: Results and Technical Aspects in 450 Consecutive Procedures
Geis WP, Crafton WB, Novak MJ, Malago M (Lutheran Gen Hosp, Park Ridge, Ill; Univ of Chicago; Christ Hosp, Cincinnati, Ohio)
Surgery 114:765–774, 1993   140-94-10–46

*Background.—*The goals of successful hernia repair with a laparoscopic approach include reduction of recurrence and postoperative discomfort, minimization of morbidity, and early return to normal and strenuous physical activity. However, the effectiveness of this approach, as well as patient outcome and technical considerations, has been controversial. This approach was evaluated by review of laparoscopic inguinal herniorrhaphies in a series of 450 consecutive patients.

*Patients and Methods.—*Hernia repairs performed in 2 medical centers over a 24-month period were included in this review (Table 1). Pa-

TABLE 1.—Distribution of
450 Laparoscopic Herniorrhaphies

Hernia	No.	(%)	Recurrence
Indirect	306	(68)	3
Direct	135	(30)	0
Primary	86	(19)	0
Recurrent	49	(11)	0
Femoral	9	(2)	0
Bilateral*	86	(19)	0
Men	77		0
Women	9		0
Incarcerated			
Chronic	9		0
Acute	4		0

* Number of patients with bilateral hernias.
(Courtesy of Geis WP, Crafton WB, Novak MJ, et al: *Surgery* 114:765-774, 1993.)

tient age ranged from 16 to 83 years. Hernias were bilateral in 19% of the patients, recurrent in 11%, giant scrotal hernias in 9%, and incarcerated in 2.8%. Synthetic mesh was used for tensionless repair, according to surgical principles of preperitoneal herniorrhaphy. Mesh was fastened to anatomical landmarks with suture or staples. The peritoneum was closed, isolating mesh from abdominal contents.

Results.—Ninety percent of the patients were discharged from the recovery area. The remaining 10% were kept in the hospital overnight (but less than 24 hours after surgery), because of urinary retention, operations performed late in the day, and evaluation with a cardiac monitor for patients with established cardiac disease. Most patients had an excellent outcome with minimal pain. Postoperative follow-up has been conducted from 6 through 30 months. Three patients experienced recurrences 2 to 4 months after surgery, and 2 of them underwent laparoscopic repair. One port site infection has been noted, although no abdominal cavity infections have occurred. No adhesive or mesh complications have been observed. Three patients have reported having chronic pain since undergoing herniorrhaphy (Table 2).

Conclusion.—Laparoscopic inguinal hernia repair is safe and effective and compares favorably with other classic approaches. Patients experience minimal morbidity and can ambulate soon after repair with little discomfort. In many patient subsets, laparoscopic herniorrhaphy should be considered the preferential approach.

▶ This report deserves respect because it is a carefully considered recitation of the (admittedly) early results of laparoscopic herniorrhaphy performed in consecutive patients by a conscientious and skilled group of surgeons using

TABLE 2.—Outcome of Laparoscopic Hernia Repair

Observation	6-30 mo
Discharge same day	327 (90%) of 364
Pain medications	
33%	None
33%	Minimal
33%	Cannot remember
Work	3-10 days
Recurrence	3
Infection	
Port	1
Mesh	0
Adhesive	0
Seroma	6
Hematoma	5
Port hernia	1
Hydrocoele	0
Nerve entrapment	2 (?)

(Courtesy of Geis WP, Crafton WB, Novak MJ, el al: *Surgery* 114:765-774, 1993.)

a standard transabdominal approach to accomplish a preperitoneal hernia repair. The results on very short-term follow-up (6 to 30 months) are as described in the abstract and must be considered quite salutary: early discharge from the recovery area in 90% of instances, a low complication rate, and only 3 proven recurrences.

The discussion of the paper is as illuminating as its substance because it outlines the essence of the ongoing debate comparing laparoscopic with open hernia repair. Is the routine use of mesh justifiable? Are there any cost advantages? Do patients actually return to work earlier? If the hernia sac is left behind, how can one accurately assess recurrences? If the hernia sac is rountinely dissected, how can the development of confined hematomas be prevented? How does one avoid the truly distressing complication of genito-femoral or lateral femoral cutaneous nerve entrapment? Should all types of groin hernias be treated similarly? Most importantly (the real essence of the issue), how durable is the laparoscopic repair compared to open techniques? Unless a well-designed prospective and randomized clinical trial of extended duration is undertaken and brought to fruition, this debate will be heated and endless but the underlying issue will never be resolved.—W.P. Ritchie, Jr., M.D., Ph.D.

Obturator Hernia: A Continuing Diagnostic Challenge
Yip AWC, AhChong AK, Lam KH (Kwong Wah Hosp, Hong Kong)
Surgery 113:266–269, 1993   140-94-10–47

Objective.—Because obturator hernia is a frequent cause of potentially lethal complications, the course of this condition was examined in 13 patients, seen in the period 1986–1991, who had 14 obturator hernias.

Patients.—All but one of the patients were women, and all were emaciated and elderly. The mean age was 82 years. All patients were seen with features of small-bowel obstruction, but only 3 had the classic Howship-Romberg sign. Five patients were given a diagnosis before exploration. Nine of the 13 patients had concomitant medical disorders.

Operative Findings and Outcome.—In all patients, the hernial sac contained small bowel, most often ileum. Ten patients had a Richter-type hernia. In 7 patients, it was necessary to resect gangrenous bowel. Five patients had postoperative complications, and 2 (15.4%) died of chest infection and septicemia. The 2 patients who died underwent surgery at 84 and 120 hours, respectively, after admission.

Conclusion.—Obturator hernia should be suspected when a thin, elderly woman is seen with small-bowel obstruction but has no history of previous abdominal surgery. Aggressive fluid resuscitation and early surgery may limit the risk of morbidity and death.

▶ It has always seemed to me that obturator hernias are encountered more frequently on board examinations than in clinical practice. This paper reminds us that these things *do* happen in real life and tells us when to be suspicious: when confronted by an emaciated, elderly woman with clinical and roentgenographic evidence of complete mechanical small-bowel obstruction, usually in the absence of previous abdominal surgery. Don't rely on the Howship-Romberg sign to help you make the diagnosis. Like hobbyhorse manure, it is more often talked about than actually seen.—W.P. Ritchie, Jr., M.D., Ph.D.

11 Oncology

Introduction

Once again, this was a very productive year with regard to manuscripts relating to oncology and basic science topics. Instead of highlighting basic science studies in a separate category, I have attempted to highlight the advances in basic science as they relate to the common clinical entities. By using molecular biological techniques and by studying basic biological mechanisms, we are able to identify both the prognostic markers and the mechanisms of oncogenesis that are so important in understanding the various aspects of different types of cancer.

With regard to breast cancer, the screening studies, especially that by Miller from Canada, have received an extensive amount of coverage in the lay press. The Canadian study may well form an objective basis for determining health care policy under the Clinton Health Plan. Although this study did not show a reduction in mortality in women younger than age 50 years, this could easily be explained on the basis of duration of follow-up or the quality of screening mammograms.

I have attempted to highlight several biological markers to demonstrate their breadth and diversity as well as their attempt to identify the various aspects of the basic mechanism of breast cancer. Some, such as *p53*, have been extensively examined, whereas others, such as angiogenesis factor, are new but show great promise in being able to predict prognosis or even response to therapy.

There were excellent clinical trials dealing with the treatment of ductal carcinoma in situ (DCIS). These trials will not only help to set the standards for treatment of this early malignancy, but they will also suggest alternative clinical trials to help define the indications for radiation therapy or extensive surgery in the treatment of DCIS. Finally, studies are highlighted for the treatment of invasive breast cancer without radiation therapy or immediate reconstruction after mastectomy.

Colorectal cancers similarly were extensively studied; these studies ranged from epidemiology (dietary fiber intake or socioeconomic class) to identifying basic biological mechanisms and markers. Much work has been done in this cancer with *p53* and *ras* oncogene, which not only builds on the work by Vogelstein, but also predicts the invasiveness and prognosis of these tumors. Once again, there was a host of excellent clinically related manuscripts dealing with diverse topics such as endorectal ultrasound, preoperative radiation therapy, adequacy of surgical margins, and sphincter-sparing techniques.

In the section on gastric cancer, I have highlighted several large trials from Milan and Germany that investigate both the importance of local regional therapy and the adequacy of lymph node dissection. There are also several excellent papers examining tissue markers and their role in the management of the patient with gastric cancer. Gastric cancer may be a particularly suitable tumor model for studying basic biological mechanisms and for using these mechanisms to select patients for experimental neoadjuvant therapies. In general, we are beginning to see that identification of the basic biological mechanisms not only provides useful tumor markers but also makes a larger presence in our everyday clinical management of many common malignancies. Additionally, we are beginning to see that some of these basic mechanisms, such as expression of *HER2/neu*, are important not only in gastric and pancreatic cancers, but also in ovarian and breast cancers. This suggests a common mechanism, and identifying the immune response to these oncogenes as well as understanding their biological mechanisms will impact on several different diseases. Future studies will be directed at two levels: first, the molecular level will examine transcriptions and translations of these oncogenes and their intermediary peptides; and second, the clinical level will be focused at either the identification of prognostic markers or the use of treatment strategies, taking into account the biological steps identified through the work of basic scientists.

Timothy J. Eberlein, M.D.

Carcinoma of the Breast

INTRODUCTION

A wide variety of manuscripts that deal with diverse topics in the diagnosis and management of breast cancer are presented. Some of these manuscripts (as will be noted) received a fair amount of publicity in the literature. Others, however, are just as important; I will attempt to discuss them under various subtopics.

The study by Crisp and co-workers (Abstract 140-94-11-1) is a large screening study of more than 25,000 women that was conducted in England. These authors show that the tumors demonstrated in this screened population tend to be smaller and have better histology and less likelihood of nodal involvement than those in members of the same population who had tumors detected clinically. This study is relatively uncontrolled because the control population consists of 71 cancers detected clinically over the same period as the screening study. It is worth note that screening was done by single-view mammography; nonetheless, like most other screening studies, this study documented a reduction in mortality and an increase in the detection of small tumors.

The Canadian National Breast Screening Study by Miller was a randomized study of more than 50,000 women having either annual mammography and physical examination or an initial physical examination followed by the usual care. Yearly mammography and breast physical examination seemed to detect smaller and more likely node-negative breast cancers in women in their forties; however, after 7 years of following the study, there did not appear to be a significant effect on the death rate from breast cancer. Obviously, this manuscript has been used by the Clinton administration as a rationale for not recommending screening mammography in the 40- to 49-year-old age group; however, the lack of a reduction in mortality as a result of the screening program simply explains the need for longer follow-up. Further studies of longer duration will be necessary to document the full effect of screening mammography (1, 2).

Timothy J. Eberlein, M.D.

References

1. Shapiro S, et al: *Am Can Soc* 39:273, 1974.
2. Tabar L, et al: *Lancet* 1:829, 1985.

SCREENING AND DIAGNOSIS

Screening for Breast Cancer Detects Tumours at an Earlier Biological Stage

Crisp WJ, Higgs MJ, Cowan WK, Cunliffe WJ, Liston J, Lunt LG, Peakman DJ, Young JR (Queen Elizabeth Hosp, Gateshead, England)
Br J Surg 80:863–865, 1993   140-94-11–1

Introduction.—The results of 2 trials suggested that with the implementation of a national screening program, the mortality rate from breast cancer in Britain could be reduced by 30% in women 50–64 years

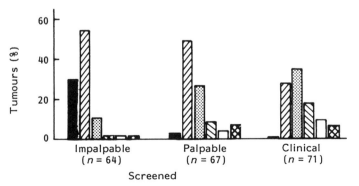

Fig 11–1.—Tumor size. *Solid bar,* less than 1 cm; *hatched to right,* from 1 to 1.9 cm; *dotted,* from 2 to 2.9 cm; *hatched to left,* from 3 to 3.9 cm; *open bar,* from 4 to 4.9 cm; *cross-hatched,* greater than 5 cm. (Courtesy of Crisp WJ, Higgs MJ, Cowan WK, et al: *Br J Surg* 80:863–865, 1993.)

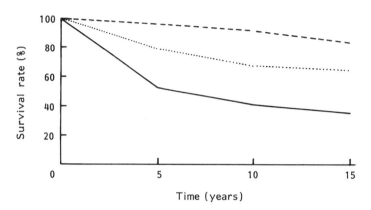

Fig 11–2.—Expected survival rate. *Solid line,* patients with tumors detected clinically; *dotted line,* patients with tumors detected by screening; *dashed line,* controls. (Courtesy of Crisp WJ, Higgs MJ, Cowan WK, et al: *Br J Surg* 80:863–865, 1993.)

of age. Another trial indicated a 14% reduction in the mortality rate at 7 years. Whether a biological difference exists between screen-detected cancers and those first seen clinically was determined.

Patients and Methods.—A total of 25,815 women in the Gateshead, Sunderland, South Tyneside, and Durham districts in England were invited to take part in the screening program. Single-view mammography in the 17,678 participants detected 131 cancers in 129 women. Sixty-seven tumors were palpable and 64 were impalpable lesions requiring guidewire localization biopsy. The morphology of cancers detected by screening was compared with that of 71 cancers seen clinically during the same period. Two consulting surgeons treated all patients. Survival was predicted from the Nottingham Prognostic Index (NPI), calculated from tumor size, grading of lesion, and lymph node status.

Survival Data for Figure 11–2

	Time (years)			
	0	5	10	15
Clinical	71 (100)	37 (52·1)	29 (40·8)	25 (35·2)
Screened				
Palpable	60 (100)	45 (75·0)	38 (63·3)	35 (58·3)
Impalpable	38 (100)	32 (84·2)	28 (73·7)	28 (73·7)
Total	98 (100)	77 (78·6)	66 (67·3)	63 (64·3)
Controls*	(100)	(96·0)	(91·0)	(83·0)

Note: Values in parentheses are percentages. **Data for controls from M.H. Galea and J.L. Haybittle, Nottingham.
(Courtesy of Crisp WJ, Higgs MJ, Cowan WK, et al: *Br J Surg* 80:863–865, 1993.)

Results.—Invasive ductal cancers made up 90% of the clinically detected tumors, 82% of the palpable screened lesions, and 31% of the impalpable screened lesions. Cancers detected at screening had a higher proportion of tumors of more favorable histologic grade and type, were smaller in size (Fig 11-1), and had less axillary node involvement than those detected clinically. Based on the NPI, patients with screen-detected tumors had an expected survival advantage of 26.5% at 5 years, 26.5% at 10 years, and 29.1% at 15 years (Fig 11-2). The expected survival rate was significantly greater for screen-detected tumors than for clinically seen tumors at 5, 10, and 15 years (table).

Conclusion.—Improvements in long-term survival depend upon detecting breast cancers with more favorable biological characteristics. It was demonstrated that tumors in a screened population are smaller, of better histologic type and grade, and have less lymph node involvement than tumors detected clinically. These findings appear to be consistent with the 30% reduction in mortality rate reported in previous trials.

Clinical Correlates of False-Negative Fine Needle Aspirations of the Breast in a Consecutive Series of 1,005 Patients
O'Malley F, Casey TT, Winfield AC, Rodgers WH, Sawyers J, Page DL (Vanderbilt Univ, Nashville, Tenn; Oschner Clinic, New Orleans, La)
Surg Gynecol Obstet 176:360–364, 1993   140-94-11-2

Background.—Although fine-needle aspiration (FNA) of the breast is useful for diagnosing breast lesions, false negative results do occur and can detract from the technique's usefulness. The clinical correlates most often associated with false negative diagnoses were evaluated.

Methods.—Of 1,005 consecutive patients undergoing FNA of the breast, 16 patients had false negative findings. Pre-FNA physical assessments and mammographic results were correlated with the gross and microscopic characteristics of these 16 patients.

Findings.—The masses in all 16 patients were palpable. Based on mammographic abnormalities, 7 cases were classified as highly suspicious for malignant tumor; 3 were indeterminate and 4 were negative. In 2 cases, mammograms were not available. The size of the carcinomas ranged from .8 to 6.5 cm, with a mean size of 1.9 (table). Of the 16 tumors 2 cm or less, histologic factors showed no special type in 6 patients and special-type carcinoma in 7 patients. The large tumor—6.5 cm—was of high grade and showed an unusual diffusely infiltrative pattern histologically, extending between normal mammary lobules. All the special-type carcinomas and 6 of the 9 of no special type were paucicellular.

Conclusion.—These results support previous findings indicating that small tumor size, paucicellularity, and special-type histologic factors contribute to false negative FNA results. Because the tumors most likely to be missed by FNA, physical examination, or mammography are slow-

Clinical Pathologic Correlates of 16 False Negative Fine-Needle Aspirations

Patient No.	Age, yrs.	Physical examination	Mammogram	FNA	Time between FNA and operation	Histology	Pathologic size, cm.	Follow-up, yrs.
1	64	Suspicious	Suspicious*†	Epithelial cells	19 mos.	NST grade I	3.6	A/W 3
2	91	Suspicious	Suspicious†	Epithelial cells	4 days	NST grade II	4.5	A/W 4
3	45	Palpable	Indeterminate	Epithelial cells	4 mos.	NST grade II	1.8	Bone mets. 3
4	48	Palpable	N/A	Epithelial cells	22 days	NST grade II	1.2	A/W 3
5	61	Thickening	Suspicious†	Connective tissue only	8 days	NST grade I	1.2	A/W 3
6	43	Ill-defined	Indeterminate	Connective tissue only	2 days	NST grade III	6.5	Dead 3
7	43	Palpable	Negative	Apocrine change	2 days	NST grade I	1.0	A/W 2
8	33	Mobile	Indeterminate	Connective tissue only	14 days	NST grade I	1.6	A/W 2
9	67	Palpable	Suspicious†	Epithelial cells	4 days	ILC	1.8	A/W 4
10	74	"Fullness"	Suspicious†	Epithelial cells	13 days	ILC	1.0	A/W 4
11	52	Suspicious	Negative	Epithelial cells	8 mos.	ICC	0.8	A/W 3
12	68	Palpable	Suspicious†	Connective tissue only	8 days	TUB	1.0	A/W 3
13	44	Palpable	N/A	Connective tissue only	10 days	Mucinous	0.8	A/W 3
14	53	Palpable	Suspicious†	Connective tissue only	5 days	NST grade I	0.8	A/W 3
15	44	Palpable	Negative	Connective tissue only	18 mos.	ILC	2.0	A/W 4
16	47	Mobile	Negative	Connective tissue only	9 mos.	ILC	1.0	A/W 4

Abbreviations: FNA, fine-needle aspiration; NST, no special type; ILC, infiltrating lobular carcinoma; *mets,* metastases; ICC, infiltrating cribriform carcinoma; TUB, tubular carcinoma; A/W, alive and well; and N/A, not available.
* Mammographic findings complicated by operation in that area.
† Highly suspicious.
(Courtesy of O'Malley F, Casey TT, Winfield AC, et al: *Surg Gynecol Obstet* 176:360–364, 1993.)

growing, a short delay in diagnosis and treatment may not adversely affect the excellent prognosis.

▶ This paper by O'Malley and colleagues from Vanderbilt University reports on a large study of FNA, but the thrust of the paper involves 16 patients who had false negative findings. These authors documented that the false negative results were associated with either small tumor size or a hypercellular type of tumor, as well as peculiar tumors that not only tend to be hypocellular but diffusely infiltrative between normal mammary lobules. In a patient with an abnormal mammogram or palpable mass and a negative FNA, incisional biopsy may still be indicated. An alternative would be a stereotactic core-needle biopsy, which has the advantage of obtaining a better pathologic sampling under mammographic guidance with minimal morbidity to the patient.—T.J. Eberlein, M.D.

BIOLOGICAL MARKERS

▶↓ Tremendous work has been done to identify various biological markers in an attempt to develop more effective prognostic indicators to evaluate the response to therapy, need for therapy, and overall survival. Understanding these basic biological mechanisms will also lead to the development of new treatment strategies for breast cancer by using antibodies to these proteins or their receptors, or perhaps by using an antisense oligonucleotide to block the expression of these peptides.—T.J. Eberlein, M.D.

---

p53 as an Independent Prognostic Marker in Lymph Node-Negative Breast Cancer Patients
Silvestrini R, Benini E, Daidone MG, Veneroni S, Boracchi P, Cappelletti V, Di Fronzo G, Veronesi U (Istituto Nazionale per lo Studio e la Cura dei Tumori, Milan, Italy; Università degli Studi, Milan, Italy)
J Natl Cancer Inst 85:965–970, 1993   140-94-11–3

Objective.—Traditional variables are generally used to make decisions about adjuvant therapy in patients with node-negative breast cancer. Some prognostic factors under study may be better able to identify patients at high risk. Expression of the mutant p53 protein encoded by the *p53* tumor suppressor gene is a reproducible, easily assessable, and independent predictor of outcome that could help in making treatment decisions. The predictive value of expression of the mutant p53 protein was studied in 256 patients with axillary lymph node–negative breast cancer.

Methods.—Expression of p53 was determined by an immunohistochemical technique using a 1:50 dilution of the monoclonal antibody PAb1801 on paraffin-embedded tumor specimens. Overexpression of p53 was defined as the presence of more than 5% positive cells from histologic sections. The [³H]thymidine labeling index was used as a measure of cell kinetics, and the estrogen receptor status was ascertained by the

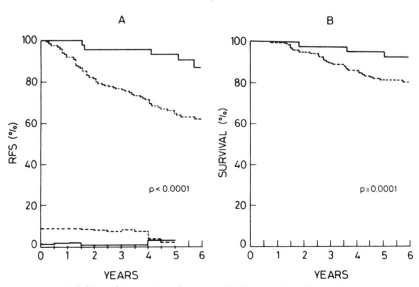

Fig 11–3.—Probability of 6-year relapse-free survival (RFS) **(A)** and overall survival **(B)** as a function of the expression of p53. At the bottom of **A**, the estimated hazard function of relapse (per 100 individuals per 6 months) is shown. *Solid line* indicates tumors with 5% or less p53-positive cells; *broken line* indicates tumors with more than 5% p53-positive cells. (Courtesy of Silvestrini R, Benini E, Daidone MG, et al: *J Natl Cancer Inst* 85:965–970, 1993.)

dextran-coated charcoal absorption technique. These 3 factors, in addition to tumor size and menopausal status, were analyzed in terms of 6-year relapse-free survival and overall survival.

Results.—Forty-four percent of the tumors showed overexpression of p53. On multiple regression analysis, the odds ratios (ORs) for 6-year relapse-free survival were 3.24 for p53 and 1.92 for the [³H]thymidine labeling index (Fig 11–3 and table). These were significantly higher than for tumor size (OR 1.49), and estrogen receptor status (OR .91). No association was noted between overexpression of p53 and menopausal status.

Conclusion.—Overexpression of p53 is an independent marker for decreased 6-year relapse-free and overall survival in patients with resectable, node-negative breast cancer. Overexpression of p53 should be used with other established factors, such as [³H]thymidine labeling index and estrogen receptor status, to further refine the prognostic assessment for these patients. The finding that expression of p53 and cell proliferation are independent at both the biological and clinical levels suggests that p53 has a biological function in addition to cell cycle regulation.

▶ This first paper by Silvestrini and colleagues at the National Cancer Institute in Milan demonstrates its point dramatically. The authors show that overexpression of the tumor suppressor gene *p53* is an independent marker for diminished relapse-free and overall survival. Of particular note was the find-

Multiple Regression Analysis of 6-Year Overall Survival

Variable	Odds ratio* (95% CL)	Wald statistic		Likelihood ratio test	
		χ^2	P	χ^2	P
p53 expression, ≤5% versus >5% positive cells†	2.61 (1.50-4.56)	11.42	.0007	14.86	.0001
[³H]thymidine labeling index, ≤3% versus >3%†	1.72 (0.99-2.99)	3.75	.052	4.12	.04
ER status, positive versus negative†	1.68 (1.01-2.77)	4.07	.04	7.96	.004

* Adjusted odds of surviving.
† Reference category.
(Courtesy of Silvestrini R, Benini E, Daidone MG, et al: *J Natl Cancer Inst* 85:965-970, 1993.)

ing that overexpression of *p53* appeared to be independent of the thymidine labeling index. This would seem to indicate the complex interaction of these various biological markers and their functions. Through large studies of many different types of patients, we will hopefully be able to identify the true biological significance of suppressor genes such as *p53*. This study, however, is very well controlled and certainly emphasizes the importance of *p53* in breast cancer.—T.J. Eberlein, M.D.

Proliferation Index As a Prognostic Marker in Breast Cancer
Veronese SM, Gambacorta M, Gottardi O, Scanzi F, Ferrari M, Lampertico P (Niguarda-Ca Granda Hosp, Milan, Italy)
Cancer 71:3926–3931, 1993   140-94-11–4

Introduction.—A number of different approaches have been taken to the study of the proliferative activity of tumors. Among these, use of the monoclonal antibody Ki-67 appears to be an easy and reliable technique. This antibody was used to study the proliferative activity of 129 primary breast cancers and the findings related to the patients' prognoses.

Methods.—The study material comprised 129 patients undergoing breast cancer surgery over 2 years. All specimens were processed by staining by the avidin-biotin complex, with diffuse or dotlike nuclear reactivity considered a positive stain for Ki-67. Patients were observed for

Relationship Between Ki-67 Proliferation Index and Probability (%) of 4-Year Survival in Lymph Nodal, Menopausal, and Nuclear Estrogen Receptor Subgroups

	No. of patients	Ki-67 index*		P value
		Low	High	
Overall	129	95.6	71.0	0.00005
Nodes				
Negative	71	98.2	82.3	0.02
Positive	58	91.9	61.9	0.003
Menopausal status				
Post	79	96.8	75.0	0.002
Pre	50	92.9	68.2	0.02
Nuclear ER				
Negative	69	88.9	66.7	0.02
Positive	60	†	†	

Abbreviation: ER, estrogen receptor.
* Ki-67 index: low < 20%; high ≥ 20%.
† All living.
(Courtesy of Veronese SM, Gambacorta M, Gottardi O, et al: *Cancer* 71:3926–3931, 1993.)

a median of 42 months, and Mantel-Cox life-table analysis was used to determine the probabilities of disease-free and overall survival.

Results.—When the Ki-67 proliferation index was greater than 20%, there was a higher 4-year probability of relapse—55% vs. 79%—and death—71% vs. 96%—compared with tumors with lower Ki-67 values. This prognostic significance persisted after stratification for lymph node involvement, menopausal status, and nuclear estrogen receptor content (table).

Conclusion.—Ki-67 determination of tumor proliferative activity appears to be a valuable indicator of disease-free and overall survival in women with breast cancer. In patient groups with a good prognosis, life expectancy is significantly better for patients with slow-growing vs. fast-growing tumors.

▶ It almost seems intuitively obvious that tumors with high proliferative activity, which, therefore, are faster growing, would tend to have a poorer prognosis. These authors did not compare a measurement using the monoclonal antibody Ki-67 with straight [^{3}H]-thymidine proliferation. This does not take away from the other prognostic factors presented in the table, such as positive nodes for estrogen receptor–negative status. Although related, these other prognostic factors may look at different aspects of the proliferating breast cancer cell.—T.J. Eberlein, M.D.

A Prospective Study of the Prognostic Value of Cathepsin D Levels in Breast Cancer Cytosol

Pujol P, Maudelonde T, Daures J-P, Rouanet P, Brouillet J-P, Pujol H, Rochefort H (INSERM U 148, Montpellier, France; Hôpital Gaston Doumergue, Nîmes, France; Parc Euromédecine, Montpellier, France)
Cancer 71:2006–2012, 1993   140-94-11–5

Background.—Cathepsin D, a lysosomal protease that is overexpressed and abnormally secreted in most breast cancer cells, has been found to be an independent prognostic factor associated with a higher risk of recurrence and shorter overall survival. Results of the first prospective study of the prognostic value of levels of cathepsin D in breast cancer cytosol are reported.

Methods.—One hundred twenty-three patients with primary breast cancer were followed for 5 years. Levels of cathepsin D in cytosol were determined by using a solid-phase sandwich immunoenzymatic assay.

Findings.—The median value of cathepsin D was 20.8 pmol/mg of protein, about half the median value found in subsequent assays done with a commercially available kit and reported in most retrospective studies. Only axillary lymph node involvement was associated with the cathepsin D status or level. According to a univariate analysis, levels of cathepsin D of more than 20 pmol of protein per mg were related to a

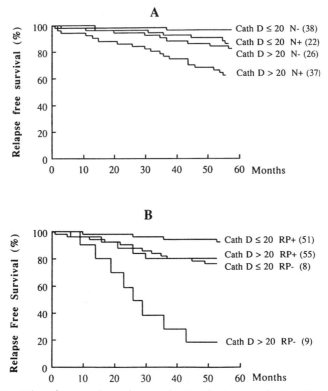

Fig 11-4.—Relapse-free survival according to cathepsin D level associated with **(A)** lymph node status or **(B)** PR status. The number of patients in each subgroup is given in parentheses. (Courtesy of Pujol P, Maudelonde T, Daures J-P, et al: *Cancer* 71:2006-2012, 1993.)

higher risk of recurrence and shorter overall survival. In a multivariate analysis, the most important variables predicting relapse-free survival were a high level of cathepsin D, a negative progesterone receptor (PR) status, and lymph node involvement (Fig 11-4). The level of cathepsin D had prognostic value in patients with node-positive disease and appeared to be especially useful in association with the PR status by isolating a high-risk subgroup of patients.

Conclusion.—The prognostic value of the level of cathepsin D, together with other major prognostic variables is confirmed (table). Future research should focus on whether the patient subgroup with high levels of cathepsin D will benefit from adjuvant treatment.

▶ These authors examine cathepsin D, a lysosomal protease often overexpressed or secreted in breast cancer. Again, cathepsin D by itself may not be an accurate representation of a complete story; however, in the context of nodal status and estrogen receptor levels, cathepsin D may help differentiate patients who might benefit from adjuvant systemic therapy. Node-positive

Correlation of Cathepsin D Levels With Other Prognostic Factors

Variables	Total (%)	Low cathepsin D level (≤ 20 pmol)	High cathepsin D level (> 20 pmol)	P value
		No. of patients		
Estrogen receptor* (n = 125)				
+	91 (73)	42	49	0.33
−	34 (27)	19	15	
Progesterone receptor* (n = 125)				
+	108 (86)	53	55	0.87
−	17 (14)	8	9	
Node status (n = 123)†				
+	59 (48)	22	37	0.01
−	64 (52)	38	26	
No. of positive lymph nodes (n = 123)				
0	64 (52)	38	26	0.05
1–3	44 (36)	17	27	
> 3	15 (12)	5	10	
Tumor size (n = 125)				
T1	33 (26)	15	18	0.87
T2	77 (62)	39	38	
T3–4	15 (12)	7	8	
Grade of Scarff and Bloom (n = 115)‡				
I	28 (24)	15	13	0.49
II	42 (36)	19	23	
III	45 (40)	20	25	
Age (n = 125) (yr)				
≤ 50	46 (37)	27	19	0.08
> 50	79 (63)	34	45	
Adjuvant therapy				
None	29 (23)	16	13	0.51
Endocrine therapy	64 (51)	28	36	
Chemotherapy +/− Endocrine therapy	32 (26)	17	15	

* Using cutoff level of 10 pmol/mg of protein.
† One patient had previous axillary lymph node clearance for melanoma and another refused it.
‡ Ten tumors were ductal comedocarcinoma.
(Courtesy of Pujol P, Maudelonde T, Daures J-P, et al: *Cancer* 71:2006–2012, 1993.)

patients appear to have higher levels of cathepsin D. Thus, overexpression of this protease in human breast cancer may well play an active role in determining tumor progression.—T.J. Eberlein, M.D.

Tumor Angiogenesis: A New Significant and Independent Prognostic Indicator in Early-Stage Breast Carcinoma
Weidner N, Folkman J, Pozza F, Bevilacqua P, Allred EN, Moore DH, Meli S, Gasparini G (Univ of California, San Francisco; Harvard Med School, Boston; St Bortolo Regional Med Ctr, Vicenza-Veneto, Italy; et al)
J Natl Cancer Inst 84:1875–1887, 1992   140-94-11–6

Introduction.—Axillary lymph node status fails to fully account for varied outcomes in patients with operable breast cancer. There is recent evidence that the density of microvessels in invasive breast cancers correlates with metastasis.

Patients and Methods.—Microvessels were counted with immunocytochemical staining for factor VIII–related antigen in a prospective, blinded study of 165 consecutive patients. The vessels were counted with light microscopy in areas of the most active neovascularization, and density was correlated with the outcome after a median follow-up of 51 months.

Results.—Forty-eight patients had recurrences during follow-up and 39 died, 28 of tumor-related causes. Microvessel density significantly predicted both overall survival and relapse-free survival in lymph node-positive and lymph node-negative (Fig 11-5) patients. Microvessel density was the only significant predictor of overall survival among lymph node–negative women. The number of positive axillary lymph nodes correlated significantly with overall survival and relapse-free survival in all patients and in lymph node–positive patients. Microvessel counts correlated with axillary lymph node involvement, tumor size, and histologic grade, but not with other prognostic indicators.

Conclusion.—The extent of angiogenesis correlates with survival in patients with breast cancer. An estimate of microvessel density could help select lymph node–negative patients at relatively high risk of having occult metastasis at presentation, and who therefore may be candidates for systemic adjuvant treatment.

▶ Axillary lymph node status, by itself, often is not a sufficient predictor of recurrence and overall survival. In this paper, the number of microvessels in node-negative patients correlates with the outcome. Several caveats regarding this technique need emphasizing. Tumors appear to be heterogeneous for angiogenic activity, and, therefore, microvessel density is determined in the most neovascular areas. Neovascularization of the primary tumor would be an early step in identifying a tumor cell that has left a primary tumor to

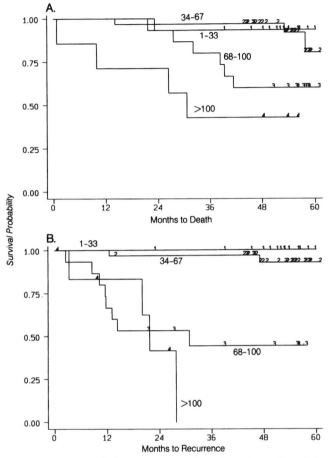

Fig 11–5.—Kaplan-Meier survival plots for node-negative patients. **A,** overall survival stratified by microvessel count. **B,** relapse-free survival stratified by microvessel count. (Courtesy of Weidner N, Folkman J, Pozza F, et al: *J Natl Cancer Inst* 84:1875–1887, 1992.)

metastasize. Thus, a new and highly predictive factor has been identified by Weidner and colleagues.—T.J. Eberlein, M.D.

Prognostic Factors in Node-Negative Breast Cancer
Johnson H Jr, Masood S, Belluco C, Abou-Azama A-M, Dee S, Kahn L, Wise L
(Long Island Jewish Med Ctr, New Hyde Park, NY; Albert Einstein College of Med , Bronx, NY; Univ of Florida Health Science Ctr, Jacksonville)
Arch Surg 127:1386–1391, 1992   140-94-11–7

Introduction.—Because some patients with axillary lymph node-negative breast cancer may benefit from adjuvant chemotherapy, an at-

Various Factors and the Relationship Between Them	
Factors	***P***
Tumor size	
S-phase fraction	.0273
HER-2/*neu* expression	.0251
S-phase fraction	
Ploidy	.0001
DNA index	.0340
Tumor size	.0273
DNA index	
Ploidy	.0001
S-phase fraction	.0001
Ploidy	
DNA index	.0001
S-phase fraction	.0001
Grade	
HER-2/*neu* expression	.0345

* Using multivariate analysis of variance.
(Courtesy of Johnson H Jr, Masood S, Belluco C, et al: *Arch Surg* 127:1386–1391, 1992.)

tempt was made to relate DNA flow cytometric parameters to other potential prognostic factors in a series of 100 lymph node–negative patients treated from 1968 to 1984. Ploidy and the S-phase fraction were determined with flow cytometry.

Results.—Survival decreased with both increasing tumor size (significantly after 3 cm) and increasing tumor grade. A major reduction in survival was noted in patients having aneuploid tumors. The S-phase fraction correlated with overall survival, which was much better when fewer than 10% of cells were in S-phase. On Cox proportional hazards analysis, tumor size was the most prominent prognostic factor, whereas tumor grade was not a significant factor in overall survival (table). Together with tumor size, the S-phase fraction and DNA index were important prognostic factors.

Conclusion.—Aneuploid breast cancers, those with an S-phase fraction of 10% or higher, and tumors more than 3 cm in diameter carry a very poor prognosis. All lymph node–negative women with infiltrating cancers should be considered for chemotherapy unless the tumor is diploid, has an S-phase fraction of less than 10%, or is 1 cm or smaller in diameter.

▶ This paper represents another example of an attempt to refine criteria to determine prognosis in patients with node-negative breast cancer. These authors again use ploidy and S-phase fraction by means of flow cytometry. As in each of the previous articles, proliferation plays a major role. These authors demonstrate that large size (greater than or equal to 3 cm), aneuploidy, and high S-phase (greater than 10%) correlate with poor prognosis.

In sum, in attempting to identify criteria for the use of systemic adjuvant therapy for the treatment of patients with node-negative breast cancer patients, we see that cathepsin D, microvessel density, and high proliferation— as well as ploidy and S-phase fraction—can be significant additions to making clinical determinations. Emphasis should be placed on patient participation in clinical trials in which specific questions may be answered to better define clinical parameters for treatment.—T.J. Eberlein, M.D.

Therapy of Small Breast Cancer: A Prospective Study on 1036 Patients With Special Emphasis of Prognostic Factors
Sauer R, Schauer A, Rauschecker HF, Schumacher M, Gatzemeier W, Schmoor C, Dunst J, Seegenschmiedt MH, Marx D (Univ of Erlangen, Germany; Univ of Göttingen, Germany; Univ of Freiburg, Germany)
Int J Radiat Oncol Biol Phys 23:907–914, 1992   140-94-11–8

Background.—The German Breast Cancer Study, a prospective multi-center trial on the treatment of early breast cancer pT1, pN0, M0 was begun in 1983. At that time, several studies had suggested that breast-conserving therapy produced the same survival figures as radical procedures. Data from the German Breast Cancer Study are presented.

Methods.—Between 1983 and 1989, 1,119 patients were recruited for the study. After exclusions, 733 underwent breast conservation and 303 had mastectomy. Although randomization was initially planned, it was found not to be feasible; almost all patients were treated according to their preference. Treatment included initial tumorectomy with microscopically free margins and lower axillary dissection, at which time pT1, pN0-stage disease was confirmed. Patients not having mastectomy were treated with adjuvant radiotherapy, 50 Gy in 25 fractions to the entire breast plus a 12 Gy electron boost. The parasternal and supraclavicular region was also treated with 50 Gy in medial tumors.

Findings.—At a median 48-month follow-up, the frequency of local recurrences, regional recurrences, and distant metastases was the same in both treatment groups. These frequencies were 4.7%, 1%, and 5.4%, respectively. Three-year disease-free survival in the breast conservation group was 90%, and in the mastectomy group it was 88%. Twenty-four patients having breast-conserving treatment with microscopically involved margins had a poorer disease-free survival than the study group. Margin width had no effect on prognosis. In univariate and multivariate analyses, other prognostic factors were tumor size and grade. Nonsignificant factors included age, menopausal status, hormone receptor status, histologic tumor type, and treatment. Transmembrane protein p185 expression, a marker of oncogene overexpression, depended on tumor grade and was the strongest prognostic factor in univariate and multivariate analyses.

Conclusion.—These findings stress the central role of tumor grade in prognosis. They also strongly suggest that the *c-erb-B2* oncogene has prognostic significance in pN0-breast cancer, challenging the assumption that it is significant only in node-negative patients.

▶ In a multicenter trial performed in Germany involving a large group of patients, Sauer and colleagues found that tumor size and grade were important prognostic factors. Associated with grade, however, was the transmembrane *p-185* expression. The expression of the oncogene *c-erb-B2* was the strongest prognostic factor in univariate and multivariate analyses. Experimental evidence from our laboratory, as well as from others, has found that the *Her2/neu* oncogene is important in recognition by the immune system (1). Studies are under way to identify the individual peptide, i.e., Her2/neu product, that is the recognition factor in breast, ovarian, gastric, and non–small-cell lung tumors. Identification of this peptide would then permit either sensitization of the immune system or creation of a vaccine to be used in the high-risk setting (2).—T.J. Eberlein, M.D.

References

1. Yoshino I, et al: *J Immunol* 152:2393, 1994.
2. Linehan D, et al: *Surg Forum* (in press).

TREATMENT OF DUCTAL CARCINOMA IN SITU (DCIS)

Ductal Carcinoma In Situ (Intraductal Carcinoma) of the Breast Treated With Breast-Conserving Surgery and Definitive Irradiation: Correlation of Pathologic Parameters With Outcome of Treatment
Solin LJ, Yeh I-T, Kurtz J, Fourquet A, Recht A, Kuske R, McCormick B, Cross MA, Schultz DJ, Amalric R, LiVolsi VA, Kowalyshyn MJ, Torhorst J, Jacquemier J, Westermann CD, Mazoujian G, Zafrani B, Rosen PP, Goodman RL, Fowble BL (Univ of Pennsylvania, Philadelphia; Univ Hosp, Basel, Switzerland; Institut Curie, Paris; et al)
Cancer 71:2532–2542, 1993   140-94-11-9

Patients.—The efficacy of breast conservation surgery and definitive radiotherapy was examined in 172 patients with pure intraductal breast carcinomas. All had unilateral malignancies staged Tis, N0, M0 by the

Fig 11–6.—Local recurrence. **A,** comparison of the histologic subtype of comedo (*solid line*) vs. noncomedo (*dashed line*) intraductal carcinoma. **B,** comparison of the presence (*solid line*) vs. the absence (*dashed line*) of the combination of the histologic subtype of comedocarcinoma plus nuclear grade 3. (Courtesy of Solin LJ, Yeh I-T, Kurtz J, et al: *Cancer* 71:2532–2542, 1993.)

(continued)

Fig 11–6 (cont).

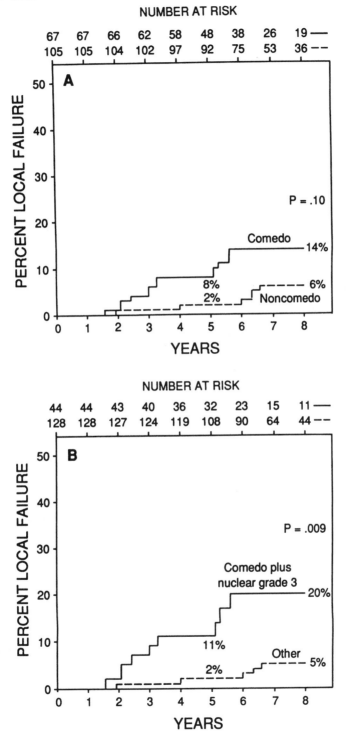

NUMBER AT RISK

American Joint Committee on Cancer system. A majority of patients had the comedo or cribriform subtype of carcinoma but papillary, micropapillary, and solid tumors were also represented.

Treatment.—Surgery included complete gross removal of the primary tumor. Twenty-four patients (14%) underwent reexcision. All 66 patients having axillary node staging were pathologically node-negative. The median total radiation dose was 6,000 cGy, and 95% of patients received 5,000 cGy or more. Nine patients received systemic treatment, usually thiotepa.

Results.—Fifteen patients had local failure, and one had both local and regional failure. All these patients were salvaged. Local recurrences correlated with a combination of comedocarcinoma and nuclear grade 3 disease (Fig 11–6), and times to recurrence were shorter in patients with these features. Actuarial survival was 98% at 5 years and 96% at 8 years. All but 4% of patients were free of distant disease at 8 years. In 7 patients (4%), carcinoma developed in the contralateral breast after a mean interval of 51 months.

Conclusion.—There are pathologic risk factors for local recurrence in women with ductal carcinoma in situ of the breast, but recurrences have not been associated with altered survival. Close follow-up of patients at increased risk of local recurrence will promote successful salvage treatment.

Ductal Carcinoma In Situ of the Female Breast: Short-Term Results of a Prospective Nationwide Study
Ottesen GL, for the Danish Breast Cancer Cooperative Group (Odense Univ Hosp, Denmark)
Am J Surg Pathol 16:1183–1196, 1992   140-94-11–10

Background.—In situ carcinoma of the breast describes a diverse array of clinical and histologic conditions requiring several different levels of therapy. Until recently, information about ductal carcinoma in situ (DCIS) has been obtained from retrospective studies involving small numbers of patients. One hundred twelve women with DCIS were studied to examine what factors were of prognostic value in predicting recurrence.

Methods.—Because Denmark has no mammography screening, all the women examined in this prospective trial were self-selected through a nationwide call for participants conducted by the Danish Breast Cancer Cooperative. The median age of the participants was 48 years. All women were treated with excisional biopsy or wide excision with the intention of free margins. Follow-up included annual mammograms and clinical examinations twice a year. Lesions were classified as microfocal, diffuse, or tumor-forming/diffuse + tumor-forming.

TABLE 1.—Occurrence of Different Histologic Subtypes in the
Individual DCIS Lesions Related to the Dominating
Histologic Subtype

Dominating histologic subtype (no. of cases)	Histologic subtypes					
	1	2	3	4	5	6
Solid (34)	6	7	11	7	3	
Clinging (31)	3	7	9	10	2	
Cribriform (40)		5	13	13	7	2
Papilliferous (7)			2	4	1	
Total (112)	9	19	35	34	13	2

(Courtesy of Ottesen GL, for the Danish Breast Cancer Cooperative Group: *Am J Surg Pathol* 16:1183-1196, 1992.)

Results.—During the median follow-up of 53 months, a crude recurrence rate of 22% was found (Table 1). Five of these patients had invasive carcinomas, whereas the remaining 20 patients had in situ carcinomas. Type of surgical intervention did not affect recurrence. Histologic growth pattern, nuclear size, and comedonecrosis were found to be significantly interrelated. Thus, tumor-forming/diffuse + tumor-forming lesions correlated with large nuclear/lesion size and comedonecrosis. Not surprisingly, these lesions also had a significantly higher rate of recurrence. A higher relapse rate was also seen in those patients who were initially seen with clinical systems, compared to those in whom DCIS was discovered incidentally or through mammography (Table 2).

Conclusion.—No microfocal lesion with a large nucleus or comedonecrosis was found. Therefore, large nuclear size and comedonecrosis may be significant prognostic indicators. These results also indicate that many women with DCIS treated by excision alone should still be considered at risk.

▶ In the paper by Solin and colleagues (Abstract 140-94-11–9), a group of patients with pure intraductal carcinoma of the breast were studied. In the majority of patients who underwent axillary node dissection, nodal status was negative. All the patients were treated with radiation therapy. Only 15 patients had local recurrence; this correlated with a combination of comedocarcinoma and high nuclear grade.

In the study by Ottesen from the Danish Breast Cancer Cooperative Group (Abstract 140-94-11–10), patients were treated with excision alone. The recurrence rate was 22%. The histologic growth, significantly large nuclear size, and comedonecrosis were most significant. Note that the rate of local recurrence was significantly higher in the Danish patients because they did not receive radiation therapy. As seen in the study of the National Surgical Adjuvant Breast Project ˈ(1), radiation therapy significantly reduces the rate

TABLE 2.—Frequency of Recurrence (N/N) Related to Growth Pattern, Primary Surgical Treatment, and Data on Specimen Margins

Growth pattern	No. of cases	Excisional biopsy (N/N)	Wide excision (N/N)	Specimen margins		
				Free (N/N)	Not free (N/N)	Unknown[a] (N/N)
Microfocal	45	4/38	0/7	0/3		4/42
Diffuse	46	4/24	9/22	6/13	1/1	6/32
Diffuse + tumor-forming	16	3/5	3/11	1/4		5/12
Tumor-forming	5	1/1	1/4	0/1	1/1	1/3
Total	112	12/68 (18%)	13/44 (30%)	7/21 (33%)	2/2 (100%)	16/89 (18%)

[a] Includes cases that were not evaluable.
(Courtesy of Ottesen GL, for the Danish Breast Cancer Cooperative Group: Am J Surg Pathol 16:1183–1196, 1992.)

of ipsilateral recurrence. This is particularly true with regard to invasive cancer. In general, patients with DCIS who are treated with conservative surgery without radiation therapy have a higher risk for local recurrence. In the study by Solin, recurrence did not adversely affect outcome, although the length of follow-up may not be conclusive. In the series by Ottesen, 5 of the patients had invasive carcinoma. Thus, one must be very careful when selecting patients for treatment without radiation therapy. Patients with comedo-type DCIS should generally be treated with radiation therapy after conservative excision.—T.J. Eberlein, M.D.

Reference

1. Fisher B, et al: N Engl J Med 328:1581, 1993.

TREATMENT OF INVASIVE CARCINOMA

▶↓ The next 5 manuscripts deal with selective topics in the management of invasive carcinoma of the breast. They address specific issues that may assist the surgeon by providing unique aspects of the care of the patient who has breast cancer.—T.J. Eberlein, M.D.

Prognosis Following Salvage Mastectomy for Recurrence in the Breast After Conservative Surgery and Radiation Therapy for Early-Stage Breast Cancer
Abner AL, Recht A, Eberlein T, Come S, Shulman L, Hayes D, Connolly JL, Schnitt SJ, Silver B, Harris JR (Harvard Med School, Boston)
J Clin Oncol 11:44–48, 1993   140-94-11–11

Background.—Randomized trials have shown that conservative surgery followed by radiation therapy in patients with early stage breast cancer results in survival rates equal to those achieved with mastectomy. However, this treatment strategy is associated with a 5-year recurrence rate of 5% to 10% and a 10-year rate of 10% to 15% in the treated breast. The prognostic factors and best treatment for patients with such recurrences were investigated.

Patients and Methods.—The study included 1,593 patients with stage I or II invasive breast cancer treated between 1968 and 1985 at the Joint Center for Radiation Therapy after gross total tumor excision. One hundred sixty-six patients, (10%), subsequently had a recurrence. One hundred twenty-three of these patients had salvage mastectomy and were further studied. Recurrent tumor was mainly invasive in 99 cases, noninvasive in 14, and focally invasive in 10. Twenty-nine patients received chemotherapy or hormonal treatment after mastectomy. The median follow-up after salvage mastectomy was 39 months.

Previous Series of Salvage Mastectomy

First Author	No. of Patients	No. of Local Recurrences	No. of Salvage Mastectomies	5-Year Survival After Salvage Mastectomy (%)	Significant Prognostic Factors at Time of Salvage Mastectomy	Prognostic Factors Examined Found Not to Be Significant
Kurtz	1,593	178	43	53	Disease-free interval (<2 vs. 2-5 years) Histologic grade Extent of recurrence	Age at diagnosis Initial stage ER status Type of salvage procedure Adjuvant therapy
Haffty	433	50	41	Not stated	Extent of recurrence (diffuse vs. local)	Disease-free interval (≤4 vs. >4 years) Method of detection
Fourquet	518	56	45	Not stated	Disease-free interval (<3 vs. ≥3 years)	

Fowble	1,030	65	52	84	Initial tumor stage	Disease-free interval (<3 vs. ≥3 years) Age at diagnosis (≤35 vs. >35 years) Nodal status Location of recurrence Method of detection Histology Adjuvant therapy
Clarke	436	24	10	81 (from time of initial diagnosis)	Nodal/dermal recurrence	
Present series	1,593	166	123	79 overall (cause-specific)	Recurrence histology	Age (≤34 vs. >35 years) Disease-free interval (<3 vs. ≥3 years) Method of detection Initial tumor stage Adjuvant therapy

Abbreviation: ER, estrogen receptor.
(Courtesy of Abner AL, Recht A, Eberlein T, et al: *J Clin Oncol* 11:44-48, 1993.)

Findings. —Overall, the 5-year actuarial rate of further local or distant relapse was 41%. None of the 24 patients with focally invasive or noninvasive tumors had a subsequent relapse, whereas the patients with predominantly invasive recurrence had a 5-year actuarial relapse rate of 52%. The risk of further relapse was not significantly associated with the method of detecting the recurrence, patient age at initial diagnosis, disease-free interval, or the location of breast recurrence. Experiences reported by other institutions are shown in the table.

Conclusion. —The histology of the recurrent tumor appears to be an important prognostic factor in the risk of further relapse. The prognosis for patients with noninvasive or focally invasive tumors after salvage mastectomy is excellent. However, those with predominantly invasive tumors are at substantial risk for further relapse.

▶ In this paper by Abner and colleagues from the Joint Center of Radiation Therapy of Harvard Medical School, although the patients had conservative surgery and radiation therapy, the prognosis after salvage mastectomy was related to the histology of the recurrence. Compared with the patients who had recurrence and underwent salvage mastectomy, the patients with noninvasive or focally invasive tumors had excellent prognoses. Those with largely invasive tumors had higher risk of systemic relapse, therefore reinforcing the need for consideration of systemic adjuvant therapy in this patient population.—T.J. Eberlein, M.D.

Cancerous Residue in Breast-Conserving Surgery
Morimoto T, Okazaki K, Komaki K, Sasa M, Mori T, Tsuzuki H, Kamamura Y, Miki H, Monden Y (Univ of Tokushima, Japan; Kunitomi Surgical Clinic, Okayama, Japan)
J Surg Oncol 52:71–76, 1993   140-94-11–12

Background. —Breast-conserving treatment for women with early-stage cancer has recently been attempted in Japan. Some problems are still unsolved, such as the presence of cancerous residues in the surgical margin and evaluation of the clinical effect of breast radiation, particularly in the presence or absence of extensive intraductal cancer. Local tumor extension was studied to assess malignancy remaining after breast-conserving surgery for early-stage breast cancer.

Methods. —A continuous series of multiple blocks of specimens obtained at mastectomy was studied. One hundred seventy-seven cases of invasive ductal carcinoma and 6 cases of noninvasive ductal carcinoma were represented.

Findings. —The histopathology in 32% of the cases corresponded to that showing extensions of more than 2.6 cm from the tumor margin. Wide extensions were also present in 17% of cases in which the tumor size was less than 2 cm. Younger patients with noninvasive ductal carcinoma had a higher incidence of wide extension. Fourteen percent of the patients with tumors less than 2 cm in size had nipple-areola extension. Breast cancers with multicentric development accounted for 3% of those with tumors less than 2 cm in size. These findings suggested that if lumpectomy is done with a margin of 2 cm for tumors 2 cm or less in size, a cancerous residue would remain in the surgical margins of 15% to 20% of the patients. In this series, the actual incidence was 23%.

Conclusion.—Breast-conserving treatment with only local resection of the primary lesion resulted in cancerous residue such as intraductal cancerous extension in about one fifth of the patients. Therefore, radiation therapy of the whole breast should be done after surgery with clear margins to control local recurrence.

▶ A study similar to that by Holland (*Cancer* 56:979, 1989) is presented in this review by Morimoto et al., in which 32% of the patients had tumor that was more than 2.6 cm from the tumor margin. In a substantial number of cases, this was true even if the primary tumor size was less than 2 cm. The conclusion that radiation therapy should be added to the treatment of patients with clear margins after excision could certainly reduce the risk of recurrence. However, there are patients who have small tumors with good prognostic features without ductal carcinoma in situ, in whom radiation therapy may be omitted.—T.J. Eberlein, M.D.

Conservative Surgery and Radiation in the Treatment of Synchronous Ipsilateral Breast Cancers
Wilson LD, Beinfield M, McKhann CF, Haffty BG (Yale Univ, New Haven, Conn)
Cancer 72:137–142, 1993   140-94-11-13

Background.—Although conservative surgery (CS) and radiation therapy (RT) are well accepted as an alternative approach to mastectomy in patients with early breast cancer, there is controversy as to their role in the patient who has 2 or more lesions in the same breast.

Methods.—An experience with CS and RT in the treatment of 13 patients with synchronous ipsilateral breast cancer (SIBC) was reviewed. The patients represented just more than 1% of 1,060 patients receiving CS and RT at one facility. In all patients, the lesions were identified macroscopically as carcinoma and confirmed microscopically. There were a total of 28 lesions, with 2 patients having 3 separate cancers. Gross excision of the cancers was followed by radiation to the breast (median tumor bed dose, 65 Gy), and to the regional lymphatic system as indicated (median dose, 48 Gy). The median follow-up was 71 months (table).

Findings.—Five-year actuarial survival among the patients with SIBC was 81%. An ipsilateral recurrence developed in 23% of patients; the 72-month actuarial recurrence rate was thus 25%, compared to 12% for the

Outcome of Patients With Synchronous Ipsilateral Breast Cancer

	Median follow-up (mo)	6-yr actuarial recurrence rate* (%)	Mean time to recurrence (mo)	5-yr actuarial survival* (%)
Patients with SIBC (n = 13) CS + RT at Yale	71	25 ± 0.16	52	81 ± 0.12
Patients with single lesions Stage I and II (n = 990) CS + RT at Yale	120	12 ± 0.02	48	85 ± 0.02

Abbreviations: CS, conservative surgery; RT, radiation therapy.
* Values are percentages ± SE.
(Courtesy of Wilson LD, Beinfield M, McKhann CF, et al: *Cancer* 72:137–142, 1993.)

patients with single lesions. At up to 135 months after diagnosis, 2 patients with recurrent disease were alive with no evidence of disease; a third died with metastatic disease at 64 months. Two of the 3 patients with local recurrence had invasive lobular histologic findings and 3 separate lesions.

Conclusion.—There was a higher local recurrence rate with CS and RT in patients with SIBC than in patients with single lesions. Further study is needed to identify specific prognostic factors for patients with SIBC. A conservative approach may be a reasonable alternative for patients who desire it.

▶ This paper represents a small series in which CS and RT were used to treat patients with SIBCs. The recurrence rate was nearly double that of patients treated for a single lesion; however, several of the patients had 3 separate lesions. Patients with SIBCs are not excluded from treatment with CS and RT, especially if the tumors are relatively close together and are confined to a single quadrant. However, the criteria for inclusion in a protocol for RT are the same as for patients with single tumors. For example, careful evaluation of the margins, the specific histology, and the presence of an extensive intraductal component are even more important when treating more than one tumor mass.—T.J. Eberlein, M.D.

Local Failure and Margin Status in Early-Stage Breast Carcinoma Treated With Conservation Surgery and Radiation Therapy
Anscher MS, Jones P, Prosnitz LR, Blackstock W, Hebert M, Reddick R, Tucker A, Dodge R, Leight G Jr, Iglehart JD, Rosenman J (Duke Univ, Durham, NC; Univ of North Carolina, Chapel Hill)
Ann Surg 218:22–28, 1993   140-94-11–14

Introduction.—Good cosmetic results from breast surgery require that as little normal tissue as possible be resected; however, at the same time, surgery should not leave behind a tumor burden that is not amenable to moderate doses of radiation. Whether microscopically positive surgical margins compromise the outcome remains uncertain.

Series.—The implications of positive surgical margins were examined in 259 consecutive women who had 262 breasts locally excised and underwent axillary dissection followed by radiotherapy. All had clinical stage I or II infiltrating ductal breast cancer. Gross tumor was totally removed with a margin.

Results.—The surgical margins were positive in 12% of operated breasts and indeterminate in another 38%. Eleven local failures occurred during a median follow-up of 44 months. Comparing actuarial rates of local failure at 5 years indicated that patients with negative margins had the best outcome (Fig 11-7). Patients who became margin-negative after reexcision did as well as those with initially negative surgical margins. Ex-

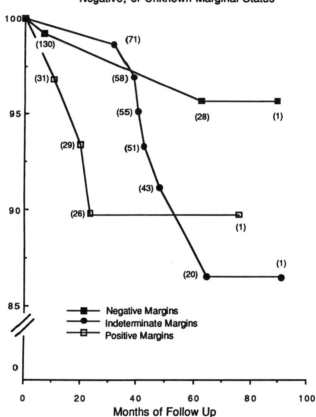

Fig 11-7.—Local control vs. marginal status. The negative margin patients did statistically better than the positive margin patients (P = .014, log rank test). Courtesy of Anscher MS, Jones P, Prosnitz LR, et al: *Ann Surg* 218:22-28, 1993.)

tensive intraductal carcinoma was not a significant predictor of local failure after controlling for marginal status. The only factor significantly influencing survival on multivariate analysis was node status.

Conclusion.—Patients having positive surgical margins after local excision of breast cancer should undergo reexcision. Isolated local recurrence in the breast appears not to compromise patient survival.

▶ In analyzing the cause of local failure in patients treated with conservative surgery and radiation therapy, the status of the margins was found to be most important. Even the presence of an extensive intraductal component was not significant as long as the margins were negative. Thus, patients who have close or positive margins—particularly if there is an association with an extensive intraductal component—should undergo a wider reexcision or perhaps a mastectomy. As in many previous series, local recurrence per se did not adversely affect survival.—T.J. Eberlein, M.D.

Partial Mastectomy Without Radiation Is Adequate Treatment for Patients With Stages O and I Carcinoma of the Breast
Hermann RE, Esselstyn CB Jr, Grundfest-Broniatowski S, Steiger E, Vogt DP, Broughan TA, Dowden RV, Hardesty I, Medendorp SV, Boyett JM (Cleveland Clinic Found, Ohio)
Surg Gynecol Obstet 177:247–253, 1993   140-94-11–15

Background.—In patients with breast carcinoma, a flexible, conservative approach to treatment is currently used. Treatment is selected on a patient-to-patient basis and is dependent upon the size and location of the tumor, evidence of multifocal disease, and histologic factors. At 1 facility, 4 types of treatment for primary, possibly curable carcinoma are used. These include modified radical mastectomy, simple mastectomy,

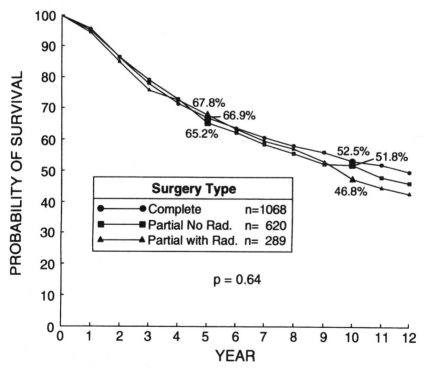

Fig 11–8.—Disease-free survival rate for patients with stages 0, I, and II disease by the type of operation performed (primary treatment given). (Courtesy of Hermann RE, Esselstyn CB Jr, Grundfest-Broniatowski S, et al: *Surg Gynecol Obstet* 177:247-253, 1993.)

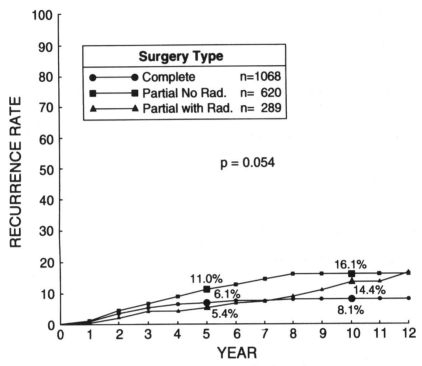

Fig 11–9.—Incidence of local recurrence. Stages 0, I, and II disease, by primary treatment given. (Courtesy of Hermann RE, Esselstyn CB Jr, Grundfest-Broniatowski S, et al: *Surg Gynecol Obstet* 177:247–253, 1993.)

partial mastectomy with postoperative adjuvant radiation therapy, and partial mastectomy without postoperative adjuvant radiation. The last treatment remains controversial and has only been investigated slightly. The largest experience with partial mastectomy without immediate radiation reported from a single institution was presented.

Patients and Findings.—A total of 2,020 patients in stages 0, I, or II who received treatment for carcinoma of the breast during a 14-year period were included. All the patients received treatment and follow-up evaluation at the clinic. An overall survival rate of 80.5% at 5 years and 63.8% at 10 years was noted. For stage 0 patients, the 5-year survival rate was 96.5%, and at 10 years it was 87.7%. A 5-year survival rate of 87.1% and a 10-year rate of 71.6% were recorded for stage I patients. Stage II patients had a 5-year survival rate of 73.2% and a 10-year rate of 54.7%. These rates merely confirm that the stage of the disease has a profound impact on survival. The type of surgery performed did not significantly affect the survival rate up to 12 years (Fig 11–8). During follow-up evaluation, 1,508 of the patients had no recurrence of breast cancer, although 512 patients did experience breast cancer recurrence. Local recurrence

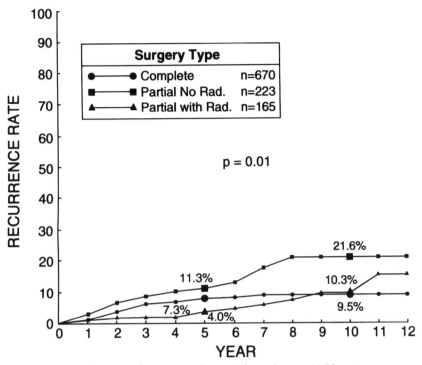

Fig 11-10.—Local recurrence for patients with stage II disease (no. = 1,058) by primary treatment given. (Courtesy of Hermann RE, Esselstyn CB Jr, Grundfest-Broniatowski S, et al: *Surg Gynecol Obstet* 177:247-253, 1993.)

was found in only 30.3% of the cases, whereas 54.1% were systemic recurrences, and only 15.6% were regional recurrences. There was no difference found in local recurrence between the patients in stage 0 or stage I who had partial mastectomy either with or without adjuvant radiation therapy (Fig 11-9). However, among stage II patients, a significant local recurrence was noted in those who did not receive radiation therapy after the partial mastectomy (Fig 11-10). In addition, patients with small tumors measuring 0-2 cm who underwent partial mastectomy without radiation had only an 11% recurrence rate at 5 years and a 14% rate at 10 years. These figures are comparable with those of patients who had a partial mastectomy followed by radiation who had a 5-year recurrence rate of 7% and a 10-year rate of 18%. Large tumors measuring 2-5 cm tended to result in higher recurrence rates.

Conclusion.—Adjuvant radiation therapy is seemingly unnecessary after surgery for patients with stage 0 or I carcinoma of the breast.

▶ This paper from the Cleveland Clinic attempts to define which patients might be treated with conservative surgery but without radiation therapy. In a large series of patients, recurrence was satisfactory as long as the tumor was small, regardless of whether the patient had radiation therapy. As the tumor got larger (for example, stage II tumor), there was a significant increase in the recurrence rate in patients treated without radiation therapy. This is one of a number of papers that attempt to identify a patient population that may be treated without radiation therapy. The tumor size per se should not be the only defining factor in determining whether a patient receives radiation therapy. Other features—such as histology, presence of an intraductal component, and other negative prognostic indicators (comedone-crosis, cathepsin D, aneuploidy, and high S-phase activity)—might well indicate the need for radiation therapy.—T.J. Eberlein, M.D.

MISCELLANEOUS

▶↓ The following several manuscripts are unique but do not conveniently fit into a separate category.—T.J. Eberlein, M.D.

Prospective Evaluation of Immediate Reconstruction After Mastectomy
Eberlein TJ, Crespo LD, Smith BL, Hergrueter CA, Douville L, Eriksson E (Harvard Med School, Boston)
Ann Surg 218:29–36, 1993 140-94-11–16

Background.—Immediate breast reconstruction after mastectomy has recently become an alternative to either mastectomy alone or delayed reconstruction. This procedure should ideally have positive psychological benefits, and it should not adversely affect the natural history of breast disease, inhibit the detection of local or regional recurrence, or increase morbidity associated with mastectomy. An experience with immediate breast reconstruction in 216 patients was evaluated.

Patients and Methods.—The 216 patients were aged 24 to 80 years. All had stage I or II breast cancer, and all underwent mastectomy with immediate reconstruction. Ninety-four procedures involved implants or tissue expanders, and 124 tissue transfers were performed.

Results.—The overall complication rate was 15.3%. Only 9% of patients who underwent autologous tissue transfers required secondary procedures. The overall rate of prosthetic loss was 8% when implants were performed. Transverse rectus abdominis musculocutaneous (TRAM) flaps were used in 101 patients. Twenty-six of the 38 patients who required transfusion were from the TRAM flap group. Partial flap loss was 7% in the TRAM flap group and was associated with a history of heavy smoking. Only 2 patients had experienced local recurrence at a median follow-up of 33.2 months. Autologous tissue transfers yielded a statistically better cosmetic result, according to patient opinion.

Conclusion.—Immediate reconstruction after mastectomy results in an excellent cosmetic outcome with limited morbidity. In addition, this procedure does not increase the risk of or a delay in the diagnosis of local recurrence and does not interfere with subsequent systemic treatment.

▶ In this large, prospective study of immediate reconstructions, the authors found that there is neither an increased risk of recurrence nor a delay in the onset of chemotherapy after immediate reconstruction, and the procedure offers the patient a high degree of satisfaction. The advantage to an immediate reconstruction is the single experience of anesthesia, whereas the disadvantage is the longer time under anesthesia as well as the extended length of stay. The overall cosmetic results are at least as good as with delayed reconstruction. In some cases in which preservation of native breast skin is possible, increased sensation may occur once healing has been completed. Unless the patient is equivocal about reconstruction or has a prohibitive anesthesia risk, immediate reconstruction offers an excellent chance for rehabilitation in the patient either choosing or requiring a mastectomy.—T.J. Eberlein, M.D.

Timing of Surgery for Breast Cancer in Relation to the Menstrual Cycle and Survival of Premenopausal Women

Nathan B, Bates T, Anbazhagan R, Norman AR (William Harvey Hosp, Ashford, England; Inst of Cancer Research, Sutton, England)
Br J Surg 80:43, 1993   140-94-11–17

Background.—A significant decrease in overall and disease-free survival rates has recently been found in studies of premenopausal women with operable breast cancer having surgery during the follicular phase of the menstrual cycle rather than the luteal phase. However, other researchers have been unable to confirm this.

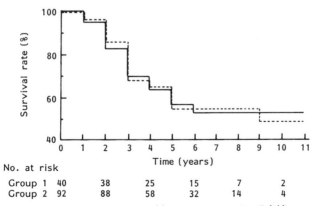

Fig 11–11.—Survival rate in relation to timing of first inpatient operation. *Solid line,* group 1 (operation between days 3 and 12 of cycle); *dotted line,* group 2 (days 0-2 or 13-33). P = .96 (log rank test). (Courtesy of Nathan B, Bates R, Anbazhagan R, et al: *Br J Surg* 80:43, 1993.)

Methods.—The data of 227 premenopausal women with operable breast cancer treated between 1979 and 1988 were reviewed. All patients had been followed regularly. Complete data were available on 132 patients. Two groups were formed: The 40 women in group 1 underwent excision or needle biopsy between days 3 and 12 of the menstrual cycle, and the 92 in group 2 between days 0 and 2 or 13 and 33.

Findings.—The 2 groups had comparable tumor stage, size, and type. Overall survival and disease-free survival were also comparable in the 2 groups (Fig 11-11). These survival rates were comparable whether the relationship to the menstrual cycle was calculated from the first intervention or from the first inpatient surgical procedure. The hazard ratio of group 1 to group 2 was .99 for overall survival and .87 for disease-free survival.

Conclusion.—These results are consistent with others, in that there is no relationship between timing of surgery in premenopausal women with operable breast cancer and survival. Before a major change in surgical practice is recommended, prospective studies are needed with biochemical analyses to determine the phase of the menstrual cycle more accurately.

▶ There has been much media coverage concerning the timing of surgery for carcinoma of the breast. This study failed to show any relationship between the timing of the surgery in premenopausal women with operable cancer and survival. A large number of studies have been conducted, and whereas some show correlation between timing of surgery and survival, others have failed to do so. Only through controlled, prospective trials in which the menstrual cycle is accurately defined and biochemical and hormonal analyses are performed might an accurate answer to this important question be obtained. In the individual patient, a delay in surgery may be warranted but is not supported by the objective data presented in this study.—T.J. Eberlein, M.D.

Axillary Biopsy Compared With Dissection in the Staging of Lymph Nodes in Operable Breast Cancer: A Randomised Trial
Christensen SB, Jansson C (Oestersund Hosp, Sweden)
Eur J Surg 159:159–162, 1993   140-94-11–18

Purpose.—Both adjuvant cytotoxic and hormonal therapy affect the prognosis in breast cancer, although the benefits are greater when the prognosis is poor. The most commonly used prognostic factor to identify patients who would benefit from aggressive adjuvant therapy is axillary lymph node involvement, but there is disagreement as to the extent of axillary clearance needed for adequate staging. Two methods of staging axillary lymph nodes in women with operable breast cancer—axillary dissection and axillary node biopsy—were compared.

TABLE 1.—Number of Patients With Histologically
Infiltrated Axillary Nodes, and Yield of Nodes in
the 2 Groups

	Axillary dissection ($n=100$)	Axillary biopsy ($n=100$)
No of patients with infiltrated nodes	43	46
Median (range) no of nodes identified*	8.5(0—16)	6(0—14)
Median(range) no of infiltrated nodes identified	2(1—14)	2(1—9)

* $P < .001$.
(Courtesy of Christensen SB, Jansson C: *Eur J Surg* 159:159-162, 1993.)

Methods.—This randomized study included 200 women in 2 different 2-year periods who were seen at 1 Swedish district hospital. One hundred patients were assigned to undergo axillary dissection, with removal of all fat from the axilla, and 100 had biopsy, including removal of the lower half of the axillary fat and obviously malignant nodes. The results were assessed in terms of the number of nodes harvested by each method and the number of metastatic nodes.

Results.—Metastatic nodes were detected in 43 patients in the dissection group and 46 in the biopsy group. The median node yield was significantly higher in the dissection group—8.5 vs. 6 (Table 1). No nodes were identified in 1 patient in each group. The distribution of recurrences among the 111 patients without histologically confirmed lymph node involvement at follow-up is shown in Table 2. A metastatic node was detected 3 months after operation in 1 patient from the biopsy group. During the last 100 operations, the surgeon's operative clinical

TABLE 2.—Distribution of Recurrences in 111 Women Who
Did Not Have Metastases in Axillary Lymph Nodes After
Dissection or Biopsy

Site of metastases	Axillary dissection ($n=57$)	Axillary biopsy ($n=54$)
Local	4	1
Axillary	0	1
Distant	1	4

(Courtesy of Christensen SB, Jansson C: *Eur J Surg* 159:159-162, 1993.)

TABLE 3.—Clinical Evaluation of Lymph Nodes During Operation Compared With Histologic Diagnosis in Last 100 Patients in Series

	Clinical judgement		
	Metastases	No metastases	Total
Histologically:			
Metastases	26(59)	18	44
No metastases	6	50(89)	56
Total	32	68	100

Note: Figures in parentheses are sensitivity and specificity.
(Courtesy of Christensen SB, Jansson C: Eur J Surg 159:159–162, 1993.)

assessment of whether the patient had involved nodes had a sensitivity of 59% and a specificity of 89% (Table 3).

Conclusion.—These 2 techniques of axillary node staging for operable breast cancer yielded similar results. A method should be chosen according to considerations such as side effects and the role of the axillary procedure in local tumor control. The surgeon's clinical judgment of node status is insufficient.

▶ This study raises several issues with regard to axillary dissection. Morbidity is clearly related to the extent of dissection, and the number of lymph nodes obtained will increase with a more complete dissection; however, determining which patients have pathologically positive nodes can be achieved by a minimal sampling. (Minimal sampling may also be used to determine the presence of any grossly involved lymph nodes, as in this study). It also appears that a change in a clinically negative axilla to a pathologically positive axilla is not significantly increased by doing a more radical dissection. However, a more complete axillary dissection will permit better definition of subgroups of node-positive patients—for example, the patient with 4 or more positive nodes. As we begin to design protocols for patients with specific numbers of involved nodes, complete axillary dissection will still be warranted. To determine a pathologically positive axilla, a minimal dissection with removal of any obvious abnormal nodes would seem sufficient.—T.J. Eberlein, M.D.

Colorectal Cancer

INTRODUCTION

During this past year, significant strides have been made in identifying the basic biology that leads to the development of colorectal cancer. We will discuss several papers that look at various oncogenes and their effects on prognosis and metastasis. Another major area of study concerns performing conservative surgery for treatment of rectal cancers. As with breast cancer, specific criteria need to be established concerning the extent of the surgery, the type of tumors treated with conservative surgery, and accurate staging, so that the treatments of selected patients can be compared between one institution and another.

Timothy J. Eberlein, M.D.

EPIDEMIOLOGY

Dietary Intake of Fiber and Decreased Risk of Cancers of the Colon and Rectum: Evidence From the Combined Analysis of 13 Case-Control Studies
Howe GR, Benito E, Castelleto R, Cornée J, Estève J, Gallagher RP, Iscovich JM, Deng-ao J, Kaaks R, Kune GA, Kune S, L'Abbé KA, Lee HP, Lee M, Miller AB, Peters RK, Potter JD, Riboli E, Slattery ML, Trichopoulos D, Tuyns A, Tzonou A, Whittemore AS, Wu-Williams AH, Shu Z (Natl Cancer Inst of Canada; Unitat d' Epidemiologia i Registre de Cancer de Mallorca, Palma de Mallorca, Spain; La Plata Natl Univ, Argentina; et al)
J Natl Cancer Inst 84:1887–1896, 1992   140-94-11–19

Introduction.—The effects of intakes of fiber, vitamin C, and β-carotene on the risk of colorectal cancer were evaluated in a combined analysis of data from 13 case-control studies previously conducted in populations with different colorectal cancer rates and dietary practices.

Methods.—Individual data records of 5,287 case subjects with colorectal cancer and 10,470 control subjects without disease were studied. The relative risks were estimated with logistic regression analysis, while adjusting for the effects of study, sex, and age.

Results.—The risk of colorectal cancer was inversely related to the intakes of fiber, vitamin C, and β-carotene. There was a monotonically decreasing dose-dependent relationship for the intake of fiber, with the highest quartile of intake (median, 31.2 g/day) having about half the risk of those with the lowest quartile of intake (median, 10.1 g/day). The inverse relationship for fiber was evident in 12 of 13 studies and was similar in magnitude for left- and right-sided colon and rectal cancers, for men and women, and for different age groups. In contrast, after adjusting for fiber intake, there was only a weak inverse relationship observed to intakes of vitamin C and β-carotene.

Conclusion.—These findings provide strong evidence for a decreasing risk of colorectal cancer with increasing intake of fiber. It is estimated that, if the United States population increased its fiber intakes from foods to at least 39 g/day, the risk of colorectal cancer would be reduced about 31% (50,000 cases annually). This dietary change would amount to an increase of about 13 g/day, or 70%, for the average individual following a typical diet.

▶ This paper by Howe et al. has received much publicity of late. It is an analysis of 13 case-control studies from populations with different colorectal cancer rates and dietary practices. More than 5,000 subjects with colorectal cancer and more than 10,000 controls were studied. The authors looked at intakes of fiber, vitamin C, and β-carotene. They showed there was an inverse relationship between an increase in fiber intake and the incidence of colorectal cancer. This was similar whether the cancer was left-sided or right-sided. When fiber intake was identified, there were only weak inverse relationships seen for the intake of vitamin C and β-carotene and the presence of colorectal cancer. These authors estimate that the incidence of colorectal cancer in as many as 50,000 people in the United States could be prevented by increasing their dietary intake of fiber. Studies such as these that focus on preventative care will be of increasing significance as the health care dollars for various treatments shrink.—T.J. Eberlein, M.D.

Influence of Socioeconomic Status on Prognosis of Colorectal Cancer: A Population-Based Study in Côte D'Or, France
Monnet E, Boutron MC, Faivre J, Milan C (Faculté de Médecine et de Pharmacie, Besancon, France; Faculté de Médecine, Dijon, France)
Cancer 72:1165–1170, 1993   140-94-11–20

Background.—The prognostic significance of the socioeconomic status of patients treated for colorectal cancer has been addressed in some investigations but remains unsettled. In a population series, the association between socioeconomic status and survival after treatment for colorectal cancer was determined.

Methods.—The study population consisted of 771 patients with colorectal cancer diagnosed from the beginning of 1976 through 1980. Socioeconomic status was determined by comfort of housing.

Findings.—Compared with patients living in comfortable houses, patients in medium- or no-comfort houses were more likely to be diagnosed at a later stage of disease and to be treated by palliative therapy. After adjusting for these factors—as well as for age, sex, place of residence, and tumor location—patients living in no-comfort situations had a twofold higher risk of dying during the 5-year follow-up than patients in comfortable situations. The relative risk for the medium-comfort category was 1.5. This effect was more pronounced in patients with early-stage disease than in those with advanced disease (table).

Conclusion.—Public health measures are needed to ensure earlier access to medical care for people of lower socioeconomic status. In addition, more research is needed to better define the host-tumor relationship.

Relationship Between Type of Housing and Prognostic Variables in Colorectal Cancer

	Comfortable (n = 421) (%)	Medium comfort (n = 325) (%)	No comfort (n = 25) (%)	P	Chi-square (df)
Age					
< 65	33.5	10.5	8.0	< 0.0001	75.2 (4)
65–74	37.8	39.4	20.0		
≥ 75	28.7	50.2	72.0		
Sex					
M	59.4	46.5	52.0	0.002	12.1 (2)
F	40.6	53.5	48.0		
Residence					
Urban	69.8	42.5	40.0	0.0001	59.7 (2)
Rural	30.2	57.5	60.0		
Tumor site					
Colon	55.1	55.7	28.0	0.03	7.3 (2)
Rectum	44.9	44.3	72.0		
Stage					
A	17.1	12.2	4.0	0.01*	11.1* (4)
B	29.0	24.9	16.0		
C	24.0	28.9	32.0		
Metastasis	20.7	21.8	28.0		
Unknown	8.3	12.3	20.0		
Treatment					
Curative	66.7	56.3	36.0	0.0005	15.1 (2)
Palliative	33.3	43.7	64.0		

Abbreviation: df, degrees of freedom.
* Test performed with grouping of medium and no comfort.
(Courtesy of Monnet E, Boutron Mc, Faivre J, et al: *Cancer* 72:1165–1170, 1993.)

▶ In a paper by Monnet and others, prognostic significance is associated with the socioeconomic status of patients with colorectal cancer. Patients in medium or no-comfort houses were not only more likely to receive a diagnosis in a more advanced stage but, when other controls were accounted for, they were also more likely to die of colorectal cancer. Again, the incidence of colorectal tumor may well be impacted by socioeconomic factors and public health measures. Thus, significant strides to decrease the incidence of colorectal tumor and its financial burden on our health care system may be made through patient education.—T.J. Eberlein, M.D.

SURVEILLANCE

Colonoscopic Surveillance Reduces Mortality From Colorectal Cancer In Ulcerative Colitis

Choi PM, Nugent FW, Schoetz DJ Jr, Silverman ML, Haggitt RC (Lahey Clinic Med Ctr, Burlington, Mass; Univ of Washington, Seattle)
Gastroenterology 105:418–424, 1993   140-94-11–21

Background.—Periodic surveillance colonoscopy with multiple biopsies is widely recommended to control the increased risk of colorectal carcinoma in patients with long-standing ulcerative colitis. However, it is not known whether this strategy reduces the number of colorectal carcinoma–related deaths.

Study Design.—Patients who had ulcerative colitis with a duration of 8 years or more and who had disease extending proximal to the sigmoid colon were enrolled in a prospective surveillance program. Colonoscopy

Dukes' Stage for Carcinoma Associated With Ulcerative Colitis
According to Method of Diagnosis

	Surveillance			No surveillance		
	Dukes' stage					
	A	B	C	A	B	C
Method of diagnosis						
Surveillance	6	5	3	—	—	—
Evaluation of symptoms	0	1[a]	1[a]	0	6	13
Operation[b]	1	2	0	3	0	0
Total[c]	7	8	4	3	6	13

* Noncompliant with the surveillance protocol.
† Cancer diagnosed incidentally at operation performed for disease control.
‡ $P = .039$ for the difference in Dukes' stage distribution between surveillance and nonsurveillance groups.
(Courtesy of Choi PM, Nugent FW, Schoetz DJ Jr, et al: *Gastroenterology* 105:418-424, 1993.)

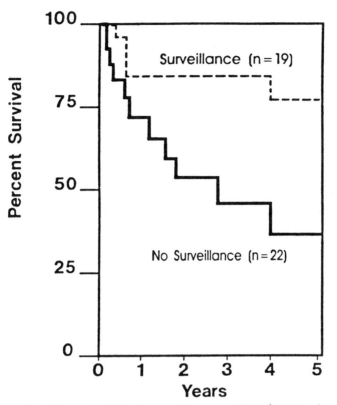

Fig 11–12.—Overall 5-year survival. The 5-year survival rates were 77.2% ± 10.1% with surveillance and 36% ± 12.7% without surveillance (P = .026). The analysis was performed using the Kaplan-Meier product limit method. (Courtesy of Choi PM, Nugent FW, Schoetz DJ Jr, et al: *Gastroenterology* 105:418–424, 1993.)

with biopsy studies was performed every 2 years after negative results were seen on 2 consecutive annual examinations.

Outcome.—Of the 2,050 patients with ulcerative colitis seen between 1974 and 1991, 41 had colorectal carcinoma. Of these, 19 were under colonoscopic surveillance and the other 22 were not. The patients who had colonoscopic surveillance had a median of 2 colonoscopies, and the diagnosis of colorectal carcinoma was made after a median of 2 years after the initial colonoscopy. Carcinoma was detected at a significantly earlier Duke's stage in these patients compared with those without colonoscopic surveillance (table). There were 4 deaths in the surveillance group and 11 deaths in the no-surveillance group. The 5-year survival rate was 77.2% for the surveillance group and 36.3% for the nonsurveillance group (Fig 11–12).

Conclusion.—Colonoscopic surveillance reduces mortality from colorectal carcinoma in patients with long-standing ulcerative colitis. This beneficial effect appears to be derived from detection of carcinoma at an earlier Duke's stage. However, it is disturbing that 3 carcinomas in the surveillance group were detected incidentally during surgery and not during previous colonoscopy, and that 3 advanced carcinomas were also detected during regular surveillance. Until a more sensitive screening method becomes available, colonoscopic surveillance with biopsies remains the best strategy for preventing the increased risk of colorectal carcinoma in patients with long-standing ulcerative colitis.

▶ This study from the Lahey Clinic, which includes a large series of patients with all types of colitis, found that those patients who underwent systematic colonoscopic surveillance and were found to have colorectal cancer, had an early Duke's stage tumor and were less likely to die of their tumor. To the casual observer, this may seem intuitively obvious; however, it raises several public health issues regarding the cost-effectiveness of surveillance vs. the definitive prevention of colorectal tumors through the increased use of ileoanal procedures. Additionally, several tumors were detected only at the time of surgery, and, in spite of surveillance, several large tumors were found. Thus, in patients with long-standing ulcerative colitis, definitive surgical removal of the colon may be preferable to surveillance.

In a related manuscript by Guillem (*Dis Colon Rectum* 35:523, 1992) from the Memorial Sloan-Kettering Cancer Center and Columbia University in New York, a study was performed involving colonoscopic screening in asymptomatic first-degree relatives of patients given a diagnosis of colon cancer. A greater proportion of the adenomas were found to be beyond the reach of flexible sigmoidoscopy. The authors concluded that, especially in males with one first-degree relative afflicted with colon cancer, there appeared to be an increased risk of the development of colonic adenoma at 40 years of age and older. Thus, this carefully controlled study suggests when one should receive colonoscopy and at what age. Obviously, these are also the patients who would probably benefit from patient education regarding dietary suggestions and other preventive measures.—T.J. Eberlein, M.D.

BASIC BIOLOGY AND TUMOR MARKERS

▶↓ In this section, several publications are grouped together, each of which attempts to define some of the basic biological mechanisms of colorectal tumors to develop markers or to relate these basic biological events to overall prognosis.—T.J. Eberlein, M.D.

---

p53 Immunoreaction in Endoscopic Biopsy Specimens of Colorectal Cancer, and Its Prognostic Significance
Yamaguchi A, Nakagawara G, Kurosaka Y, Nishimura G, Yonemura Y, Miyazaki I (Fukui Med School, Japan; Kanazawa Univ, Japan)
Br J Cancer 68:399–402, 1993   140-94-11-22

Objective.—Materials from 203 colorectal cancers were analyzed immunohistochemically with the use of the PAb1801 mouse anti-p53 MAb to determine the expression of the p53 protein. Elevated levels of p53 protein have been found in many human-derived cell lines.

Patients and Methods.—Seventy-eight of the colorectal tumors were well differentiated, 111 were moderately differentiated, 5 were poorly differentiated adenocarcinomas, and 9 were mucinous carcinomas. By the Duke's classification, 25 patients had stage A tumors, 68 had stage B, 55 had stage C, and 55 had stage D. Resected specimens were fixed in 10% formalin overnight and embedded in paraffin.

Results.—There were 121 cancers (59.6%) with evidence of p53 protein overexpression. Reactivity was localized in the nuclei. No correlation was found between p53 protein expression and histologic classification, wall invasion, lymphatic invasion, venous invasion, lymph node metastases, or peritoneal metastasis. The p53 protein–positive rate was higher for tumors with liver metastasis (72.7%) than for tumors without liver metastases (56%). The prognosis was significantly poorer for patients with p53-positive tumors than for those with p53-negative tumors; the 5-year survival rate was 58.1% for the former group and 76.3% for the latter. Differences in survival associated with p53 immunoreactivity were particularly marked among patients with Duke's stage C tumors. Patients with p53-positive tumors also had higher rates of recurrence. Flow cytometric analysis yielded no correlation between the p53 immunoreactivity and the DNA ploidy pattern.

Conclusion.—Several recent studies have indicated a close correlation between p53 immunoreactivity and the prognosis of several malignant tumors, and the findings of this study confirm such a correlation in colorectal cancers. The p53 immunoreactivity detected by PAb1801 is a useful prognostic indicator and would allow preoperative analysis of biopsy specimens.

▶ In this article by Yamaguchi, the results were extended to endoscopic biopsy specimens. Again, a correlation with survival was identified, with p53 expressors having a worse prognosis. However, the paper points to the fact that preoperative identification of p53 is possible. Only through large-scale prospective studies will its true significance be correlated with potential therapeutic interventions such as preoperative radiation therapy or neoadjuvant chemotherapy.—T.J. Eberlein, M.D.

Determination of Tumor Aggressiveness in Colorectal Cancer by K-*ras*-2 Analysis

Finkelstein SD, Sayegh R, Bakker A, Swalsky P (Brown Univ, Providence, RI)
Arch Surg 128:526–532, 1993   140-94-11–23

Introduction.—Point mutations of the well-studied K-*ras*-2 gene appear to be especially important in colorectal cancer. Specific mutations in this gene might be useful in predicting the aggressiveness of colorectal cancer, allowing individualization and optimization of oncologic therapy.

Methods.—The presence and specific type of K-*ras*-2 point mutation in formalin-fixed, paraffin-embedded tissue blocks of 247 primary, 5 anastomotic recurrent, and 161 metastatic colorectal adenocarcinomas were evaluated. To do this, morphologic analysis and topographic tissue selection, DNA amplification, and direct sequencing (a technique designed to be applicable to large as well as needle biopsy–sized specimens) were used.

Findings.—The cancers showed either a normal K-*ras*-2 gene or 1 of 7 types of point mutations resulting in unique amino acid substitution at the 12th or 13th codon. In no case was a mutation acquired in a metastatic deposit whose primary tumor showed a normal K-*ras*-2 gene. About one third of the primary tumors contained mutations, with T3 and T4 tumors having a 42% rate of mutation, not significantly higher than the 30% for the more superficial tumors. The mutation rate was significantly lower for anastomotic recurrent and transcoelomic implants than for primary tumors (19% vs. 37%). For patients with morphologically similar primary tumors, the course was more likely to be limited to local or transcoelomic growth. Tumors with a normal K-*ras*-2 gene were more likely to have spread by the hematogenous route than were tumors having codon 13–aspartic acid or codon 12–valine substitutions. Visceral metastasis occurred in only 2 of 23 patients with normal K-*ras*-2 primaries.

Conclusion.—The K-*ras*-2 status of colorectal adenocarcinomas was examined in this study. The data can be used in a genotypic classification to predict tumor aggressiveness. This classification will have to be validated in both experimental and prospective clinical studies. This approach to studying these mutations may be useful in the study of other potentially important point mutations.

▶ Finkelstein studied point mutations of the K-*ras*-2 gene in colorectal cancers. No definitive correlation was identified between a particular mutation and a particular subgroup of patients; however, larger tumors tended to have higher expression of the mutation. Additionally, primary tumors with a normal K-*ras*-2 gene were more likely to spread by the hematogenous route and were less likely to have visceral metastasis. Through large prospective trials using this gene, specific correlations that would allow for the selection of patients for adjuvant chemotherapy may be made. These authors report this novel system of tissue sampling to study the point mutations of this gene. They are also currently working within the Cancer and Leukemia Group B to correlate expression of the K-*ras*-2 gene and responsiveness to systemic therapy.—T.J. Eberlein, M.D.

Site-Specific Differences in pp60^{c-src} Activity in Human Colorectal Metastases

Termuhlen PM, Curley SA, Talamonti MS, Saboorian MH, Gallick GE (MD Anderson Cancer Ctr, Houston)
J Surg Res 54:293–298, 1993   140-94-11-24

Purpose.—In patients with primary colorectal carcinoma, progression to hepatic metastasis may involve the c-src proto-oncogene. The protein product of the c-src proto-oncogene is pp60^{c-src}, and its protein tyrosine kinase activity is 1 of the regulatory molecules altered during malignant transformation of colonic epithelial cells. Whether increased pp60^{c-src} tyrosine kinase activity is a colon-specific phenomenon in all colorectal metastases was determined.

Observations.—Tyrosine kinase activity was measured by immune complex kinase assay, and immunoblotting was used to determine protein levels. The pp60^{c-src} activity of colorectal liver metastases was increased an average of 2.2 times over that of the normal mucosa. Liver

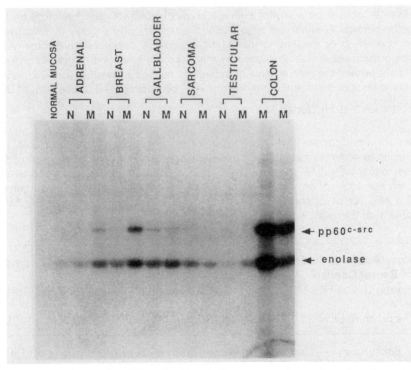

Fig 11–13.—Activity of pp60^{c-src} tyrosine kinase in liver metastases from various primary human tumors. The pp60^{c-src} was immunoprecipitated from equal amounts of total cellular protein from lysates made from human tissue specimens of liver metastasis (M) and adjacent normal liver (N). The origin of the primary tumor is indicated along the top of the figure. (Courtesy of Termuhlen PM, Curley SA, Talamonti MS, et al: *J Surg Res* 54:293–298, 1993.)

metastases from other primary tumors, however, showed only minimal pp60$^{c\text{-}src}$ activity (Fig 11–13). The pp60$^{c\text{-}src}$ activity of extrahepatic colorectal metastases was even higher, averaging nearly 13 times higher than that of normal mucosa and 6 times higher than that of colon liver metastasis. The findings were confirmed by examination of multiple synchronous colon carcinoma metastases.

Conclusion.—Increases in specific activity of pp60$^{c\text{-}src}$ were documented in colon carcinoma liver metastases, and little such activity was seen in liver metastases from other primary sites. There are also site-specific differences in the magnitude of activity. These findings suggest that tyrosine kinase inhibitors such as herbimycin A may be useful in controlling or preventing metastasis in patients with colon cancer.

▶ Termuhlen and colleagues from M.D. Anderson Cancer Center looked at the c-*src* proto-oncogene and its role in the development of hepatic metastasis. Specifically, they measured tyrosine kinase activity (pp60$^{c\text{-}src}$). They found that activation of pp60$^{c\text{-}src}$ was unique to colon metastasis, and although its activity was significantly increased, site-specific differences and the magnitudes of activity were evident. The primary therapy for metastatic colorectal disease focuses on adjuvant chemotherapy. Tyrosine kinase inhibitors such as herbimycin A, which are specifically directed at pp60$^{c\text{-}src}$, may be effective in controlling or preventing metastatic disease in colorectal carcinoma. As the protein substrates correlated by this gene are identified, further information regarding the mechanisms of activation, as well as avenues for new diagnostic tests or therapeutic intervention, will be obtained.—T.J. Eberlein, M.D.

ENDORECTAL ULTRASOUND

▶↓ As more conservative treatments for rectal cancer become available, a means to accurately stage the disease is necessary not only to be able to select patients, but to compare results. Endorectal ultrasound has become a common tool not only in the selection of patients for conservative surgery, but also for preoperative radiation therapy. The following articles address several of these issues.—T.J. Eberlein, M.D.

How Accurate Is Endorectal Ultrasound in the Preoperative Staging of Rectal Cancer?
Herzog U, von Flüe M, Tondelli P, Schuppisser JP (St Claraspital, Basel, Switzerland)
Dis Colon Rectum 36:127–134, 1993   140-94-11–25

Background.—The depth of tumor infiltration in rectal cancer and its metastatic involvement of lymph nodes are important prognostic factors. Previous studies have shown that clinical staging can predict the depth of tumor infiltration in 60% to 80% of cases and that CT shows infiltration by tumor in 53% to 94% of cases. Neither method can predict nodal in-

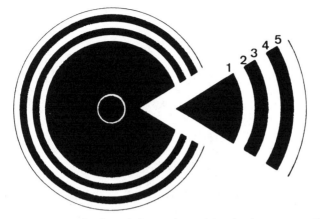

Fig 11–14.—Interpretation of endorectal ultrasound scan. *1,* interface between water-filled balloon and mucosal surface; *2,* mucosa and muscularis mucosae; *3,* submucosa; *4,* muscularis propria; *5,* interface between muscularis propria and perirectal fat or serosa. (Courtesy of Herzog U, von Flüe M, Tondelli P, et al: *Dis Colon Rectum* 36:127-134, 1993.)

volvement or distinguish between early and late tumor stages. The accuracy of endorectal ultrasonography (EUS) for the preoperative staging of rectal cancer was assessed in a prospective study.

Methods.—On EUS, the rectal wall shows 5 layers, of which 3 are hypoechoic, and 2 are hyperechoic (Fig 11-14). The fourth layer is hypoechoic and it may be divided into 2 layers separated by a fine hypere-

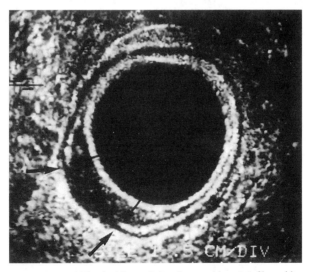

Fig 11–15.—uT2 carcinoma. The third hypoechoic submucosal layer is infiltrated by tumor. *Arrows* show disruption of submucosal layer. (Courtesy of Herzog U, von Flüe M, Tondelli P, et al: *Dis Colon Rectum* 36:127-134, 1993.)

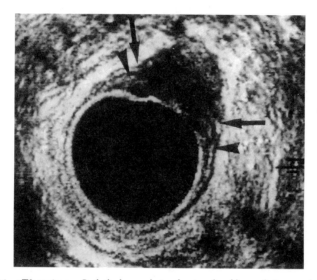

Fig 11–16.—uT3 carcinoma. Both the hyperechoic submucosal and hypoechoic muscularis layers are destroyed by the rectal carcinoma. *Arrowheads* show disruption of the submucosal layer. *Arrows* show disruption of muscularis propria. (Courtesy of Herzog U, von Flüe M, Tondelli P, et al: *Dis Colon Rectum* 36:127–134, 1993.)

choic layer. In the TNM classification adjusted for ultrasonography, a uT1 lesion is confined to the mucosa and submucosa, a uT2 lesion infiltrates the muscularis propria but does not penetrate the rectal wall (Fig 11–15), a uT3 lesion invades perirectal fat (Fig 11–16), and a uT4 lesion infiltrates the surrounding organs. Lymph nodes in perirectal fat are considered as metastases if they are hypoechoic.

Patients.—During a 3-year period, 58 men and 60 women, aged 40–93 years, who had histologically proved rectal cancer or rectal adenoma,

TABLE 1.—Preoperative Staging With CT
and EUS: Results in 87 Patients

	CT (%)	EUS (%)
Accuracy	74.7	90.8
Sensitivity	68.9	98.3
Specificity	86.2	75
PPV	90.9	89.2
NPV	58.1	95.4

Abbreviations: PPV, positive predictive value; NPV, negative predictive value.
(Courtesy of Herzog U, von Flüe M, Tondelli P, et al: *Dis Colon Rectum* 36:127–134, 1993.)

TABLE 2.—Overall Accuracy of EUS in the Preoperative Staging
of Rectal Cancer (Depth of Infiltration)

Literature	No. of Patients	No. with Correct Diagnosis	Accuracy (%)
Rifkin *et al.*	101	61	60
Saitoh *et al.*	88	79	90
Orrom *et al.*	77	58	75
Glaser *et al.*	86	76	88
Accarpio *et al.*	54	51	94
Beynon *et al.*	89	82	92
Hildebrandt *et al.*	98	87	89
Jochem *et al.*	50	40	80
Present study	118	105	89

(Courtesy of Herzog U, von Flüe M, Tondelli P, et al: *Dis Colon Rectum* 36:127–134, 1993.)

underwent EUS. Eighty-seven patients also had preoperative CT. One hundred five patients had a laparotomy and 13 were treated by local excision.

Results.—According to the EUS findings, there were 20 uT1 lesions, 20 uT2 lesions, 75 uT3 lesions, and 3 uT4 lesions. Pathologic tumor examination identified 22 pT1, 26 pT2, 68 pT3, and 2 pT4 carcinomas. The overall accuracy in staging depth of infiltration was 89%. Twelve tumors (10.2%) were overstaged and 1 (.8%) was understaged. Incorrect staging occurred for 9 of 54 tumors (16.7%) in the lower third of the rectum, 3 of 45 tumors (6.7%) in the middle third of the rectum, and 1 of 19 tumors (5.3%) in the upper third of the rectum. The overall accuracy for predicting depth of tumor infiltration was 74.7% for CT and 90.8% for EUS (Table 1). For staging lymph nodes, EUS had an overall diagnostic accuracy of 80.2%, a sensitivity of 89.4%, a specificity of 73.4%, a positive predictive value of 71.2%, and a negative predictive value of 90.4%. The overall accuracy of EUS for staging rectal cancer fell within the previously reported range (Table 2).

Conclusion.—Endorectal ultrasonography is a safe, inexpensive, and accurate method for the preoperative staging of rectal cancer. It provides information on both depth of tumor infiltration and nodal status.

▶ Herzog studied a group of 118 patients and showed that EUS was more accurate at predicting the depth of tumor infiltration than was CT scanning. The overall accuracy of lymph node staging was about 80%, but the negative predictive value was 90%. Thus, EUS is certainly safe, inexpensive, and accurate.—T.J. Eberlein, M.D.

Endorectal Ultrasound for Control of Preoperative Radiotherapy of Rectal Cancer

Glaser F, Kuntz C, Schlag P, Herfarth C (Univ of Heidelberg, Germany)

Ann Surg 217:64–71, 1993   140-94-11–26

Background.—Endorectal ultrasound (EUS) is a reliable method for preoperative staging of rectal tumors. Preoperative radiation therapy reduces the risk of local tumor recurrence, but it should only be used in cases where there is high risk of local recurrence. Endorectal ultrasound is used to identify those high risk cases. In this study, EUS was used to select patients with rectal cancer for preoperative radiation therapy and was then performed again after radiation therapy. The effectiveness of EUS in monitoring the results of preoperative radiation therapy was evaluated.

Study Design.—A series of 154 patients with rectal carcinoma was examined by EUS. Of these patients, 17 with large T3 or T4 tumors received preoperative radiation therapy with follow-up EUS. Tumor infiltration depth, lymph node localization, echostructure of tumor and lymph nodes, and maximal tumor size were determined before and after radiation therapy. All patients underwent surgery within 5 weeks of radiation treatment. After surgery, the EUS results were compared to histologic examination of the surgical specimen.

Results.—Radiation induced a decrease in the size of the tumor. The echopattern of the tumor changed after radiation therapy to more hyperechoic gray levels. There was a loss of the normal architecture in the rectal wall. The lymph nodes either disappeared or became echorich. However, there was no downstaging of the tumor by EUS after radiation therapy (table). The EUS preoperative staging was wholly correct in 13 of these 17 patients.

Conclusion.—Endorectal ultrasonography is an effective, reliable method for selecting patients for preoperative radiation therapy. Because radiation treatment alters the sonographic image of the tumor, rectal wall, and lymph nodes, EUS is most effective when used both before and after radiation therapy. This also permits the effects of the radiation therapy to be assessed.

▶ In the work by Glaser and colleagues, EUS is used to select patients with rectal cancer for preoperative radiation therapy. The authors emphasize, however, the need for comparing the ultrasound pattern before and after radiation therapy. No downstaging of the tumor by EUS after radiation therapy was found.—T.J. Eberlein, M.D.

Patients Staged by Endorectal Ultrasound Before and After Radiation Therapy

Patient No.	Sex	Age	Total Dose/Single Dose (Gy)	Time Interval (wk)	Tumor Size Before/After Radiation Therapy (cm)		Staging by EUS Before Radiation	Staging by EUS After Radiation	Histologic Type
1	F	48	40/2	4	3,7	3,4	uT4, N+	uT4, N+	pT4, N3, M0
2	F	59	40/2	5	4,5	3,2	uT3, N+	uT3, N+	pT3, N0, M1
3	F	72	40/2	4	4,2	3,8	uT4, N+	uT4, N+	pT4, N2, M0
4	F	52	40/2	5	4,1	2,0	uT3, N-	uT4, N+	pT4, N1, M0
5	F	45	40/2	5	3,4	2,0	uT3, N-	uT3, N-	pT3, N1, M0
6	M	58	40/2	4	3,0	2,2	uT4, N+	uT4, N+	pT4, N3, M1
7	M	41	40/2	4	4,2	2,3	uT3, N+	uT3, N+	pT3, N2, M0
8	F	84	40/2	4	3,0	2,4	uT3, N+	uT3, N-	pT3, N0, M0
9	M	74	40/2	4	4,1	3,2	uT3, N+	uT3, N+	pT3, N1, M0
10	F	69	40/2	4	3,6	2,5	uT3, N+	uT3, N+	pT3, N1, M0
11	F	72	40/2	5	3,0	2,1	uT3, N+	uT3, N+	pT3, N1, M0
12	M	57	40/2	4	4,6	3,5	uT4, N+	uT4, N+	pT3, N2, M0
13	M	51	40/2	5	4,1	3,7	uT3, N-	uT3, N-	pT3, N0, M0
14	F	69	40/2	5	2,8	2,4	uT3, N+	uT3, N+	pT3, N1, M0
15	F	72	40/2	5	3,1	2,3	uT3, N+	uT3, N-	pT3, N0, M0
16	M	56	40/2	5	2,9	2,8	uT3, N+	uT3, N+	pT3, N2, M0
17	M	69	40/2	4	3,1	2,4	uT4, N+	uT4, N+	pT3, N0, M0

(Courtesy of Glaser F, Kuntz C, Schlag P, et al: *Ann Surg* 217:64–71, 1993.)

Endorectal Ultrasonography for Staging Small Rectal Tumors: Technique and Contribution to Treatment

Detry RJ, Kartheuser A, Kestens PJ (Univ of Louvain-en-Woluwe, Belgium; St-Luc Hosp, Brussels, Belgium)

World J Surg 17:271–276, 1993   140-94-11-27

Objective.—The value of endorectal ultrasonography (EUS) for evaluating small rectal tumors was examined in 17 men and 14 women with a mean age of 67 years who had a tumor in the lower two thirds of the rectum that was considered suitable for local resection. The series included 18 sessile villous adenomas and 13 invasive cancers 3 cm or less in size.

Findings.—Twenty-seven of the 31 tumors (87%) were correctly staged by EUS when compared with the pathologic findings. Sonography had a positive predictive value of 93% for distinguishing between stage T1 and T2/T3 tumors and 100% in differentiating between T1/T2 and T3 lesions. The respective negative predictive values were 94% and 93%. In 17 patients with cancer, EUS predicted lymph node involvement with a sensitivity of 75% and a specificity of 91% (table).

Conclusion.—Staging small rectal tumors by EUS can accurately gauge the depth of penetration in most cases, and it can help select small cancers that may be amenable to local treatment. The finding of involved nodes contraindicates local excision. The chief problem in using EUS for staging early rectal cancers is in correctly evaluating the state of the regional lymph nodes.

▶ Detry used EUS to select patients for local treatment. Again, the limitation of EUS is in the prediction of lymph node involvement, which will be made more accurate only by improvements in the equipment and more experience with large numbers of patients. Because of the potential for inaccuracy in evaluating lymph node status, patients selected for local treatment will need careful follow-up, optimally in a protocol setting.—T.J. Eberlein, M.D.

Overall Results

All cases (no.)

EUS type	T1	T2	T3
uT1	15	1	—
uT2	1	9	2
uT3	—	—	3

All cancers (no.)

EUS type	pN0	pN1	Unknown
uN0 ($n = 13$)	10	1	2
uN1 ($n = 4$)	1	3	—

(Courtesy of Detry RJ, Kartheuser A, Kestens PJ: *World J Surg* 17:271–276, 1993.)

TREATMENT OF RECTAL CANCER

Phase I/II Trial of Pre-Operative Radiation Therapy and Coloanal Anastomosis in Distal Invasive Resectable Rectal Cancer
Minsky BD, Cohen AM, Enker WE, Sigurdson E (Mem Sloan-Kettering Cancer Ctr, New York)
Int J Radiat Oncol Biol Phys 23:387–392, 1992   140-94-11–28

Introduction.—Patients with invasive rectal cancer who cannot tolerate a low anterior resection commonly have an abdominoperineal resection (APR), which produces a permanent colostomy. The preliminary phase I toxicity outcome and phase II local control and survival data of patients who received preoperative radiation therapy in addition to an APR and coloanal anastomosis procedure were reported.

Methods.—Of the 22 patients with invasive, resectable, primary distal rectal adenocarcinoma, all had preoperative radiation therapy by means of an external-beam device and underwent presurgical staging. The patients were observed weekly during radiation therapy and for 2–3 weeks thereafter. Four to 5 weeks after radiation treatment completion, the patients had surgery.

Results.—Downstaging occurred upon preoperative radiation therapy, with 10% of the patients having a complete pathologic response, and 90% became able to successfully undergo the APR plus coloanal anastomosis. The crude failure rate for all patients was 5% local, 9% abdominal, and 0% distal. The 4-year actuarial survival rate was 61% in this population. No patients sustained radiation toxicity requiring hospitalization. Of the 19 patients undergoing the low APR and coloanal anastomosis, 1 did not have the diverting colostomy reversed because of a postsurgical cerebrovascular complication. Of the 18 patients who had this procedure, 1 had a partial disruption of the anastomosis. Thus, 16 of 18 patients experienced a good or excellent functional outcome of this operation.

Conclusion.—The combination of preoperative radiation therapy, APR, and coloanal anastomosis produced good local control of the cancer and 4-year survival rates. These rates appear similar to those obtained for the APR alone.

▶ Patients who have invasive rectal cancer that is too low for anterior resection generally undergo APR with a permanent colostomy. These authors look at preoperative radiation therapy with subsequent performance of an APR and coloanal anastomosis. The local failure and survival rates were similar to those of standard APR, although one of the patients had excellent bowel sphincter function. Several caveats need emphasizing. First, preoperative radiation successfully downstaged patients; however, nearly half had positive pelvic nodes at the time of surgery. These results are directly related to the skill of the surgical team as well as to their skill in the selection of patients, which will have an important impact on local failure and overall survival.—T.J. Eberlein, M.D.

Patterns of Recurrence Following High-Dose Preoperative Radiation and Sphincter-Preserving Surgery for Cancer of the Rectum

Mohiuddin M, Marks G (Thomas Jefferson Univ Hosp, Philadelphia)
Dis Colon Rectum 36:117–126, 1993   140-94-11-29

Background.—One alternative to abdominoperineal resection and permanent colostomy in patients with distal and unfavorable rectal cancers is high-dose preoperative radiation with new sphincter-preserving surgical options. Patterns of recurrence seen after this alternative form of management were analyzed.

Methods.—One hundred sixty-one patients with rectal cancer were enrolled in a program of high-dose preoperative radiation and radical sphincter-preserving surgery from 1976 to 1989. All had unfavorable tumors located at a low level in the rectum. A minimum dose of 4,000 to 4,500 cGy was delivered over 4½ weeks in fractions of 180 to 250 cGy. Patients with tumor fixation received an additional 1,000 to 1,500 cGy, for a total of 5,500 to 6,000 cGy. A coned-down field was used. Surgery was done 4–8 weeks after irradiation. One hundred forty-seven patients had radical curative surgery with sphincter preservation. Combined abdominotransacral resection was done in 63 patients, transanal-abdominal-transanal resection in 53, and anterior resection in 31. The median follow-up was 5 years.

Patterns of Recurrence by Level in the Rectum

Level	Local	Local + Distant	Distant
0–3 cm (n = 58)	2 (3%)	6 (10%)	6 (10%)
4–6 cm (n = 52)	5 (10%)	4 (8%)	10 (19%)
≥7 cm (n = 37)	1 (3%)	0	9 (24%)
Total	8 (6%)	10 (7%)	25 (17%)

B. Patterns of Recurrences by Mobility

Clinical Stage	Local	Local + Distant	Distant
Mobile (n = 75)	1 (1%)	5 (7%)	8 (11%)
Fixed (n = 72)	7 (10%)	5 (7%)	17 (24%)
Total	8 (6%)	10 (7%)	25 (17%)

(Courtesy of Mohiuddin M, Marks G: *Dis Colon Rectum* 36:117–126, 1993.)

Outcomes.—No perioperative deaths occurred. Three patients had anastomotic failure; 2 were reconstituted. In another 10 patients, late diversion was needed, mainly for recurrent disease. One hundred thirty-four of the 147 patients (91%) had long-term normal sphincter function. Eighteen patients had pelvic-perineal recurrence; 12 of the 18 had fixed tumors below the 6-cm level of the distal rectum. The median time to local recurrence was 24 months. Thirty-five patients had distant metastasis with or without local recurrence; 22 of the 35 had fixed tumors below the 6-cm level of the rectum. Patterns of failure by tumor level and mobility in the rectum are shown in the table. Distant metastasis occurred at a median of 17 months. Forty-three patients have died, 32 of their disease. The overall 5-year actuarial survival was 79%, with a disease-free survival of 73%.

Conclusion.—High-dose preoperative radiation combined with radical sphincter-preserving surgical techniques results in excellent local control and improved survival. Furthermore, the quality of life, with retention of normal anal sphincter function, is enhanced.

▶ In a study by Mohiuddin from Thomas Jefferson University, a large number of patients were treated with high-dose preoperative radiation therapy and radical sphincter-preserving surgery. More than 90% of the patients had long-term normal sphincter function, which again emphasizes the technical skill of the operator and its effect on the outcome. Overall and disease-free survival were excellent, although this was a highly selected patient population. In the opinion of these authors, sphincter preservation should not be restricted by any prescribed length of distal margin or pretreatment assessment of tumor fixation. In fact, as long as an adequate dose of radiation has been delivered, they use a margin of 5 mm distally. Again, emphasis needs to be placed on the experience of these authors regarding patient selection criteria, individualized radiation dose, and the use of special surgical techniques in obtaining their excellent results.—T.J. Eberlein, M.D.

Surgical Lateral Clearance in Resected Rectal Carcinomas: A Multivariate Analysis of Clinicopathologic Features
Ng IOL, Luk ISC, Yuen ST, Lau PWK, Pritchett CJ, Ng M, Poon GP, Ho J
(Univ of Hong Kong; Queen Mary Hosp, Hong Kong)
Cancer 71:1972–1976, 1993   140-94-11–30

Background.—In patients with rectal carcinomas, incomplete removal of tumors is the main cause of local recurrence. This often occurs at the lateral aspects devoid of peritoneum. An attempt was made to find a reliable method for detecting lateral resection margin (LRM) involvement by these tumors and to identify pathologic factors that may be important prognostically.

Methods.—Eighty resected rectal carcinoma specimens were examined prospectively. In each specimen, the whole tumor was embedded, and

Parameters Influencing Survival Rates of Patients With Resected
Rectal Carcinoma: Overall Data With Univariate Survival Analysis

Parameters	No. of patients	Median survival (days)	P value
Clearance (mm)			
≤ 1	16	431	< 0.0001
> 1	63	> 812	
Dukes staging			
A	9	> 684	0.004
B	29	> 812	
C	33	798	
D	8	393	
Cellular differentiation			
Good	7	> 805	< 0.001
Moderate	66	798	
Poor	6	329	
Tumor size (cm)			
≤ 6	63	> 812	0.005
> 6	16	463	
Depth of tumor penetration			
≤ 10	50	> 812	< 0.001
> 10	29	482	
No. of lymph nodes involved			
0	38	> 812	< 0.001
1	13	798	
≥ 2	29	> 601	
Venous permeation			
Absent	56	> 812	0.001
Present	23	482	
Lymphatic permeation			
Absent	43	> 812	0.002
Present	36	526	
Peritoneal involvement			
Absent	73	> 812	0.005
Present	6	419	

(Courtesy of Ng IOL, Luk ISC, Yuen ST, et al: *Cancer* 71:1972-1976, 1993.)

whole-mount sections of the tumor and surrounding mesorectum were assessed after serial transverse slicing. The distance between the LRM and outermost part of the tumor was measured.

Findings.—Eight percent of the specimens showed LRM involvement in the single slice macroscopically seen to have the deepest tumor invasion. Twenty percent of the specimens were found to have LRM involvement after all slices were examined microscopically. Surgical clearance was strongly inversely related to Duke's staging and depth of tumor invasion. Local recurrence rates were 28% overall and 53% in patients with LRM involvement. Survival rates were associated with macroscopic and microscopic features of the specimens. Three of the 9 pathologic characteristics identified—surgical clearance, cellular differentiation, and number of involved pericolic lymph nodes—were found to be favorable independent prognostic variables (table).

Conclusion.—Local recurrence is closely associated with LRM involvement. The only reliable and satisfactory way to evaluate LRM is by embedding and examining the entire tumor and mesorectum. Detailed pathologic assessment of the resected tumor is important when determining prognosis.

▶ This paper represents clinical pathologic analysis of the LRM in rectal cancers. These authors make an excellent point that the LRM is important in minimizing local recurrence and that only the detailed and systematic pathologic study of the resection specimen will adequately assess the LRM. This would also be important in assessing prognoses.—T.J. Eberlein, M.D.

GASTRIC CANCER

▶↓ Two major directions are emphasized in the selection of papers for this section. The first is the extent of lymph node dissection (Abstract 140-94-11–31), which has been popularized in the specific studies by J.P. Kim and others; the second (Abstracts 140-94-11–32 and 140-94-11–33) deals with the basic biology of prognostic factors, as well as the methodology for selecting patients for adjuvant therapy.—T.J. Eberlein, M.D.

Extensive Versus Limited Lymph Node Dissection for Gastric Cancer: A Comparative Study of 320 Patients
Pacelli F, Doglietto GB, Bellantone R, Alfieri S, Sgadari A, Crucitti F (Università Cattolica del Sacro Cuore, Rome)
Br J Surg 80:1153–1156, 1993   140-94-11–31

Introduction.—The value of extensive regional lymph node dissection in the treatment of gastric adenocarcinoma remains controversial. More radical types of gastrectomy are commonly performed in Japan but have not been widely used in the West because of 25-year-old research that reported unfavorable results. The results of extended lymphadenectomy were compared with those of limited lymph node dissection in 320 patients with adenocarcinoma of the stomach.

Patients and Methods.—The patients underwent resection from 1981 to 1990. Two surgical teams at 1 institution adopted different policies, with one routinely performing extended lymph node dissection and the other a limited procedure. In the extensive group, 157 patients under-

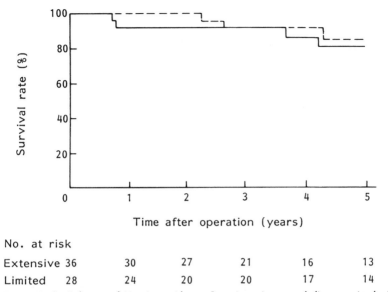

Fig 11–17.—Survival curves of 64 patients with stage I gastric carcinoma, excluding operative deaths. *Broken line,* extensive lymph node dissection; *solid line,* limited lymph node dissection. P = .60 (Mantel-Cox test) (Courtesy of Pacelli F, Doglietto GB, Bellantone R, et al: *Br J Surg* 80:1153-1156, 1993.)

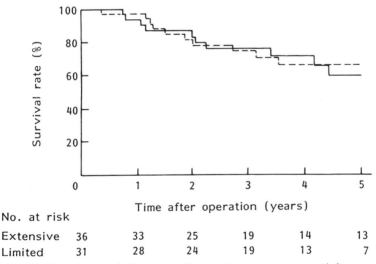

Fig 11–18.—Survival curves of 67 patients with stage II gastric carcinoma, excluding operative deaths. *Broken line,* extensive lymph node dissection; *solid line,* limited lymph node dissection. P = .82 (Mantel-Cox test) (Courtesy of Pacelli F, Doglietto GB, Bellantone R, et al: *Br J Surg* 80:1153-1156, 1993.)

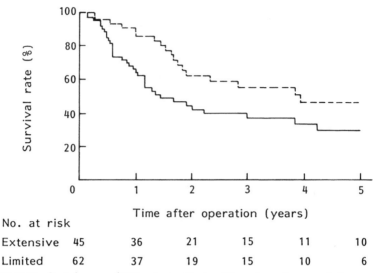

No. at risk					
Extensive	45	36	21	15	11	10
Limited	62	37	19	15	10	6

Fig 11–19.—Survival curves of 107 patients with stage III gastric carcinoma, excluding operative deaths. *Broken line*, extensive lymph node dissection; *solid line*, limited lymph node dissection. P = .02 (Mantel-Cox test) (Courtesy of Pacelli F, Doglietto GB, Bellantone R, et al: *Br J Surg* 80:1153–1156, 1993.)

went total gastrectomy with R_3 lymphadenectomy and 63 underwent distal subtotal gastrectomy and R_2 lymphadenectomy extended to the hepatic pedicle and retropancreatic nodes. The 163 patients in the limited group underwent R_1 gastrectomy. The data recorded included length of operation, intraoperative blood loss, postoperative morbidity, hospital mortality, and 5-year survival after curative resection.

Results.—The 2 groups were similar in age and sex distribution and pathologic features. The mean number of lymph nodes dissected per operative specimen was 37 in the extensive group and 12.4 in the limited group. Nodal involvement was found in 59.2% of the extensive dissection group and in 64.4% of the limited dissection group. In the extensive group, 35.7% had positive N1 nodes, 11.5% had N2 involvement, and 12.1% had N3 involvement. The limited group had only N1 (44.8%) and N2 (19.6%) involvement. Patients undergoing extensive lymphadenectomy had a longer mean operating time and greater intraoperative blood transfusion requirements than patients who had the limited procedure, but the incidence of postoperative complications and the rate of hospital mortality were similar in the 2 groups. The 5-year survival after curative resection was 65.4% in the extensive group and 50.1% in the limited group. The survival advantage for extensive dissection was observed for patients with stage I disease (Fig 11–17), stage II disease (Fig 11–18), and stage III disease (Fig 11–19).

Conclusion.—Lower rates of postoperative morbidity and mortality and a similar rate of survival have been reported for limited vs. extensive nodal dissection in the treatment of gastric carcinoma. The immediate results, however, support the value of the extensive procedure. Multivariate analysis identified the extent of lymphadenectomy as an independent prognostic factor for survival.

▶ This paper examines the value of extensive regional lymph node dissection. These authors conclude that lymph node involvement and radical lymphadenectomy are independent prognostic factors for survival. Although the incidence of this type of tumor is diminishing in the United States, locoregional resection seems to offer the best chance of survival.—T.J. Eberlein, M.D.

A Prognostic Score for Patients Resected for Gastric Cancer

Marubini E, Bonfanti G, Bozzetti F, Boracchi P, Amadori D, Folli S, Nanni O, Gennari L (Istituto Nazionale dei Tumori, Milano, Italy; Ospedale GB Morgagni—L Pierantony di Forli', Italy; Istituto Oncologico Romagnolo, Forli', Italy)
Eur J Cancer 29A:845–850, 1993   140-94-11-32

Partial Scores for Categories of Prognostic Factors and
Classification of Patients in 3 Risk Groups

Variables	Partial score	Variables	Partial score
Age (years)		Tumor site	
≤ 60	0	Lower third	0
> 60	1	Other	1
		Upper third	4.5
Wall invasion			
pT1	0	Nodal status	
pT2	2.5	N −	0
pT3–4	3.5	N +	3

Risk groups	Total score
I: 5 year survival probability ≥ 70%	≤ 3.5
II: 5 year survival probability 30%–69%	3.6–7
III: 5 year survival probability < 30%	> 7

Note: Total score = age score + wall invasion score + tumor site score + nodal status score.
(Courtesy of Marubini E, Bonfanti G, Bozzetti F, et al: *Eur J Cancer* 29A:845–850, 1993.)

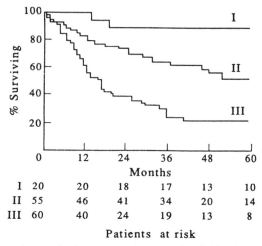

I 20 20 18 17 13 10
II 55 46 41 34 20 14
III 60 40 24 19 13 8

Patients at risk

Fig 11–20.—Survival curves for the 3 groups of patients identified by the prognostic score in the table for 1 series of patients (Kaplan-Meier estimates). (Courtesy of Marubini E, Bonfanti G, Bozzetti F, et al: *Eur J Cancer* 29A:845–850, 1993.)

Background.—In patients with gastric cancer, a knowledge of prognostic factors is very important in clinical practice. The construction, validation, and use of a simple prognostic score that can be used to predict survival among patients undergoing curative gastric resection were described.

Methods.—Two hundred thirteen patients were recruited in a multicenter trial. The prognostic significance of age, sex, tumor site, disease stage, surgical treatment, and histologic type was assessed. Death from all causes was used as outcome. A Weibull multiple regression model was adopted for assessing the combined effect of these factors on survival. A backward selection procedure was applied to the full model to produce a parsimonious model.

Findings.—Based on the final model, the prognostic score included age, wall invasion, tumor site, and nodal status (table). Three patient groups with different 5-year survival probabilities were identified (Fig 11-20). The reliability of the score in predicting survival was confirmed in an independent institution.

Conclusion.—Assessing prognosis in individual patients apparently cured of a cancer has always been challenging. This simple scoring system can be used to classify patients undergoing radical surgery for gastric cancer into different, well-discriminated prognostic groups.

▶ This study by the National Cancer Institute in Milan formed a prognostic score for patients with radical resection for gastric cancer. Although their prognostic score is, in fact, reproducible, it emphasizes the basic tumor biology associated with gastric cancer. Age, depth of wall invasion, tumor site in the upper or lower third, and the presence of positive lymph nodes made up the total score. Other than age, tumor spread again predicted survival. Emphasis is placed on the importance of adequate locoregional therapy for gastric cancer.—T.J. Eberlein, M.D.

Prognostic Factors in Gastric Carcinoma: Results of the German Gastric Carcinoma Study 1992
Roder JD, Böttcher K, Siewert JR, Busch R, Hermanek P, Meyer H-J, and the German Gastric Carcinoma Study Group (Technische Universität München, Germany; Universität Erlangen, Germany; Medizinische Hochschule Hannover, Germany)
Cancer 72:2089–2097, 1993   140-94-11–33

Introduction.—The prognosis of patients with gastric carcinoma is determined by tumor- and patient-associated factors, some of which can be influenced by therapy. In a prospective, multicenter study, the prognostic factors and postoperative course were studied in patients who underwent resection for gastric carcinoma between 1986 and 1989.

Study Design.—The resection technique, extent of lymph node dissection, and histopathologic assessment of specimens were standardized at all 19 participating medical centers in Germany and Austria. The study included 1,654 patients, with a median follow-up of 48 months. Multivariate analysis was used to evaluate prognostic factors.

Results.—In the total patient population, there was an independent prognostic effect of nodal status, an International Union Against Cancer (UICC)-R0 resection, distant metastases, the pT category, 3 or more risk factors at preoperative analysis, and postoperative complications. In the subgroup of patients who had a UICC-R0 resection, the nodal status was the major independent prognostic factor.

Conclusion.—It appears that the prognosis of patients undergoing gastrectomy for carcinoma can be improved by a complete resection of the primary tumor and its lymphatic drainage, a UICC-R0 resection. A detailed preoperative risk analysis and meticulous attention to surgical detail to avoid postoperative complications may also improve the prognosis for these patients.

▶ Similar results were identified by the German Gastric Carcinoma Study Group in their study of 1,654 patients. This large cooperative group confirms that nodal status, depth of tumor invasion, extent of lymph node dissection, and the presence of residual tumor were independent prognostic factors in patients with gastric carcinoma. They also found, however, that the presence of postoperative complications served as an independent prognostic factor. Although surgery does not obviously have any impact on nodal status or depth of invasion, complete resection of the primary tumor and all of its lymphatic drainage will improve survival.—T.J. Eberlein, M.D.

p53 Mutation in Gastric Cancer: A Genetic Model for Carcinogenesis is Common to Gastric and Colorectal Cancer

Uchino S, Noguchi M, Ochiai A, Saito T, Kobayashi M, Hirohashi S (Natl Cancer Ctr Research Inst, Tokyo; Oita Med Univ, Japan)

Int J Cancer 54:759–764, 1993   140-94-11–34

Background.—The human *p53* gene on chromosome 17p13 is a tumor-suppressor gene whose inactivation may be a factor in carcinogenesis in various organs. Because most early gastric cancers are surgically curable, greater knowledge of differences in genetic status between early and advanced cancers, or between slow and rapidly growing tumors, would help in making treatment decisions.

Objective and Methods.—Mutations of *p53* in exons 5 through 8 were examined by polymerase chain reaction/single strand conformation polymorphism analysis and direct sequencing in 118 cases of gastric cancer. Fifty-nine early cancers, with invasion limited at the laminaris submucosa, were compared with 59 advanced tumors.

Findings.—Mutations were detected in 37% of 41 early gastric cancers of the cohesive type and in 42% of 59 advanced cancers of this type (Table 1), which is not a significant difference. No mutations were detected in 18 early cancers of the noncohesive type. The frequency of *p53* mutations in cohesive-type cancers could not be related to the macroscopic classification, node involvement, or the depth of tumor invasion (Table 2). A majority of the mutations in advanced cancers were accompanied by allele loss at the *p32* gene locus. The spectrum of mutations was similar to that observed in colorectal cancer.

Conclusion.—That *p53* mutations occur at the intramucosal stage in cohesive-type gastric cancers and that the range of mutations resembles that of colorectal cancer suggest that these mutations may be critical at a relatively early stage of gastric carcinogenesis.

TABLE 1.—Histopathologic Classification and *p53* Mutation in Primary Gastric Cancer

Histopathological classification*	Mutation in early gastric cancer		Mutation in advanced gastric cancer	
Papillary adenocarcinoma	1/2 (50%)		1/3 (33%)	
Well-differentiated tubular adenocarcinoma	8/24 (33%)	15/41	8/15 (53%)	25/59
Moderately differentiated tubular adenocarcinoma	5/13 (42%)	(37%)	10/20 (50%)	(42%)
Poorly differentiated adenocarcinoma with solid nests or focal tubular structures	1/2 (50%)		6/21 (29%)	
growing in a scattered manner	0/2 (0%)			
Signet-ring-cell carcinoma	0/15 (0%)	0/18		
Mucinous adenocarcinoma	0/1 (0%)			
Total	15/59 (25%)		25/59 (42%)	

* According to the classification of the General Rules for Gastric Cancer Study of the Japanese Research Society for Gastric Cancer.

(Courtesy of Uchino S, Noguchi M, Ochiai A, et al: *Int J Cancer* 54:759-764, 1993.)

TABLE 2.—Histopathologic Parameters and *p53* Mutation in Gastric
Cancer of the Cohesive Type

Histopathological parameters	*p53* mutation (%)
Macroscopic classification	
Early gastric cancer	
protruded type	2/10 (20)
depressed type	7/19 (37)
protruded and depressed type	6/12 (50)
Advanced gastric cancer	
Borrmann I	2/6 (33)
Borrmann II	15/31 (48)
Borrmann III	5/16 (31)
Borrmann IV	3/6 (50)
Lymph-node metastasis	
Early gastric cancer	
presence	4/7 (57)
absence	11/34 (31)
Advanced gastric cancer	
presence	17/40 (43)
absence	8/19 (42)
Depth of tumour invasion	
intramucosa	4/17 (24)
submucosa	11/24 (46)
muscularis propria or subserosa	15/32 (47)
beyond serosa	10/27 (37)

(Courtesy of Uchino S, Noguchi M, Ochiai A, et al: *Int J Cancer* 54:759–764, 1993.)

▶ This article by Uchino from Japan shows a correlation between *p53* mutation in early gastric cancers of cohesive type, as well as advanced cancers.
No mutations were seen in early cancers of the noncohesive type. This suggests that these mutations may be critical during the early stages of gastric
carcinogenesis. First, these authors classify gastric cancers into cohesive and
noncohesive subtypes, which roughly correspond to differentiated and undifferentiated histologic types. They emphasize, however, the differences in ge-
netical alterations of oncogenes or tumor-suppressor genes corresponding
well to these histopathologic classifications. Thus, gastric carcinomas of
these 2 types are considered to arise through different genetic pathways and
show differences in pathologic activity, e.g., tumor cell proliferation or tumor
invasion. Identification of these genetic changes would, therefore, help in the
selection of patients for adjuvant treatment.

A similar relationship exists with *C-erb-B2* protein expression. A study has
shown similar findings using this different oncogene. *C-erb-B2* expression
was associated with virtually all of the poor prognostic features, e.g., lymph
node involvement, tendency for deep invasion, and aggressive growth pattern. Identification studies are currently under way to identify the peptide
product of *HER2/neu,* which may be capable of sensitizing the immune sys-

tem to react against it, or to perform the foundation of a vaccine-based trial. Thus, identification of these genetic markers has short-term benefit in defining prognosis, but with further research it may have longer range therapeutic potential.—T.J. Eberlein, M.D.

Hepatocellular Carcinoma

INTRODUCTION

Hepatocellular carcinoma is a rare tumor in the United States, and much of the world literature comes from the countries of the Pacific Ocean. These 2 articles are no exception. Hepatic resection is still the most effective treatment for hepatocellular carcinoma. Liver transplantation remains an effective treatment for incidental small hepatocellular carcinomas associated with advanced cirrhosis or for nonresectable fibrolamellar carcinoma. Until more improved chemotherapies become available, a combination of judicious resection, postoperative chemotherapy, and liver transplantation will be the primary treatments for hepatocellular carcinoma.

Timothy J. Eberlein, M.D.

Rationale of Surgical Management for Recurrent Hepatocellular Carcinoma
Matsuda Y, Ito T, Oguchi Y, Nakajima K, Izukura T (Otemae Hosp, Osaka, Japan)
Ann Surg 217:28–34, 1993   140-94-11–35

Introduction.—Surgery for recurrent hepatocellular carcinoma (HCC) usually is more difficult than that for primary HCC because of technical problems and reduced hepatic functional reserve. Nevertheless, conservative measures are usually ineffective against recurrent cancers. The role of repeat surgery, including hepatectomy, was examined in a series of 100 patients undergoing surgery for primary HCC from 1979 to 1991.

Patients and Methods.—Ninety-one surviving patients were followed for a mean of 32 months. Recurrent HCC developed in 36 patients 2 to 81 months after initial hepatectomy; the mean interval was 23 months. Twenty-two patients underwent repeat surgery, and 16 of them underwent hepatic resection. These 19 men and 3 women had a mean age of 63 years at the time of the second operation. Most patients had had partial liver resection initially. Twelve had partial resection at repeat surgery, 3 had segmentectomies, and 1 had lobectomy. The second hepatectomy was done with curative intent in 13 cases and palliatively in 3. Four patients had a third hepatectomy.

Results.—The mean disease-free interval was 793 days for the 22 patients having a second operation and 514 days for 14 patients not having a second operation. One patient each had liver failure and bacterial peritonitis postoperatively. Patients with recurrent disease who underwent a second operation had significantly higher survival rates than those who did not. Fifteen patients remain alive up to 92 months after initial resection, 8 of them without disease.

Discussion.—Early detection is the key to curatively resecting hepatic cancers. Aggressive surgical management of recurrent HCC will enhance the overall prognosis.

▶ Matsuda reports on a highly selected series of patients with recurrent HCC who underwent hepatic resection. In most series, the tumors of more than 50% of the patients are deemed inoperable. In this series, recurrence developed in 36 patients, 22 patients underwent exploration, and 16 patients underwent resection. As might be predicted, the patients who had recurrent disease and who underwent a second operation had a higher survival rate. This most likely is the result of a combination of early detection and patient selection for aggressive treatment because of the biological behavior of the tumor at the time the recurrence was detected.—T.J. Eberlein, M.D.

Experience With Liver Resection After Hepatic Arterial Chemoembolization for Hepatocellular Carcinoma

Yu Y-Q, Xu D-B, Zhou X-D, Lu J-Z, Tang Z-Y, Mack P (Shanghai Med Univ, China; Singapore Gen Hosp, Republic of Singapore)
Cancer 71:62–65, 1993   140-94-11–36

Introduction.—Percutaneous transcatheter hepatic arterial chemotherapy and embolization (THACE) is increasingly used to treat primary liver cancer. Patients with moderate and advanced disease have improved overall survival, and some initially unresectable tumors have become resectable.

Patients and Methods.—Thirty patients with liver cancers greater than 5 cm in diameter underwent resection after preliminary treatment with THACE. The tumors were either too bulky to be resected or were at the hepatic hilus. The mean patient age was 49 years. A majority of the patients had tumors in the right lobe of the liver. The mean tumor diameter was 8.1 cm. Cirrhotic change was variable.

The femoral artery was catheterized percutaneously for administration of cisplatin, mitomycin C, and 5-fluorouracil. In addition, ethiodized oil or an absorbable gelatin sponge was used to embolize all tumor vessels. Chemoembolization was repeated at 4- to 6-week intervals up to 5 times, the mean number of sessions being 3. Partial or segmental liver resection ensued, except for 2 patients who underwent left trisegmentectomy.

Results.—All patients were symptomatic and had varying degrees of hepatic dysfunction after THACE. Seven patients regained normal α-fetoprotein levels. The tumor diameter decreased by 32% on average after treatment. All the patients had hepatocellular carcinoma. With 5 exceptions, tumor cells were still identifiable beneath the intact liver capsule. One patient died of acute pulmonary embolism after treatment for a tumor embolus in the portal vein. Five patients died of recurrent cancer. Survival rates were 89% at 1 year and 77% at both 2 and 3 years.

Conclusion.—Resection is the primary treatment for relatively small and resectable liver cancers. A promising approach to large, advanced liver cancers that formerly would have been considered unresectable is THACE followed by resection.

▶ Yu reports alternatives to primary resection using THACE. A combination of cisplatin, mitomycin C, and 5-fluorouracil was administered. This type of treatment may be used as primary therapy in the palliation of unresectable hepatocellular carcinoma; however, because a majority of patients will have shrinkage of tumor (almost 25% of this series had normalization of their α-fetoprotein levels), patients treated with arterial chemotherapy and embolization may then become resectable. If resection is performed, postoperative chemotherapy may be considered, depending on the surgical margins.—T.J. Eberlein, M.D.

PANCREATIC CARCINOMA

▶↓ Pancreatic carcinoma remains one of the most difficult types of tumors to treat. Early diagnosis and efficient surgery with low morbidity have been the mainstay of treatment strategy. New directions, such as the identification of biological markers and mechanisms for this deadly disease that might suggest alternative treatment are in progress.—T.J. Eberlein, M.D.

Intraoperative Fine Needle Aspiration of Pancreatic and Extrahepatic Biliary Masses
Earnhardt RC, McQuone SJ, Minasi JS, Feldman PS, Jones RS, Hanks JB (Univ of Virginia, Charlottesville)
Surg Gynecol Obstet 177:147–152, 1993   140-94-11–37

Background.—Intraoperative fine-needle aspiration (IFNA) provides a means of rapid tissue diagnosis in patients with masses of the pancreas and the extrahepatic biliary system, with many fewer complications than occur with wedge or large-bore needle biopsies.

Series.—Ninety-nine IFNA procedures were carried out from 1981 to 1991: 75 on the pancreas, 17 on the extrahepatic biliary system, and 7 on the ampulla. All aspirations were done after directly visualizing or palpating the tumor, making several passes with a 22-gauge needle.

Results.—Diagnostic readings were made in 90 cases. Thirty-four of 43 patients with confirmed pancreatic carcinoma had positive cytologic findings. Three cases were considered "suspicious," and 6 specimens were unsatisfactory (table). All but 1 of 18 confirmed cancers of the am-

Confirmed Intraoperative Fine-Needle Aspirations with Positive or Negative Readings

	Sensitivity		Specificity		Accuracy		Positive Predictive value		Negative Predictive value	
	No.	Percent	No.	Percent	No.	Percent	No.	Percent	No.	Percent
Pancreas	34/39	87	14/14	100	48/53	91	34/34	100	14/19	74
Extrahepatic	12/13	92	1/1	100	13/14	93	12/12	100	1/2	50
Ampulla	5/5	100	2/2	100	7/7	100	5/5	100	2/2	100
Total	51/57	90	17/17	100	68/74	92	51/51	100	17/23	74

Note: *Sensitivity*, true positives/(true positives + false negatives); *Specificity*, true negatives/(true negatives + false positives); *Accuracy*, (true positives + true negatives)/(true positives + true negatives + false positives + false negatives); *Positive Predictive Value*, true positives/(true positives + false positives); and *Negative Predictive Value*, true negatives/(true negatives + false negatives).

(Courtesy of Earnhardt RC, McQuone SJ, Minasi JS, et al: *Surg Gynecol Obstet* 177:147–152, 1993.)

pulla or extrahepatic biliary tract were detected by IFNA. The sensitivity of diagnostic IFNA procedures was 90% and their specificity was 100%, for an overall accuracy of 92%. The procedure had a positive predictive value of 100% and a negative predictive value of 74%.

Conclusion.—In evaluating masses of the pancreas, extrahepatic biliary tract, and ampulla, IFNA is accurate. Positive findings are a reliable guide to deciding on surgery, but a negative result does not definitively exclude carcinoma.

▶ In this study examining IFNA, sensitivity was 90% and specificity was 100%. The negative predictive value was only 74%. These data rely on a competent cytologist who is skilled in examining specimens from the pancreas and extrahepatic biliary tract. There seems to be no doubt that this type of procedure can be done with less morbidity than either wedge or large-bore needle biopsies.—T.J. Eberlein, M.D.

One Hundred and Forty-Five Consecutive Pancreaticoduodenectomies Without Mortality
Cameron JL, Pitt HA, Yeo CJ, Lillemoe KD, Kaufman HS, Coleman J (Johns Hopkins Med Insts, Baltimore, Md)
Ann Surg 217:430–438, 1993   140-94-11–38

Background.—In the past, pancreaticoduodenectomy carried high hospital morbidity and mortality, and in the 1970s some suggested that

TABLE 1.—Indications for
Pancreaticoduodenectomy

Disease	Patients
Adenocarcinoma	
Pancreas	53
Ampulla	18
Distal bile duct	13
Duodenum	8
Cystic neoplasm	11
Islet cell tumor	4
Metastatic tumor	3
Villous adenoma	2
Chronic pancreatitis	22
Trauma	1
Miscellaneous	10
	145

(Courtesy of Cameron JL, Pitt HA, Yeo CJ, et al: *Ann Surg* 217:430–438, 1993.)

TABLE 2.—Complications of Pancreaticoduodenectomy
in 145 Patients

Postoperative Complications	Patients	%
Delayed gastric emptying	52	36
Pancreatic fistula	28	19
Intraabdominal abscess	13	9
Wound infection	11	8
Pancreatitis	9	6
Bile leak	8	6
Cholangitis	7	5
Pneumonia	1	1
Small bowel obstruction	1	1
Dehiscence	1	1
None	70	48

(Courtesy of Cameron JL, Pitt HA, Yeo CJ, et al: *Ann Surg* 217:430–438, 1993.)

the procedure should be abandoned. In recent years, however, there have been marked reductions in both morbidity and mortality with this operation.

Series.—The outcome of pancreaticoduodenectomy was examined in 145 consecutive patients with a mean age of 59 years who underwent surgery between August 1988 and April 1991. Thirty-seven patients were aged 70 years or older, and 4 were older than age 80. The most common indication was pancreatic adenocarcinoma (Table 1).

Surgery.—The mean operating time exceeded 7 hours, and blood loss averaged 970 mL. Patients received a mean of 1.4 units of blood replacement. Only 9 patients had total pancreatectomy. The pylorus was preserved in 117 cases. Eight patients underwent partial resection of the portal or superior mesenteric vein with reanastomosis. The mean postoperative hospital stay was 19 days.

Outcome.—Fifty-two percent of the patients had postoperative complications, most frequently delayed gastric emptying or formation of a pancreatic fistula (Table 2). None were life-threatening. Two patients required reoperation during the initial hospitalization. No patient died within a month of surgery. The incidence of complications in the younger and older age groups was not significantly different.

Conclusion.—Given proper patient selection, pancreaticoduodenectomy may be done in patients of any age, with benign or malignant disease and with minimal risk of hospital mortality.

▶ Cameron reports on 145 consecutive pancreaticoduodenectomies. More than 20% of the patients studied were older than age 70 years. This series underscores the importance of surgery as a primary treatment of pancreatic cancer. In this highly selected series, patients younger than 70 had the same morbidity as those over 70. The authors attribute their superb results to better anesthesia, improved intensive care units, and improvements in critical care surgery; however, perhaps the specialization within surgery was most important. This resulted in a shortening of the operative time, decreased operative blood loss, and more familiarity with the anatomy and management of intraoperative and postoperative complications. Until other treatment strategies, such as neoadjuvant therapy and better chemotherapies, are developed, surgery will remain the standard treatment of pancreatic cancer. This emphasizes the importance of centers like Johns Hopkins, where they are performed exceedingly well.—T.J. Eberlein, M.D.

Overexpression of HER2/*neu* Oncogene in Human Pancreatic Carcinoma

Yamanaka Y, Friess H, Kobrin MS, Büchler M, Kunz J, Beger HG, Korc M
(Univ of California, Irvine; Univ of Ulm, Germany; Nippon Med School, Tokyo)
Hum Pathol 24:1127–1134, 1993   140-94-11-39

Background.—Pancreatic carcinoma is an aggressive neoplasm with a generally poor prognosis. The growth advantage of pancreatic cancer cells appears to be related to various molecular alterations. Previous research has reported overexpression of the epidermal growth factor receptor, a high frequency of Ki-*ras* oncogene mutations, and mutations of the *p53* tumor suppressor gene in human pancreatic carcinomas. The HER2/*neu* expression in the normal and cancerous pancreas was examined.

Methods.—Pancreatic cancer tissue samples were obtained from 76 patients with surgically resectable disease. Twelve organ donors provided normal pancreatic tissues. The tumor samples were classified according to the tumor-node-metastasis (TNM) classification. Tissue samples were fixed and paraffin embedded for histologic analysis; those designated for DNA and RNA extraction were frozen in liquid nitrogen immediately on surgical removal.

Results.—In samples from normal pancreas, HER2/*neu* immunostaining was observed on the surface and/or in the cytoplasm of some acinar and ductal cells. In 34 of 76 pancreatic carcinomas, HER2/*neu* immunoreactivity was expressed. A significant correlation existed between tumors with well-differentiated histology and HER2/*neu* expression. In the normal pancreas, HER2/*neu* messenger RNA (mRNA) expression was demonstrated both in acinar and ductal cells. The levels of HER2/*neu* mRNA expression were elevated in 52% of tumors in comparison with the normal tissues. These tumors demonstrated a strong but heterogeneous distribution of mRNA grains by in situ hybridization; Southern blot analysis revealed no HER2/*neu* gene amplification. Postoperative survival, examined in 53 patients, did not differ significantly between HER2/*neu* oncoprotein-positive and oncoprotein-negative groups.

Conclusion.—The HER2/*neu* protein was found to be synthesized in the normal exocrine pancreas and was often overexpressed in well-differentiated adenocarcinomas of the pancreas, a result of increased HER2/*neu* mRNA levels. This factor, together with previously observed molecular alterations, may account for rapid tumor progression in human pancreatic carcinoma.

▶ This report details the overexpression seen in association with well-differentiated adenocarcinoma of the pancreas. Because the HER2/*neu* protein is found to be synthesized by the normal exocrine pancreas, its overexpression in cancer may explain one mechanism for the proliferation of this tumor. The HER2/*neu* oncogene is not the only oncogene expressed in human pancreatic tumors; EGF receptor, transferrin growth factor-α, Ki-*ras*, and *p53* mutations also occur. That the EGF receptor is also overexpressed may help to explain the autonomous growth behavior of human pancreatic cancer cells. Because EGF and EGF receptor, as well as HER2/*neu*, are increased, therapeutic modalities that interrupt only one of these activated pathways may be insufficient to arrest tumor growth.—T.J. Eberlein, M.D.

MELANOMA: NEW MODALITIES OF THERAPY

▶↓ This section is divided into 2 broad categories. The first deals with the clinical aspects of melanoma treatment. There were several significant manuscripts published during this past year. Melanoma, however, has also been an excellent model for the study of basic immunobiology. Thus, the second half of this section deals specifically with the basic mechanisms of tumor identification and enhancement of immune response to melanoma. A more thorough understanding of the immune system and tumor interaction, using melanoma as a model, will not only aid in the therapy of metastatic disease but will also form a basis which could potentially apply to other human malignancies as well.—T.J. Eberlein, M.D.

Efficacy of 2-cm Surgical Margins for Intermediate-Thickness Melanomas (1 to 4 mm): Results of a Multi-Institutional Randomized Surgical Trial
Balch CM, Urist MM, Karakousis CP, Smith TJ, Temple WJ, Drzewiecki K, Jewell WR, Bartolucci AA, Mihm MC Jr, Barnhill R, Wanebo HJ (M D Anderson Cancer Ctr, Houston; Univ of Alabama, Birmingham; Roswell Park Cancer Inst, Buffalo, NY; et al)
Ann Surg 218:262–269, 1993   140-94-11-40

Background.—The incidence of melanoma is increasing at an alarming rate. The surgical management of this disease is, therefore, becoming more important. In a prospective, multi-institutional, randomized study, it was determined whether the excision margins for intermediate-thickness melanomas can be safely reduced from the standard 4-cm radius.

Methods.—Four hundred eighty-six patients with localized melanoma, with thicknesses of 1 to 4 mm, were enrolled in the study. The melanomas were located on the trunk or proximal extremities. By random assignment, the patients received either a 2- or 4-cm surgical margin. The median follow-up was 6 years.

Findings.—The local recurrence rates for the 2- and 4-cm-margin groups were .8% and 1.7%, respectively. The respective rates of in-transit metastases were 2.1% and 2.5%. Five of the six patients with local recurrences have died. The recurrence rates were uncorrelated with surgical margins, even among patients stratified for melanoma thickness. The overall 5-year survival rate was 79.5% for patients receiving 2-cm margins and 83.7% for those receiving 4-cm margins. The need for skin grafting was decreased with 2-cm margins from 46% to 11%. Mean hospital stays were 7 days for patients in the 4-cm-margin group and 5.2 days for those in the 2-cm-margin group, a reduction mainly caused by the decreased need for skin grafting.

Conclusion.—Excision margins can be safely reduced from 4 to 2 cm for patients with melanomas of intermediate thickness. The narrower margins significantly decreased the need for skin grafting and shortened the length of hospitalization.

▶ In this large intergroup study, patients with truncal or proximal extremity melanoma were randomized to receive either 2- or 4-cm surgical margins. There was no significant difference in the overall 5-year survival rate. Thus, it appears that more is not necessarily better. The other half of the same intergroup study is the randomization to prophylactic lymphadenectomy. The analysis of this portion of the study is still ongoing, but it should be published soon.—T.J. Eberlein, M.D.

Elective and Therapeutic Regional Lymph Node Dissection for Cutaneous Malignant Melanoma: Experience of the British Columbia Cancer Agency, 1972 to 1981
Carmichael VE, Robins RE, Wilson KS (Univ of Victoria, BC, Canada; Univ of British Columbia, Vancouver, Canada)
Can J Surg 35:600–604, 1992   140-94-11–41

Background.—The value of surgery in patients with clinically malignant or equivocal regional lymph nodes at the time of diagnosis of primary malignant melanoma or later at recurrence is established. However, there is controversy regarding the benefit of removing clinically normal regional lymph nodes when the primary lesion is diagnosed.

Methods and Findings.—A 10-year review of patients undergoing lymph node dissection for malignant melanoma was performed. Pathologic findings in regional lymph nodes were associated with primary site, growth pattern, depth of invasion, and Clark's level. Two hundred

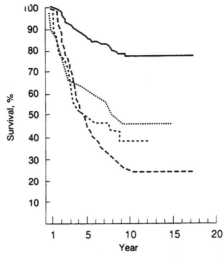

Fig 11–21.—Ten-year disease-specific survival rates in patients with negative ELND (*solid line*); positive ELND (*short dashed line*), positive TLND (*dotted line*), and RTLND (*long dashed line*). (Courtesy of Carmichael VE, Robins RE, Wilson KS: *Can J Surg* 35:600-604, 1992.)

twenty-three patients had elective lymph node dissection (ELND). In this group, the overall positivity rate was 16%. Survival rates for patients with ELND were compared with rates for patients not undergoing ELND and for patients at a different institution. Patients who had ELND had thicker and more frequently ulcerated primary tumors than patients with stage I disease not undergoing ELND. However, survival was better in the group that had ELND. When all potential prognostic variables were assessed in a multivariate analysis, ELND proved to be a nonsignificant factor in prognosis. Fifty patients underwent therapeutic lymph node dissection (TLND) at the time of primary tumor diagnosis. Lymph node involvement was found in 36 of these patients. Of 525 patients with clinical stage I disease not undergoing ELND, 119 had recurrence in the regional lymph nodes, 86 of whom had TLND for recurrence (RTLND). The median survival rate from time of primary tumor diagnosis for patients with positive nodes at ELND was 4.2 years; for those with positive nodes on TLND, it was 2.7 years; and for those having RTLND, it was 4.4 years. These differences were nonsignificant (Fig 11–21).

Conclusion.—In this series, patients with positive nodes on ELND and TLND and patients undergoing RTLND had comparable median survival rates. These rates compare favorably with those from other published series. All of the current findings underscore the need for new therapy for patients with lymph node–positive melanoma.

▶ The paper addresses regional lymph node dissection. Several important points are emphasized. Although survival was better in the group that had lymph node dissection, when other prognostic variables were assessed in multivariate analysis, ELND proved to be a nonsignificant factor in prognosis. The second major point to be emphasized is that patients who had positive nodes from ELND tended to do no better than patients who underwent TLND or those who had TLND for recurrence after ELND. Thus, only a very small number of patients who have microscopic disease confined to the lymph nodes will undergo ELND. Patients with microscopic diseases, however, or those patients who already have systemic disease would benefit little. More effective systemic treatment for melanoma remains to be developed.—T.J. Eberlein, M.D.

Multiple Primary Melanoma: Incidence and Risk Factors in 283 Patients
Slingluff CL, Vollmer RT, Seigler HF (Duke Univ Med Ctr, Durham, NC; Durham VA Med Ctr, NC)
Surgery 113:330–339, 1993   140-94-11-42

Background.—Malignant melanoma is associated with a high incidence of regional recurrence and systemic metastasis. There is also an increased risk of a second primary lesion after one primary tumor has been diagnosed. One patient series treated for malignant melanoma was reviewed.

Patients and Findings.—Two–nine primary lesions were identified in 283 of 7,816 patients with malignant melanoma (3.6%). Eighty-two percent of the 283 patients had 2 lesions, 11% had 3, and 3% had 4. Sixty-four percent of the lesions were metachronous. The 10-year actuarial risk of a second primary lesion was 5%. A third of that risk was expressed within 3 months of the initial diagnosis, plus a subsequent risk of .38% per year. A family history of melanoma, thin primary lesions, male sex, Celtic complexion, and a history of another cancer were risk factors

Multivariate Analysis of Risk of Multiple Primary Melanoma	
Variable	*p Value*
Family history	<0.001
Thickness	0.002
Sex	0.007
Celtic	0.021
Other cancers	0.035
Age	0.067*

* Difference not significant.
(Courtesy of Slingluff CL, Vollmer RT, Seigler HF: *Surgery* 113:330–339, 1993.)

for multiple primary lesions (table). Univariate and multivariate analyses showed no survival disadvantage for patients with multiple primary lesions. In both groups, 51.7% and 50.5% were disease free at 3.7 and 4.8 years, respectively. The respective mortality rates were 31% and 25%.

Conclusion.—Identifying patients at high risk for multiple primary tumors may enable earlier diagnosis and better outcomes. Treatment decisions and prognostic assessments are appropriately based on the specific risk factors of each individual lesion.

▶ This study identifies patients at high risk of having multiple primary melanoma. However, there were no survival disadvantages for patients with multiple primary lesions. The point to be emphasized is that this population represents only a small percentage of patients with the diagnosis of malignant melanoma. Therapeutic decisions need to be made based on the specific risk factors and the circumstances of each new lesion.—T.J. Eberlein, M.D.

Enhanced Expression of HLA Molecules and Stimulation of Autologous Human Tumor Infiltrating Lymphocytes Following Transduction of Melanoma Cells With τ-Interferon Genes

Ogasawara M, Rosenberg SA (Natl Cancer Inst, Bethesda, Md)
Cancer Res 53:3561–3568, 1993   140-94-11–43

Introduction.—Gene therapy for cancer is presently under clinical evaluation. The treatment involves tumor-infiltrating lymphocytes (TILs) or tumor cells modified by the insertion of genes coding for interleukin-2 or tumor necrosis factor-α.

Objective and Methods.—The feasibility of transducing human tumor cells with genes coding for γ-interferon (IFN-γ) or α-interferon (IFN-α) was investigated. Tumor cells from 12 patients with melanoma and 2 with renal cell carcinoma were transduced with retroviral vectors containing the gene for IFN-γ. The ability of HLA DR+ melanoma cells transduced with the IFN-γ gene to stimulate specific cytokine release by autologous CD4+ TILs also was examined.

Results.—Northern blot analysis revealed IFNγ transcripts only in cells transduced with the IFN-γ gene. The increase in expression of HLA class I and class II molecules after transduction was greater in tumor lines secreting IFN-γ. Two melanoma cell lines were successfully transduced with an IFN-α retroviral factor. Transduced cells secreted large amounts of IFN-α. The expression of HLA class II molecules was not increased in these transduced cells. Specific secretion of cytokine by TILs was observed when TILs and IFN-γ gene-transduced tumor cells were cultured together, but not when TILs were cultured alone.

Conclusion.—It appears that the HLA DR molecules newly expressed on IFN-γ gene-transduced tumor cells promoted antigen presentation and T-cell responses against the transduced tumor cells. Inserting the

IFN-γ gene into melanoma cells may prove useful for active immunization against melanoma and also for generating TILs for use in adoptive immunotherapy.

▶ Novel experiments by Ogasawara and Rosenberg demonstrate the effect of an IFN-γ transduction into human melanoma or renal cell carcinoma. Transduction of IFN-γ increased HLA class I and class II expression. Most importantly, melanoma cells transduced with IFN-γ genes that expressed HLA DR were able to cause a release of cytokines when cultured with autologous CD4+-positive TILs. These findings would suggest 2 possible approaches to therapy. The first alternative would be to transduce IFN-γ genes into melanoma cells to promote an active immunization against melanoma by increasing HLA expression. The second alternative would be to perform transduction in the HLA DR–positive melanoma cell to generate more effective TILs. Subsequent adoptive transfer of these TILs would be expected to render an enhanced antitumor response.—T.J. Eberlein, M.D.

Recognition of Human Melanoma Cells by HLA-A2.1-Restricted Cytotoxic T Lymphocytes Is Mediated by at Least Six Shared Peptide Epitopes
Slingluff CL, Cox AL, Henderson RA, Hunt DF, Engelhard VH (Univ of Virginia, Charlottesville)
J Immunol 150:2955–2963, 1993   140-94-11–44

Introduction.—Lymphocytes from melanoma-bearing patients, after stimulation in vitro with recombinant interleukin-2 and autologous melanoma cells, develop a melanoma-specific cytotoxic response. Most effector lymphocytes are CD8+ cytotoxic T cells restricted by class I MHC molecules. The HLA-A2 molecule is an effective restricting element for the melanoma-specific cytotoxic T-lymphocyte (CTL) response. To identify clinically relevant melanoma-specific epitopes, it is necessary to show that peptides comprising these epitopes can be extracted from melanoma cells and that they are shared by different melanoma cell lines. A study involved extracting HLA-A2.1–associated peptides from 2 melanoma cell lines and using them to reconstitute epitopes for HLA-A2.1–restricted melanoma-specific CTLs.

Methods.—The CTLs were generated from tumor-bearing lymph nodes by in vitro stimulation with autologous melanoma cells and, subsequently, allogeneic A2.1+ melanoma cells. HLA-A2.1 molecules were purified from human melanoma cell lines with immunoaffinity column chromatography. Peptides bound to these molecules were acid-eluted and fractioned, and the fractions were examined for their ability to reconstitute melanoma-specific epitopes when added to an HLA-A2.1+ antigen-processing mutant.

Results.—The CTLs generated from tumor-involved lymph nodes lysed autologous melanoma as well as 4 allogeneic A2.1+ melanomas, 1 of which was an HLA-A2.1–transfected melanoma. Melanomas negative for HLA-A2 and nonmelanomas positive for HLA-A2 were not lysed. Two distinct reconstituting peptides were identified within one peak. In all, at least 6 distinct peptides recognized by melanoma-specific CTLs were found associated with different melanoma lines.

Conclusion.—Multiple peptide-defined CTL epitopes are shared by unrelated human melanoma cell lines. The estimate of 6 peptides is a minimum. They could be peptides derived from distinct endogenous proteins, or more than 1 epitope might derive from the proteolysis of a smaller number of proteins. It may be that multiple transformation-related gene products are expressed in melanoma cells and could serve as targets. Sequencing of the peptides and identifying the proteins from which they derive may allow the development of novel peptide-based synthetic tumor vaccines.

▶ It has been shown that HLA-A2 is a restricting element from melanoma-specific CTL response. However, the CTLs are not specifically recognizing HLA-A2 but, rather, a peptide sitting in the HLA-A2 cleft. Cross-reacting peptides were found in this elegant paper by Slingluff and colleagues. After using immunoaffinity column chromatography, peptides were eluted with acid and the reactivity of the peptides to the CTLs was fractionated. There are multiple possibilities as to the ideology of these peptides. They could be distinct and endogenous proteins representing tumor antigens. They also may be intermediary peptides produced from endogenous peptides by proteolysis. Identification of a single purified peptide in sequencing this peptide will then provide the ability to sensitize lymphocytes to tumor or to use the peptides in a vaccine-based treatment. Several groups are currently working on this peptide purification step, which is significant in obtaining the purified antigenic peptide(s) in melanoma.—T.J. Eberlein, M.D.

Evidence for *in Situ* Amplification of Cytotoxic T-Lymphocytes With Antitumor Activity in a Human Regressive Melanoma

Mackensen A, Ferradini L, Carcelain G, Triebel F, Faure F, Viel S, Hercend T (Institut Gustave Roussy, Villejuif, France)
Cancer Res 53:3569–3573, 1993   140-94-11–45

Background.—Previous research on lymphocytes from a patient with regressive melanoma yielded a series of T-cell receptor (TCR) α/β-dependent, HLA-B14–restricted cytotoxic T-lymphocyte clones that were reactive against autologous tumor cells. The patient, a woman aged 65 years, had a primary melanoma with both clinical and histologic signs of tumor regression.

Objective.—The tumor-reactive cytotoxic T-lymphocyte clones were analyzed, and the sequences of the TCR transcripts in the clones compared with those expressed in tumor tissue.

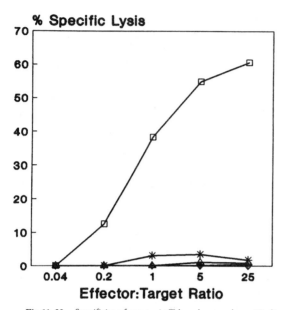

% Specific Lysis

Effector:Target Ratio

- ⊟ autologous melanoma
- ✚ allogeneic melanoma
- ✳ autologous EBV-B
- △ allogeneic EBV-B
- ◇ K562

Fig 11–22.—Specificity of cytotoxic T-lymphocyte clone 5G directed against autologous melanoma cells. The cytolytic activity was measured in a 4-hour ^{51}Cr release assay on autologous and allogeneic melanoma cells, autologous and allogeneic EBV-B cells, and K562. Values represent means of triplicates (SD < 5%) at E:T ratios of 25:1, 5:1, 1:1, 2:1, and .04:1. *White box*, autologous melanoma; *line*, allogeneic melanoma; *asterisk*, autologous EBV-B; *white triangle*, allogeneic EBV-B; *white diamond*, K562. (Courtesy of Mackensen A, Ferradini L, Carcelain G, et al: *Cancer Res* 53:3569–3573, 1993.)

Findings.—Analysis of TCR gene expression revealed that all the clones represented unique cells that expressed a Vβ13.1/Jβ1.1 gene segment. Comparison of the TCR transcripts expressed in the cloned cells with those present in uncultured tumor tissue showed that the specific cytotoxic T-lymphocyte clones characterized in vitro were selected and amplified in vivo at the lesion site (Fig 11–22 and table).

Implication.—The association of a specific cytotoxic T-lymphocyte with regression of melanoma in this case strongly suggests that effector T-cells contributed to regression.

▶ This paper looks at the other side of the lymphocyte-tumor interaction when compared with the Slingluff paper. The authors studied the TCR response to melanoma in a patient with a regressing melanoma. They identified a specific TCR gene rearrangement consisting of Vβ13.1/Jβ1.1. Although this specific TCR gene rearrangement is applicable only in this patient with a regressing melanoma, it clearly suggests a mechanism whereby a specific TCR is associated with antitumor reactivity. In similar work in a totally different system (1), specific Vβ gene rearrangements are seen in antiovarian carcinoma reactivity. These studies obviously suggest specific mechanisms to select for highly reactive T cells and optimize for an antitumor reactivity.—T.J. Eberlein, M.D.

Proliferative Responses of Cytotoxic T-Lymphocyte Clone 5G to Autologous and Allogeneic Tumor and EBV-B Cells

	Clone	Autologous tumor	Allogeneic tumor	Autologous EBV-B	Allogeneic EBV-B
None	2,520 ± 214	2,572 ± 142 *	2,633 ± 206	3,958 ± 502	3,779 ± 402
Medium		6,969 ± 338	1,967 ± 112	3,642 ± 305	3,300 ± 285
IL-2 †	2,657 ± 401	12,877 ± 1,133	2,514 ± 199	3,936 ± 197	3,717 ± 601

* Results are expressed as mean cpm ± standard deviation for [^{3}H] thymidine incorporation by clone 5G for triplicate cultures with a responder:stimulator ratio of 2:1.
† 5 units/mL.
(Courtesy of Mackensen A, Ferradini L, Carcelain G, et al: *Cancer Res* 53:3569–3573, 1993.)

Reference

1. Peoples GE, et al: *J Immunol* 151:5472, 1993.

In Vitro and In Vivo Targeting of Gene Expression to Melanoma Cells
Vile RG, Hart IR (Biology of Metastasis Laboratory, London)
Cancer Res 53:962–967, 1993   140-94-11–46

Introduction.—Gene therapy for cancer usually entails removing tumor cells, culturing them in vitro to allow gene transfer to take place, and reintroducing the altered cells. Problems in targeting genes to tumor cells in situ may be overcome by using tumor cell–specific promoters to direct the expression of a therapeutic gene.

Methods.—Two promoters that are preferentially active in melanocytic cells—the 5′-flanking regions of the tyrosinase and tyrosinase-related protein (TRP)-1 genes—were used to direct gene expression to melanoma cells in vitro and in vivo. Specific melanin synthesis is partly dependent on the melanocyte-specific transcription of both these genes.

Results.—As few as 769 base-pairs of the 5′-flanking regions of the tyrosinase gene and 1.4-kb pair of the TRP-1 gene sufficed to direct expression of the β-galactosidase gene to human and murine melanoma cells and melanocytes. High levels of activity were noted in 12 of 14 melanoma cell lines, whereas only basal levels of activity were observed in various other cell types. Cell-type specificity was noted when the construct was delivered physically to cells or by including the expression cassette in a retroviral vector. When DNA encoding the β-galactosidase gene expressed from either of the promoters was injected directly into established melanoma in syngeneic mice, about 10% of tumor cells expressed the gene after 10 days. The reporter gene was expressed in both melanoma cells and some normal melanocytes.

Conclusion.—Safe and specific gene therapy for solid tumors may be possible by combining a tissue-specific promoter driving a therapeutic gene with delivery of the construct directly to sites of tumor growth in vivo. Either direct injection of DNA or retroviral infection is feasible.

▶ In this paper, a technique of in situ gene transfer is described. This work is complicated by the difficulty that inserting a gene into a tumor in situ could be hazardous unless it is specific. The alternative of removing the tumor, inserting a gene, and then reinjecting the tumor presents many technical and ethical problems. The authors describe 2 promoters that are preferentially active in melanoma cells. By means of these promoters, the gene was preferentially inserted into sites of established melanoma in syngeneic mice. There are additional difficulties with this approach; one is the expression of the transfected gene in normal melanocytes, and the second is control of the transfected gene in the tumor cell once it has been transfected. Future developments in this area will address these issues; however, understanding the basic biological mechanisms of tumorigenesis, as well as the oncogenes and growth factors involved, will suggest which gene to transfect into a tumor cell. This type of in situ transfection made with specific promoters holds more promise than simple transfections of a lymphocyte.—T.J. Eberlein, M.D.

SARCOMA

Lymph Node Metastasis From Soft Tissue Sarcoma in Adults: Analysis of Data From a Prospective Database of 1772 Sarcoma Patients
Fong Y, Coit DG, Woodruff JM, Brennan MF (Memorial Sloan-Kettering Cancer Ctr, New York)
Ann Surg 217:72–77, 1993   140-94-11–47

Background.—Because lymph node metastasis is rare in soft tissue sarcomas, its natural history is not well documented. The natural history of lymph node metastasis from sarcomas and the use of treatment lymphadenectomy were reported.

Methods.—The clinical histories of all adults prospectively identified from a sarcoma database were studied. The patients were initially seen between 1982 and 1991. Forty-six of the 1,772 patients, or 2.6%, had lymph node metastasis. The median follow-up from diagnosis of metastasis was 12.9 months.

Findings.—Nonsurvivors had a median survival of 12.7 months. Tumor types associated with the greatest incidence of lymph node metastasis were angiosarcoma, embryonal rhabdomyosarcoma (ERMS), and epithelial sarcoma. A very poor prognosis was associated with lymph node metastasis from visceral primary and malignant fibrous histiocytomas.

Factors That Adversely Influenced Survival After Lymph Node Metastasis From Sarcoma

Factor	No.	p
Age < 30 yr	11/46	0.19
Male sex	24/46	0.55
Lymph node metastasis		
at time of primary	21/46	0.79
Nonextremity lesion	20/46	0.93
Visceral lesion	3/46	0.004*
Embryonal rhabdomyosarcoma	12/46	0.84
Malignant fibrous histiocytoma	8/46	0.006*
Noncurative surgery	15/46	0.003*

* $P < 0.05$.
(Courtesy of Fong Y, Coit DG, Woodruff JM, et al: *Ann Surg* 217:72-77, 1993.)

Thirty-one patients received radical lymphadenectomy with curative intent, and 15 had less than curative procedures. Patients not receiving radical lymphadenectomy had a median survival of 4.3 months. Those treated with radical lymphadenectomy had a 16.3-month median survival. The only long-term survivors had undergone radical lymphadenectomy (table).

Conclusion.—Lymph node metastasis from sarcoma in adults is rare, but vigilance is indicated, particularly in cases of angiosarcoma, ERMS, and epithelioid subtypes. Radical lymphadenectomy is appropriate for patients with isolated metastasis to regional lymph nodes and may lengthen survival.

▶ Lymph node metastasis associated with soft tissue sarcoma is exceedingly rare. The group from the Memorial Sloan-Kettering Cancer Center reports on a series in which lymph node metastasis occurred. The metastases were more commonly associated with angiosarcoma, ERMS, and epithelial sarcoma. The treatment is radical lymphadenectomy, which may extend survival. The incidence is not high enough to recommend routine lymphadenectomy; however, vigilance is necessary to detect the patient who may have lymph node metastasis, because an increase in survival can be anticipated with appropriate therapy.—T.J. Eberlein, M.D.

Call Mosby Document Express at **1 (800) 55-MOSBY** to obtain copies of the original source documents of articles featured or referenced in the YEAR BOOK series.

12 Plastic, Reconstructive, Head/Neck Surgery

Introduction

In an effort to provide information derived from the field of head and neck surgery, as well as from plastic and reconstructive surgery, that would directly impact on the reader's practice, we have selected papers in 4 broad categories: head and neck, breast, burn reconstruction, and general reconstruction. In some instances, although the paper may reflect a tenor of basic science, the choice has been made to provide the reader with the contemporary developments in a particular aspect of that field.

Approximately one half of the publications selected for perusal were in the broad category of head and neck surgery. In turn, several subdivisions, or classes, of papers were chosen. First, in the area of diagnosis are 2 papers on fine-needle aspiration (FNA) of parotid masses (Abstracts 140-94-12-1 and 140-94-12-2). These 2 groups of authors bring somewhat different perspectives to the use of FNA and arrive at somewhat different conclusions as well. The controversy about neck node biopsy, in regards to its necessity and its potential detrimental effect, continues; however, as the authors of the paper on neck node biopsy and nasopharyngeal carcinoma (Abstract 140-94-12-3) conclude, biopsy is rarely necessary.

If the treatment of patients with head and neck cancer is to be individualized in the future, particularly with regard to the emerging role of adjuvant therapy, better prognostic indices are needed. A paper on tumor thickness and soft palate carcinoma (Abstract 140-94-12-4) attempts to accomplish that goal; however, further work is needed. This deficiency in our knowledge is certainly evident in the review of management of squamous cell carcinoma of the tongue, as outlined in 2 additional papers (Abstracts 140-94-12-5 and 140-94-12-6). The emphasis in one is a review of the oncologic considerations; in the other, it is efforts at restoration of function. Both will provide the reader with an update on the management of this difficult problem in head and neck surgery.

More outcome studies are needed in head and neck surgery to guide the magnitude of the resection, such as the criteria for orbital preservation in maxillectomy seen in Abstract 140-94-12-8. This paper summarizes an extensive experience and provides some specific guidelines for indications of long-term occular functioning with irradiation. With respect to irradiation, the preoperative use, either planned or for surgical salvage, can adversely affect soft- and hard-tissue healing. One decision that must be reached is whether reconstruction can be successfully accomplished in the heavily irradiated patient. The paper by Bengtson et al. from the M.D. Anderson Cancer Center (Abstract 140-94-12-9) answers this question quite conclusively. Another problem with irradiation is the possible development of osteoradionecrosis in retained mandibles. Is hyperbaric oxygen an appropriate treatment modality for this complication? We have selected a paper to address that issue (Abstract 140-94-12-10). Reconstruction of head and neck defects has passed from the phase of simply "filling the hole" to an effort to provide sufficient refinement to achieve better functioning. One of the criteria for successful mandibular reconstruction is prosthetic rehabilitation. Zlotolow and his co-authors examine that topic in patients who have had microvascular free flap mandibular reconstruction (Abstract 140-94-12-11).

An additional topic in head and neck surgery is lentigo maligna melanoma. This variant has often and traditionally been considered a more benign lesion. The paper on that subject included in the collection (Abstract 140-94-12-12) may raise some substantial questions as to whether this is an appropriate and valid view of the behavior of lentigo maligna. The final paper in this series of head and neck subjects is an examination of the placement of a tracheotomy in an intensive care unit setting compared to the operating room (Abstract 140-94-12-13).

Two difficult problems in burn reconstruction are those of closure of burns of the foot and successful skin grafting of particular anatomical areas of difficult skin graft "take," such as the posterior shoulder and back and perineum. The paper on the use of fibrin glue (Abstract 140-94-12-14) may be a good technical addition for management of some of these more difficult anatomical regions. The second paper included in the burn reconstruction group reports on a technique of management of foot burns that worked quite well for the authors (Abstract 140-94-12-15).

Again this year, the area of breast reconstructive surgery was dominated by the silicone gel issue. Included for consideration are 4 papers on various aspects of this topic. Two papers examine the issue of the detection of breast cancer after augmentation mammaplasty; one is an epidemiologic study (Abstract 140-94-12-16), and the other is a report on the relative radiolucencies of different breast implant filler materials (Abstract 140-94-12-17), an impetus to develop some material besides silicone gel for breast implants. Another paper examines the relationship between silicone gel and the incidence of autoimmune disease in patients who have had breast reconstruction after mastectomy (Abstract 140-94-12-18). The last paper in this group is an interesting examination of the relationship between the age of implants and the probability of rupture (Abstract 140-94-12-19).

Some procedures performed by plastic surgeons sit in the gray zone between reconstruction and aesthetic. Reduction mammaplasty is one of these procedures. Justification for the performance of reduction mammaplasty as a reconstructive procedure hinges on addressing specific problems, and outcome studies of their medical effectiveness must be performed by surgeons in the future. Included in the series of articles on the breast is a study of the preoperative and postoperative clinical findings in reduction patients, which should demonstrate the efficacy of the procedure (Abstract 140-94-12–20).

The transverse rectus abdominis musculocutaneous (TRAM) flap has evolved—particularly with the advent of the silicone gel controversy—as a frequently selected option for breast reconstruction after mastectomy. What may be particularly advantageous is an opportunity not only for immediate reconstruction at the time of the mastectomy with a TRAM flap but, also, for the use of microvascular technique or a "free" flap. The study on this subject (Abstract 140-94-12–21) is a large series, perhaps the largest, of immediate breast reconstruction with the use of autologous tissue in the TRAM flap technique. The authors make a compelling argument for the use of this technique.

The collection of general reconstruction papers was chosen to illustrate a variety of points. A paper selected from the *Canadian Journal of Surgery* (Abstract 140-94-12–22) is an excellent description and review of contemporary head and neck reconstructive techniques, including some of the "cutting-edge" methods drawn from related fields such as craniofacial surgery. Minimally invasive surgery may soon be incorporated into the field of reconstructive plastic surgery, and no better example exists than the endoscopic harvest of omentum for free flap reconstruction, as outlined in a study by Saltz and his co-workers (Abstract 140-94-12–23). Other contemporary methods of reconstruction include not only the salvage of limbs by the use of tissue transfer techniques in oncologic surgery but, also, the next plateau, i.e., restoration of function. Doi and his co-authors from Japan have taken a big step in this direction with a considerable-sized series of patients so managed (Abstract 140-94-12–24). In fact, the reconstructive challenge in cancer surgery is often simply how to accomplish wound closure in massive defects. A paper that addresses this topic includes a review of the inherent complication rate (Abstract 140-94-12–25). Finally, in the group of papers on general reconstruction is a review of management of war wounds drawn from Croatia, the first such published experience in well over a decade (Abstract 140-94-12–27). The authors have taken a considerably more aggressive approach to closure of these wounds than others have in the past.

Edward A. Luce, M.D.

Fine-Needle Aspiration of Parotid Masses

Zurrida S, Alasio L, Tradati N, Bartoli C, Chiesa F, Pilotti S (Istituto Nazionale Tumori, Milano, Italy)
Cancer 72:2306–2311, 1993   140-94-12–1

Introduction.—Open biopsy provides reliable information about the nature of intraparotid swellings whereas clinical examination and imaging studies cannot. However, the invasiveness of open biopsy contraindicates the procedure. There is debate over the value of fine-needle aspiration biopsy (FNAB) in these patients. The findings of preoperative FNAB in 246 consecutive patients with carotid lumps were compared with the histopathologic diagnoses in surgically resected specimens.

Patients.—Fine-needle aspiration biopsy was performed on a total of 692 parotid swellings during an 11-year period; in 246 cases, surgery and subsequent histologic examination of the surgical specimen were performed. There were 126 female patients (mean age, 48 years) and 120 male patients (mean age, 52 years).

Findings.—Ninety-two percent of the 173 benign tumors were correctly diagnosed by FNAB, and more than 60% were correctly typed. Sixty-one percent of 36 malignant tumors were also recognized by FNAB. Fine-needle aspiration biopsy gave false negative results in 9 cases and an unsatisfactory specimen in 5. All 4 cases of metastatic cancer were correctly typed, but only 2 of 7 cases of lymphoma were. In all patients with non-neoplastic disease, the cytologic and histologic findings agreed. The overall accuracy of FNAB in this sample was 87%.

Conclusion.—Fine-needle aspiration biopsy is an accurate diagnostic procedure for patients with parotid masses. The procedure requires a certain level of skill, both in obtaining and evaluating the cytologic material. Primary malignancies of the salivary glands may pose a difficult diagnostic challenge, although metastatic intraparotid tumors are easy to diagnose.

▶ Fine-needle aspiration biopsy is a valuable diagnostic tool in masses of the head and neck and can provide us with important preoperative information for planning and patient counseling. Fine-needle aspiration diagnosis of salivary gland masses, done in the hands of a skilled cytopathologist, can effect treatment plans in 10% to 20% of the instances.—E.A. Luce, M.D.

Value of Fine Needle Aspiration Biopsy of Salivary Gland Masses in Clinical Decision-Making

Heller KS, Dubner S, Chess Q, Attie JN (Long Island Jewish Med Ctr, New Hyde Park, NY)
Am J Surg 164:667–670, 1992   140-94-12–2

Background.—Many surgeons do not routinely use fine-needle aspiration biopsy (FNAB) in the diagnosis of salivary gland masses, in part because they assume that the biopsy results will not affect the management approach to the patient. The effects of FNAB on salivary gland masses on patient management were examined in a retrospective study.

Methods.—The analysis was based on records of 101 patients who had FNAB as part of their initial evaluation for major salivary gland masses over a 4½-year period. Although not all patients with salivary gland masses had FNAB during this period, 52 consecutive patients of 2 of the investigators did undergo FNAB. The physician's initial clinical impression was compared with the FNAB findings and the final diagnosis.

Results.—Forty patients were believed on clinical grounds to have benign, non-Warthin's salivary tumors. The FNAB confirmed this impression in only 17 patients, whereas 13 patients were able to have either lesser or no surgery. The clinical diagnosis of Warthin's tumor was confirmed by FNAB in 14 patients, 8 of whom were managed by follow-up only. In 9 cases, FNAB proved a diagnosis other than Warthin's tumor. Of 10 patients with clinically suspected cancers, 1 had sialadenitis and another had lymphoma. Overall, FNAB allowed surgery to be avoided in 27% of cases and permitted a lesser procedure to be performed in 8%. In 3 cases, inadequate surgery might have been performed on the basis of FNAB findings.

Conclusion.—Fine-needle aspiration biopsy may alter the management approach for about one third of patients with salivary gland masses. It is a highly accurate diagnostic procedure, although not in differentiating various types of malignancies, and it has a low complication rate. It is essential to read the results of FNAB in terms of the patient's history, physical examination findings, and course of illness. Routine use of FNAB as part of the initial evaluation for patients with major salivary gland masses is recommended.

▶ Although FNAB modified the management of the authors' patients in one third of the instances, we have not ascertained that magnitude of impact on the treatment plan of patients with parotid masses. In our hands, the principal value of FNAB has been preoperative counseling of the patient. The results of this technique are extremely specific and dependent on the cytopathologist. As the authors emphasized, considerable experience with the use of FNAB must be accrued in the diagnosis of salivary gland masses before accuracy is achieved. Nevertheless, the technique is simple and has an extremely low complication rate.—E.A. Luce, M.D.

Pretreatment Neck Node Biopsy, Distant Metastases, and Survival in Nasopharyngeal Carcinoma

Leung SF, Teo PML, Foo WWL, Van Hasselt CA, Shiu WCT, Ting CL, Lau JTF (Chinese Univ of Hong Kong; Queen Elizabeth Hosp, Hong Kong)
Head Neck 15:296–299, 1993   140-94-12-3

Background.—Patients with nasopharyngeal carcinoma (NPC) commonly have cervical node metastases. In many cases, the presenting symptom is a neck mass, and node biopsy may be performed before the primary tumor is detected. There is controversy as to the association between node biopsy and the subsequent course of disease in patients with NPC.

Methods.—To explore this relationship, 422 patients with newly diagnosed NPC and cervical node metastases were reviewed. Fifty of them underwent biopsy of the lymph nodes of the neck before receiving definitive treatment. Nodal biopsy was performed in 8% of patients with stage N1 nodal involvement, 14% of those with stage N2 involvement, and 14% of those with stage N3 involvement. Treatment was by a standardized radiotherapy regimen, and patients were followed for a median of 53 months.

Findings.—At 5 years, patients with and without node biopsy had no significant differences in probability of distant metastases (60% vs. 68%, respectively) or survival (40% vs. 39%, respectively). Neither end point was significantly affected by the performance of pretreatment node biopsy in either sex. Node biopsy did not predict tumor recurrence in the neck on multivariate analysis.

Conclusion.—There apparently is no association between pretreatment neck node biopsy and subsequent metastasis or survival in patients with NPC. However, node biopsy is rarely necessary to make the diagnosis of NPC, as long as a diligent examination of the nasopharynx is performed. If there is any doubt, fine-needle aspiration of the cervical node is often sufficient. Node biopsy delays the definitive diagnosis and therapy.

▶ The literature presents conflicting views regarding the association between pretreatment neck node biopsy and the rate of locoregional control in patients with NPC as well as other primaries of the upper aerodigestive tract. The argument as to whether biopsy should be performed may be moot. The contemporary management of NPC is a diligent examination, including the use of fiberoptic endoscopy, and then a fine needle aspirate to establish the diagnosis. Nodal biopsy or removal would only be indicated if a diagnosis of lymphoma is entertained and/or more tissue is needed than is provided by fine needle aspiration for tumor typing.—E.A. Luce, M.D.

Significance of Tumor Thickness in Soft Palate Carcinoma

Baredes S, Leeman DJ, Chen TS, Mohit-Tabatabai MA (VA Med Ctr, East Orange, NJ; Univ of Medicine and Dentistry of New Jersey–New Jersey Med School, Newark)

Laryngoscope 103:389–393, 1993   140-94-12-4

Introduction.—In patients who have tumors outside of the upper aerodigestive tract—including cutaneous melanoma, colorectal carcinoma, and cervical carcinoma—tumor thickness and depth of invasion are useful indicators of prognosis. Some reports have suggested that tumor thickness may also be a valuable indicator for tumors of the upper aerodigestive tract. The associations between tumor thickness and nodal disease and survival were studied in 44 patients with soft palate epidermoid carcinoma (table).

Observations.—Tumor thickness was measured in blinded fashion with an ocular micrometer, in most cases from biopsy material. Thicknesses ranged from 0.3 to 6.4 mm, with a mean of 2.9 mm. Cervical adenopathy was present in none of the 24 patients with tumors of less thickness than approximately 2.9 mm, and in none of them did palpable metastases develop after initial treatment. In contrast, palpable adenopathy was present in all patients with lesions with a thickness of 3.1 mm or greater. The correlation of tumor thickness with nodal disease was more direct than the correlation with T stage. The 3-year unadjusted survival rate was 79% for patients with tumors measuring 1.62 mm or less, 52% for tumors measuring 1.63 to 2.7 mm, 43% for tumors measuring 2.71 to 4.26 mm, and 37% for tumors measuring 4.27 to 6.40 mm.

Conclusion.—These findings suggest the potential prognostic importance of tumor thickness in head and neck cancers. Techniques of measuring thickness should be standardized, with a greater emphasis on as-

Distribution of T and N Stages in 44 Patients With Soft Palate Carcinoma				
	N0	N1	N2	N3	Total
T1	6	1	0	0	7
T2	11	1	1	1	14
T3	8	3	4	1	16
T4	2	4	1	0	7
Total	27	9	6	2	44

sessing thickness from biopsy material. This study was unable to evaluate the ability of tumor thickness to predict subsequent neck disease.

▶ Decisions regarding dissection of the regional nodes in the N0 neck usually hinge on the size of the tumor (T stage) and, to some degree, the site. Because tumor size, particularly for smaller tumors, is at best a crude estimate of the likelihood of occult nodal metastasis, head and neck surgery awaits more specific criteria. Tumor thickness may be just one of those, but this article falls short in that the majority of the necks in stage N0 (drawn from a relatively small number of patients, anyway) were managed with radiotherapy. The success of the predictive value of thickness in melanoma arose because of a pathologic correlation established between tumor thickness and the presence of occult metastases in nonpalpable nodes. This type of controlled study will further elucidate the usefulness of tumor thickness in carcinoma of the upper aerodigestive tract.—E.A. Luce, M.D.

Surgical Management of Squamous Cell Carcinoma of the Base of the Tongue

Kraus DH, Vastola AP, Huvos AG, Spiro RH (Mem Sloan-Kettering Cancer Ctr, New York)
Am J Surg 166:384–388, 1993   140-94-12-5

Background.—Treatment alternatives for patients with squamous cell carcinoma of the base of the tongue include surgery and external-beam radiation therapy, with or without brachytherapy implantation or induction chemotherapy. Few studies have addressed the effects of the various treatments on the patient's speech and swallowing.

Patients and Treatment.—The analysis included 100 patients who underwent resection for squamous cell carcinoma of the base of the tongue. Thirty-six patients were women. Stage III or IV disease was present in 80% of patients, and the neck was clinically involved in 62%. Surgery was done by mandibulotomy in 59 patients, composite resection in 15, a transcervical approach in 13, a transhyoid approach in 8, and a peroral approach in 5. Sixteen patients had supraglottic laryngectomy, and 20 had laryngectomy for either direct laryngeal invasion or risk of aspiration. Eighty-four patients underwent primary repair, with a pectoralis major myocutaneous flap in 16.

Neck dissection was comprehensive in 71 patients, supraomohyoid in 8, bilateral radical in 5, bilateral supraomohyoid in 4, and radical and supraomohyoid in 1. In 11 patients, the cervical lymphatics were managed by observation. Sixty-three patients received adjunctive radiotherapy. The patients were followed for a median of 3 years.

Outcomes.—Twenty-one patients had positive surgical resection margins. Forty-one had some type of complication, most commonly wound problems and pulmonary compromise, but none died in the postoperative period. The 5-year cumulative survival rate was 55%, and the 5-year cause-specific survival rate was 65%. Locoregional recurrence, with or without distant metastasis, developed in 28 patients. Treatment achieved local control in all but 18 patients.

Conclusion.—In well-selected patients with squamous cell carcinoma of the base of the tongue, surgical treatment can achieve good local control and survival. It is usually possible to resect the larger, well-defined tumors while preserving the mandible and larynx. The authors prefer a median or paramedian mandibulotomy approach to these tumors; defining the extent of the tumors can be difficult, however.

▶ Carcinoma of the base of the tongue is seen in an advanced stage of the disease. In this group of patients, postoperative radiotherapy was given to two thirds, 1 in 5 had positive resection margins of the primary, and complications occurred in 40%. The results, both in terms of function and survival, were excellent. Twenty percent of the group required a laryngectomy, either for oncologic reasons or because of the risk of aspiration. If the epiglottis can be retained in patients even with a subtotal glossectomy, in the majority of such cases, a laryngectomy can be avoided.

What is needed in reports such as this one, however, is some objective measurement of the essential functions of speech and deglutition. No longer can we judge results solely in terms of locoregional recurrence and survival.—E.A. Luce, M.D.

Tongue Reconstruction: Concepts and Practice
Haughey BH (Washington Univ, St Louis, Mo)
Laryngoscope 103:1132–1141, 1993   140-94-12–6

Background.—Partial or complete removal of the tongue leads to dysfunction of the oral cavity, posing a threat to quality of life and life itself. Resection of the tongue is necessary in patients with cancer of the tongue, which is the most common subsite of cancer of the oral cavity. Few previous reports have focused on the problems and techniques of tongue reconstruction. A new technique of tongue reconstruction, total or subtotal, has been developed and used in 14 patients.

Patients.—The retrospective analysis included 15 patients who had resection of at least the entire anterior two thirds of the tongue because of malignant tumors. The glottic larynx was preserved if possible. Fourteen of these patients had reconstruction using latissimus dorsi myocutaneous flaps.

Technique.—In this surgical procedure, the latissimus dorsi flap was harvested with the muscle fibers oriented transverse to its long, skin component axis. This allowed creation of a contractile muscle sling to raise the reconstructed tongue toward the palate for use in speech and swallowing. After transfer to the oral defect, the flap was sutured to the remaining muscles of mastication at the level of the mandibular angle. The free flap was anastomosed using conventional microvascular technique. The hypoglossal nerve stump was then reanastomosed end-to-end to the latissimus dorsi nerve. The skin component of the flap was placed in the floor of the mouth, with anterior resection of a curved wedge creating a mound to help in articulation.

Outcomes.—At a median of 3 weeks after surgery, the decannulation rate in the 14 patients was 80%. Seventy percent of patients were able to take at least pureed food by mouth. Video swallowing studies demonstrated upward motion of the flap in 2 cases. Especially good results were achieved in terms of articulation. Seven patients are still alive, with a median survival of 22 months.

Conclusion.—For patients who have had total or subtotal glossectomy, the innervated latissimus dorsi flap described in this study is a useful method of tongue reconstruction. It can permit decannulation, oral nutrition, and intelligible speech in some patients. Further study is needed to define the eventual role of this technique in total tongue reconstruction.

▶ The reader must be careful of 2 variables that have been mixed into the results of this study of a small series of patients. One was the author's use of the static suspension and the careful orientation of the muscle fibers of the donor flap (latissimus) transversely, such that a sling could be constructed to the remaining muscles of mastication. The other variable, of course, was the nerve anastomosis to the hypoglossal, and no evidence was provided that reinnervation occurred. In fact, such was unlikely, because the recovery of the patients who were successfully decannulated and obtained deglutition was shorter than one would anticipate for neural regeneration. Regardless, the authors are on target with their emphasis on the importance and necessity of demonstrating functional results after subtotal and total tongue resection and reconstruction. Little has been published on this topic.—E.A. Luce, M.D.

Verrucous Carcinoma of the Larynx: Role of Human Papillomavirus, Radiation, and Surgery
Hagen P, Lyons GD, Haindel C (Louisiana State Univ, New Orleans)
Laryngoscope 103:253–257, 1993   140-94-12-7

Introduction.—Confusion continues regarding verrucous cancer of the larynx, which occurs as a well-differentiated variant of squamous cell carcinoma that frequently recurs and undergoes anaplastic transformation after radiation therapy. The lesion lacks typical cytologic features of malignancy and is difficult to diagnose from a superficial biopsy specimen.

Methods.—Between 1977 and 1987, a total of 12 new cases of verrucous carcinoma of the larynx were diagnosed at the authors' institution.

Tumor registry files, patient records, and pathologic slides for this disorder were studied.

Results.—The 12 cases made up 2.2% of the 552 primary laryngeal cancers diagnosed during the 10 study years. The 11 men and 1 woman had a mean age of 57 years. All patients had had hoarseness for 1 month to 4 years. Two patients had dyspnea and upper airway blockage that required tracheotomy. All patients had glottic primaries. Five of the 6 patients with T1a lesions had surgery. Two patients with T2 lesions initially had laryngofissure and cordectomy, but 1 of these patients had stomal recurrences that were treated with successive carbon dioxide laser excisions. There was no response to cobalt radiation therapy for palliation of overwhelming diseases and the patient had died at 6-year follow-up. The 3 patients with T3 lesions had a total laryngectomy and are alive and disease-free at 3–6 years of follow-up. Two patients had primary radiation treatment; 1 remains alive and free of disease at 12-year follow-up. Overall, the series yielded an 83% disease-free survival rate at 3 to 12 years of follow-up.

Conclusion.—Surgery appears to be preferable to radiation therapy in treating patients with verrucous cancer of the larynx. The carbon dioxide laser excision offers the best results for removing T1 lesions, but hemilaryngectomy or laryngofissure with cordectomy is recommended for stage T2 lesions, and total laryngectomy is recommended for stage T3 and T4 tumors.

▶ The controversy regarding the appropriate treatment of verrucous carcinoma of the oral cavity has been heightened by recent challenges to the tenets first advanced by Ackerman; these challenges recommend that such a lesion should be resected rather than irradiated. The second most common site for verrucous carcinoma in the upper aerodigestive tract is the larynx. This paper nicely summarizes the literature and clearly defines, at least in regards to the larynx, that radiation therapy has a 50% failure rate and is complicated by anaplastic transformation in an unacceptably high number of patients. Old lessons sometimes have to be relearned.—E.A. Luce, M.D.

Orbital Preservation in Maxillectomy
Stern SJ, Goepfert H, Clayman G, Byers R, Wolf P (Univ of Arkansas, Little Rock; MD Anderson Cancer Ctr, Houston)
Otolaryngol Head Neck Surg 109:111–115, 1993   140-94-12–8

Objective.—The poor results of treatment for squamous carcinoma of the maxillary sinus (SCMS) probably result as much from unrecognized involvement of contiguous structures and the biological characteristics of the tumor as from the advanced stage of the tumor at recognition. In recent years, the trend in treatment has been toward orbital preservation during maxillectomy; however, little attention has been given to the fate of the eye in such cases. The results in 28 patients with SCMS who had maxillectomy with preservation of the orbital contents were evaluated.

Patients.—The patients, all previously untreated, underwent surgery from 1971 to 1986. The orbital floor was resected either in part or completely in 18 patients; reconstruction was with a split-thickness skin graft. Nine patients received 50–60 Gy of radiotherapy; 9 had surgery only. The orbital floor was retained in 10 patients, 4 of whom received radiotherapy and 6 of whom did not. The ocular results in these patients were compared with those in a group of 25 patients who had maxillectomy with exenteration in terms of local control and survival.

Outcomes.—Only 3 of the 18 patients with resection of the orbital floor retained significant function of the ipsilateral eye. The local recurrence rate was 44%, regardless of whether the patient received postoperative radiotherapy. Ten of the 18 patients died of their disease. The 10 patients with preservation of the orbital floor had few eye problems as long as the eye was not included in the radiation field. All patients receiving radiation therapy and half of those not receiving radiation therapy died of their disease. Local control and survival were no different for patients with and without exenteration of the eye, although this finding may have resulted from selection bias.

Conclusion.—In patients with SCMS, orbital floor resection yields very poor operative function. Eye problems are relatively few for patients in whom the orbital floor is preserved, as long as the eye is not in the radiation field. It may be that preservation of the orbit is merely converting a subset of patients with earlier, potentially controllable disease into a group with more advanced disease who require exenteration for tumor clearance.

▶ Preservation of the eye in maxillectomy for malignancy has become more widely adopted, but what function remains? The evidence presented in this paper indicates that if the orbital floor is resected, the eye is preserved, and the patient is given postoperative radiotherapy, then a nonfunctional eye will almost uniformly result. Preservation of the floor, with or without radiation therapy, did not result in dysfunction in the vast majority of patients who received that treatment. One would anticipate that this last group of patients would do well because their maxillectomy was of the infrastructure type.

One problem with the results of this study is that the orbital floor resection patients had no reconstruction. Perhaps primary reconstruction would have permitted the use of postoperative radiotherapy without the extremely detrimental result observed.—E.A. Luce, M.D.

Influence of Prior Radiotherapy on the Development of Postoperative Complications and Success of Free Tissue Transfers in Head and Neck Cancer Reconstruction
Bengtson BP, Schusterman MA, Baldwin BJ, Miller MJ, Reece GP, Kroll SS,

Robb GL, Goepfert H (MD Anderson Cancer Ctr, Houston)
Am J Surg 166:326–330, 1993   140-94-12-9

Introduction.—Although radiation has demonstrated effects on vascular and perivascular tissues, there is no clinical evidence that the histologic changes observed translate into higher postoperative complication rates for patients undergoing reconstructive surgery. The effects of preoperative radiotherapy on the rates of complication or flap loss in patients with head and neck cancer who were undergoing reconstructive surgery with microvascular free tissue transfers were evaluated.

Methods.—Three hundred fifty-four consecutive patients, who underwent a total of 368 free tissue transfers in the head and neck in a 4-year period, were identified by a prospective database. Preoperative radiotherapy was used in 167 patients and was not used in 187. The average follow-up was 26 months. Postoperative complications in patients who did and did not receive preoperative radiotherapy were compared.

Results.—The 2 groups showed no significant difference in complication rates or flap loss. About 5% of each group had total flap loss. The rates of partial flap loss were 4.1% in the irradiated group and 2.5% in the nonirradiated group. Additional surgery was required because of major wound complications in 16% of the irradiated group vs. 11% of the nonirradiated group. The irradiated group also had a slightly higher incidence of minor wound complications not requiring additional surgery (21% vs. 18%). Failed flaps were no different than successful flaps in terms of timing or dose of radiation, previous neck dissection, and type of anastomosis.

Conclusion.—Preoperative radiation therapy does not appear to increase flap loss or the complication rate in patients with cancer receiving free tissue transfers to the head and neck. Radiation therapy, as well as previous surgery, can make for a more technically demanding dissection and microvascular anastomosis. However, as long as meticulous planning and surgical technique are used, complication rates are no higher for patients who have received radiation therapy.

▶ The selection of options in the reconstruction of head and neck defects is often couched in terms of the "reconstructive ladder," meaning a hierarchy of options from the most simple (direct closure) to the more complex (muscle-skin flap) to the more sophisticated (free tissue transfer). Actually, free tissue transfer has become sufficiently consistent and reliable that very frequently microvascular reconstruction is the option of choice. As the defect becomes more complex—for example, combined lining and bone components—reconstruction with a free tissue technique (osteocutaneous flap) is the preferred and most widely used method. The authors have convincingly demonstrated that an irradiated recipient site does not affect the outcome.—E.A. Luce, M.D.

Role of Hyperbaric Oxygen Therapy in the Management of Mandibular Osteoradionecrosis

Mounsey RA, Brown DH, O'Dwyer TP, Gullane PJ, Koch GH (Toronto Hosp)
Laryngoscope 103:605–608, 1993   140-94-12-10

Background.—It was formerly thought that mandibular osteoradionecrosis (ORN) occurs when soft tissue trauma allows oral pathogens to enter demineralized bone, followed by the development of osteomyelitis in irradiated bone. It now seems likely that micro-organisms are the contaminants in ORN, and the role of trauma also has been questioned. Irradiation may lead to tissue hypoxia, hypocellularity, and hypovascularity; as a result, the tissue loses its ability to repair and heal.

Patients.—The value of hyperbaric oxygen (HBO) was examined in 41 patients with ORN of the mandible who had failed to respond to local wound care alone. Nearly all the patients had received 50 to 55 Gy of external-beam radiation, given with single-daily-dose fractionation. Three patients received radioactive implants as well. Complications other than ORN were relatively few, and none were major. Osteoradionecrosis most often involved the mandibular symphysis.

Treatment.—Patients were treated in a hyperbaric chamber at 2.0 ATA daily. Treatment lasted 141 minutes, and the patients breathed oxygen for three 40-minute periods during this time. Each course of HBO consisted of 40 treatments (Fig 12–1).

Results.—Osteoradionecrosis resolved completely after HBO alone in 6 patients (15%), and another 28 patients (68%) improved significantly, for a total response rate of 83%. Thirty-five patients had surgery to remove sequestra and enhance healing. The 7 patients who failed to benefit from HBO had evidence of dead bone; they later underwent major

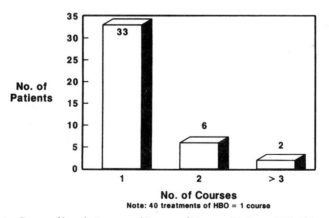

No. of Patients

No. of Courses
Note: 40 treatments of HBO = 1 course

Fig 12–1.—Courses of hyperbaric oxygen. (Courtesy of Mounsey RA, Brown DH, O'Dwyer TP, et al *Laryngoscope* 103:605–608, 1993.)

mandibular resection and received HBO after operation. Antibiotics were used inconsistently.

Conclusion.—Hyperbaric oxygen therapy is an effective approach to the management of mandibular ORN.

▶ Hyperbaric oxygen has been advocated for some time as the nonsurgical treatment of choice for ORN. More recently, HBO has been trumpeted as a method to successfully address chronic wounds. The common denominator of the rationale for these approaches is increased oxygen delivery to the tissues as well as promotion of neovascularization. This editor always has some sense of guilt because of his failure to routinely use HBO in chronic wound management. However, the expense is substantial and the efficacy is not proven.

An example is this study. Although all patients had pain, only 3 of the 41 patients had fistula, and little information is given about the extent of the ORN. Nevertheless, the patients were given a minimum of 40 treatments, each lasting more than 2 hours. The approximate cost at our institution would be $8,000. In addition, a number of other modalities were used, including surgery, wound care, and oral hygiene. We need a more scientific demonstration of the efficacy of HBO in ORN before we can move onward to chronic wounds.—E.A. Luce, M.D.

Osseointegrated Implants and Functional Prosthetic Rehabilitation in Microvascular Fibula Free Flap Reconstructed Mandibles
Zlotolow IM, Huryn JM, Piro JD, Lenchewski E, Hidalgo DA (Mem Sloan-Kettering Cancer Ctr, New York)
Am J Surg 165:677–681, 1992   140-94-12-11

Background.—Immediate mandibular reconstruction using the microvascular fibula free flap can improve the mandibulectomy deformity. Conventional and maxillofacial prosthetic rehabilitation, which fails to reestablish the bony foundation and soft tissues, has offered only limited success. The records of 7 patients who received reconstructive surgery and osseointegrated implants, were reviewed, with emphasis placed on a discussion regarding prosthetic design and preservation of tissues.

Patients and Methods.—The patients, 4 men and 3 women, had a median age of 45.3 years and various types of head and neck cancer. All had mandibulectomies with microvascular free flap reconstruction. After allowing time for primary bony healing at the osteotomy sites, the patients were evaluated for soft tissue thickness over the new bony foundation. Mounted maxillary and mandibular study casts were evaluated to determine implant placement and design. After implant fixtures were placed, 4 to 6 months were allowed for osseointegration of the titanium fixture with the new bone before recovery of the fixtures and insertion of the transmucosal abutments. Panoramic photographs were taken to ensure that each fixture and abutment collar was securely fastened.

Results.—All 7 patients were free of disease after 4.2 to 20.7 months of follow-up and have achieved functional and cosmetic rehabilitation. None of the 23 osseointegrated fixtures had to be removed because of complications or infection. Periimplantitis, which occurred in 1 patient after stage II procedures, resolved with antibiotic treatment and placement of longer abutment collars. None of the 4 patients who underwent resection of the condyle with reattachment to the fibula by means of miniplates and screws reported pain, malocclusion, or temporomandibular joint disorders after the implant prostheses were completed.

Conclusion.—The fibula provides an excellent foundation for osseoimplants; the osseointegrated implant offers functional and cosmetic benefits to patients who have undergone mandibular dissection. The results in these patients are far superior to those previously obtained with nonreconstructed mandibles and removable appliances.

▶ The authors eloquently establish the point that to reconstruct a mandible with free tissue transfer is not sufficient. Whatever flap is chosen, sufficient bone stock must be available to perform dental rehabilitation by the use of a permanent functional prosthesis (osseointegrated implants). The results are vastly superior to reconstruction without prosthetic rehabilitation and are certainly superior to the use of removable appliances without reconstruction.—E.A. Luce, M.D.

Lentigo Maligna Melanoma of the Head and Neck
Langford FPJ, Fisher SR, Molter DW, Seigler HF (Duke Univ, Durham, NC)
Laryngoscope 103:520–524, 1993   140-94-12-12

Introduction.—Traditionally, it has been thought that lentigo maligna melanoma (LMM) has a better prognosis than other histologic types and that wide local excision can be curative. Prompted by reports of LMM recurrences, a retrospective review of a melanoma database was done to evaluate LMM of the head and neck.

Patients.—From 1,067 patients with head and neck melanomas who were followed at Duke University Medical Center, 156 (59%) had LMM, including 143 with stage I LMM. Of all patients with LMM, 56% were seen with lesions deeper than .76 mm and 8% were seen with stage II or III disease. Primary treatment of all stage I head and neck LMM consisted of wide local excision. Seventeen percent of patients underwent elective lymph node dissection, and 58% underwent immunotherapy.

Results.—Recurrent disease developed in 47% of patients with stage I LMM over a mean follow-up of 6 years. The recurrences were local in 39%, in the regional nodal basis in 33%, and distant in 28%. The median disease-free interval for stage I head and neck LMM was 6 years, and the median survival time was 10 years. Recurrence significantly shortened survival, for a median survival of 4 years after recurrence. Univariate analysis indicated that thickness, ulceration, and sex significantly affected the disease-free interval. Histologic subtyping had little prognostic significance.

Conclusion.—Contrary to previous notions, LMM should not be considered a "favorable" histologic classification of melanoma. Treatment should primarily be based on depth of invasion, not histologic subtype.

▶ The paper debunks the myth of LMM being more of a benign lesion rather than a garden-variety melanoma. The patients had recurrence with a dismaying frequency (45%) in stage I disease, and more than one half of the lesions were deeper than .76 mm, which is the usual line of division between "thin" and "immediate" lesions. Without dispute, the appropriate treatment for LMM is wide local excision, but what margin?—E.A. Luce, M.D.

The Safety and Efficacy of Bedside Tracheotomy
Futran ND, Dutcher PO, Roberts JK (Univ of Rochester, NY)
Otolaryngol Head Neck Surg 109:707–711, 1993   140-94-12-13

Introduction.—In many institutions, it is policy that tracheotomy, one of the most common operations done in critically ill patients, be performed in the operating room. However, for critically ill patients who are receiving life support, transfer to the operating room is difficult, labor intensive, and potentially hazardous. An experience with bedside tracheotomy in nearly 1,000 patients was analyzed.

Patients.—A total of 1,088 tracheotomies were performed as isolated procedures in critically ill patients at the study institution from 1983 through 1991. The patients' age range was 1 week to 94 years, with a mean of 68 years. Ninety-three percent of the procedures were performed in the intensive care unit (ICU) and the remainder in the operating room. Patients who were undergoing tracheotomy in the ICU all had endotracheal tubes in place. The indications for doing the procedure in the operating room were lack of intubation, a coagulation profile 25% or more above normal, abnormal thyroid gland, nonpalpable cricoid cartilage, and morbid obesity. The 2 groups of patients, as well as 346 patients who underwent tracheotomy in the operating room in conjunction with other head and neck procedures, were compared for incidence of intraoperative, early, and late complications.

Findings.—All tracheotomies in the ICU group were successfully completed in the ICU. There was 1 intraoperative complication each in the ICU group and in the patients undergoing isolated tracheotomy in the operating room. Bleeding within 48 hours and stomal infection occurred in about 2% of all 3 groups. The rate of tube dislodgement was 1% or less in all 3 groups, and all patients were successfully recannulated.

Conclusion.—There is no significant difference in complication rates when tracheotomy is done at the bedside rather than in the operating room. Tube dislodgement is the most common cause of life-threatening morbidity, both early and late, and is preventable. Performing the procedure in the ICU rather than the operating room not only avoids the dangers of moving the critically ill patient, it also saves the additional costs of the operating room.

▶ The authors convincingly demonstrate that intraoperative, immediate postoperative, and late postoperative (2 weeks) complications are not increased by the performance of tracheotomy in the ICU. Remember, however, that all the patients in the ICU were intubated. The most frequent early postoperative complication, the dislodgement of the tracheotomy tube, could have been prevented in 4 of the 5 instances in the ICU group by suturing the tracheotomy. A portable headlight is also a nice adjunct if the tracheotomy is to be performed in the ICU.—E.A. Luce, M.D.

Fibrin Glue: Its Use for Skin Grafting of Contaminated Burn Wounds in Areas Difficult to Immobilize
Vedung S, Hedlund A (Akademiska sjukhuset, Uppsala, Sweden)
J Burn Care Rehabil 14:356–358, 1993   140-94-12-14

Purpose.—Conjugation between burn wounds and skin grafts can be difficult to achieve in certain areas, including the axillae, side of the trunk, perineum, and gluteal folds. Human fibrin glue is of proven use for a variety of plastic and reconstructive surgical procedures. Its use was evaluated in patients with burns after failure of skin grafts. Fibrin glue was used for the dual objective of hemostasis and stable fixation of the graft to avoid dead space and loosening.

Methods.—Fibrin glue was used to repair skin grafts on 29 granulating wounds in 23 patients. The grafts were located on the sides of the trunk in 11 cases, the shoulder in 9, the perineum in 5, and the gluteal folds in 4. The fibrin adhesive system consisted of 2 components: a highly concentrated human fibrinogen solution combined with factor XIII, fibronectin, and aprotinin, and a combination of thrombin and calcium chloride. The glue is lysed into soluble fibrin degradation products during the process of wound healing.

Findings.—The wounds were contaminated in every case, although they appeared clear after revision at the time of skin grafting. The use of fibrin glue between the graft and the wound eliminated dead space and provided a safe anchor for the graft. Healing occurred in 28 of the 29 sites, with nearly complete take of the skin grafts.

Discussion.—Fibrin glue was successfully used for skin grafting of burn wounds in difficult areas. The glue does not impair vascularization, and little remains in the wound after 2 weeks of healing. There is some risk of disease transmission because the fibrinogen is made from pooled human plasma; it is hard to obtain as much fibrinogen and adhesive strength with autologous tissue glue, however.

▶ This is a description of a nifty little technical maneuver that can be used to successfully graft those areas that are infamous for "poor take": the posterior shoulder, flank, and perineum. In burns covering a larger body surface area, these areas are always the last to be closed because of poor take and past efforts at closure of the burn wound. Fibrin glue has evolved into a prominent role in many reconstructive procedures.—E.A. Luce, M.D.

Early Ambulation and Discharge in 100 Patients With Burns of the Foot Treated by Grafts
Grube BJ, Engrav LH, Heimbach DM (Univ of Washington, Seattle)
J Trauma 33:662–664, 1992   140-94-12–15

Background.—Burns to the foot or ankle, which often involve only a miniscule proportion of the total injured body surface area, are frequently fraught with complications that prolong recovery. In 1982, it was suggested that aggressive surgery and early ambulation could decrease hospital stay and morbidity. Since that time, excision and grafting have been used, with early application of an Unna (dome paste) boot and normal ambulation 4 hours later. The patient is then discharged if there are no other reasons for hospitalization. The results of treating 92 patients with this protocol were reported.

Patients.—Ninety-two of 100 patients with burns of the foot, ankle, or distal leg were treated with Unna boots, including 7 with bilateral injuries. The mean patient age was 28.8 years, and the mean burn size was 3.7% of total body surface area. The most common cause of injury was scalding. Excision and grafting were done a mean of 6 days after the burn. Sheet grafts were used in 64% of cases and narrowly meshed autografts were used in 36%; the take rates were 96% and 97%, respectively. The Unna boot was applied either in the operating room or the morning after surgery, the latter being more common for patients receiving sheet grafts. The patient was discharged within 3 days in 64% of cases.

Outcomes.—Eighty five patients had an excellent result and 10 had a satisfactory result, but 3 required another graft. The mean time to return to work was 4.7 weeks among 43 patients employed at the time of injury.

Conclusion.—Good results have been obtained with early postoperative ambulation and discharge for patients with burns of the foot or ankle. Early grafting is followed by application of an Unna boot, ambulation without crutches, discharge, application of a second Unna boot at 1 week after discharge, and application of a support stocking at 2 weeks.

This treatment provides excellent graft take, early discharge, and rapid functional recovery for patients who have sustained a major injury.

▶ The authors have provided us with a follow-up of their previous report of a group of patients with foot burns treated by early ambulation and discharge. In this era of medical cost-consciousness, we need to challenge traditional methods that may not have a solid therapeutic foundation. As the authors note, a survey of burn centers indicates that more than two thirds permit ambulation only after postoperative day 5 for skin grafts applied to the foot and leg. Clearly, hospitalization would be even longer.

This method would be best applied to early burn wound excision and is probably not appropriate for late grafting of granulating wounds. Because foot and lower leg burns tend to be deep and slowly healing, early tangential excision with grafting (using the method described) is an appealing alternative.—E.A. Luce, M.D.

The Detection of Breast Cancer After Augmentation Mammaplasty
Carlson GW, Curley SA, Martin JE, Fornage BD, Ames FC (MD Anderson Cancer Ctr, Houston)
Plast Reconstr Surg 91:837–840, 1993   140-94-12–16

Background.—Delayed detection of cancer in women with augmentation mammaplasty is of concern. One experience with patients seen between 1975 and 1990 was reviewed.

Patients and Findings.—Thirty-five patients treated for 37 breast cancers after augmentation mammaplasty were included in the review. All augmentations had been done with silicone gel implants at a mean pa-

Breast Cancer After Augmentation Mammaplasty:
Mammographic Evaluation

Type			
Xeromammography	27		
Plain-film mammography	4		
Findings			
Mass	12		
Calcifications	5		
Mammogram type			
Xeromammography	15	55.6%	
Plain-film mammography	2	50%	NS*
Implant location			
Subglandular	17/27	63%	
Subpectoral	0/4	0%	$p = 0.03$†
Overall	17	54.8%	

* NS indicates not significant.
† Fisher exact test.
(Courtesy of Carlson GW, Curley SA, Martin JE, et al: *Plast Reconstr Surg* 91:837–840, 1993.)

tient age of 38 years. The mean interval from augmentation to cancer detection was 7.5 years. A palpable breast mass was found on physical examination in 95% of the cases. Pathologic staging was in situ in 8%, local in 49%, and nonlocal in 43%. Thirty-one patients underwent standard mammography before breast biopsy. Abnormalities were seen in 54.8%. Palpable lesions were visualized in only 38.7% of the patients. Ultrasonography was successfully performed in 3 patients with palpable lesions to guide fine-needle aspiration biopsy (table).

Conclusion.—The sensitivity of standard 2-view mammography for detecting palpable cancers is low in women who have had augmentation mammaplasty. The value of ultrasonography as a routine adjunctive screening method in such patients should be assessed. The pathologic staging in this group suggests that the clinical detection of breast cancer was not delayed.

▶ This report was drawn from the experience at M.D. Anderson Cancer Center and defines the difficulty of mammographic visualization in the augmented patient. Virtually all of the patients in this series had a palpable mass, but mammography fell far short of the desired end point in terms of detection, even in the 4 patients with subpectoral implants. The authors are careful to note that only standard techniques—not special views or displacement methods—were used. However, at least for the future, the answer may be a different filler material. See reference 1.—E.A. Luce, M.D.

Reference

1. Young VL, et al: *Plast Reconstr Surg* 91:1066, 1993.

The Relative Radiolucencies of Breast Implant Filler Materials
Young VL, Diehl GJ, Eichling J, Monsees BS, Destouet J (Washington Univ, St Louis, Mo)
Plast Reconstr Surg 91:1066–1072, 1993   140-94-12–17

Introduction.—Silicone gel has been the most commonly used breast implant filler for the past 3 decades. Substantial drawbacks of this material are its radiodensity and its lack of biocompatibility. Because silicone gel is radiopaque, there is inadequate visualization of breast tissue during standard mammography. The radiolucencies of various breast implant filler materials were compared.

Methods.—Standard mammography equipment was used to evaluate silicone gel, saline, breast tissue equivalent, triglycerides (peanut oil), and polyvinylpyrrolidone (Bio-Oncotic gel). Mammographic images of a breast phantom with simulated microcalcifications and soft-tissue masses were obtained through the different materials. To better reflect the clinical setting, one set of images was generated using the filler materials

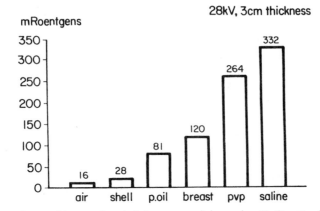

Fig 12–2.—Peanut oil is approximately 3 times more radiolucent than Bio-Oncotic gel (*pvP*) and 4 times more radiolucent than saline. The breast tissue equivalent is closest to peanut oil. (Courtesy of Young VL, Diehl GJ, Eichling J, et al: *Plast Reconstr Surg* 91:1066–1072, 1933.)

within implant envelopes. The x-ray dosage required to create each mammographic image was measured.

Results.—As expected, silicone was nearly radiopaque and was 9 times more radiodense than the next nearest material, saline. Peanut oil was approximately 4 times more radiolucent than Bio-Oncotic gel and 4 times more radiolucent than saline (Fig 12-2). The breast tissue equivalent was closest to peanut oil in radiolucency. Clearest visualization of the artifacts in the phantom were provided, in order, by peanut oil, breast equivalent, Bio-Oncotic gel, saline, and silicone gel. When the various materials were placed in a flask over the phantom, the peanut oil allowed all artifacts except for some fine microcalcifications to be identi-

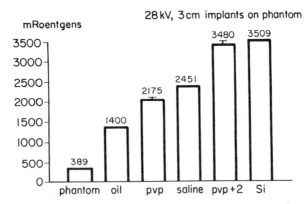

Fig 12–3.—Relative radiodensities of implants combined with phantom. Note the 46% increase in exposure to radiation needed to improve visualization through the Bio-Oncotic gel (PVP) and that this reaches the dosage needed to penetrate silicone. (Courtesy of Young VL, Diehl GJ, Eichling J, et al: *Plast Reconstr Surg* 91:1066–1072 1993.)

fied. There were no discernible artifacts with silicone gel in a flask over the phantom (Fig 12–3).

Conclusion.—The optimal breast implant material would be radiolucent, biocompatible, nontoxic, noncarcinogenic, nonteratogenic, and affordable. A radiopaque implant such as silicone gel interferes with the ability to image the breast properly. Use of the modified compression technique does not entirely solve this problem. Of the alternatives to silicone gel that were evaluated, triglycerides appear to be the most radiolucent and require the least radiation exposure.

▶ Recent concerns about the efficacy of silicone breast implants have centered not only on biocompatibility, but also on radiolucency and the interference with detection of breast cancer by mammographic techniques. Silicone gel is highly radiodense and obscures much of the breast tissue with standard mammography. Even with a specialized approach (Eklund views), the images obtained can be compromised, particularly in the presence of capsular or scar contracture. The winner in this paper was peanut oil as the most radiolucent. The next question is: Is peanut oil biocompatible?—E.A. Luce, M.D.

Incidence of Autoimmune Disease in Patients After Breast Reconstruction With Silicone Gel Implants Versus Autogenous Tissue: A Preliminary Report

Schusterman MA, Kroll SS, Reece GP, Miller MJ, Ainslie N, Halabi S, Balch CM (MD Anderson Cancer Ctr, Houston)
Ann Plast Surg 31:1–6, 1993   140-94-12–18

Introduction.—Since autoimmune arthritis was first described in patients who were given injections of paraffin for breast augmentation in the mid-1960s, a wide range of disorders allegedly caused by a variety of injected substances has been described. In addition to paraffin, these have included liquid silicone of varying grade and purity, silicone gel, silicone elastomer, and Marlex mesh.

Objective.—The development of autoimmune disease was compared in 250 women who, from 1986 to 1992, received 308 silicone gel implants with or without a latissimus dorsi flap, and 354 patients having a total of 408 reconstructions using autogenous tissue. Both latissimus dorsi and transverse rectus abdominis flap reconstructions were performed in the latter group.

Findings.—More than 600 person-years of follow-up were accumulated in each group. In 1 patient in each group, an autoimmune syndrome requiring treatment developed; this represented an overall incidence of less than .5%. Both patients were mildly affected and required only low-dose steroid therapy, which is no longer necessary.

Conclusion.—Autoimmune disease appears not to be more frequent in mastectomy patients given silicone gel implants than in those having autogenous tissue reconstruction without an implant.

▶ The breast implant controversy rages on. The plastic surgeons at M. D. Anderson Cancer Center perform a huge volume of breast reconstructions and, thus, could complete this comparative study. Virtually all the information and evidence regarding the relationship between silicone implants and immunologic disease or disorder has been anecdotal, as the authors point out. In fact, the discussion in this paper is worthwhile reading to put the controversy into perspective. However, the average follow-up in this series of patients was relatively short when viewed in the context of possible long-term problems with implants. Please see the next paper by Donna de Camara and her co-authors.—E.A. Luce, M.D.

Rupture and Aging of Silicone Gel Breast Implants
de Camara DL, Sheridan JM, Kammer BA (Carle Clinic Assoc, Urbana, Ill)
Plast Reconstr Surg 91:828–836, 1993   140-94-12-19

Purpose.—Rupture of breast implants appears to be an uncommon problem that has not been directly associated with aging of the implant. However, one recent study did find some decrease in the strength of implants over time. A retrospective study sought to evaluate the condition of aging silicone gel implants.

Methods.—A total of 51 silicone gel implants that were removed from 31 women 1 to 17 years after insertion were examined. They assessed the age and condition of each implant, reviewed any history of capsulotomy or trauma, and examined the mammograms which were available in 13 patients.

Findings.—There were 27 ruptured implants with visible tears in the implant shell, 7 leaking implants with no apparent tears, and 17 intact implants (table). Implants in 16 of 20 breasts in the ruptured group, which were evaluated retrospectively by mammography, showed abnormal findings. Mammography usually showed the rupture on the lateral

Distribution of Removed Implants by Implantation Time and Condition

Years Implanted	Group I: Ruptured	Group II: Leaking	Group III: Intact	Total
1 to 9	10	2	16	28
10 to 17	17	5	1	23
TOTAL	27	7	17	51

(Courtesy of de Camara DL, Sheridan JM, Kammer BA; *Plast Reconstr Surg* 91:828–836, 1993.)

surface, with extravasation toward the axilla. On microscopic examination, the capsule around the intact implants showed fibrous tissue with some mild inflammation. The capsule around leaking implants showed inflammation and a foreign-body tissue reaction; this response was more intense—including calcification—in the ruptured-implant group. Treatment consisted of removal of the implants and silicone gel, capsulectomy, and new implant insertion. No infections or inflammations were recorded postoperatively.

Discussion.—The condition of silicone gel implants may deteriorate over time. The original quality of the shell appears to be an important variable; shells have become thicker, and possibly stronger, in recent years. The cause of silicone leakage remains to be determined. Some "bleed" is expected in older implants, and leakage may progress to rupture. Mammography may have to be done cautiously in women with older implants. Closed capsulotomy is another potential cause of rupture. An editorial comment on this article points out that implant rupture should be suspected when the implant is over 10 years old and the capsule is contracted.

▶ Although this is not a large series (31 patients), a statistical significance could be demonstrated because of the small number of intact implants found after 10 years. In fact, the authors did not remove an implant older than 10 years that was intact and in good condition.

What can be learned from this paper is that patients who are seen with complaints about implants that have been in place for more than a decade and who have hardness of the breast caused by capsular contracture need to be investigated carefully for rupture. Currently, no consensus has been reached regarding the best imaging approach for the diagnosis, but in our hands, ultrasound has been as effective as any technique. Due consideration needs to be given to removal of the implants as well as the capsule to ensure complete removal of the silicone gel.—E.A. Luce, M.D.

Reduction Mammaplasty Improves Symptoms of Macromastia
Gonzalez F, Walton RL, Shafer B, Matory WE Jr, Borah GL (Univ of Massachusetts, Worcester)
Plast Reconstr Surg 91:1270–1276, 1993   140-94-12-20

Background.—Much has been written about breast reduction techniques, but little has been said about the effects of reduction mammaplasty in reducing the adverse symptoms associated with large breasts. Specific diagnostic criteria are not currently available to describe macromastia. The symptoms in patients with macromastia were determined, and the relief brought by reduction mammaplasty was assessed.

Method.—Patients who volunteered for mammaplasty completed a study questionnaire and examination. They rated symptoms, including headache, neck pain, breast pain, and hand numbness, as mild, moderate, or severe. All underwent bilateral reduction mammaplasty and, after full recovery, completed a questionnaire and underwent an examination identical to the preoperative one. A control group of 40 women with a bra cup size of A or B, who had never had breast surgery, completed identical questionnaires.

Results.—An average of 753 g of tissue was removed from each breast. Follow-up data were obtained from 85% of the patients in an average follow-up of 8.6 months. Preoperatively, all patients complained of at least one symptom, and 97% had 3 or more pain symptoms. Reduction mammaplasty reduced the incidence of headache, neck pain, shoulder pain, and back pain to levels lower than those in the control group. Problems with fitting clothing, sleeping, maintaining posture, and intertrigo, common in patients with breast hypertrophy, were also significantly reduced after surgery. Overall, pain symptoms were markedly diminished by breast reduction. There was no correlation between cumulative symptom improvement and body type when the change in symptom severity sum was analyzed as a function of patient height/weight ratio.

Conclusion.—Macromastia has been ill-defined in the past. This study indicates that to diagnose this condition adequately, it is necessary to look at the degree of upper body pain symptoms rather than simply the degree of breast hypertrophy. The incidence and severity of headache, neck pain, shoulder pain, back pain, breast pain, and painful bra strap grooves in these patients were greater by 3 standard deviations than in the control group. It is suggested that the pathologic condition macromastia be defined as a chronic pain complex affecting at least 3 anatomical upper body areas in a patient with bilateral breast hypertrophy.

▶ The "cosmetic" pall still looms over the procedure of reduction mammaplasty. Extremely large breasts are a significant problem for such patients—not only in terms of clothes fit, but with the more straightforward physical problems of shoulder, back, and breast pain, all of which are alleviated by the procedure, as these authors convincingly demonstrate.

How do you define large? The mean resected weight in this series was 1,506 grams or 750 grams per breast, a substantial but not massive resection. The average patient weighed 150 lbs. What is needed, perhaps, is another series of smaller resection weights, perhaps 350–400 grams; however, this paper is convincing.—E.A. Luce, M.D.

Immediate TRAM Flap Breast Reconstruction: 128 Consecutive Cases

Elliott LF, Eskenazi L, Beegle PH Jr, Podres PE, Drazan L (Atlanta Plastic Surgery, Ga)

Plast Reconstr Surg 92:217–227, 1993   140-94-12–21

Ipsilateral Pedicle   **Contralateral Pedicle**

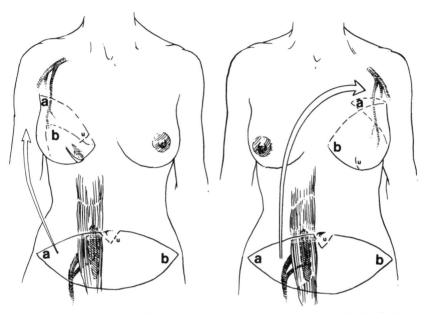

Fig 12–4.—**Left,** note that the flap is only turned approximately 30 degrees and that the distal portion of the flap (*b*) is tucked under to increase projection. **Right,** the flap is turned 180 degrees in a counterclockwise manner when the contralateral pedicle is used. Projection is increased by closing the umbilical V. This site is designated by the letter *u*. (Courtesy of Elliott LF, Eskenazi L, Beegle PH Jr, et al: *Plast Reconstr Surg* 92:217-227, 1993.)

Introduction.—Because of its clinical and psychological advantages, more and more women with breast cancer are choosing to have immediate breast reconstruction at the time of mastectomy. As surgeons have become more familiar with the transverse rectus abdominis musculocutaneous (TRAM) flap, it has become more widely used as an immediate reconstructive option.

Patients.—A series of 128 consecutive patients undergoing immediate TRAM flap breast reconstruction during a 5-year period was examined (Fig 12–4). Eighty-six patients had conventional TRAM flap reconstruction, whereas 40 had free TRAM flap reconstruction; the remaining 2 patients had "supercharged" TRAM flap breast reconstruction. Reconstruction was bilateral in 62 patients. The patients were followed for an average of 23 months.

Findings.—Use of the free TRAM flap was associated with a shorter hospitalization time and a decreased incidence of fat necrosis. There was no apparent association between immediate reconstruction and an increased chance of local recurrence. Chemotherapy had to be delayed because of healing problems after immediate reconstruction in only 1 patient. In comparison with previously reported series, operative time and complication rates appeared to be improving.

Conclusion.—The transverse rectus abdominis musculocutaneous flap is a good choice of immediate breast reconstruction after mastectomy. The free TRAM flap carries fewer complications, probably because of its more robust blood supply, than the conventional pedicled TRAM flap. Used unilaterally or bilaterally, the free TRAM flap has the potential to become the new standard for immediate reconstruction.

▶ With their report on the TRAM flap, these authors have published one of the largest studies of immediate breast reconstruction with the use of autologous tissue. Their data indicate that not only can immediate breast reconstruction be accomplished without an increase in the rate of complications, but, even more to the point, the free flap with microvascular anastomosis in the immediate setting had a lower complication rate than the conventional or pedicle flap. Vascularization of the flap by reinstitution of blood flow to the *inferior* deep epigastric vessels by microvascular means enhances flap viability compared with pedicle flaps based on the *superior* deep epigastric vessels. These results were obtained with a 50% increase in operative time, but the improved results and the smaller muscle harvest that was needed probably justified such an investment.—E.A. Luce, M.D.

Reconstruction of Composite Facial Defects: The Combined Application of Multiple Reconstructive Modalities
Antonyshyn OM, Paletz JL, Wilson KL (Univ of Toronto; Dalhousie Univ, Halifax, NS, Canada)
Can J Surg 36:441–452, 1993   140-94-12-22

Purpose.—Until recently, there were few options for the reconstruction of composite facial defects, which involve combined deficiency of multiple tissues (including skin, muscle, fat, bone, and mucosal lining). Innovations in surgical technique and imaging have brought major advances in facial reconstructive surgery in recent years. Three case reports illustrate the combined use of various reconstructive techniques for the repair of composite facial defects.

Assessment and Reconstruction.—The complexity of composite facial defects warrants a comprehensive, multidisciplinary preoperative assessment, including neurologic, ophthalmologic, and dental examinations; anthropometric analysis; prosthodontic assessment; CT; and, most recently, computer graphics. Craniofacial exposure is achieved according to the basic principles established by Tessier. Skeletal reconstruction aims to create a stable, 3-dimensional bony structure to provide a supportive framework for the soft tissues. Bone grafting is used, as needed, for restoration of bony continuity and increased stability, and rigid internal fixation is routinely used to position and immobilize osseous segments. Tissue expanders are used to create local tissue for wound closure and resurfacing of soft tissue defects. They are increasingly used for resurfacing of the cheek and neck, in reconstruction of the neck, and for coverage of craniofacial defects in preference to distant flaps. Functional replacement of deficient tissues can be achieved by microsurgical techniques of free tissue transfer. Among the main uses of this technique are to create a lining for intraoral defects, to obliterate cavities and exposed sinuses, to provide vascularized cover for the cranial base, and to augment subcutaneous tissue deficits.

Discussion.—The integrated use of these modalities is illustrated in 3 patients with composite facial defects: a 15-year-old boy with a self-inflicted shotgun wound to the face, a 23-year-old man with Treacher-Collins syndrome, and a 55-year-old woman with a post-traumatic composite defect of the central midface. These cases demonstrate the ways in which the surgeon can use craniofacial skeletal reconstruction, tissue expansion, and free tissue transfer to tailor reconstruction to the patient's specific functional and anatomical needs. An integrated team approach is essential for optimizing the results of reconstruction.

▶ This paper was selected primarily because the text contains an excellent description of contemporary head and neck reconstructive techniques; the emergence of technology for craniofacial surgery includes the use of wide operative exposure and rigid skeletal fixation. When the tissue transfer techniques of free flaps and tissue expansion are added, quite complex defects of a composite (soft tissue and bone) nature, whether post-traumatic, extirpative, or congenital, can be successfully addressed. In particular, the use of rigid internal fixation has become a standard method of facial skeletal reconstruction. The newer technology of small plates and screws provides the basis for 3-dimensional reconstruction. What needs to be accomplished now is further refinement in the aesthetics, or appearance, of the soft tissue transfer.—E.A. Luce, M.D.

Laparoscopically Harvested Omental Free Flap to Cover a Large Soft Tissue Defect

Saltz R, Stowers R, Smith M, Gadacz TR (Med College of Georgia, Augusta)
Ann Surg 217:542–547, 1993   140-94-12-23

Objective.—Many standard surgical procedures can now be done by laparoscopy. A laparoscopic technique in reconstructive surgery that involved harvesting an omental free flap for coverage of a soft tissue defect was applied.

Case Report.—Man, 61, sustained severe trauma and third-degree burns to the right lower leg. He was an obese smoker with a history of hypertension. After knee fusion and several skin grafts, he was referred with graft failure and infection resulting in a large wound with exposed bone and chronic drainage. He had

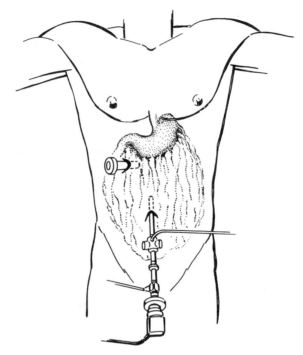

Fig 12–5.—The position of the cannulas and laparoscopic instruments for harvesting the omentum. (Courtesy of Saltz R, Stowers R, Smith M, et al: *Ann Surg* 217:542–547, 1993.)

a sensate foot but could not ambulate; arteriography showed a patent but calcified popliteal artery with 3 patent vessels to the leg and foot.

The patient was managed with a laparoscopic omental free flap approach, developed and refined in a dog model. One surgical team harvested the omentum under laparoscopic guidance, and the other prepared the recipient site (Fig 12–5). A large segment of omentum based on the gastroepiloic vessels was taken. The end-to-side microvascular anastomosis was performed using 9-0 absorbable sutures. A skin graft was placed over the granulating omental bed 3 days later. The procedure was well tolerated, and the patient was healed and ambulatory at 10 months' follow-up.

Discussion.—The successful application of a laparoscopically harvested omental free flap to cover a large soft tissue defect of the leg was reported. This flap provides long, large vessels to simplify the anastomosis and avoid the use of vein grafts in complicated reconstructive cases. It may prove to be a very useful technique for reducing the morbidity of reconstructive surgery.

▶ The use of the omentum is an extremely valuable tool for difficult defects in the armamentarium of the reconstructive surgeon for a number of reasons, including the length of the vascular pedicle (for microvascular purposes), and the vascularity, bulk, and pliability. The principal limitation has been the necessity of laparotomy for harvest, particularly in the compromised patient.

This paper probably heralds the advent of minimally invasive surgery into the arena of reconstruction. Some surgeons might validly argue that the 8-cm incision used would have been sufficient to exteriorize, ligate, and harvest the omentum but, with experience, this technique will be truly modified to be "minimally invasive."—E.A. Luce, M.D.

Reinnervated Free Muscle Transplantation for Extremity Reconstruction

Doi K, Sakai K, Ihara K, Abe Y, Kawai S, Kurafuji Y (Yamaguchi Univ, Ube, Japan)

Plast Reconstr Surg 91:872–883, 1993   140-94-12-24

Purpose.—For patients with severe injuries of the extremities, motor function may be recovered by reinnervated free muscle transplantation. A method of successful reconstruction of more than one function in patients with brachial plexus palsy, as well as restoration of function after muscle loss secondary to extirpation of malignant soft tissue tumors, is presented.

Patients.—Forty-six patients underwent a total of 58 reinnervated free muscle transplants. The 39 men and 7 women were followed for an average of 26 months after operation. Simultaneous reconstruction of 2 functions, such as finger and elbow flexion, was performed in 24 patients with severely injured extremities and brachial plexus palsy. Double muscle transplantation was performed in 12 patients; free muscle transplantation for limb salvage after tumor excision was performed in 15; transplantation to replace traumatic muscle loss was done in 6; and reconstruction of finger flexion was performed in 1 patient after poliomyelitis. The donor muscles were the latissimus dorsi in 26 transplants, the gracilis in 25, and the rectus femoris in 7.

Outcomes.—Muscles reinnervated by the spinal accessory nerve took a mean of 3 months to electromyographic evidence of reinnervation, compared with a mean of 5 months for muscles reinnervated by the intercostal nerves. The time to reinnervation did not vary significantly among different types of muscle transplant. Patients with brachial plexus palsy had an average range of elbow motion of -25 degrees in extension to 90 degrees in flexion, with grade 3 to 4 power on the Highet scale. Elbow flexion power was equally good with the different muscles reinnervated by the spinal accessory nerve. The patients with tumor resection gained power and range of motion gradually with reinnervation. For patients with brachial plexus palsy who were younger than age 50 years, there was no significant relationship between age and time to reinnervation or final functional recovery. Recovery of function was not affected by postoperative chemotherapy.

Conclusion.—For patients with brachial plexus palsy, traumatic muscle loss, or radical excision of soft tissue malignancies, free muscle transplantation is a consistently successful procedure that offers restoration of extremity function. The speed and extent of reinnervation depend on the recipient nerve, patient age, and postoperative vascular complications. Recovery is quickest with neurotization by the spinal accessory or posterior interosseous nerve.

▶ The use of microsurgical transfer of tissue has extended the limits and frontiers of oncologic surgery and resection. "Limb salvage" surgery refers to the radical resection of extremity tumors with preservation of the limb, often by tissue transfer techniques done to fill the defect and close the wound. This technique, although laudable, often results in a functionally impaired limb. The next step in the evolution is not only the closure of the defect but, also, restoration of function. One should observe that the authors could not clearly separate the residual function of native muscles that remain in the extremity after resection from that added by the transplantation and reinnervation. More sophisticated studies (including electromyography and individual muscle testing) will be necessary for that to occur, but this advance is the correct approach conceptually.—E.A. Luce, M.D.

Immediate Flap Coverage in the Treatment of Large Surgical Defects After Tumor Resection

Anthony JP, Mathes SJ, Hoffman WY (Univ of California, San Francisco)
Surg Gynecol Obstet 176:355–359, 1993   140-94-12-25

Objective.—Patients with cancer often require extensive resections that leave huge defects of 50 to 100 cm^2 or more. Such defects can rarely be managed by primary or random flap closure. Recent advances in reconstructive surgery allow coverage of large defects in all parts of the

Most Frequent Flap Choices by Location

Wound location	Flap utilized	No.	Percent
Head and neck	Free latissimus dorsi	7	54
	Other muscle flaps	2	15
	Other skin, fascial flaps	4	31
Trunk and perineum .	Rectus abdominis	11	24
	Other muscle flaps	18	39
	Other skin, fascial flaps	16	35*
Extremity and groin . .	Rectus abdominis	3	38
	Other muscle flaps	5	62
	Other skin, fascial flaps	0	

* One trunk was covered with a pedicled omental flap.
(Courtesy of Anthony JP, Mathes SJ, Hoffman WY: *Surg Gynecol Obstet* 176:355–359, 1993.)

body. Such immediate coverage permits wide oncologic resection, resection and coverage in a single procedure, and radiation therapy beginning shortly after surgery. Fifty-one patients with massive surgical defects that were managed by immediate flap coverage were reviewed.

Experience.—The patients were treated from 1984 to 1990. The defects, measuring 100 to 1,050 cm², all resulted from tumor resection. The tumor was located in the perineum in 32 patients, the head and neck in 12, and the extremity and groin in 7. Radiation therapy had failed as primary treatment in 17 patients. Eleven of the defects were managed with free flaps, and the rest were managed with rotation of pedicled skin, muscle, or fasciocutaneous flaps (table). Two flaps were needed for coverage in 13 patients.

Results.—Three patients had complete flap loss; 2 of these patients had had free flaps. Eight additional patients had other extensive complications requiring surgery, and 22 patients had some type of complication. Barring complications, healing occurred in an average of 2 weeks. Healing time extended to 9 weeks for patients with lesser complications and 19 weeks for those with extensive complications.

Conclusion.—This experience supports the use of immediate flap coverage of massive surgical defects after tumor resection. Modern reconstructive techniques allow the characteristics of the malignancy itself, rather than the resulting wound, to determine resectability. Immediate coverage promotes healing while restoring or preserving function.

▶ In this era of oncologic treatment using combined modalities with the frequent use of postoperative radiation, composite tissue closure of the wound has advantages over that of skin grafts alone. The price paid is a significant complication rate, because although flap necrosis was distinctly uncommon in this study, major complications occurred in 22% of these patients. The defects, however, were massive (an average of 260 cm² for the group as a whole and 160 cm² in the head and neck subgroup). Simpler options probably would not have been sufficient for even wound closure, but the provision of flap coverage enables the oncologic surgeon to take the most aggressive approach feasible. Although free flaps were used in only 15% of the patients in this group, free tissue transfer is selected with increasing frequency—even in the majority of instances in some plastic surgery units.—E.A. Luce, M.D.

Extracorporeal Circulation for Tissue Transplantation (In the Case of Venous Flaps)

Maeda M, Fukui A, Tamai S, Mii Y, Miura S (Omiwa Hosp, Nara, Japan; Nara Med Univ, Japan)
Plast Reconstr Surg 91:113–126, 1993   140-94-12–26

Introduction.—The anastomosis of vessels in free tissue transplantation may be difficult when recipient vessels are crushed or damaged by

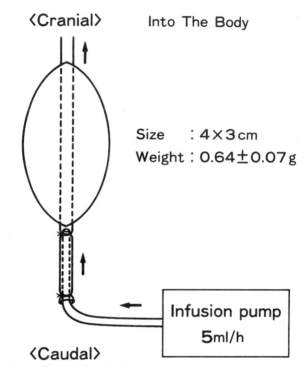

⟨Cranial⟩   Into The Body

Size   : 4×3 cm
Weight : 0.64±0.07 g

Infusion pump
5ml/h

⟨Caudal⟩

Fig 12–6.—Venous flap including the thoracoepi-gastric vein as the flow-through vein. The value of flap weight is mean ± standard deviation. (Courtesy of Maeda M, Fukui A, Tamai S, et al: *Plast Reconstr Surg* 91:113–126, 1993.)

trauma or radiotherapy. To avoid the need for postoperative reexploration and thrombectomy, a method allowing free tissue transplantation to sites with damaged, or even absent, recipient vessels was sought.

Methods.—Experiments involving venous flaps were performed in male Japanese White rabbits. The flaps, located on the cranial side of the abdomen without covering the thorax, were spindle-shaped and 4 × 3 cm in size. A 24-gauge silicone tube was inserted into the caudal thoracoepigastric vein in the flap and fixed in position for infusion (Fig 12-6). Perfusates of the flaps were stabilized hemoglobin, lactated Ringer's solution, whole blood collected using CPD solution, and plasma. Each perfusate was injected at a rate of 5 mL/hr continuously for 3 days in good recipient sites and for 7 days in poor recipient sites. Three of the experiments were conducted to determine the speed of optimal inflow of the perfusate, the optimal duration of perfusion, and whether the flaps were viable despite a poor recipient site for perfusion of plasma. Flaps were examined histologically and electron microscopically, and microangiography was performed in the plasma group to observe blood circulation between the flap and surrounding tissue.

Results and Conclusion.—Flap survival was seen in all cases in which the plasma group had good recipient beds. There was no survival in the other cases, in which degeneration of the endothelial cells was detected before edema. The tissue viability of a venous flap can persist for at least 3 days by perfusion of plasma. In the case of good recipient sites, blood circulation between flap and surrounding tissue may recur during this time. Also, at a good recipient site, oxygen may not be important for the viability of a comparatively thin venous flap with little subcutaneous fat. Development of a satisfactory artificial blood is expected to make transplantation of flaps and other tissues possible at any site, even without vascular anastomoses.

▶ The capacity of microsurgical free tissue transfer for reconstruction/closure of defects is considerably limited by hostile recipient beds with few, if any, vessels. If transplanted tissues could be maintained for a sufficient period to allow vascular ingrowth and permanent viability, outcome could be enhanced in situations in which results, at present, are marginal. The authors have permitted us a peek at such a possibility.

Numerous technical and conceptual questions remain, some of which are elucidated by Dr. James W. May, Jr. in his discussion that follows the article. In addition (and unfortunately), tissue viability was maintained in "good" recipient beds and not well in poorly vascularized beds—the very hostile environment that is the present enigma for the reconstructive surgeon.—E.A. Luce, M.D.

High-Energy War Wounds: Flap Reconstruction
Stanec Z, Škrbić S, Džepina I, Hulina D, Ivrlač R, Unušić J, Montani D, Prpić I
(Univ of Zagreb, Croatia)
Ann Plast Surg 31:97–102, 1993   140-94-12-27

Objective.—As a result of the Croatian War, surgeons in Croatia have had to confront the problems of treating war wounds, most of which are caused by high-energy missiles. To understand the pathophysiology of these wounds, the surgeon must have some knowledge of terminal ballistics. Writing from Zagreb, surgeons review their experience in treating 75 patients with high-energy war wounds.

Methods.—The patients (average age, 30 years) all had massive soft tissue loss and associated open fractures, vascular injury, or nerve injury. The patients were divided into 3 groups, depending on the time of flap closure. Nine patients (group I) had reconstruction within 5 days of injury. In 14 patients (group II), reconstruction was done 6–15 days after injury. The remaining 54 patients (group III) did not have reconstruction until more than 15 days after injury.

On admission, patients underwent immediate surgical exploration with excision of wounds while under general anesthesia. The primary excision was evaluated after 24 hours to determine whether it was sufficient. Patients initially treated elsewhere were also evaluated to determine whether they needed additional débridement.

Findings.—Sixty-six percent of the injuries involved the lower extremities, 38% involving the lower leg. Fractures were present in nearly two thirds of the patients. Microsurgical technique and distant flaps were used for closure in about 40%. Nine percent of free flaps failed completely, and in 9% of local flaps, partial necrosis developed. More than three fourths of the patients in group I needed only 1 or 2 débridements, and 67% were discharged in less than 20 days. Although two thirds of group II patients needed only 1 or 2 débridements, they had a 14% incidence of flap failure. More than half of group III patients needed 3 or more débridements, and 82% remained hospitalized for more than 21 days.

Discussion.—In patients with high-energy war wounds, early reconstruction is a desirable goal that is only attainable with radical primary treatment. Even very small wounds can pose reconstruction problems because of the lack of sufficient skin and soft tissue cover. The subacute phase appears to be the worst time for reconstruction, in part because of the high rate of bacterial colonization at that time. Giving conservative treatment while waiting for granulation tissue to grow prolongs the hospital stay and risks contracture and functional loss of the extremity.

▶ Patients injured by material from warfare never seem to be lacking, despite "world peace." This series was derived from the conflict in Croatia and demonstrates the efficacy of the application of current reconstructive techniques of free tissue transfer and myocutaneous and fasciocutaneous flaps in the closure of high-velocity wounds. Eighty-five percent of the flaps used for wound closure/reconstruction involved 1 of these 3 techniques. The other point persuasively made by the authors is the necessity for achieving primary excision and closure of the wound in the early (3–5 days) postinjury period. How this concept meshes with the military practice of transporting soldiers with more complex wounds to rear hospitals is another issue. Extremity wounds, and especially upper extremity wounds, have a much better functional outcome if closed early, rather than allowing the formation of granulation tissue and eventual skin graft closure.—E.A. Luce, M.D.

13 Noncardiac Thoracic Surgery

Introduction

Surgical therapy remains the foundation of the treatment of solid tumors in the United States. For the thoracic surgeon, the diagnosis, staging, and therapy of lung cancer remains the centerpiece of clinical practice. Indeed, the incidence of lung cancer continues to escalate; it has now become the Number 1 killer in both women and men. Approximately 180,000 new cases of lung cancer were diagnosed in 1993, with an increase in incidence expected through the year 2000. Smoking remains the Number 1 cause of bronchogenic carcinoma. Unfortunately, although the incidence among adults has continued to decrease during the past decade, the incidence of smoking among young people, particularly females, continues to escalate. This proves to be of continued importance to the thoracic surgeon, because smoking is the principal cause of non–small-cell lung cancer and is exclusively the cause of small-cell cancer in the United States. The rising incidence of adenocarcinoma in nonsmoking females is also of note. Carcinoma now is a prime suspect in any nonsmoking female seen with a solitary mass in the lung.

Because of the importance of lung cancer in the everyday practice of a thoracic surgeon and because of its changing demographics, we have selected several papers that review the early diagnosis, staging, and therapy of bronchogenic carcinoma in a variety of stages. New molecular markers and clinical markers used in the staging of patients are reviewed by a variety of groups. The use of flow cytometry and monoclonal antibodies is addressed in several of the articles. These new markers may lead to early detection of patients who are at risk for local and distant recurrence. Every attempt has been made to keep the reader abreast of each of these new markers, as they are the subject of credible reports.

Of interest is the prognosis of lung cancer in young patients younger than 40 years of age. The efficacy of surgical and adjuvant intervention, as well as the primary use of radiotherapy, are examined in stages I, II, and III as well as in inoperable carcinoma. In patients with end-stage cancer, a variety of palliative techniques meant to alleviate symptomatology, including the use of laser and brachyradiography as well as some new palliative maneuvers, are reviewed.

Thoracoscopy in video-assisted thoracic surgery continues to be a focus of thoracic surgical investigation. In the papers reviewed in this year's

YEAR BOOK OF SURGERY, we note a progression from single-institution case reports to the emergence of comparison studies involving conventional techniques and thoracoscopic video-assisted approaches. We have selected a number of articles that appear to advance the field with meaningful study in well-controlled patient populations. The integration of these new techniques into the management scheme of patients is beginning to occur, as opposed to the simple replacement of operative technique with thoracoscopic approaches. We believe the articles reviewed in the section on thoracoscopy demonstrate this fact very nicely.

The surgeon's role in the treatment of metastatic disease to the pulmonary tree is reviewed in several articles contained in this YEAR BOOK. Decisions regarding indications and surgical intervention in patients with metastatic disease to the lung will depend on the surgeon's enhanced understanding of tumor biology, which varies from cell type to cell type. The selected papers reveal the differences in clinical behavior among various metastatic tumors. Each of these differences will tend to modulate the aggressiveness of the thoracic surgeon asked to evaluate patients for pulmonary metastasectomy. A variety of surgical approaches are evaluated and illustrated in these reports. It is hoped that this constellation of articles will assist the surgeon in the formation of a clinical plan and operative approach to this challenging group of patients.

The last section of this YEAR BOOK review contains several articles that illustrate recent advances in the understanding of the surgeon's role in a variety of malignancies of the chest. The treatment of patients with mesothelioma—a group of patients who often are difficult to approach surgically—is reviewed, providing new information that may be valuable to the thoracic surgeon in the management of these cases. Characterization of primary mediastinal lymphoma and the patterns of involvement, as well as the clinical behavior of pulmonary lymphoma, are presented and reviewed, because these cases often are not totally understood by the thoracic surgeon and the oncologic team. Finally, thymic carcinoma, which is a particular technical challenge to the thoracic surgeon, is reviewed in light of the application of multimodality therapy.

In the next decade, the thoracic surgeon will need to acquire a thorough understanding of the molecular markers of prognostic significance in a variety of tumors, as well as an understanding of the differences in the biological behavior of tumors of different cell types. This enhanced understanding will be required, because further decision-making will depend on this information. Selection of patients for adjuvant chemotherapy and radiotherapy, as well as the use of induction chemotherapy and radiotherapy, will depend on this understanding. It is hoped that this review will provide the basis for further study in this field, as well as provide practical information for today's thoracic surgeon as he or she makes clinical decisions on a daily basis.

David J. Sugarbaker, M.D.

The Treatment of Lung Cancer

EARLY DIAGNOSIS AND PROGNOSTIC FACTORS

Screening for Lung Cancer: The Mayo Lung Project Revisited

Flehinger BJ, Kimmel M, Polyak T, Melamed MR (T J Watson Research Ctr, Yorktown Heights, NY; Rice Univ, Houston; New York Med College, Valhalla)
Cancer 72:1573–1580, 1993   140-94-13-1

Background.—Lung cancer, the most significant cause of cancer death in the United States, is usually diagnosed when the disease is advanced and incurable. Early, asymptomatic lung cancer can be detected by the chest radiograph and sputum cytologic examination. The Mayo Lung Project (MLP) compared lung cancer incidence and mortality in a population offered these tests every 4 months and a population offered only the advice to undergo annual examination. Frequent screening was not associated with any mortality benefit. Whether a tangible potential benefit from radiographic screening might have been overlooked was determined.

Methods.—The MLP participants were men older than 45 years of age without known lung cancer who smoked at least 1 pack of cigarettes daily. They were randomized to undergo screening tests at intervals of 4 months for 6 years (4,618 patients) or to undergo yearly chest x-ray examinations and sputum tests (4,593 patients). At follow-up, 151 cancer cases (115 non–small-cell) were found in the patient group, and 121 cancer cases (87 non-small-cell) were found in the control group. There were 80 lung cancer deaths during the 7-year period in the patient group and 70 in the control group; non–small-cell cancer accounted for 50 and 43 deaths, respectively. Thus, the group with frequent screening actually had more cancer deaths.

Results.—A mathematical model of the progression kinetics of lung cancer in a population screened periodically for disease was developed. The mean duration of stage I non–small-cell lung cancer was found to be at least 4 years. The rates of stage I detectability and curability are less than 25% and 35%, respectively. Because the results of the MLP showed no benefit associated with screening, simulation techniques were used to explore the sample sizes and trial durations that would be necessary to demonstrate benefit. A program of 10,000 participants screened from age 45 until age 80 years or death might show a modest reduction in lung cancer mortality, ranging from 0% to 13%. Only 40% of the cancers would be found by screening.

Conclusion.—The benefits of frequent screening with chest radiographs and sputum tests would not be great. The methods of detection and treatment must be vastly improved before mortality from lung cancer can be reduced by more than 50%.

▶ The authors have reexamined a study with a very timely topic. They sought to review previous studies that have demonstrated no value for the screening of lung cancer by conventional plain chest radiography. The review and reanalysis of this project comes when the incidence of lung cancer in men and women continues to escalate.

Reanalysis (1) of both the Mayo Clinic (2, 3) and Memorial Sloan-Kettering (4, 5) lung cancer screening project reports has yielded conclusions that differ from those of the original reports. Strauss et al. (6) report a possible significant benefit in screening for lung cancer with plain chest films. Further analysis will need to be undertaken, and it is the belief of this author that soon plain chest x-ray films will be in routine use, particularly in the subset of patients with smoking histories or in current smokers.—D.J. Sugarbaker, M.D.

References

1. Flehinger BJ, et al: *Cancer* 72:1573, 1993.
2. Fontana RS, et al: *Am Rev Respir Dis* 130:561, 1984.
3. Fontana RS, et al: *J Occup Med* 28:746, 1986.
4. Melamed MR, et al: *Chest* 86:44, 1984.
5. Flehinger BJ, et al: *Am Rev Respir Dis* 130:555, 1984.
6. Strauss G, et al: *Proc Am Soc Clin Oncol* 12:329, 1993.

Blood Vessel Invasion by Tumor Cells Predicts Recurrence in Completely Resected T1 N0 M0 Non-Small-Cell Lung Cancer
Macchiarini P, Fontanini G, Hardin MJ, Chuanchieh H, Bigini D, Vignati S, Pingitore R, Angeletti CA (Univ of Pisa, Italy; Univ of Alabama at Birmingham)
J Thorac Cardiovasc Surg 106:80–89, 1993   140-94-13-2

Background.—The success or failure of surgery for early-stage non-small-cell lung cancer (NSCLC) has traditionally been estimated in terms of survival or disease-free interval, which may overestimate or underestimate the therapeutic index of the surgery. A number of parameters—including tumor size, histology, and location—have been identified as prognostic indicators of the natural history of NSCLC. In this study, traditional, as well as newer, tumor cell–related biological parameters were investigated.

Methods.—Ninety-five consecutive patients with T1, N0, M0 NSCLC were studied. All had had surgery alone between 1975 and 1985. The median follow-up was 8.3 years.

Findings.—The overall survival was 75% at 5 years, 69% at 10 years, and 61% at 15 years. Twenty-two patients died of local or systemic recurrent disease. Five died of causes unrelated to cancer, 2 died of new primary lung cancer, and 1 died of an extrathoracic cancer. According to multivariate analysis, blood vessel invasion by tumor cells and mitotic count independently predicted survival. By contrast, only blood vessel invasion affected disease-free survival. The relative risk of death from recurrent NSCLC for 79 low-risk patients was 13.3 times lower than that of the 16 patients at high risk. High-risk patients had a relative risk of recurrent disease manifesting as distant metastasis that was 25.6 times higher than that of low-risk patients.

Conclusion.—In completely resected T1, N0, M0 NSCLC, the presence or absence of intratumoral or peritumoral blood vessel invasion by cancer cells indicates high or low risk, respectively. Patients with a good prognosis may be considered for close monitoring without adjuvant treatment, because most of these patients can be cured by surgery alone. Patients at high risk may benefit from adjuvant systemic chemotherapy or new therapeutic interventions.

▶ This report is a follow-up of a previously published report by Macchiarini et al. With these patients added to the previous number reported in *Lancet* (1), the authors have further confirmed their original finding. That blood vessel invasion predicts for survival in T1, N0, M0 NSCLC in their series offers the foundation for further therapeutic studies.

Adjuvant therapy in the form of current chemotherapeutic agents or in the form of antiangiogenic factors, such as are currently available (Folkman, personal communication), may provide new strategies in the often disappointing therapy of stage I NSCLC. The potential importance of tumor size in predicting prognosis is particularly relevant to the use of neoadjuvant therapies. However, the need for biopsy tissue to elucidate various molecular, histologic, and genetic markers of recurrence precludes the use of neoadjuvant therapy in most instances.

Potential interest in tumor size as a predictor of stage I survival could be used as an indicator for the use of mediastinoscopy in cases in which the computerized tomogram of the chest does not show mediastinal node involvement. Previous studies (1, 2) have looked at the incidence of occult mediastinal nodes in patients with T2 and T3 lesions. These studies have confirmed an increased incidence of involved mediastinal nodes in patients with T2 or T3 lesions as opposed to T1. This has led some to suggest that mediastinoscopy might be considered based on the presence of T2 or T3 lesions despite a negative chest CT scan.

Of interest is the fact that the rate of differentiation and DNA ploidy pattern appeared to be the predominate prognostic factors in these patients with pathologic stage I NSCLC. The authors found the T size to be marginally significant ($P < .08$). This study needs to be interpreted in the light of previous studies indicating the potentially greater importance of tumor size.—D.J. Sugarbaker, M.D.

References

1. Macchiarini P, et al: *Lancet* 340:145, 1992.
2. Sugarbaker DJ, Strauss GM: *Semin Oncol* 20:163, 1993.

Prognostic Significance of Flow Cytometry in Non-Small-Cell Lung Cancer

Rice TW, Bauer TW, Gephardt GN, Medendorp SV, McLain DA, Kirby TJ (Cleveland Clinic Found, Ohio)
J Thorac Cardiovasc Surg 106:210–217, 1993   140-94-13–3

Background.—Disease stage is the most important prognostic factor for patients with non–small-cell bronchogenic carcinoma. The prognosis varies within staging groups, however, and there has been no way to identify patients at risk of recurrence. The value of DNA ploidy analysis was investigated in 272 patients with primary non–small-cell lung cancer (NSCLC).

Methods.—All study patients were previously untreated and had an adequate cancer specimen for flow cytometric analysis. The 179 men and 93 women had a mean age of 65.5 years. Thirty-nine percent had adenocarcinoma, 37% had squamous cell carcinoma, 21% had large cell carcinoma, 3% had adenosquamous carcinoma, and less than 1% had giant cell carcinoma. Histologic grade at diagnosis was I in 6%, II in 37%, and III in 58%; the American Joint Committee on Cancer (AJCC) stage was I in 56%, II in 14%, III in 27%, and IV in 3%.

Results.—Flow cytometry detected no aneuploidy in 18% of tumors and aneuploid populations in 82%. Overall, the 1-year survival rate was 74% and the 3-year survival rate was 52%. On multivariate analysis of the nonsquamous cell tumors, factors independently associated with poor outcome were increasing AJCC stage, male sex, and histologic grades II and III. However, presence of DNA aneuploidy, classification of the DNA histogram, DNA index, and results of cell cycle analysis in aneuploid tumors showed no prognostic significance. On multivariate analysis of the squamous cell tumors, the independent (negative) prognostic factors were increasing AJCC stage and increasing DNA index. Aneuploidy was not a significant factor, although patients with hypertetraploid tumors tended to have decreased survival.

Conclusion.—Only limited prognostic value of flow cytometry for DNA quantification of NSCLC was found in this study. The DNA index does appear to be a significant predictor of decreased survival in squamous cell tumors. Future refinements in DNA analysis may produce more useful prognostic information.

▶ The prognostic significance of flow cytometry in NSCLC has been the subject of study in several recent publications. This useful technique can provide a quantitative reproducible analysis of specific cellular characteristics. It is automated and can examine samples of tumor of 10^5 cells in minutes. Studies can be performed on fresh tumors or those obtained from paraffin blocks. This technique identifies 2 cellular characteristics that have prognostic significance: the DNA content of tumor cells or ploidy, and the fraction of cells in specific phases of the cell cycle. Specifically, this means the content of DNA in tumor cells is determined to be either greater than normal or normal, i.e., aneuploid or diploid, and the fraction of cells in the S phase is taken to indicate the tumor's mytotic activity.

The interesting aspect of this particular paper is the comparison of nonsquamous to squamous tumors of the lung. In nonsquamous tumors, in addition to the AJCC staging, male gender and histologic grades II and III were of independent prognostic significance; the presence of aneuploidy, classification of the DNA histogram, and the results of cell cycle analysis in tumors with no aneuploidy were of no prognostic significance. In contrast, squamous cell lung cancers demonstrated, via multivariate analysis, that in addition to the AJCC stage, an increase in the DNA index was of negative prognostic significance.

It is of additional interest that male gender was a negative prognostic factor in this study. The study has confirmed previous reports that showed no prognostic significance for the use of analysis by flow cytometry in patients with NSCLC; however, it demonstrated a significant correlation between the content of DNA, as determined by flow, and patient survival. The exact prognostic significance and role of flow cytometry in NSCLC remains to be elucidated. Disappointing results from surgical therapy alone continue to prompt reexamination of this readily available technique as, hopefully, its potential and prognostic therapeutic impact are continually reexamined. See reference 1 for further information.—D.J. Sugarbaker, M.D.

Reference

1. Merkel DE, et al: *J Clin Oncol* 5:1690, 1987.

---

bcl-2 Protein in Non–Small-Cell Lung Carcinoma

Pezzella F, Turley H, Kuzu I, Tungekar MF, Dunnill MS, Pierce CB, Harris A, Gatter KC, Mason DY (John Radcliffe Hosp, Oxford, England)
N Engl J Med 329:690–694, 1993   140-94-13–4

Background.—The *bcl-2* proto-oncogene participates in the 14;18 translocation, a chromosomal abnormality found in 70% of follicular lymphomas and in 20% of diffuse B-cell lymphomas. It may be that the oncogene is also expressed in basal epithelial cells, such as those of the skin and intestine, serving to aid the survival of stem cells while preventing the excessive accumulation of differentiated cells. Persistent expression of *bcl-2* might provide a mechanism of neoplastic cell growth.

Objective and Methods.—Samples of tumor tissue were collected from 122 patients having primary lung cancers resected. Immunochemical analysis using a monoclonal antibody specific for *bcl*-2 was used to detect the protein and quantify the extent of gene expression. Eighty squamous cell carcinomas and 42 adenocarcinomas were evaluated. Follow-up data were available for 115 patients during a median of 34 months.

Results.—One fifth of the tumors were found to have *bcl*-2 protein. Basal cells in areas of normal epithelium adjacent to the tumor stained positively, but columnar cells did not. Expression of *bcl*-2 could not be related to the grade of tumor differentiation, T stage, or N stage. No major difference in survival was noted according to whether the protein was present. When only the patients with squamous cell cancer were analyzed, however, *bcl*-2 status was a better predictor of survival than was the state of the regional nodes. Patients aged 60 years and older who had *bcl*-2-positive tumors had the best outlook.

Conclusion.—Some non–small-cell lung cancers (NSCLCs) express *bcl*-2 to an abnormal degree, and the extent of expression may have prognostic import.

▶ This study is of importance because it has identified a potentially positive prognostic factor in patients with NSCLC. The proto-oncogene *bcl*-2 encodes for a protein that prevents apoptosis (programmed cell death). It is normally found in the basal cells of human epithelium. The authors have noted that the presence of *bcl*-2 in patients with NSCLC was correlated with an improved survival. This was particularly true in patients older than 60 years of age. It was true in patients with squamous cell carcinoma as well as all other patients. Cox regression analysis revealed that the presence of *bcl*-2 was a stronger predictor of survival than node status in patients with squamous cell cancers. The mechanism by which the presence of the *bcl*-2 proto-oncogene is associated with enhanced survival remains to be elucidated.—D.J. Sugarbaker, M.D.

IMPROVED TECHNIQUES FOR PREOPERATIVE STAGING

NR-LU-10 Monoclonal Antibody Scanning: A Helpful New Adjunct to Computed Tomography in Evaluating Non-Small-Cell Lung Cancer

Rusch V, Macapinlac H, Heelan R, Kramer E, Larson S, McCormack P, Burt M, Martini N, Ginsberg R (Mem Sloan-Kettering Cancer Ctr, New York; New York Univ)

J Thorac Cardiovasc Surg 106:200–204, 1993   140-94-13–5

Background.—Although it is useful in the noninvasive staging of lung cancer, CT is unable to differentiate benign and malignant lesions. The new, radiolabeled murine immunoglobulin G2b antibody NR-LU-10 recognizes a 40-kD glycoprotein expressed in lung and other epithelial cancers. The use of this antibody as an adjunct to CT in detecting malignant primary lung tumors and lesions of the mediastinal nodes was investigated.

Methods.—A prospective, single-arm trial included 24 patients with known or suspected non–small-cell lung cancer (NSCLC) who were scheduled to undergo mediastinoscopy or thoracotomy. All had potentially resectable tumors. Each patient underwent whole body and single-photon emission CT 14 to 17 hours after intravenous infusion of NR-LU-10, 20–30 mCi. The complete mediastinal node map obtained at mediastinoscopy or thoracotomy was used to confirm the CT findings.

Results.—There were no adverse reactions to antibody administration. High-quality images were obtained in all patients but one, in whom there was interference from a previous ventilation-perfusion scan. Antibody uptake was noted in all 22 primary malignant tumors; one lung nodule that later proved to be benign showed no uptake. Surgical correlation of mediastinal node involvement was obtained in 21 patients. Five of these patients had false positive results with NR-LU-10, and one had a false negative result. With CT, 6 had false positive results and one had a false negative result.

Conclusion.—These promising results of NR-LU-10 monoclonal antibody scanning for detecting primary NSCLC await confirmation in larger clinical trials. The technique is safe and easy to perform, and it produces good images of the lung and mediastinum. Its value in mediastinal staging must be studied further, especially as an adjunct to CT for distinguishing malignant from benign lesions.

▶ The authors from this large cancer center have an excellent opportunity to evaluate new staging techniques in NSCLC. Development of monoclonal antibodies to specific cell surface tumor antigens has been the subject of study in many malignancies. The ability to accurately detect the presence of neoplastic disease in the mediastinum before surgical resection would have tremendous usefulness in the neoadjuvant therapy of patients with NSCLC.

If the technique, as described by the group from Memorial Sloan-Kettering, were to be validated clinically by other centers, it could be used as a means of assessing the presence of malignant disease and solitary pulmonary nodules, as well as detecting the presence of active disease in patients treated in neoadjuvant protocols. Specifically, this study could heavily impact on the clinicians' decision to watch solitary pulmonary nodules in follow-up or to proceed immediately with a surgical resection or fine-needle aspiration. Additionally, particularly protocols using induction therapy for lymph node stage IIIA and IIIB NSCLC could use such a technique to assess the adequacy of induction therapy before a surgical resection. The number and composition of conventional chemotherapeutic approaches, as well as the use of preoperative radiotherapy, could be determined based on such techniques should they ultimately be validated in multi-institutional trials.

The traditional problem with monoclonal antibodies to cell surface tumor antigens has been their nonspecificity and nonsensitivity. The group from

Memorial Sloan-Kettering may have identified a particular antibody in NR-LU-10 that has a higher sensitivity and specificity to this particular disease. A positron emission tomography scanner has also been used to detect the presence of neoplastic cells based on the uptake of sugars before scanning. See also reference 1.—D.J. Sugarbaker, M.D.

Reference

1. Patz EF Jr, et al: *AJR* 159:961, 1992.

The Role of Mediastinoscopic Biopsy in Preoperative Assessment of Lung Cancer
Funatsu T, Matsubara Y, Hatakenaka R, Kosaba S, Yasuda Y, Ikeda S (Kyoto-Katsura Hosp, Kyoto, Japan)
J Thorac Cardiovasc Surg 104:1688–1695, 1992   140-94-13-6

Background.—Mediastinal lymph node involvement strongly affects prognosis in patients with lung cancer. Appropriate treatment relies on the accurate preoperative determination of mediastinal lymph node involvement. The role of mediastinoscopic biopsy in the preoperative evaluation of lung cancer was investigated.

Methods and Findings.—Mediastinoscopy and thoracotomy were performed on 619 patients with lung cancer seen at 1 clinic between 1970 and 1989. When analyzed by lymph node location, mediastinoscopy was most sensitive for the left paratracheal nodes and least sensitive for

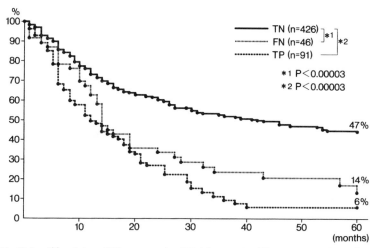

Fig 13–1.—*Abbreviations:* TN, true negative; FN, false negative; TP, true positive. Survivals according to results of mediastinoscopy, excluding patients whose thoracotomies were only exploratory. (Courtesy of Funatsu T, Matsubara Y, Hatakenaka R, et al: *J Thorac Cardiovasc Surg* 104:1688–1695, 1992.)

nodes at the bifurcation. Those sensitivities were 95.7% and 64%, respectively. According to the results of mediastinoscopy, the 5-year survival rates were 47% for patients with negative results, 14% for those with false negative results, and 6% for those with positive results. The 5-year survival rate was significantly higher at 28% in 13 patients with positive mediastinoscopic findings who had complete resection of the primary tumor and all involved nodes than in the 78 patients who had incomplete resection (Fig 13-1).

Conclusion.—Mediastinoscopy has a role in the assessment of lung cancer before treatment, not in the selection of patients for thoracotomy. Patients with positive mediastinoscopic findings should not always be excluded from thoracotomy treatment.

▶ This is an interesting study from an historical standpoint. Dr. Dwight Harken (1), of the Peter Bent Brigham Hospital in Boston, first described the possible prognostic significance of mediastinal lymph nodes obtained via a cervical mediastinal exploration. This work was later corroborated by Dr. Kern (2) and Dr. Pearson (3, 4). In the Toronto experience (3, 4), patients with a positive mediastinoscopy before surgical resection did significantly worse than those whose mediastinum was either negative or falsely negative by mediastinoscopy.

The study abstracted here, which has a more recent cohort of patients, confirms the findings of the Toronto experience. However, the authors' conclusion that mediastinoscopy has a role in the assessment of lung cancer before treatment but not in the patients selected for treatment with surgery alone, is somewhat preposterous. I believe the more demonstrated efficacy of neoadjuvant or induction chemoradiotherapy in the treatment of patients with positive mediastinal nodes warrants all of these patients being treated in such a fashion, given the poor overall survival in the group with surgery alone (approximately 20% for all N2 patients with positive nodes in this study). This rather dismal outlook compares poorly with phase II and early phase III trials of neoadjuvant therapy (5).—D.J. Sugarbaker, M.D.

References

1. Harken DE, et al: N Engl J Med 251:1041, 1954.
2. Kern JA, et al: Cancer Res 50:5184, 1990.
3. Pearson FG: J Thorac Cardiovasc Surg 49:11, 1965.
4. Pearson FG: J Thorac Cardiovasc Surg 55:617, 1968.
5. Rosell R, et al: N Engl J Med 330:153, 1994.

REPORTS OF STAGE-RELATED THERAPIES AND TREATMENTS

Primary Lung Cancer in Young Patients: A Study of 82 Surgically Treated Patients
Icard P, Regnard J-F, de Napoli S, Rojas-Miranda A, Dartevelle P, Levasseur P
(Marie-Lannelongue Hosp, Le Plessis Robinson, France)
Ann Thorac Surg 54:99–103, 1992   140-94-13-7

Background.—Lung cancer in individuals younger than 40 years of age is thought to have a poorer prognosis than lung cancer in older patients. The prognosis for resected cancers in young patients, however, is not well documented.

Methods.—Eighty-two patients younger than 40 years of age who had surgery between 1982 and 1990 were studied to determine prognosis. Fifty-nine percent of the patients had smoked for more than 20 pack-years. Forty-two percent had adenocarcinoma; 28% had epidermoid carcinoma; 16% had mixed cell carcinoma; 8.5% had small cell carcinoma; and 6% had undifferentiated large cell carcinoma. Sixty-nine tumors were resected. Twenty-two of those were stage I, 10 were stage II, 32 were stage IIIa, and 5 were stage IIIb.

Outcomes.—Resection was considered complete and curative in 68% and noncurative in 32%. The overall actuarial 5-year survival rate was 41%. For those who had complete resection, the actuarial 5-year survival rate was 56%. The actuarial 5-year survival rates were 70% for patients in stage I; 54% in stage II; 28% in stage IIIa; and 0% in stage IIIb. Patients having exploratory thoracotomy only had a survival rate of 18% (Fig

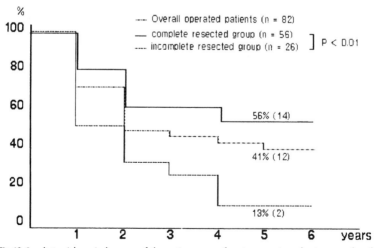

Fig 13–2.—Actuarial survival curves of the entire group of patients, patients having complete (curative) resection, and those having incomplete (palliative) resection. (Courtesy of Icard P, Regnard J-F, de Napoli S, et al: *Ann Thorac Surg* 54:99–103, 1992.)

13–2). Those rates are comparable to rates in patients older than 40 years of age with similar stages of disease. Sex, age younger than 30 years, smoking status, and histologic type did not affect survival. Survival depended primarily on extent of disease.

Conclusion.—These findings suggest that, at similar disease stages, resection is associated with a survival rate that is at least as high in younger patients as in older ones. The prognosis for younger patients seems to be related more to disease extent than to particularly aggressive cancer behavior.

▶ This interesting paper looks at a problem that every thoracic surgeon in our society faces. It is clear from our own practice, as well as from discussions with other surgeons, that the median age of patients with carcinoma of the lung continues to decrease. Of note is the similar survival, on a stage-by-stage basis, of patients younger than 40 years of age compared with previous reports of older patient populations.

It is of particular interest that there has been some suggestion in previous literature that genetic tendencies have led to the earlier development of lung cancer in certain populations. It was thought that this genetic predisposition could lead to a poor prognosis.

Also of note is that 59% of the patients in this study who were younger than 40 years of age had smoked for more than 20 pack-years. This is an indication of earlier smoking habits, which are now documented in society.

This paper suggests that patients younger than 40 years should be staged aggressively from a surgical standpoint, because one cannot expect these patients to do any better, based on their age, than the older populations. This importance of age is often used by surgeons as an excuse for overly aggressive surgical intervention. It is clear from this paper that patients in this series, as in previous reports, do better when complete surgical resection is achieved.—D.J. Sugarbaker, M.D.

Clinical Stage II Non-Small Cell Lung Cancer Treated With Radiation Therapy Alone: The Significance of Clinically Staged Ipsilateral Hilar Adenopathy (N1 Disease)
Rosenthal SA, Curran WJ Jr, Herbert SH, Hughes EN, Sandler HM, Stafford PM, McKenna WG (Fox Chase Cancer Ctr/Univ of Pennsylvania, Philadelphia)
Cancer 70:2410–2417, 1992   140-94-13–8

Background.—The role of radiation therapy in the treatment of patients with unresected non–small-cell lung carcinoma (NSCLC) is still debated. The prognosis associated with clinical stages N1 and II NSCLC treated with radiation therapy alone has not been well documented.

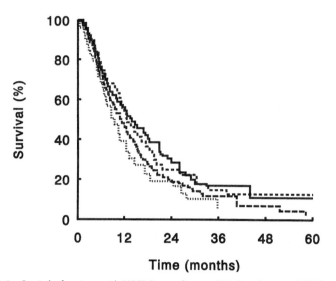

Fig 13–3.—Survival of patients with NSCLC according to clinical node stage. *Solid line indicates* N0; *short-dashed line*, N1; *long-dashed line*, N2; *dotted line*, N3. (Courtesy of Rosenthal SA, Curran WJ Jr, Herbert SH, et al: *Cancer* 70:2410–2417, 1992.)

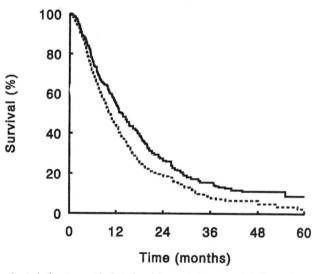

Fig 13–4.—Survival of patients with clinical nodal stage 0–1 vs. stage 2–3 disease (P = .0006). *Solid line* indicates N0-1; *dashed line*, N2-3. (Courtesy of Rosenthal SA, Curran WJ Jr, Herbert SH, et al: *Cancer* 70:2410–2417, 1992.)

Methods.—The records of 758 patients with stages I–III NSCLC were reviewed. All had undergone radiation therapy. Sixty-two patients had clinical stage II NSCLC, and 126 had stage N1 disease.

Findings.—Patients with stage II disease had a median survival of 17.9 months. Overall actuarial survival rates at 1, 2, 3, and 5 years were 70%, 33%, 20%, and 12%, respectively. The survival of patients with stage II disease was significantly better than that of 389 patients with stage IIIA and 267 with stage IIIB disease. However, it was comparable to that of 40 patients with clinical stage I tumors. Patients with a performance status of 0–1 lived longer than patients with a status of 2 or more. The median survival was 13.7 months for patients with stage N0 disease, 12.6 months with stage N1, 10.9 months with stage N2, and 9.1 months with stage N3. The median survival of patients with stage N0–1 disease was significantly longer than that of patients with stage N2–3 disease (Figs 13–3 and 13–4).

Conclusion.—Clinical stage and clinical N stage are significant prognostic factors for patients with NSCLC treated with radiation therapy. Definitive radiation therapy can be used to treat clinical stage II disease in patients who cannot or will not undergo surgery.

▶ This report is of interest in that surgeons rarely get a look at the results of radiation therapy as primary treatment in NSCLC. Radiation is often an alluring alternative, particularly for patients with traditional risk factors for thoracic surgery. It is of note that the median survival rate for all stages at 5 years was 12%. It is clear that without surgical staging, the distinction between stage I, II, and III disease, based on radiographic evidence of nodal disease, is highly inaccurate. This is because of the incidence of benign lymphadenopathy in this subgroup of patients.

What appears to be clear from this paper is that radiotherapy has a very small role to play in the therapy of stage III disease, based on the numbers reported in this study. One can expect a salvage in patients with stage I and II disease treated with radiation therapy or chemotherapy when surgical resection is prohibited. It may be that with the advent of new, less invasive means of surgical resection, the disease in many of these patients will be considered resectable.—D.J. Sugarbaker, M.D.

Adjuvant Chemotherapy After Radical Surgery for Non-Small-Cell Lung Cancer: A Randomized Study

Niiranen A, Niitamo-Korhonen S, Kouri M, Assendelft A, Mattson K, Pyrhönen S (Helsinki Univ; North Karelia Central Hosp, Finland)
J Clin Oncol 10:1927–1932, 1992   140-94-13–9

Background.—There has been renewed interest in the use of preoperative or postoperative chemotherapy in patients with non–small-cell lung cancer (NSCLC) in the past 10 years. The efficacy and toxicity of adjuvant chemotherapy in patients undergoing radical surgery for NSCLC were investigated.

Methods.—One hundred ten patients treated from 1982 through 1987 were included in the study. After surgery, 54 patients were randomly assigned to receive adjuvant chemotherapy with cyclophosphamide, 400 mg/m^2; doxorubicin, 40 mg/m^2; and cisplatin, 40 mg/m^2 for 6 cycles; 56 patients were assigned to receive no treatment.

Findings.—Ten years after initiation of the study, 61% of the patients in the chemotherapy group were alive, compared with 48% in the control group. The recurrence rates were 31% and 48%, respectively. The 5-year survival rates in the chemotherapy and control groups were 67% and 56%, respectively. Patients in the treatment group who completed therapy had a slightly better 5-year survival rate than patients stopping chemotherapy. Gastrointestinal toxicity of grade 3–4, occurring in 63%, was the main reason for stopping chemotherapy.

Conclusion.—Adjuvant chemotherapy in patients with radically resected NSCLC merits further study. Patients in such studies should be stratified in groups according to surgical extent before randomization. Effective antiemetic treatments are needed to improve compliance with chemotherapeutic regimens.

▶ The use of adjuvant chemotherapy in patients with stage II or microscopic stage III NSCLC is without significant evidence for efficacy in the literature. The single largest prospective, randomized trial conducted by the Lung Cancer Study Group demonstrated no efficacy in the use of CAP chemotherapy (cyclophosphamide, doxorubicin, and cisplatin) in patients with N1 or microscopic N2 disease who had undergone complete surgical resection. This study, therefore, runs counter to current thinking and may represent a significant advance in our understanding of the use of adjuvant chemotherapy in the treatment of NSCLC. Its examination of patients with T1–3 N0 NSCLC who had undergone surgical resection demonstrates that the real efficacy of chemotherapy may be in the earlier stages of disease. The 13% difference in 10-year survival between the 2 study groups would represent a large number of patients if one extrapolated it to the incidence of NSCLC in the United States.

Nevertheless, the importance of improved survival in patients with stage I disease receiving adjuvant chemotherapy, as documented in this report, would certainly demand multi-institutional prospective randomized trials to confirm its efficacy. This could lead to a change in the way patients with NSCLC who are undergoing surgical resection are routinely treated in the United States. Surgeons should be on the lookout for new studies currently being done by the National Institutes of Health, within the Cancer and Leukemia Group B and other cooperative groups.—D.J. Sugarbaker, M.D.

Role of Systematic Mediastinal Dissection in N2 Non-Small Cell Lung Cancer Patients

Nakahara K, Fujii Y, Matsumura A, Minami M, Okumura M, Matsuda H
(Osaka Univ, Japan)
Ann Thorac Surg 56:331–336, 1993   140-94-13-10

Introduction.—Several workers believe that even N2 lung cancer calls for extensive mediastinal dissection, because skip metastases and multilevel metastases frequently are found in the mediastinal nodes. It is possible that a reason for the apparently poor outlook of patients with N2 disease is that some who died of recurrent disease shortly after surgery may actually have had N3 disease.

Series.—The operative results were reviewed in 26 patients with primary lung cancer who had confirmed N2 disease on the basis of histologic assessment of suspicious lymph nodes but did not undergo systematic mediastinal dissection (PI group). Another 50 patients (R2 group) did have systematic mediastinal dissection, and 17 patients (R3 group) underwent bilateral mediastinal dissection. Four of the latter patients were N3-positive and 13 were N3-negative.

Observations.—The PI and R2 groups had respective 5-year survival rates of 8% and 16%, which is not a significant difference. All 4 patients in the R3 group who were N3-positive died of recurrent disease within 14 months of surgery. Patients in the R3 group who were N3-negative had a 3-year survival rate of 51% compared with 33% for the R2 group, also not a significant difference. The PI group had a 3-year survival rate of only 24%. Patients with N2 metastases in 2 stations or less did better than those with 3 or more N2-positive stations.

Conclusion.—Bilateral mediastinal dissection provides important prognostic information in patients with N2 non–small-cell lung cancer. It is especially important when 3 or more stations are N2-positive.

▶ Through the years, the role of systemic mediastinal node dissection has been a source of debate among thoracic surgeons. The routine use of radical mediastinal node dissection has been favored by some groups, whereas the selective use of radical node dissection in certain clinical situations has been noted by others, particularly those using routine mediastinoscopy.

This particular study is of note because it demonstrates the overall lack of therapeutic efficacy of systemic nodal dissection in patients with N2 disease. The overall survival rate quoted in this paper is dismal, again pointing out the need to identify these patients before surgical resection in the hope of extending their survival with the use of induction chemotherapy protocols. Indeed, the advent of prospective randomized trials confirming the efficacy of systemic neoadjuvant chemotherapy makes much of the discussion in this paper and similar ones moot. See also references 1 and 2.—D.J. Sugarbaker, M.D.

References

1. Rosell R, et al: N Engl J Med 330:153, 1994.
2. Strauss GM, et al: J Clin Oncol 10:829, 1992.

Surgical Resection of Stage IIIA and Stage IIIB Non-Small-Cell Lung Cancer After Concurrent Induction Chemoradiotherapy: A Southwest Oncology Group Trial
Rusch VW, Albain KS, Crowley JJ, Rice TW, Lonchyna V, McKenna R Jr, Livingston RB, Griffin BR, Benfield JR (Mem Sloan-Kettering Cancer Ctr, New York; Loyola Univ Chicago, Maywood, Ill; Southwest Oncology Group Statistical Office, Seattle; et al)
J Thorac Cardiovasc Surg 105:97–106, 1993   140-94-13-11

Background.—For patients with stage IIIA non–small-cell lung cancer (NSCLC) there is evidence that preoperative induction chemotherapy, with or without radiotherapy, can improve resectability and survival. Associated morbidity and mortality can be considerable. The potential benefits of this approach have not been examined in stage IIIB NSCLC.

Methods.—A multicenter phase II study of concurrent preoperative chemoradiotherapy for 146 patients with stage IIIA or IIIB NSCLC was reported. Complete data for evaluation were available for 75 patients, two thirds of them men. The median patient age was 58 years. All patients had pathologically confirmed T1 to T4, N2 to N3 disease without pleural effusions. All received induction chemotherapy with cisplatin, 50 mg/m² on days 1, 8, 9, 29, and 36; VP-16, 50 mg/m² on days 1 to 5 and 29 to 33; and concurrent radiotherapy, 4,500 cGy in 180 cGy fractions. Patients with at least a stable response underwent attempted resection 3 to 5 weeks after induction therapy. All patients underwent complete nodal mapping at the time of thoracotomy.

Results.—Ninety-one percent of patients were eligible for surgery, and 84% went through with thoracotomy. Complete resection was possible in 73%, including 12 of 16 patients with a stable response. There was a 6% postoperative mortality rate. One third of patients needed some type of complex resection, such as lobectomy plus chest wall or spine resection. However, mean operating time was about 3 hours and mean blood loss was less than 1,000 mL for patients with stage IIIA or IIIB disease. Of the 53 patients on whom complete pathologic data were available, 21% were completely tumor free and 30% had rare microscopic cancerous foci. In both tumor stages, the 2-year survival rate was 40%.

Conclusion.—Good response and resectability rates with preoperative induction chemotherapy and radiation were reported in patients with stage IIIA and IIIB NSCLC. The induction chemotherapy was generally well tolerated, and survival better than in historic controls. The foundations for future phase III clinical trials of concurrent induction chemoradiotherapy have been laid.

▶ It is of interest that of the 146 patients entered in the protocol, only 75 were eligible for data analysis. This is presumed to be the result of difficulty in obtaining clinical records. This substantial reduction in the number of patients eligible for data analysis makes further conclusions somewhat difficult. The use of the authors' therapeutic approach in stage IIIB disease represents new ground in the use of surgical resection in locally advanced NSCLC. It is not clear how patients with stage IIIb disease were successfully resected. Nevertheless, this study does represent the type of thoracic surgical research we are looking for, i.e., a National Institutes of Health–sponsored multi-institutional prospective trial. The precise placement of particular modalities needs to be further validated in prospective randomized trials in multi-institutional settings. See the references.—D.J. Sugarbaker, M.D.

References

1. Kirn DH, et al: *J Thorac Cardiovasc Surg* 106:696, 1993.
2. Strauss GM, et al: *J Clin Oncol* 10:829, 1992.
3. Sugarbaker DJ, Strauss GM: *Semin Oncol* 20:163, 1993.

▶↓ The following reports will conclude our discussion of advanced non–small-cell lung cancer (NSCLC). Each deals with traditionally unresectable (T4) lesions that have led investigators to innovative surgical, radiotherapeutic, chemotherapeutic, and technical approaches. These papers are included to highlight that in patients with advanced NSCLC, treating physicians are often ready to discontinue further treatment without exploring a palliative treatment option.—D.J. Sugarbaker, M.D.

Anterior Transcervical-Thoracic Approach for Radical Resection of Lung Tumors Invading the Thoracic Inlet
Dartevelle PG, Chapelier AR, Macchiarini P, Lenot B, Cerrina J, Ladurie FLR, Parquin FJF, Lafont D (Paris-Sud Univ, Le Plessis Robinson, France)
J Thorac Cardiovasc Surg 105:1025–1034, 1993   140-94-13-12

Introduction.—The combination of preoperative radiotherapy and radical resection has become the standard treatment of bronchogenic carcinomas of the superior pulmonary sulcus situated in the thoracic inlet. However, when such tumors have extensive involvement of adjacent structures above the thoracic inlet, the classic posterior thoracic approach cannot be used. An original, anterior, transcervical-thoracic approach for the surgical treatment of non–small-cell lung cancer (NSCLC) invading the thoracic inlet was studied.

Patients and Methods.—The technique described was used in 29 of the more than 3,000 patients who underwent surgery for lung cancer at the study institution between January 1980 and June 1991. Most (83%) of these patients were men; the median age was 56 years. Through a large L-shaped incision and after removal of the internal half of the clavicle, the steps performed might include dissection or resection of the subclavian vein, section of the anterior scalenus muscle and resection of the cervical portion of the phrenic nerve (if invaded), exposure of the subclavian and vertebral arteries, dissection of the brachial plexus up to the spinal foramen, section of invaded ribs, and en bloc removal of chest wall and lung tumor. In 20 cases, an additional posterior thoracotomy was required for resection of the chest wall below the second rib. Twelve patients had vascular involvement, which included either alone or in various combinations, the subclavian artery, the subclavian vein, and the vertebral artery.

Results.—Fourteen patients had wedge resections, 14 had lobectomies, and 1 required pneumonectomy. Twenty-five patients had postoperative radiotherapy (11 in combination with adjuvant chemotherapy). There were no operative or hospital deaths. With a median follow-up of 2.5 years, the overall 2-year survival was 50% and 5-year survival was 31%. Twelve patients were alive and free of carcinoma at 4 to more than 137 months. Neither univariate nor multivariate analysis revealed any clinical, pathologic, or surgical characteristics influencing survival.

Conclusion.—Long-term survival was encouraging in this series of patients who underwent radical resection of NSCLC involving the thoracic inlet by means of the transcervical-thoracic approach. Such patients represent a very small fraction of those with lung carcinoma, but they would otherwise be considered inoperable.

▶ This group from Hôpital Marie-Lannelongue, Paris-Sud University, Le Plessis Robinson, France, has made many contributions to the understanding of a therapeutic option in advanced NSCLC. The anterior transcervical-thoracic approach for radical resection of thoracic inlet tumors is well illustrated.

This surgical technique should only be attempted by those surgeons who are well experienced in Pancoast and extended Pancoast resections. A potential for extreme surgical morbidity is present in this approach. The need for the preoperative informed consent of patients who may experience a complete loss of the function of the arm as a result of transection of the brachial plexus, as described by Dr. Dartevelle, makes a complete understanding of this clinical situation imperative for each patient.

Nevertheless, the survival probability, as noted in this study, should mandate that this therapeutic option at least be contemplated. Moreover, the wider use of induction chemoradiotherapy in patients with large tumors in the apex may provide further rationale for surgical resection in these specific cases. See also reference 1.—D.J. Sugarbaker, M.D.

Reference

1. Harpole DJ Jr, et al: *Chest* 1994, in press.

Hypofractionated Radiation Therapy in Unresectable Stage III Non-Small Cell Lung Cancer

Slotman BJ, Njo KH, de Jonge A, Meijer OWM, Karim ABMF (Free Univ Hosp, Amsterdam)

Cancer 72:1885–1893, 1993   140-94-13–13

Background.—In patients with non–small-cell lung cancer (NSCLC), the highest cure rates are achieved by surgery, although not many patients are eligible for curative resection. Thus, most patients are treated via radiation therapy. In patients with advanced NSCLC, this treatment is considered to be of palliative benefit. At one institution, hypofractionation is the current radiation therapy for patients with stage III and IV NSCLC, as this treatment decreases inconvenience for patients, particularly those in poor condition or those having to travel long distances. The results of treatment using 3 hypofractionated radiation programs in patients with stage III NSCLC were evaluated.

Patients and Methods.—A total of 301 patients with unresectable stage III disease were included in a nonrandomized study. Of these, 90 patients were treated with a 40-Gy split course given in 3 weeks; 128 received 30–32 Gy in 6 fractions, and 83 were given 24 Gy in 3 fractions. No patient was lost to follow-up, which occurred at a minimum of 25 months.

Results.—Patients with stage IIIA disease treated with the 40-Gy split course had longer survival and lower local relapse rates compared with those receiving 24–32 Gy. Survival for stage IIIA patients treated with 40 Gy for 1-, 2-, and 5-years comprised 47%, 22%, and 7%, respectively. For patients with stage IIIB disease, no correlations between the radiation program used and survival and relapse rates was seen. In these patients, survival rates were 30%, 9%, and 2% for treatment intervals of 1, 2, and 5 years, respectively. Patients tolerated the radiation programs well, with no severe complications.

Conclusion.—Survival rates similar to those obtained using standard radiation therapy were found in stage IIIA patients treated with a 40-Gy split-course radiation program. In addition, patients with stage IIIB and IV NSCLC treated with 24 Gy in 3 weekly fractions achieved survival rates similar to those obtained when higher doses given in more fractions are used. For patients in poor general condition or with tumors too advanced for radical treatment, treatment inconveniences should be minimized. Thus, a short course of radiation therapy (e.g., the 24-Gy in 3 weekly fractions) may be used.

▶ This paper confirms a suspicion that many surgeons have had through the years, i.e., that in patients undergoing palliative radiation therapy, the treatment schedule itself can be onerous for a patient with limited life expectancy. The use of limited courses of radiotherapy with larger fractions given in weekly doses would appear to be an important option for patients and treating physicians.

The methodology of this paper is fairly clear and rational. It appears that prospective, randomized multi-institutional trials would now be in order for documenting the efficacy of hypofractionation in unresectable stage III NSCLC.—D.J. Sugarbaker, M.D.

Hypotonic Cisplatin Treatment for Carcinomatous Pleuritis Found at Thoracotomy in Patients With Lung Cancer: In Vitro Experiments and Preliminary Clinical Results
Ichinose Y, Hara N, Ohta M, Asoh H, Yano T, Maeda K, Yagawa K (Natl Kyushu Cancer Ctr, Fukuoka, Japan; Kyushu Univ, Fukuoka, Japan)
J Thorac Cardiovasc Surg 105:1041–1046, 1993   140-94-13–14

Introduction.—The finding of carcinomatous pleuritis at thoracotomy in patients with non–small-cell lung cancer (NSCLC) is considered a contraindication to surgical resection. Because these lesions will eventually become symptomatic, an intraoperative intrapleural treatment for the control of pleural disease has been developed.

Methods.—In vitro experiments were followed by a trial of the treatment in 7 patients with pleural carcinomatosis. Three different cell lines were used as a model of malignant pleural effusion. The cells were exposed to cisplatin in either phosphate-buffered saline solution (PBS) or distilled water for .5 to 5 minutes. After a 3-day culture, cell growth and viability were examined. The procedure performed in the patients consisted of washing out the thoracic cavity with saline solution and distilled water and exposing the entire thoracic cavity for 10–15 minutes to cisplatin (50 μg/mL) in prewarmed distilled water.

Results.—Exposure of the cells to distilled water and cisplatin induced a significantly higher growth inhibition than exposure to cisplatin in PBS. The viability of tumors obtained by resection of NSCLC and exposed to hypotonic cisplatin (50 μg/mL) for 10 minutes was markedly decreased after a 3-day culture. In all 7 patients, no clinically detected pleural effusion, growth of disseminated tumor, or relevant chest pain was observed during follow-up ranging from 6 to 29 months. The administration of cisplatin was not associated with bone marrow suppression, abnormal data on renal function, or intestinal symptoms. Four patients are alive with no evidence of disease at 6 to 16 months and 3 have died of disease.

Conclusion.—Cisplatin is known to be one of the most effective drugs against lung cancer, and distilled water can damage cells, including tumor cells. The combination was shown to have an antitumor effect when used at thoracotomy in patients with lung cancer.

▶ The use of sterile water to lavage wounds after surgical resection of malignant tumors has long been a standard practice in operating rooms. The cytolytic efficacy of hypotonic sterile water has largely been of a theoretical nature. This report seems to document the effects of sterile water when used in the setting of prewarmed cisplatin lavage.

This paper is notable in the outstanding results the authors claim in 7 patients with malignant pleural effusions, of whom 4 are alive with no evidence of disease at 6–16 months; 3 of the 7 died of disease after lavage with a cisplatin/sterile water combination. I believe this very interesting report merits further investigation in larger single institutional and multi-institutional trials. The question as to the efficacy of sterile water preparations in causing cytolysis and inhibiting growth of implanted cells needs further study.—D.J. Sugarbaker, M.D.

Survival of Patients Undergoing Nd:YAG Laser Therapy Compared With Nd:YAG Laser Therapy and Brachytherapy for Malignant Airway Disease
Shea JM, Allen RP, Tharratt RS, Chan AL, Siefkin AD (Univ of California, Sacramento)
Chest 103:1028–1031, 1993   140-94-13–15

Introduction.—Laser treatment is used for palliative therapy in patients with symptomatic recurrent endobronchial malignant neoplasms.

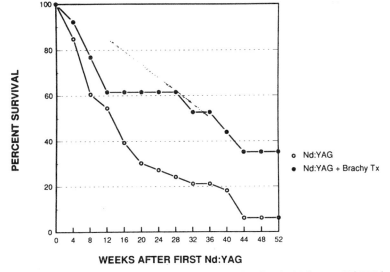

WEEKS AFTER FIRST Nd:YAG

Fig 13–5.—Comparison of survival between patients treated with Nd:YAG laser vs. Nd:YAG laser and endobronchial brachytherapy for squamous cell carcinoma from the time of the first Nd:YAG laser treatment. *Open circles*, Nd:YAG laser; *filled circles*, Nd-YAG laser and endobronchial brachytherapy. (Courtesy of Shea JM, Allen RP, Tharratt RS, et al: *Chest* 103:1028-1031, 1993.)

There is a risk of massive hemorrhage with the laser, however, and frequent procedures may be necessary. The combination of brachytherapy with the Nd:YAG laser is reported to add to the quality and duration of the palliative period in these patients. The length of survival of patients who had undergone Nd:YAG laser therapy either alone or in combination with brachytherapy was examined.

Patients and Methods. —A review of the records of patients with inoperable squamous cell carcinoma involving the airway for a 3-year period identified 13 such patients who had previously been treated with the Nd:YAG laser and who underwent the bronchoscopic placement of a hand-loaded, low-dose brachytherapy catheter. Custom-fabricated sources of ^{192}Ir with a dose rate that delivered between 51 and 133 cGy/hr at 1 cm were used. That group of patients was compared with 33 patients who had undergone Nd:YAG therapy alone during an earlier 5-year period.

Results. —The two groups were similar in age; those also treated with brachytherapy had fewer laser treatments performed. Patients treated with Nd:YAG laser and brachytherapy survived longer than those treated with laser alone (Fig 13-5). One complication was related to brachytherapy; multifocal atrial tachycardia developed in the patient while the catheter was being placed, but the arrhythmia resolved with intravenous administration of verapamil.

Conclusion. —The addition of brachytherapy to Nd:YAG laser therapy increased survival in patients with squamous cell carcinoma involving the airway. This effect is thought to be the result of improved airway patency and a reduction in the incidence of obstructive pneumonitis and respiratory distress. Although no data were available on the patients' symptomatic improvement, a good-to-excellent response to the palliative treatment has been reported in other studies.

▶ The palliative use of endobronchial laser resection has become popular in patients with adenoidcystic and obstructive non–small-cell lung cancers. Alternative methods of treatment for endobronchial tumors not amenable to surgical resection have also included the use of afterloading catheters. This aforementioned population of patients can be particularly challenging for the thoracic surgeon or pulmonologist managing the palliative stages of these patients' disease. This study demonstrates the superiority of using combination brachytherapy with laser treatment during the palliative period of patients with recurrent endobronchial tumors. Our own suggestion would be to use brachytherapy at the second, staged endobronchial resection (1).—D.J. Sugarbaker, M.D.

Reference

1. Sugarbaker DJ, et al: *Otolaryngol Head Neck Surg* 3:93, 1992.

Expandable Wallstent for the Treatment of Obstruction of the Superior Vena Cava
Watkinson AF, Hansell DM (Royal Brompton Natl Heart and Lung Hosp, London)
Thorax 48:915–920, 1993   140-94-13–16

Background.—Percutaneous intravenous stent placement, including use of the Gianturco stent and the Palmaz stent, have been reported for treatment of superior vena cava obstructions. The self-expanding metallic Wallstent has been used in arterial and hepatobiliary work, and has also been described as treatment for malignant superior vena cava obstruction in 2 instances. An initial experience with the Wallstent in treating superior vena cava obstructions was reported.

Patients and Methods.—A total of 5 patients, 4 with advanced mediastinal malignancy previously treated via radiotherapy and 1 with fibrosing mediastinitis, were studied. All patients underwent balloon angioplasty of the stricture and percutaneous insertion of an expandable Wallstent endoprosthesis across the stricture site.

Results.—All patients had rapid symptomatic relief after surgery. In addition, 3 of the 5 achieved complete symptom alleviation throughout 7 weeks, 9 weeks, and 24 weeks of survival, respectively. The remaining 2 surviving patients were symptom-free at 8- and 9-month follow-up evaluations, respectively.

Conclusion.—The Wallstent endoprosthesis is a useful treatment option after standard therapy has failed to yield desired results. In addition, this method provides rapid symptom relief to patients with obstruction of the superior vena cava.

▶ The use of an expandable stent within the lumen of the superior vena cava to relieve obstruction from advanced mediastinal malignancies is well described in this report. This treatment option would appear to be a relatively straightforward one for the patient with superior vena cava syndrome and advanced disease. The routine use of radiotherapy in this disorder is of interest in that studies have demonstrated a lack of patency of the vena cava after radiation therapy, despite its demonstrated ability to ameliorate symptoms.—D.J. Sugarbaker, M.D.

Thoracoscopy: Evolution and Evaluation

INTRODUCTION

Video-assisted thoracoscopy and pure thoracoscopic surgery remain the focus of much clinical/surgical investigation and evaluation. In the 1993 YEAR BOOK OF SURGERY, we reviewed a number of initial reports on the use of video-assisted thoracic surgery in the performance of diagnostic and some therapeutic thoracic surgical procedures. We are now beginning to see the natural evolution of this technique as surgeons begin to find new roles for thoracoscopy as a tool in the diagnosis, staging, and treatment of disease. In some instances, we are beginning to see thoracoscopy changing the way in which tumors are diagnosed, evaluated, staged, and treated based on thoracoscopic technique and intervention.

The first of the following abstracts looks at conventional bronchoscopy in the workup and diagnosis of the solitary pulmonary nodule (Abstract 140-94-13-17). It is precisely in this clinical situation where thoracoscopic resection may provide a meaningful alternative to the options of watch and wait, fine-needle aspiration, bronchoscopic evaluation, and standard operative surgical resection.

Thoracic surgeons need to remain vigilant and highly critical of reports using thoracoscopic and video-assisted techniques in the performance of routine therapeutic thoracic surgical procedures. Each advantage should be proven with prospective randomized trials and each disadvantage documented and clearly understood.

Given the potential advantages to the patient in terms of pain and morbidity, surgeons need to be ever mindful that it is the therapeutic advantage seen in 1-, 2-, 3-, and 5-year survival rates that must remain of paramount importance in the treatment of thoracic malignancies. Nevertheless, thoracoscopic staging of intrathoracic malignancies, as well as selected use of therapeutic maneuvers, may provide real alternatives for patients with limited pulmonary reserve or medical comorbidities. Particularly in elderly patients in whom surgical resection has not been an option in the past, thoracoscopic surgery may provide a real therapeutic option for this select high-risk group of patients.

David J. Sugarbaker, M.D.

The Utility of Fiberoptic Bronchoscopy in the Evaluation of the Solitary Pulmonary Nodule
Torrington KG, Kern JD (Walter Reed Army Med Ctr, Washington, DC)
Chest 104:1021–1024, 1993   140-94-13-17

Background.—Patients with solitary pulmonary nodules (SPNs) are screened with fiberoptic bronchoscopy at many institutions before undergoing curative surgery. The records of all patients with SPNs who underwent fiberoptic bronchoscopy at Walter Reed Army Medical Center during a 4-year period were retrospectively examined to assess the value of routine, preoperative fiberoptic bronchoscopy for diagnosis and treatment of SPNs.

Methods.—The medical records of 191 patients were studied before selecting 91 for evaluation. Of these, 72 had bronchogenic carcinomas (BCs), 7 had carcinoid tumors, and 12 had benign tumors. Solitary pulmonary nodules were radiographically defined as less than or equal to 6 cm peripheral pulmonary lesions completely encompassed by pulmonary parenchyma. The remaining 100 records were ruled out for evaluation purposes for various reasons.

Results.—One unsuspected vocal cord carcinoma and no occult synchronous BCs were shown via fiberoptic bronchoscopy. Submucosal or endobronchial tumors were seen in 5 patients, and BC was found in 4 of 5 tumors from which specimens were taken. Cytologic evaluations of bronchial brushings or washings diagnosed BC in 4 of 66 instances. Nine of 30 transbronchial lung biopsy specimens revealed BC in patients shown to have BC at surgery. In the patients who underwent biopsies under fluoroscopic guidance, no improvement in diagnostic yield of the transbronchial lung biopsy specimens was seen. The 16 fiberoptic bronchoscopy specimens found to be positive for BC concurred with the surgical specimens 100% of the time. Fiberoptic bronchoscopy findings did not preclude the need for surgery, and they did not alter the surgical stage of BC. A preoperative malignant diagnosis did not affect operative time or procedure, as many patients needed frozen-section biopsy of mediastinal lymph nodes before undergoing lung resection.

Conclusion.—Routine, preoperative fiberoptic bronchoscopy did not significantly benefit patients with SPNs.

▶ This paper confirms the authors' suspicion that the use of preoperative fiberoptic bronchoscopy in the majority of patients with lesions in the parenchyma of the lung is of limited clinical value. I believe it remains only a matter of time before third-party payers and managed care plans will no longer pay for routine bronchoscopic evaluation in patients seen with a peripleural SPN. As is noted in the following 2 papers (Abstracts 140-94-13–18 and 140-94-13–19), the use of thoracoscopy in the diagnosis of the indeterminant SPN would appear to have significant clinical and, possibly, financial advantages to physician and patient alike.—D.J. Sugarbaker, M.D.

Thoracoscopy for the Diagnosis of the Indeterminate Solitary Pulmonary Nodule

Mack MJ, Hazelrigg SR, Landreneau RJ, Acuff TE (Med City Dallas; St Luke's Med Ctr, Milwaukee, Wis; Univ of Pittsburgh, Pa)
Ann Thorac Surg 56:825–832, 1993   140-94-13–18

Background.—In diagnosing the indeterminate solitary pulmonary nodule, standard nonoperative approaches include bronchoscopy and percutaneous needle biopsy, both of which are minimally invasive. However, each method may fail to identify the small, peripheral nodule. In such situations, open thoracotomy is frequently necessary to obtain a diagnosis, although this method is associated with significant morbidity. With the recent broader application of thoracoscopic techniques, however, most peripheral pulmonary nodules can now be removed using thoracoscopic resective methods. The use of thoracoscopy as the primary diagnostic modality for indeterminate single pulmonary nodules was assessed.

Patients and Findings.—During a 1.5-year period, 242 patients underwent thoracoscopic excisional biopsy as the primary diagnostic method. Wedge excisions of the nodules were conducted via thoracoscopic techniques. An endoscopic stapler alone was used in 72%, an Nd:YAG laser was used in 18%, and both methods were used for 10% of the patients. Definite diagnoses were obtained for all patients. In 2 patients, conversion to thoracotomy was necessary to locate each nodule, both of which were malignant. Benign and malignant diagnoses were obtained in 127 and 115 patients, respectively. Of those patients with malignant diagnoses, 51 were primary lung cancer and 64 were metastases. Twenty-nine of the patients with primary lung cancer, all of whom had adequate pulmonary reserve, underwent formal open lung resection during the same procedure. Significant morbidity comprised atelectasis in 3 patients, pneumonia in 2, and prolonged air leak for more than 7 days in 4. There was no mortality. For 213 patients undergoing thoracoscopy only, the average hospital stay was 2.4 days, with a range of 1–12 days.

Conclusion.—Because of its being virtually 100% sensitive and specific, with no mortality and minimal morbidity, thoracoscopy has advantages over standard diagnostic methods. In addition, thoracoscopy is a minimally invasive method, and has the added benefits of both time and cost effectiveness. Thoracoscopy may play an important role in the diagnostic management of indeterminate solitary pulmonary nodules.

▶ This report is the first detailed look at the diagnostic accuracy of thoracoscopy in the decision analysis of patients with an indeterminate solitary pulmonary nodule. The paper is well thought out and would appear to indicate that thoracoscopy is a definite alternative to open thoracotomy, the watch and wait approach, or fine-needle aspiration. In fact, it appears to have a significant advantage in terms of giving a definitive diagnosis with a limited morbidity and mortality.

There are some problematic parts to the paper, particularly as they relate to the use of conventional lobectomy in the treatment of patients with suspected carcinoma of the lung. Ten of the patients with malignant tumors were noted to have adenocarcinoma of the breast, and 5 had adenocarcinomas of unknown primaries. It is not clear whether these patients underwent standard lobectomy. In my institution, it is impossible to distinguish, even on permanent sections, an adenocarcinoma occurring in the lung as primary carcinoma and one representing a solitary metastasis from the breast or other sites of primary adenocarcinoma.

From a clinical standpoint, the existence of a solitary lesion in the lung makes one highly suspicious that it represents a primary bronchogenic malignancy. Therefore, it would appear that these patients should have undergone therapeutic lobectomy if, from a therapeutic standpoint, the benefit of the doubt is to be given to the patient when there is pathologic uncertainty as to the etiology of the tumor. From a review of the literature, it would appear that it is more likely for the patient to have a primary bronchogenic malignancy with a cell type of adenocarcinoma than it is for them to have a solitary pulmonary metastasis from a primary adenocarcinoma of some other visceral site (1). Nevertheless, this report demonstrates that thoracoscopy is now becoming a tool whose appropriate place is to be defined and one which is no longer a technical stunt.—D.J. Sugarbaker, M.D.

Reference

1. Todd TR: *Chest* 103(suppl):401S, 1993.

Thoracoscopic Surgery for Diseases of the Lung and Pleura: Effectiveness, Changing Indications, and Limitations
Daniel TM, Kern JA, Tribble CG, Kron IL, Spotnitz WB, Rodgers BM (Univ of Virginia, Charlottesville)
Ann Surg 217:566–575, 1993   140-94-13–19

Background.—To date, no research has compared the value of video-assisted thoracic surgery (VATS) with advanced video systems and instrumentation to that of thoracoscopic surgery (TS). Such a study has now been done in patients with lung and pleural diseases.

Methods.—The results of procedures performed from 1981 to 1992 were analyzed retrospectively. Thoracoscopic surgery or VATS was performed for pleural fluid problems, diffuse lung disease, lung masses, and pneumothorax. Eighty-nine TS procedures were performed from 1981 to 1990, and 64 VATS procedures were performed from 1991 to 1992.

Findings.—Thoracoscopic surgery successfully resolved pleural fluid problems in 85% of the cases, and VATS was successful in 90%. Before 1991, diffuse lung disease was diagnosed by TS using a cup biopsy on end stage patients in respiratory failure. Since that time, VATS using stapled wedge excisions has been done to establish diagnoses in ambulatory patients. Surgical mortality decreased from 33% to 9%; the postoperative stay decreased from 16.6 to 8.2 days. With TS, lung masses were diagnosed completely by incisional biopsies. Diagnosis was made in 83% of cases, with a mean postoperative length of hospitalization of 5.3 days. Using VATS, excisional biopsies were done, enabling diagnosis in 100% of cases and a shortened postoperative stay of 3 days. However, in 20% of these patients conversion to thoracotomy was required to find the subpleural mass. Thorocoscopic surgery was done for spontaneous pneumothorax in only 26% of patients compared with 67% with VATS.

Conclusion.—Video-assisted thoracic surgery is as effective as TS in the treatment of pleural fluid problems and has greatly increased safety, efficacy, and indications for lung mass biopsy. It has also resulted in earlier surgical diagnostic intervention in diffuse lung disease and earlier treatment in primary pneumothorax states.

▶ This paper seeks to compare the use of VATS with traditional pleurascopic surgery or TS using a mediastinoscope. It clearly demonstrates the enhanced visualization of intrathoracic lesions by means of video-assisted techniques. The techniques include the use of a limited thoracotomy (utility thoracotomy), and this study demonstrates the superiority of this technique both in diagnostic procedures and in procedures with therapeutic intent. Conclusions regarding the improved length of stay are difficult in a longitudinal study such as this. This really represents a comparison of the 2 phases of TS. The limitations of current instrumentation are again highlighted in this report.—D.J. Sugarbaker, M.D.

Effects of Insufflation on Hemodynamics During Thoracoscopy
Jones DR, Graeber GM, Tanguilig GG, Hobbs G, Murray GF (West Virginia Univ, Morgantown)
Ann Thorac Surg 55:1379–1382, 1993   140-94-13–20

Background.—Thoracic techniques that once required open thoracotomy can now be done with video-assisted thoracoscopy. Some have advocated creating an artificial pneumothorax by carbon dioxide insufflation under positive pressures to visualize the intrathoracic structures adequately. However, positive-pressure insufflation during thoracoscopy may significantly compromise hemodynamics.

Methods.—Monitoring lines and a thoracoscope were placed in 8 healthy female pigs under general endotracheal anesthesia. Baseline hemodynamic measurements were obtained at 0 mm Hg. Measurements were randomly taken at 5, 10, and 15 mm Hg using carbon dioxide insufflation after stabilization at each pressure.

Findings.—Insufflation pressures of 5 mm Hg or more significantly reduced cardiac index, mean arterial pressure, stroke volume, and left ventricular stroke work index. Central venous pressure increased. Heart rate changes were nonsignificant.

Conclusion.—The routine use of positive-pressure insufflation during thoracoscopy is not recommended. Significant hemodynamic compromise was associated with the procedure in the animal model used. If positive-pressure insufflation is to be used, more invasive monitoring than electrocardiographic and noninvasive blood pressure instrumentation needs to be initiated.

▶ This is one of the first studies reporting on the negative effects of intrathoracic insufflation during thoracoscopy. Although the use of routine insufflation is fraught with complications, particularly those involving hemodynamic compromise and tamponade-like effects, there is a role for limited insufflation in our thoracic practice. This is in situations in which patients (1) are to undergo closed lung biopsy because of severe acute interstitial disease, and (2) require very high levels of forced inspiratory oxygen. In these patients, single-lung ventilation is not feasible. We have, therefore, had limited success with the use of partial insufflation causing a moderate amount of atelectasis, allowing enough room between the chest wall and parenchyma for successful closed-lung biopsy for rapid diagnosis and therapy.—D.J. Sugarbaker, M.D.

▶↓ The localization of intraparenchymal nodules during thoracoscopic surgery remains a challenge for the thoracic surgeon. In addition to localizing the lesion, preserving an adequate margin in cases where further resection is not a therapeutic option, based on the patient's pulmonary function, is of concern to the surgeon. Abstracts 140-94-13–21, 140-94-13–22, and 140-94-13–23 deal with this problem in a variety of ways.—D.J. Sugarbaker, M.D.

Localization of Peripheral Pulmonary Nodules for Thoracoscopic Excision: Value of CT-Guided Wire Placement

Shah RM, Spirn PW, Salazar AM, Steiner RM, Cohn HE, Solit RW, Wechsler RJ, Erdman S (Jefferson Med College, Philadelphia; Beilinson Med Ctr, Tel Aviv, Israel)
AJR 161:279–283, 1993   140-94-13–21

Purpose.—Video-assisted thoracoscopy is being used as an alternative to thoracotomy for an expanding range of indications, including resection of peripheral lung nodules. Preoperative localization is needed for nodules considered too small or too far from the pleural surface to be detected by visual inspection or palpation. The use of percutaneous spring hookwire placement for prethoracoscopic localization of such nodules was reported.

Methods.—Under CT guidance, 17 nodules in 14 patients were localized before operation with the Kopans breast lesion localization system. In 3 patients with solitary nodules, previous transthoracic needle biopsy or transbronchial biopsy had failed. In another 4 patients with lesions measuring less than 8 mm in diameter, transthoracic fine-needle aspiration biopsy was not considered likely to be diagnostic. The remaining 7 patients underwent therapeutic wedge resection of limited metastases or a second bronchogenic carcinoma. The mean diameter of these nodules was 10 mm, and their mean distance from the costal pleura was 9 mm. All wire placements were confirmed by CT.

Results.—A hookwire was successfully placed in all 17 lesions. In 1 patient, the wire was dislodged before thoracoscopy, but only after a 6-hour preoperative delay and extreme bending of the wire during induction of anesthesia. In this case, the bloodstain on the pleura was sufficient to guide the resection. In all cases but one, the surgeon believed the nodule could not have been localized thoracoscopically without the hookwire. A second wire was needed for 1 nodule that was located across a major fissure. Two patients had serious pain related to wire placement, and 5 had clinically insignificant pneumothorax. One large pneumothorax had to be drained before a second nodule in the same lung could be localized. Presumed local bleeding was noted on CT in 6 cases.

Conclusion.—Percutaneous placement of spring hookwires appears to be a safe, simple, and effective procedure for prethoracoscopic localization of lung nodules. This procedure increases the chances of successful thoracoscopic resection for lesions that could not otherwise be detected.

▶ The use of wire placed in lesions transcutaneously and under CT guidance is evaluated in this study. We have found that this procedure represents a significant logistical challenge before planned surgical resection. Although it is an accurate way of assessing a lesion's location, the practicality of this approach may not be shared equally in all institutions.

However, the ability to place a wire under CT guidance should remain in the armamentarium of the thoracic surgeon for those cases in which thoracoscopic resection is of paramount importance to the therapeutic success of a procedure, particularly for patients with limited pulmonary reserve in whom therapeutic thoracoscopic resection represents the only therapeutic alternative.—D.J. Sugarbaker, M.D.

Intraoperative Transthoracic Ultrasonographic Localization of Occult Lung Lesions
Shennib H, Bret P (Montreal Gen Hosp; McGill Univ, Montreal)
Ann Thorac Surg 55:767–769, 1993   140-94-13-22

Introduction.—Video-assisted thoracoscopic surgery has become an increasingly useful means of approaching a variety of intrathoracic problems. One of the chief indications is wedge resection of peripheral lung lesions, for either diagnostic or therapeutic purposes. The need to localize the lesion has been a major limitation to the use of thoracoscopic methods.

A New Approach.—Intrathoracic video-assisted ultrasonography was performed intraoperatively in 2 patients to localize lung tumors before removing them.

Case Report.—Man, 67 years, with severe emphysema, had a central left upper lobe cancer that responded to radiotherapy, but a 2-cm peripheral nodule was present in the apical part of the right upper lobe 1.5 years later when there was also radiation pneumonitis in the left lung. A second primary lung cancer was diagnosed by transthoracic needle aspiration of the nodule. A 21-gauge needle was inserted into the tumor under CT guidance and, during surgery, ultrasonography using a transvaginal transducer and convex probe clearly defined the tumor and its margins and allowed accurate positioning of a stapling device. The same technique was successfully used to localize a peripheral lung tumor in a frail woman, 83, except that a rectal probe with a side transducer was used.

Conclusion.—Intraoperative intrathoracic ultrasonography may be used to localize peripheral lung tumors, which then are resected by video-assisted thoracoscopy. The patient is taken to the radiology suite just before surgery, and the lesion is localized by methylene blue dye and a wire under CT guidance. Intraoperative ultrasonography then is used to confirm the site of the tumor and to guide stapler application or laser resection.

▶ The use of intraoperative ultrasound is an intriguing possibility for the localization of intraparenchymal lesions. This has been particularly difficult for us and for others because of the presence of air in the lung, which precludes an accurate ultrasonographic localization. This approach demonstrates that localization of occult lung lesions by transthoracic ultrasound is possible. However, its routine use will depend on larger studies documenting its practicality. It appears we will see more in the technical development of ultrasound devices for localization of tumors in patients undergoing thoracoscopic resection.—D.J. Sugarbaker, M.D.

Techniques for Localization of Pulmonary Nodules for Thoracoscopic Resection
Mack MJ, Shennib H, Landreneau RJ, Hazelrigg SR (Humana Hosp, Dallas; Montreal Gen Hosp; Univ of Pittsburgh, Pa; et al)
J Thorac Cardiovasc Surg 106:550–553, 1993   140-94-13–23

Objective.—Recent surgical and technologic advances have made it possible to perform pulmonary resection as a thoracoscopic procedure. However, with such thoracoscopic techniques, the loss of manual palpation makes it impossible to identify a nodule that is too small or too deep beneath the pleural surface. Techniques used in detecting occult pulmonary nodules in 300 thoracoscopic pulmonary resections were reported.

Localization Techniques.—The preoperative chest CT scan is reviewed to assess the likelihood of finding the localized nodule at thoracoscopy. For nodules deeper than 1 cm beneath the pleural surface or smaller than 1 cm in size, greater difficulty in detection can be anticipated. Subtle findings on the CT scan, such as puckering or inflammatory changes, may facilitate detection. Nodules adjacent to fissures are easily detected visually at thoracoscopy. Preoperative or fluoroscopic needle localization can be performed if problems are anticipated.

Intraoperative Techniques.—Nodules on the pleural surface are almost always visible during thoracoscopy. Those in the subpleural areas may be located by effacement of the parenchyma around the nodule as the lung collapses. Carbon dioxide insufflation may enhance this effacement. Palpation with a blunt instrument may succeed where visual inspection fails. Partial insufflation of the lung, allowing digital palpation, may be necessary if the nodule remains undetected. Localizing wires placed before operation are easy to find at thoracoscopy; even if they have come dislodged, the site can usually be found by the methylene blue stain or the subtle subpleural hematoma in the area.

Intraoperative Ultrasound.—Intraoperative ultrasound of the collapsed lung is another useful technique, which is easily performed by placing a 12-mm probe with a 5-MHz transducer through the slightly enlarged trocar site. Carbon dioxide insufflation and placement of fluid in the thoracic cavity to submerge the lung may help in achieving complete collapse.

Discussion.—Using these techniques, all target nodules were successfully located in the last 200 thoracoscopic lung resections performed. With greater experience, less reliance on needle localization is expected. Nodules more than 2 cm below the pleural surface can be approached with more confidence as experience with laser lung resection grows.

▶ This paper dealing with techniques of localization of pulmonary nodules demonstrates one practical point. This is that digital palpation of the lesion is the most accurate and easiest way to identify its location before thoracoscopic resection. The placement of a port directly over the suspected location of the lesion, based on the CT scan, is the quickest way to digitally palpate it and confirm its location.

It is of particular note that with atelectasis there often is a dislocation of the nodule from the location seen by CT scan. We have found that reinflating the lung will, in many instances, restore the anatomical location of the lesion such that it can be easily palpated with another review of the CT scan.—D.J. Sugarbaker, M.D.

Accuracy of Lung Imaging in Metastases With Implications for the Role of Thoracoscopy

McCormack PM, Ginsberg KB, Bains MS, Burt ME, Martini N, Rusch VW, Ginsberg RJ (Mem Sloan-Kettering Cancer Ctr, New York)
Ann Thorac Surg 56:863–866, 1993   140-94-13-24

Background.—Interest in using thoracoscopy for wedge resection of lung metastasis is rapidly increasing. However, although this technique provides excellent lung surface exposure, it does not allow lung palpation. Thus, there are concerns that surgeons using this method may not be able to identify and remove all metastatic lesions. To determine the accuracy of imaging techniques, the number of lesions seen on chest roentgenogram or CT scan was compared with the final pathologic report in a sample of resected patients.

Patients and Methods.—The charts, chest roentgenograms, CT scans, and pathologic findings of 144 patients who had undergone resection of lung metastases from colorectal primary tumor during a 23-year period were retrospectively examined. Chest roentgenograms were performed as the initial diagnostic test to detect metastases in all patients, and 72 patients also had CT scans of the lung. Pathologic reports were available on all 144 patients.

Results.—In 17 of 72 patients, chest roentgenograms and CT findings differed with respect to the number of nodules reported. Of these, 3 of the chest roentgenograms revealed more nodules than the CT scans. In 57 of the 144 patients, chest roentgenograms differed from pathologic findings at surgery. Of these, 26 had more and 31 had fewer lesions than were found on chest roentgenograms. In 30 of 72 patients, CT scans differed from pathologic results. If 1 or 2 lesions were imaged, fewer cancers were noted for 12 patients (some lesions were benign) and 18 had more cancers than noted via CT. Computed tomographic scans were in error 28% of the time.

Conclusion.—When using the thoracoscope alone, the surgeon is unable to adequately palpate the entire lung. Thus, the ability to determine whether resection of all lesions has been done is markedly impaired. Other than for diagnosis, the validity of using thoracoscopic resection in the management of metastatic disease is seriously debatable.

▶ This very interesting paper by McCormack et al. demonstrates the potential inadequacy of thoracoscopy in resection of lesions that are only visible by CT scan or digitally palpable. Twenty-six patients had more lesions than the chest roentgenogram detected; 31 patients had fewer, with computerized tomography erroring in 28% of cases.

Complete cytoreduction in surgery for metastatic disease has remained the goal for the surgeon for the last decade, and Martini et al. (1) present a well-illustrated article. Although it is clear that digital bimanual palpation of the lung remains the most accurate way of detecting intraparenchymal metastases, it is not clear that resecting only those lesions that are of sufficient size to be seen by CT scan and leaving the smaller lesions for subsequent surgery in any way detracts from overall survival. An interesting prospective trial would compare thoracoscopic resection of all nodules radiographically visible by high-resolution CT vs. mediastinotomy and bimanual/bilateral palpation. Demonstration of the therapeutic efficacy in such a trial of bimanual/bilateral palpation would be of importance.—D.J. Sugarbaker, M.D.

Reference

1. Martini N, et al: *Ann Thorac Surg* 12:271, 1971.

Video Thoracoscopic Management of Benign and Malignant Pericardial Effusions

Mack MJ, Landreneau RJ, Hazelrigg SR, Acuff TE (Humana Hosp Med Ctr, Dallas; Montefiore Univ Hosp, Pittsburgh, Pa; St Luke's Med Ctr, Milwaukee, Wis)

Chest 103:390S–393S, 1993   140-94-13–25

Background.—Pericardial effusion may pose difficult management challenges, especially in patients with cancer and in those with limited life expectancy. All surgical approaches have specific associated disadvantages. The use of video-assisted thoracoscopic (VATS) pericardiectomy as a means of extensive resection with reduced operative morbidity was reported.

Patients and Technique.—The VATS technique has been used in 22 patients with medically refractory, effusive, nonconstrictive pericarditis. Thirteen patients had inflammatory pericarditis, and 9 had pericardial effusions resulting from malignancy. Fourteen had failed therapeutic pericardiocentesis. The VATS technique used general anesthesia with double-lumen endotracheal intubation to provide for ipsilateral pulmonary collapse. A 3-portal technique was used for the video camera and endoscopic instruments. The pericardium was resected by endoscopic electrocautery and scissors. Drainage of associated pleural effusion or chemical pleurodesis was performed as indicated. Chest tubes were placed after the resection.

Results.—All patients had pericardial resection equivalent to that achieved by anterolateral thoracotomy. The surgery provided symptomatic control in all cases. Ipsilateral pleural effusions were successfully managed in 11 patients. The mean duration of chest tube drainage was 2 days in all patients; the mean hospital stay was 4 days in patients with benign disease. All of the latter patients were alive and recurrence-free an average of 7.5 months postoperatively.

Conclusion.—The VATS technique may be a useful alternative to lateral thoracotomy or the subxiphoid pericardial window for patients with pericardial effusion, whether benign or malignant. It is well tolerated, even by very ill patients with cancer.

▶ The immediate application of therapeutic VATS surgery would appear to be in those situations in which limitation in morbidity and mortality are paramount and yet therapeutic efficacy is dependent upon intrathoracic resections that do not require a clear margin or other evidence of complete resection. Therefore, VATS pericardiectomy would be an excellent application of these techniques. This is well documented in this report. The safety and efficacy of this technique should obviously be compared to more traditional approaches, including a subxiphoid approach.—D.J. Sugarbaker, M.D.

Thoracoscopic Pleurectomy for Treatment of Complicated Spontaneous Pneumothorax

Inderbitzi RGC, Furrer M, Striffeler H, Althaus U (Univ of Berne, Switzerland)
J Thorac Cardiovasc Surg 105:84–88, 1993   140-94-13–26

Introduction.—Parietal pleurectomy has offered the best long-term results in the treatment of complicated spontaneous pneumothorax. Several newer thoracoscopic procedures have been recommended, however, in the past decade. A recently developed method, the thoracoscopic parietal pleurectomy, was studied.

Patients and Methods.—The method, which uses videoendoscopy and specially designed equipment, was successful in treating 12 patients with spontaneous pneumothorax. The patients ranged in age from 23 to 64 years; 9 were men and 1 had cystic fibrosis. In the remaining 11 patients, the indication for endoscopic pleurectomy was based on pathologic findings verified as stage 4 (numerous large bullae) in Vanderschueren's classification. The operation is performed under general anesthesia. Incisions are made triangularly in the third, fourth, and fifth intercostal spaces. A straight telescope connected to the video camera is inserted via the trocar and the procedure is transmitted to a television monitor. The picture facilitates insertion of the 2 other 7-mm trocars. Pliable silicone tubes and instruments with a 25-degree angle were designed for the procedure, the steps of which are detailed in the study.

Results.—The operative procedure lasted for a mean of 55 minutes. There was no surgical morbidity. In all patients, radiologic evaluation on the first postoperative day revealed an open, infiltration-free lung without effusion or residual pneumothorax. Patients were hospitalized for a mean of 3.3 days after the procedure, and all had resumed normal activity within 3 weeks. At an average follow-up of 7.5 months, there was no relapse of pneumothorax.

Conclusion.—Videoendoscopy allows unrestricted visualization of the pleural cavity, accurate assessment of the lung, and clear delineation of the extension of pleural resection. The application of the thoracoscopic technique meets all requirements of successful pneumothorax management: elimination of the causative lesion, rapid and full expansion of the lung, minimal risk of recurrence, low morbidity and cost, and a short hospital stay.

▶ Video-assisted thoracic surgical techniques have principally been used for the treatment of uncomplicated spontaneous pneumothorax. The placement of trocars medically and laterally has been described by our group and others as a way of performing apical pleurectomy and pleurodesis. This group from the University of Berne has very nicely demonstrated that more difficult cases of resistant pneumothorax with recurrent atelectasis can be successfully treated with thoracoscopic pleurectomy. One needs to be mindful of adhesions along the pleura in assessing patients for a possible thoracoscopic approach. In addition, resection of the pleura at the apex can be complicated by injury to the brachial plexus and major arteries if care is not taken.—D.J. Sugarbaker, M.D.

Comparison of Open Versus Thoracoscopic Lung Biopsy for Diffuse Infiltrative Pulmonary Disease
Ferson PF, Landreneau RJ, Dowling RD, Hazelrigg SR, Ritter P, Nunchuck S, Perrino MK, Bowers CM, Mack MJ, Magee MJ (Univ of Pittsburgh, Pa; St Luke's Med Ctr, Milwaukee, Wis; Humana Hosp, Dallas)
J Thorac Cardiovasc Surg 106:194–199, 1993   140-94-13–27

Introduction.—Patients with diffuse pulmonary infiltrates often require a biopsy for diagnosis. Open wedge resection via thoracotomy is the standard procedure, but it carries significant morbidity. The morbidity and length of hospital stay may be reduced by closed thoracoscopic wedge resection. Results of using the 2 techniques were compared in 75 patients with diffuse pulmonary infiltrates.

Methods.—All patients who needed mechanical ventilation and high levels of pressure support before biopsy were excluded from the study. From March 1987 to April 1991, open wedge resection via thoracotomy was done in 28 patients. Thereafter, thoracoscopic resection was done in 47. The 2 groups were comparable in terms of age, sex, immunosuppression, and final diagnosis.

Findings.—Both techniques provided sufficient tissue for diagnosis in every case. The operating surgeons reported that visualization of the entire lung was better with the thoracoscopic procedure. Although mean operative time was longer for thoracoscopic biopsy (93 vs. 69 minutes), the mean length of hospital stay was significantly shorter (5 vs. 12 days). There was no significant difference in mean duration of chest tube drainage. Complications occurred after 50% of the open biopsies compared with 19% of the closed biopsies. Six patients in the open biopsy group died compared with 3 in the closed biopsy group; this difference was not significant.

Conclusion.—For patients undergoing biopsy for diffuse infiltrative lung disease, thoracoscopic biopsy can significantly reduce the length of hospital stay and morbidity, compared with standard open biopsy techniques. Thoracoscopic visualization of the lung is excellent, and sufficient tissue can be obtained for pathologic diagnosis.

Comparison of Video Thoracoscopic Lung Biopsy to Open Lung Biopsy in the Diagnosis of Interstitial Lung Disease
Bensard DD, McIntyre RC Jr, Waring BJ, Simon JS (Univ of Colorado, Den-

ver; Rose Med Ctr, Denver)
Chest 103:765–770, 1993   140-94-13–28

Background.—Diffuse infiltrative disease of the lung is difficult to diagnose, necessitating that one third of these patients undergo lung biopsy. The most accepted method of lung biopsy is open lung biopsy (OLB). However, new technology now permits video thorascopic lung biopsy (VTLB) to be performed. The efficacy and safety of VTLB were compared to those of OLB in the diagnosis of interstitial lung disease.

Surgical Technique.—The anesthetized patient is placed in the lateral decubitus position, and a pneumothorax is created. A 2-cm chest wall incision posterior to the scapula is created, and a 12-mm trocar is inserted. The videoscope is introduced into the pleural cavity. Two other trocars are then inserted. A suitable biopsy site is chosen, and the biopsy is obtained and removed through the 12-mm port.

Methods.—From December 1990 to January 1992, 43 patients were referred for diagnostic lung biopsy. In a retrospective study, 22 consecutive patients who underwent VTLB and 21 consecutive patients who underwent OLB were compared.

Results.—The operation time for VTLB was similar to that for OLB. The same number of biopsies were performed per patient using these 2 methods, and the same amount of material was obtained per biopsy. The diagnostic accuracy of the 2 methods was comparable. However, there was a significant reduction in pleural drainage and hospital stay in patients undergoing VTLB. Complications occurred in 9% of the VTLB patients and in 19% of the OLB patients. There was 1 death in the OLB group.

Conclusion.—Video thorascopic lung biopsy provides similar biopsy specimens and diagnostic accuracy as OLB, without increasing operation time or complications. In addition, VTLB reduces pleural drainage and hospital stay. These results indicate that VTLB is a safe and effective alternative to OLB in the diagnosis of interstitial lung disease.

▶ This study represents the second generation of thoracoscopic evaluations. We are now beginning to see trials that compare minimally invasive surgical techniques and standard operative approaches. Abstract 140-94-13–28 confirms my own clinical suspicion that closed lung biopsy will soon become an outpatient procedure as techniques of resection are improved and control of postresection air leak is improved.

Both of these studies (Abstracts 140-94-13–27 and 140-94-13–28) suffer from being retrospective analyses and, therefore, do not represent a prospective, randomized phase III trial. They lend a great degree of credence to thoracoscopic surgery, but they do not obviate the need for prospective, randomized trials in the validation of these new techniques.—D.J. Sugarbaker, M.D.

Current Indications and Efficacy of Pulmonary Metastasectomy

INTRODUCTION

The following 5 papers (Abstracts 140-94-13-29 through 140-94-13-33) were selected because of the variety of patients presented in terms of tumor cell type as well as the conclusions developed by the authors as a result of the data analysis. Indications for pulmonary metastasectomy remain in a state of flux, as is noted when one reviews these articles. The efficacy of pulmonary metastasectomy will be influenced by more effective adjuvant therapies and by the advent of new immunologic treatments of these tumors.

David J. Sugarbaker, M.D.

Extended Resection of Pulmonary Metastases: Is the Risk Justified?
Putnam JB Jr, Suell DM, Natarajan G, Roth JA (MD Anderson Cancer Ctr, Houston)
Ann Thorac Surg 55:1440–1446, 1993   140-94-13-29

Introduction.—Complete resection of pulmonary metastases (PM) isolated to the parenchyma enhances survival, regardless of the histology of the primary neoplasm. Extended resection, however, of multiple PM or PM involving more than lung parenchyma may carry increased risk in some patients. The safety and efficacy of these more extensive operations were examined in a review of data on 38 patients.

Patients and Methods.—The 38 cases represented about 3% of all operations for PM performed at one study institution between 1981 and 1992. The patients ranged in age from 13 to 77 years and had a variety of primary tumors. Nineteen underwent pneumonectomy, 11 had some type of pulmonary resection with en bloc chest wall excision for PM, and 8 had resection of lung with some other thoracic structure. For survivors, the median follow-up is 18 months; all others were followed until death.

Results.—Resection was complete in 33 of the 38 patients. Two patients, both of whom underwent right pneumonectomy, died within 30 days of operation. There were 6 cases of minor morbidity and 4 of major morbidity, including postpneumonectomy pulmonary edema, recurrent laryngeal nerve paralysis, empyema, and pneumonia. The overall median postresection actuarial survival was 27 months; 5-year survival was 25.4%. Patients treated with pneumonectomy tended to have an improved survival, compared with those who underwent other extended resections. The median survival was 28 months for patients who had extended resection as the initial operation for PM and 14 months for patients who had a previous resection of PM before the extended resection.

Conclusion.—The biological characteristics of neoplasms that selectively metastasize to the lungs generally enable resection of these metastases to improve survival. Extended resection of PM by pneumonectomy or in continuity with chest wall or other thoracic structures may be performed safely, and survival may approach that of patients with more limited resections of PM that involve lung parenchyma alone.

▶ This study reports on the efficacy of extended pulmonary resections in the treatment of PM. From reviewing this data, it appears that extended pulmonary metastasectomy, which may include pneumonectomy, can be expected to yield higher perioperative morbidity and mortality rates than standard resections. Two of 19 patients who were undergoing pneumonectomy died in this series, for a mortality rate of approximately 10.5%. The major morbidity reported in 4 patients and the minor morbidity in 6 patients also are not insignificant. In addition, complete resection was achieved in only 33 of 38 patients.

This group's overall 5-year survival rate was 25.4%. However, surgeons should be mindful that extended resection of PM can be expected to be accompanied by increased perioperative mortality and morbidity and, therefore, patients should be selected accordingly.—D.J. Sugarbaker, M.D.

Aggressive Pulmonary Metastasectomy for Soft Tissue Sarcomas
Ueda T, Uchida A, Kodama K, Doi O, Nakahara K, Fujii Y, Komatsubara Y, Ono K (Osaka Univ, Japan)
Cancer 72:1919–1925, 1993   140-94-13–30

Objective.—Because pulmonary metastases (PM) remains the major cause of death from soft tissue sarcomas and several reports have documented long-term survival after resection of isolated PM, an aggressive policy of pulmonary metastasectomy was evaluated in 23 patients with metastatic soft tissue sarcoma.

Patients.—The 14 female and 9 male patients were aged 13–68 years at the time PM were resected. A large majority of patients had primary tumors in the lower extremities. Synovial sarcoma and alveolar soft part sarcoma were the most frequent histologic diagnoses. Twenty-one patients had multiple, bilateral metastases, and 2 had solitary lesions. Fourteen patients had both primary disease and PM.

Management.—Patients with solitary lesions or a small number of metastases on 1 side underwent lateral thoracotomy, whereas those with bilateral lesions had median sternotomy. If recurrent metastases were present on both sides, patients had staged lateral thoracotomies. The Nd:YAG laser has recently been used in an effort to preserve uninvolved lung tissue. Fifteen of the 23 patients received adjuvant chemotherapy postoperatively.

Outcome.—A total of 41 thoracic explorations were performed for PM with no perioperative deaths, and with only 3 complications. Actuarial survival was 50% at 2 years, compared with 10% for patients whose metastases were unresectable. One fourth of the patients who underwent resection but none of the patients in the unresectable disease were alive at 5 years. Patients with alveolar soft part sarcoma did better than those with synovial sarcoma. Histologic grade also was a significant factor in survival, but the number of nodules resected was not. The performance of laser surgery and the absence of locally recurrent disease were favorable prognostic factors, as was the absence of extrapulmonary metastases before pulmonary metastasectomy.

Conclusion.—Aggressive resection of PM can potentially prolong the survival of patients with soft tissue sarcoma, even those with extensive metastases.

▶ This paper proposes to report on the efficacy of using pulmonary metastasectomy for soft tissue sarcomas. Actuarial survival of 50% at 2 years was compared to actuarial survival at 10% for those patients in whom the metastasectomy was not possible. Any conclusions based on that comparison between resectable and unresectable patients are fragile at best. Previous studies have reported on the prognostic significance of the number of nodules resected. This was not noted in this study. Soft tissue sarcomas did better than synovial sarcomas in this series, which is at odds with the results from previous reports. The use of laser surgery in this report appeared to have no substantive effect on the outcome. This study, as do most studies of pulmonary metastasectomies, suffers from the lack of a nonsurgical control.—D.J. Sugarbaker, M.D.

Resection of Lung Metastases From Soft-Tissue Sarcomas: A Multivariate Analysis
Verazin GT, Warneke JA, Driscoll DL, Karakousis C, Petrelli NJ, Takita H (Roswell Park Cancer Inst, Buffalo, NY)
Arch Surg 127:1407–1411, 1992   140-94-13–31

Objective.—There is considerable debate regarding the significant prognostic variables in patients who have undergone removal of pulmonary metastases (PM) from soft tissue sarcomas. Prognostic factors were analyzed in a group of 78 patients, with tumors representing a variety of histologic types, who were treated aggressively for PM.

Patients and Methods.—The patient group of 41 males and 37 females had a mean age of 33 years. The location of the primary sarcoma was the extremity in 65% of the patients, the retroperitoneum in 19%, and other sites in 15%. Complete pulmonary resections were performed in 61 patients, 29 of whom subsequently underwent 2 or more thoracic explorations for recurrent PM. Follow-up data were available for 92% of the patients.

Results.—Patients who had a complete resection had a significantly longer median survival (21 months) than patients who had an incomplete resection (8 months). Local recurrence associated with PM had poor prognostic implications, as did a shorter disease-free interval. Neither the histologic type of the sarcoma nor the number of metastases resected had a significant impact on survival. There was a trend, however, toward a higher 10-year disease-free survival in patients with 5 or fewer metastases. And patients who underwent multiple thoracotomies had longer survival.

Conclusion.—More than half of the patients with a diagnosis of soft tissue sarcoma will have isolated PM as the initial site of recurrence. The findings of this study should help to identify patients who would benefit from surgical removal of these metastases. Results of multivariate analysis using Cox's proportional-hazards model emphasize the prognostic importance of complete resection, local control of the primary tumor, and disease-free interval.

▶ This article makes an important point. Twenty-eight of the patients reported in this series underwent multiple thoracotomies in the linear treatment of their pulmonary metastatic sarcomas. The use of multiple thoracotomies to control multiple recurrent metastatic lesions in the lung highlights that many sarcomas are pneumotropic. Indeed, many sarcomas metastasize to pulmonary parenchyma exclusively. Therefore, it appears that surgeons should not be hesitant to perform second, and even third, operative procedures if substantial intervals of disease-free status are obtained after each procedure. Our own cut-off point is 6 months to 1 year. If surgical control is able to gain at least a 12-month interval from a required second thoracotomy, we would proceed. This is particularly true in younger patients in whom the quality of life can be maintained with reduced pulmonary function.—D.J. Sugarbaker, M.D.

Lung Resection for Colorectal Metastases: 10-Year Results
McCormack PM, Burt ME, Bains MS, Martini N, Rusch VW, Ginsberg RJ
(Mem Sloan-Kettering Cancer Ctr, New York)
Arch Surg 127:1403–1406, 1992   140-94-13–32

Introduction.—Of patients undergoing curative resection for primary colorectal carcinoma, only 2% to 4% have metastases only to the lungs. There is controversy regarding the use of metastasectomy in such patients. A total of 144 cases of patients undergoing complete resection of pulmonary metastases (PM) from colorectal cancer were reviewed.

Patients.—The patients underwent a total of 170 operations at a single cancer center over 23 years. There were 89 men and 55 women, ranging in age from 26 to 83 years. Preoperatively, all patients were carefully evaluated to ensure that there were no metastases elsewhere in the body, particularly the liver. All but 4 patients were available for follow-up.

Outcomes.—Eighty-three percent of patients had metastases in 1 lung only, and 55% had a single lesion. Overall survival, as calculated by the Kaplan-Meier method, was 44% at 5 years and 26% at 10 years. There was no difference in survival between patients with 1 vs. multiple completely resected metastases. On comparison by log-rank analysis, patients with solitary lesions and a short disease-free interval tended to have better 5-year survival.

Conclusion.—Long-term survival is possible with complete resection of PM from colorectal carcinoma. Survival is poor with incomplete resection. Metastasectomy should be offered to appropriately selected patients.

▶ This study illustrates that there exists a unique patient population among patients who have recurrent colorectal carcinoma. These are patients whose tumors are exclusively pneumotropic in their metastatic pattern. It is of note that of the 89 men and 55 women reviewed in this report, none had evidence of systemic metastases elsewhere in the body, particularly the liver.

It is important to identify this subset of patients with pulmonary metastatic colorectal carcinoma. It is important because we believe that these patients should be candidates for secondary thoracotomies for resection of recurrent intraparenchymal disease. In rare instances, we have performed a third thoracotomy to resect recurrent disease. Again, it is of note that all of these patients, throughout the linear treatment of their pulmonary metastatic disease, did not have systemic metastases develop elsewhere. This unique tumor biology predisposing to a pulmonary metastatic pattern in colorectal carcinoma should be identified by the clinician so that appropriate referral and treatment may be done.—D.J. Sugarbaker, M.D.

Results of Surgical Resection of Pulmonary Metastases of Squamous Cell Carcinoma of the Head and Neck
Finley RK III, Verazin GT, Driscoll DL, Blumenson LE, Takita H, Bakamjian V, Sako K, Hicks W Jr, Petrelli NJ, Shedd DP (Roswell Park Cancer Inst, Buffalo, NY)
Am J Surg 164:594–598, 1992   140-94-13–33

Background.—Distant metastases of squamous cell carcinoma of the head and neck are found in 11% to 23% of the patients. Most metastases occur in the lung. A retrospective review was done to assess the value of pulmonary resection in patients with pulmonary metastases (PM) of squamous cell carcinoma of the head and neck.

Methods.—Fifty-eight patients treated from 1970 through 1989 were included in the analysis. The patients were 46 men and 12 women with a median age of 62 years at diagnosis of primary tumor.

Findings.—Factors predicting survival in patients with PM were pulmonary resection, locoregional control of primary tumor at the diagno-

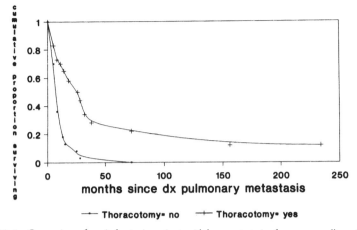

months since dx pulmonary metastasis

—•— Thoracotomy• no   —+— Thoracotomy• yes

Fig 13-6.—Comparison of survival rates in patients with lung metastasis of squamous cell carcinoma of the head and neck who had thoracotomy or who did not. Diagnosis is indicated by *dx*. (Courtesy of Finley RK III, Verazin GT, Driscoll DL, et al: *Am J Surg* 164:594-598, 1992.)

sis of PM, TNM stage of the head and neck primary tumor, a single nodule on radiography, and disease-free interval (DFI) from diagnosis of primary tumor of 2 or more years. Twenty-four patients had thoracotomy for resection of metastases. Seventeen percent of those patients had a second primary tumor in the lung. Of the 20 patients having exploratory surgery for possible pulmonary resection, 90% had complete resection of all malignant disease. That group had an estimated 5-year survival rate of 29%. A DFI of less than 1 year in that group was associated with a 5-year survival of 0%, whereas a DFI of 1-2 years carried a 5-year survival rate of 43%, and a DFI of 2 years or more had a 5-year survival rate of 33%. The number of malignant pulmonary nodules resected ranged from 1 to 5 and did not significantly predict survival. Four of 8 patients undergoing resection of more than 1 malignant pulmonary nodule survived 2 years, but none survived 5 years (Fig 13-6).

Conclusion.—Resecting a solitary PM from squamous cell carcinoma of the head and neck can result in long-term survival in selected cases. Important prognostic variables are locoregional control of the primary tumor, number of nodules seen on chest radiograph, TNM stage of the primary tumor, and the DFI of the head and neck primary tumor. The value of resection in patients with more than 1 malignant pulmonary nodule has yet to be established.

▶ This report is of interest because it highlights the differences in tumor biology among various tumor cell types. The patients with squamous cell carcinomas exhibited a variety of factors that appeared to affect their survival, factors that have not been noted to be consistent factors affecting survival in other tumor cell types. The DFI, for example, which was significant in this study, has not been significant in the assessment of other PM from other tumors. In addition, the effect that the stage and locale of the primary tumor has on the survival of these patients is significant.

Finally, it is of note that 17% of the patients taken to thoracotomy were found to have new primary bronchogenic carcinomas. One cannot overstress that patients with head/neck tumors have a high incidence of primary bronchogenic carcinoma and vice versa. Follow-up of these patients requires vigilance for the development of these related primary lesions. This report is an excellent review of the field of pulmonary metastasectomy, including its current indications and efficacy.

As minimally invasive surgical techniques are applied to pulmonary metastasectomy, indications may change. The equation that relates postoperative morbidity to therapeutic efficacy can be altered if morbidity is lessened via these new techniques. In addition, we can expect improvement in chemotherapeutic agents to increase the number of patients who will become candidates for cytoreductive surgery. The primary goal in each of these situations is complete control and complete cytoreduction of these lesions. Recognition of specific and unique tumor biologies that metastasize exclusively to the pulmonary parenchyma should be remembered, and all attempts should be made to spare pulmonary parenchyma during metastasectomy. Indeed, the sparing of pulmonary parenchyma, particularly in the young patient, can lead to improved long-term survival, as depletion of pulmonary reserve is often the limiting factor leading to a patient's demise.—D.J. Sugarbaker, M.D.

Challenging Problems in Thoracic Malignancies

INTRODUCTION

This last section deals with a variety of thoracic malignancies that often pose diagnostic and therapeutic challenges for the thoracic surgeon. The treatment of mesothelioma has been changing during the past 3–5 years. Included is a report using multimodality therapy in this malignancy (Abstract 140-94-13-34). Large-cell immunoblastic lymphomas of the mediastinum are often an interesting diagnostic challenge for thoracic surgeons. Abstract 140-94-13-35 was chosen because it gives some feedback for thoracic surgeons as to the prognosis of these patients presenting with primary disease in the mediastinum. Occasionally, surgeons will resect primary pulmonary lymphoma in the context of a malignant tumor. One paper is selected for its documentation of interesting patterns of involvement as possible prognostic factors in this disease. The last paper (Abstract 140-94-13-37) involves treatment of invasive thymoma, which is often a difficult technical challenge for the thoracic surgeon. This report again emphasizes the use of multimodality therapy in the treatment of this thoracic malignancy.

David J. Sugarbaker, M.D.

Node Status Has Prognostic Significance in the Multimodality Therapy of Diffuse, Malignant Mesothelioma

Sugarbaker DJ, Strauss GM, Lynch TJ, Richards W, Mentzer SJ, Lee TH, Corson JM, Antman KH (Brigham and Women's Hosp, Boston; Dana-Farber Cancer Inst, Boston; Harvard Med School, Boston)

J Clin Oncol 11:1172–1178, 1993   140-94-13–34

Background.—Little is known about the prognostic value of cell type and node status in malignant mesothelioma. In other primary intrathoracic malignancies, cell type and stage predict survival and dictate treatment. In a current series of patients with malignant pleural mesothelioma, a multimodality approach to treatment was used.

Methods.—Fifty-two selected patients were treated from 1980 to 1992. Treatment consisted of extrapleural pneumonectomy; cyclophosphamide, doxorubicin, and cisplatin (CAP) chemotherapy; and radiation therapy. The patients had no medical contraindications and potentially resectable mesothelioma on CT scanning.

Findings.—Perioperative morbidity was 17% and mortality was 5.8%. The median survival was 16 months. Among the 32 patients with epithelial histologic variants, survival rates were 77% at 1 year, 50% at 2 years,

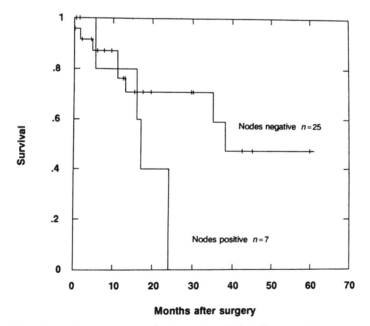

Fig 13–7.—Kaplan-Meier survival curve of patients with epithelial cell tumors with negative or positive nodes, as determined by pathologic review of resected specimens. Patients with negative nodes tended to have longer survival durations. (Courtesy of Sugarbaker DJ, Strauss GM, Lynch TJ, et al: *J Clin Oncol* 11:1172-1178, 1993.)

Proposed Staging System for Patients With Mesothelioma Based on
Survival of 52 Patients

Stage	Definition
I	Disease confined to within capsule of the parietal pleura: ipsilateral pleura, lung, pericardium, diaphragm, or chest-wall disease limited to previous biopsy sites
II	All of stage I with positive intrathoracic (N1 or N2) lymph nodes
III	Local extension of disease into: chest wall or mediastinum; heart, or through diaphragm, peritoneum; with or without extrathoracic or contralateral (N3) lymph node involvement
IV	Distant metastatic disease

Note: Butchart stage II and III patients are combined into stage III. Stage I represents resectable disease in patients with negative nodes. Patients with stage II disease are resectable but have positive nodal status.

(From Sugarbaker DJ, Strauss GM, Lynch TJ, et al: *J Clin Oncol* 11:1172-1178, 1993. Modified from Butchart EG, Ashcroft T, Barnsley WC, et al: *Thorax* 31:15-24, 1976.)

and 42% at 3 years. The 1- and 2-year survival rates of patients with mixed and sarcomatous cell disease were 45% and 7.5%, respectively. None of the patients in that group lived longer than 25 months. Positive regional mediastinal lymph nodes were found in 13 cases at resection. Patients with positive lymph nodes had poorer survivals than those with negative nodes. Patients with epithelial variant and negative mediastinal lymph nodes had a 5-year survival rate of 45% (Fig 13–7).

Conclusion.—In selected cases, this multimodality treatment has acceptable rates of morbidity and mortality. Patients with epithelial histologic variant and negative mediastinal lymph nodes had a prolonged survival. The findings provide the rationale for a revised staging system for malignant pleural mesothelioma and enable patient stratification into groups likely to benefit from aggressive multimodality therapy (table).

▶ The appropriate use of extrapleural pneumonectomy in the treatment of malignant pleural mesothelioma has been the subject of great debate during the past decade. During the past 3–5 years, there have been reports of lower operative morbidity/mortality with improved techniques and perioperative care (1, 2). The treatment of this disease has continued to move toward a primarily multimodal approach (3, 4). This particular report is of importance because, for the first time, we are given prognostic factors that may help to select patients for a very aggressive multimodal approach. Epithelial cell type and node status were shown to be predictors of prognostic significance.

With the use of minimally invasive techniques, it may be that preresectional node status can be determined pathologically and, therefore, a patient could be selected or excluded for this more aggressive approach. A revised staging system, which provides a rationale for further aggressive treatment based on node status and technical resectability, is presented.—D.J. Sugarbaker, M.D.

References

1. Sugarbaker DJ, et al: *J Thorac Cardiovasc Surg* 102:10, 1991.
2. Sugarbaker DJ, et al: *Ann Thorac Surg* 54:941, 1992.
3. Rusch VW: *Chest* 103:382S, 1993.
4. Sugarbaker DJ, et al: *Chest* 103:377S, 1993.

Large-Cell and Immunoblastic Lymphoma of the Mediastinum: Prognostic Features and Treatment Outcome in 57 Patients
Kirn D, Mauch P, Shaffer K, Pinkus G, Shipp MA, Kaplan WD, Tung N, Wheeler C, Beard CJ, Canellos GP, Shulman LN (Brigham and Women's Hosp, Boston; Dana-Farber Cancer Inst, Boston; Beth Israel Hosp, Boston; et al)
J Clin Oncol 11:1336–1343, 1993   140-94-13–35

Background.—The prognosis of patients with large-cell lymphoma of the mediastinum after chemotherapy and radiation therapy is not well defined. The value of radiation therapy remains unclear. Furthermore,

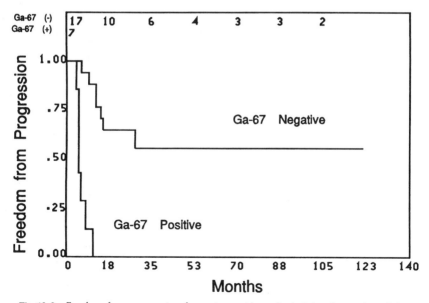

Fig 13–8.—Freedom from progression for patients with mediastinal lymphoma depended on whether ⁶⁷Ga avidity persisted in the area of known lymphoma midway through or after initial chemotherapy. Patients who underwent autologous bone marrow transplantation are censored at time of transplant. (Courtesy of Kirn D, Mauch P, Shaffer K, et al: *J Clin Oncol* 11:1336–1343, 1993.)

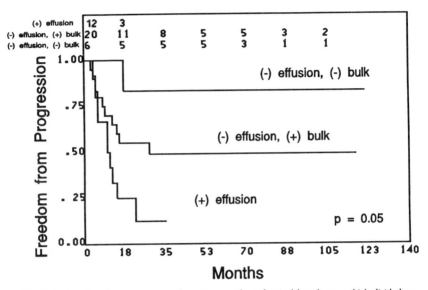

Fig 13–9.—Freedom from progression for patients with mediastinal lymphoma, which divided patients into 3 prognostic groups: patients with pleural effusion and tumors of any bulk, patients without pleural effusion and with bulky tumors, and patients without pleural effusions and with nonbulky tumors. Bulky tumors are defined on plain chest x-ray tests as those with a tumor diameter of $\geq$ 10 cm or an area of $\geq$ 60 cm². (Courtesy of Kirn D, Mauch P, Shaffer K, et al: *J Clin Oncol* 11:1336–1343, 1993.)

prognostic factors have not been documented. The clinical characteristics and treatment outcomes of patients with large cell and immunoblastic lymphoma of the mediastinum were determined.

Methods.—Fifty-seven patients seen with primary, mediastinal, large-cell, and immunoblastic lymphoma between 1979 and 1991 were included in the analysis. Initial sites of disease, radiologic features, treatment, outcomes, and prognostic factors were noted.

Findings.—Almost all patients had disease confined to sites above the diaphragm. In these patients, bulky disease and extensive intrathoracic infiltration were common. All patients underwent intensive chemotherapy. Forty-four percent underwent chest irradiation. The overall survival at 5 years was estimated to be 50%, with a freedom-from-relapse rate of 45%. Factors predicting disease relapse after chemotherapy were the presence of a pleural effusion, a number of involved extranodal sites, a lactic dehydrogenase (LDH) ratio of more than 3.0, and an incomplete treatment response as evidenced by a residual mass on a chest radiograph or persistent gallium 67 avidity after chemotherapy. Factors predicting reduced survival included the presence of pleural effusion, the number of involved extranodal sites, and a positive ^{67}Ga scan after therapy (Figs 13–8 and 13–9).

Conclusion.—After initial treatment, patients with large-cell lymphoma of the mediastinum have about a 50% chance of surviving without disease. The presence of pleural effusion at the initial assessment was associated with a very poor outcome. Bulk disease in itself was a negative predictive factor only in patients without pleural effusions compared with patients without bulk disease. All patients with the involvement of 2 or more extranodal sites had relapses after standard chemotherapy.

▶ The presence of a pleural effusion in these patients with primary mediastinal lymphoma is the single most important predictor of poor outcome. In addition, involvement of extranodal sites is important if 2 or more sites are involved.

It is important that surgeons approach patients with variegated or lobular masses in the anterior mediastinum with preoperative biopsy. There has been some discussion in the literature (1) that has suggested that mediastinal masses not be biopsied to avoid pleural seeding, particularly of thymic carcinoma.

On the other hand, the CT scan and MRI of the mediastinum are helpful in determining whether typical thymomas are to be encountered or whether one might expect a hemopoietic disorder. The safest route: When in doubt, do a biopsy of a mediastinal mass before full sternotomy and surgical resection.—D.J. Sugarbaker, M.D.

Reference

1. Wilkins EW Jr: Thymus:Myasthenia Gravis and Thymoma, in Grillo HC, (eds): *Current Therapy In Cardiothoracic Surgery* Toronto, B.C. Decker Inc. 1989, pp 117–121.

Primary Pulmonary Lymphomas: A Clinical Study of 70 Cases in Nonimmunocompromised Patients
Cordier J-F, Chailleux E, Lauque D, Reynaud-Gaubert M, Dietemann-Molard A, Dalphin JC, Blanc-Jouvan F, Loire R (Claude Bernard Univ, Lyon, France; Univ Hosp, Nantes, France; Univ Hosp, Toulouse, France; et al)
Chest 103:201–208, 1993   140-94-13-36

Introduction.—Primary non-Hodgkin's lymphomas of the lung are rare extranodal lymphomas that generally have a more favorable prognosis than nodal lymphomas. A retrospective study was designed to obtain a current clinical view on the course and treatment of primary pulmonary lymphomas.

Methods.—With the use of strict clinical criteria, 70 patients with primary pulmonary lymphoma diagnosed between 1970 and 1990 were identified. Pathologic slides of pulmonary or bronchial specimens were reviewed and survival of patients estimated from the time of pathologic diagnosis. The cases were separated into 2 groups: low-grade (LG) or high-grade (HG) lymphomas.

Results.—The patient group consisted of 35 men and 35 women with a mean age of 58.4 years. Thirty-nine were nonsmokers and 27 were smokers or ex-smokers. Low-grade lymphomas accounted for 87% of the pulmonary lymphomas. Symptoms included cough, dyspnea, chest pain, and hemoptysis, although 41% of the patients with LG lymphomas had no pulmonary symptoms at diagnosis. Chest x-ray films, tomograms, and CT scans identified localized alveolar opacities, diffuse infiltrative opacities, atelectasis, and pleural effusions. Biopsy specimens revealed lymphomatous infiltration in 12 cases. Forty-two patients underwent surgical exeresis and 16 had cytostatic treatment as their primary therapy. Overall survival of the patients with LG lymphoma was 100% at 2 years and 93.6% at 5 years. Prognoses did not differ significantly according to the treatment modalities. The patients with HG lymphomas were all symptomatic. Localized opacities were seen on radiographs in 6 patients, and inflammatory changes occurred in 7 of the 9 cases. Survival for that group was significantly worse than that of the LG group. At the close of the study, 5 patients had died, 2 were in complete remission, and 2 were relapsing.

Conclusion.—Findings confirm the favorable course of LG primary pulmonary lymphomas. The progression of these lymphomas in the lung is very slow. In contrast, HG lymphomas are aggressive malignancies, probably requiring polychemotherapy as do nodal HG lymphomas. Clinical and imaging features are often suggestive of the diagnosis of primary pulmonary lymphomas.

▶ This important paper outlines the appropriate postoperative care of patients given a diagnosis of primary pulmonary lymphoma. The majority of these (87%) were LG lymphomas. The high survival rate of 93.6% at 5 years is indicative of the excellent prognosis in these patients who were treated in a variety of ways. Of note is the distinction in prognosis between LG lymphomas in which the prognosis was excellent to HG lymphomas in which the prognosis was more guarded and the use of adjuvant therapy was indicated. The operative approach for the diagnosis of pulmonary lymphoma would depend on the radiologic pattern. It is important to understand that an open or closed lung biopsy would be appropriate for the alveolar pattern of lung involvement as opposed to surgical resection or biopsy in the bronchovascular lymphogenic pattern or nodule pattern of involvement by malignant lymphoma. The clinical course of these patients will be linked to their clinical and radiographic presentation at diagnosis. Indeed, the diagnostic procedure of choice will depend on the pattern of clinical presentation.—D.J. Sugarbaker, M.D.

Chemotherapy and Operation for Invasive Thymoma
Rea F, Sartori F, Loy M, Calabrò F, Fornasiero A, Daniele O, Altavilla G (Univ

of Padua, Italy)
J Thorac Cardiovasc Surg 106:543–549, 1993   140-94-13–37

Background.—Radical surgery has been used as a primary measure in patients having invasive malignant thymoma, but involvement of local structures often precludes radical resection and allows only "debulking" of the tumor. The use of radiotherapy, chemotherapy, or both in these cases remains controversial.

Objective.—A prospective trial evaluating neoadjuvant chemotherapy was done in 16 patients with invasive stage III/IVA thymoma. All the tumors were considered unresectable after initial staging.

Treatment.—Patients received cycles of cisplatin (50 mg/m²) and doxorubicin (40 mg/m²) on day 1, vincristine (.6 mg/m²) on day 3, and cyclophosphamide (700 mg/m²) on day 4. At least 3 cycles were administered at 3-week intervals. Resection was done after chemotherapy. Patients in whom radical surgery was not feasible and those with residual disease in a biopsy specimen received radiotherapy.

Results.—Seven of the 16 patients had a complete remission when given combination chemotherapy, and 9 others had a partial response. Resection of the thymoma was possible in all but 1 of the patients, and 11 of them—including all patients with a complete response—underwent radical resection. Five of 11 patients who had persistent tumor and were given radiotherapy had a relapse. Ten patients were alive at last follow-up and 6 had died, all but 1 of them with evidence of disease. The median survival was 5.5 years, and the 3-year survival rate was 70%. Eight of the 11 patients having radical resection survived.

Conclusion.—Surgery after adjunctive combination chemotherapy can be an effective approach to patients having highly invasive thymoma.

▶ The relatively low incidence of malignant thymoma will certainly preclude a prospective, randomized trial in the evaluation of therapeutic strategies for this disease. Therefore, reports such as this one will need to be used to develop effective treatment strategies for this group of malignancies. The use of neoadjuvant chemotherapy in such patients who are considered to have unresectable thymoma after surgical expiration did convert a number of patients and allowed a complete or incomplete surgical debulking of the tumor (1). Resection of malignant thymomas is a technical challenge. We have found the use of MRI important in the preoperative assessment of these patients and in the determining of their resectability. Magnetic resonance imaging can provide improved visualization of the great vessels and the tumor before surgical resection and has replaced the phlebogram, which was used in this study in many centers. Induction chemotherapy can often complicate the resection, but from this report, it appears to be a viable therapeutic strategy in selected cases. See also references 2–4.—D.J. Sugarbaker, M.D.

References

1. Salgia R, et al: *Hosp Physician* January:33, 1994.
2. Kirn DH, et al: *J Thorac Cardiovasc Surg* 106:696, 1993.
3. Strauss GM, et al: *J Clin Oncol* 10:829, 1992.
4. Sugarbaker DJ, Strauss GM: *Semin Oncol* 20:163, 1993.

14 Vascular Surgery

Introduction

Recent publications have helped to resolve some clinically important issues in the management of patients with peripheral vascular disease. Publication of the VA Cooperative trial on the "Efficacy of Carotid Endarterectomy for Asymptomatic Carotid Stenosis" has partially clarified the role of carotid endarterectomy in the treatment of this problem. Surgical therapy was shown to significantly reduce the risk of stroke plus transient ischemic attacks, and a strong trend ($P < .06$) in favor of reduction of the risk of stroke alone in patients undergoing carotid endarterectomy was also seen. Thus, the surgical management of patients with asymptomatic, high-grade carotid stenosis appears appropriate if low ($< 2\%$) rates of perioperative morbidity and mortality can be achieved. In contrast, recurrent carotid stenosis after carotid endarterectomy appears to be a benign lesion that requires neither repeat endarterectomy nor routine duplex surveillance.

Although some advocate repair of small (< 5 cm) aortic aneurysms, demonstration of a clear-cut benefit in this group of patients remains elusive, and the majority of published studies do not recommend such an approach. Similarly, although cardiac disease is a primary cause of morbidity after aortic reconstruction, whether preoperative cardiac evaluation of patients undergoing aortic reconstruction identifies patients who are likely to have significant postoperative cardiac complications remains unproven. Unfortunately, other attempts at reducing cardiac morbidity after arterial reconstruction, such as the use of epidural anesthesia, have also proven ineffective. Fortunately, contrary to what was previously thought, the risk of cardiac complications after aortic procedures is relatively low, and patients undergoing aortic reconstruction are at lower risk for cardiac complications than are those undergoing peripheral vascular reconstruction procedures.

Endovascular therapy, including balloon angioplasty and the use of endoluminal stents, is becoming a standard part of therapy for peripheral arterial occlusive disease, particularly in patients with disease in the iliac arteries. As more is known about the long-term results of these procedures, selection of patients with lesions appropriate for endovascular therapy becomes easier. Patients with focal lesions in the iliac arteries and symptoms of claudication respond well to endovascular treatment. In contrast, those with multiple iliac artery lesions indicating diffuse disease and those with critical ischemia appear to do poorly after balloon angioplasty and probably should not undergo this procedure. Use of metallic endoluminal stents after iliac artery balloon angioplasty appears to improve the initial and, potentially, the long-term clinical results of the procedure, but use of metallic stents in the femoral popliteal arteries appears to produce poorer results than balloon angioplasty alone.

Technical perfection of an infrainguinal bypass procedure and the quality of the vein used for that bypass remain critically important determinants of long-term graft patency. However, vein graft stenosis likely resulting from intimal hyperplasia remains a problem, and graft surveillance using color-flow Doppler imaging is prudent in that "failing" grafts that can be repaired can be detected. Patient selection for infrainguinal reconstruction also remains a critical step in improving outcome after reconstructive procedures. Recognition of subsets of patients, such as those undergoing dialysis who have diabetes and those who do poorly after any type of reconstructive procedure, will allow these patients to avoid essentially doomed attempts at arterial reconstruction.

A better understanding of the management of phlegmasia cerulea dolens and traumatic venous injuries should allow better outcome in patients with these difficult problems. In addition, the long-term results of the use of intracaval devices for the prevention of pulmonary emboli are finally being published to enable easier selection from among the various devices available for the management of patients at risk for pulmonary emboli. Finally, efforts to contain the cost of treatment of patients with peripheral vascular disease are rapidly moving forward. Hopefully this will not mean that, in the future, noninvasive vascular testing, which has been so instrumental in the understanding and management of patients with peripheral vascular disease, will no longer be available.

James M. Seeger, M.D.

Efficacy of Carotid Endarterectomy for Asymptomatic Carotid Stenosis

Hobson RW II, Weiss DG, Fields WS, Goldstone J, Moore WS, Towne JB, Wright CB, and the Veterans Affairs Cooperative Study Group (Veterans Affairs Cooperative Studies Program Coordinating Ctr, Perry Point, Md)
N Engl J Med 328:221–227, 1993   140-94-14–1

Background.—Randomized trials have failed to confirm benefit for carotid endarterectomy in patients with asymptomatic carotid stenosis, notwithstanding the fact that surgery is often performed in such patients.

Methods.—A multicenter trial was conducted at 11 VA medical centers, where 444 men having at least 50% carotid stenosis were randomly assigned to receive either optimal medical care alone or medical care plus carotid endarterectomy. Medical management included aspirin in an initial dose of 650 mg twice daily. The mean follow-up was 4 years.

Results.—Ipsilateral neurologic events occurred in 8% of surgically treated patients and 21% of the medical group, for a relative risk of 0.38. First ipsilateral stroke and transient ischemic attacks were substantially more prevalent in the medical patients. Strokes were half as frequent in the surgical group. The rates of postoperative stroke and death did not differ significantly. Coronary atherosclerosis was the predominant cause of death in this series.

Conclusions.—Carotid endarterectomy lowered the risk of ipsilateral neurologic events in men with asymptomatic carotid stenosis. The combined rates of stroke and death did not differ significantly, but a modest effect was not excluded. Coronary atherosclerosis remains the chief cause of death in this population. A low rate of perioperative complications is necessary whenever a program of operative intervention is under consideration.

▶ The management of patients with significant carotid atherosclerosis continues to evolve. This report suggests the potential of carotid endarterectomy in reducing the risk of stroke in patients with asymptomatic carotid stenosis; however, because of the study's size and patient selection, this benefit was not confirmed statistically. This study also demonstrates that the margin of benefit for carotid endarterectomy is far narrower in asymptomatic patients than in symptomatic patients, reemphasizing the need for very low postoperative morbidity and mortality rates when carotid endarterectomy is done for asymptomatic disease.—J.M. Seeger, M.D.

Early and Late Outcome of Surgical Repair for Small Abdominal Aortic Aneurysms: A Population-Based Analysis
Hallett JW Jr, Naessens JM, Ballard DJ (Mayo Clinic and Found, Rochester, Minn)
J Vasc Surg 18:684–691, 1993   140-94-14-2

Background.—It remains uncertain whether abdominal aortic aneurysms (AAAs) 5 cm or less in diameter should be repaired at an early stage promote late survival.

Methods.—In a population-based study done in Olmsted County, Minnesota, patients given a clinical diagnosis of AAA in 1951–1984 were targeted to learn the reasons for surgery, the perioperative mortality, and the late survival.

Results.—The 195 aneurysms less than 5 cm in size when initially diagnosed represented 53% of the total. The incidence of small AAAs increased 30-fold during the review period, and the trend toward repairing these aneurysms also increased. One third of the small aneurysms eventually were repaired. There were no particular indications for surgical consultation and operation other than the presence of an aneurysm in half the cases. The major specific indications were expansion on serial examination and the presence of nonspecific symptoms in the abdomen or back. Operative mortality was 2.6% for patients with small aneurysms and 5.5% for those with large lesions. Only 62% of the patients with small AAAs were alive 5 years after repair compared with an expected survival of 83%. The relative survival rates were similar for patients having small and large aneurysms repaired. In both groups, myocardial infarction was the primary cause of death.

Conclusions.—The early results of elective repair of small AAAs are excellent, but coronary heart disease continues to limit the late survival of these patients. At present, most small AAAs should be closely watched and repaired electively when they approach—or reach—5 or 6 cm in size and the patient is a good operative risk.

▶ Although elective repair of small (< 5 cm) AAA is associated with low perioperative mortality rates, it does not appear that such procedures improve long-term survival. Thus, the argument for elective repair, rather than observation, of these small aneurysms remains unconvincing.—J.M. Seeger, M.D.

◢

Routine Postendarterectomy Duplex Surveillance: Does It Prevent Late Stroke?

Mackey WC, Belkin M, Sindhi R, Welch H, O'Donnell TF Jr (Tufts Univ; New England Med Ctr, Boston)
J Vasc Surg 16:934–940, 1992   140-94-14-3

Background.—Fewer than half of late postendarterectomy strokes are related to recurrent carotid stenosis, a finding that brings into question the practice of routine postoperative duplex surveillance for the prevention of late strokes.

Methods.—The results of postoperative duplex ultrasound studies were correlated with the clinical outcome in 258 patients having a total of 1,053 examinations of 348 carotid arteries. The average follow-up interval was 53 months.

Results.—Recurrent carotid stenosis exceeding 50%, or occlusion of the common or internal carotid, was observed in 16% of vessels. Only 2 of these stenoses directly led to unexpected stroke. Eight other patients had a preventive reoperation, whereas 8 had reoperation for transient ischemia. Eight vessels became occluded without a stroke developing. If it is assumed that each patient who had prophylactic reoperation would have had a stroke otherwise, and that the 2 unheralded strokes would have been prevented by closer follow-up, routine duplex examination might have prevented late stroke in 4% of all patients.

Conclusion.—Routine duplex ultrasonography is not an efficient means of preventing late strokes related to recurrent carotid stenosis.

▶ Although recurrent carotid stenosis after CEA is not uncommon, these recurrent stenoses are, for the most part, benign. Because of this, routine postendarterectomy surveillance does not appear to be necessary, and it likely will not be reimbursed in the increasingly cost-conscious health care environment.—J.M. Seeger, M.D.

Does the Clinical Evaluation of the Cardiac Status Predict Outcome in Patients With Abdominal Aortic Aneurysms?
Lachpelle K, Graham AM, Symes JF (Royal Victoria Hosp; McGill Univ, Montreal)
J Vasc Surg 15:964–971, 1992   140-94-14–4

Background.—The repair of nonruptured abdominal aortic aneurysms (AAA) is now a relatively safe procedure. Because operative mortality after aneurysm repair is low, properly selecting patients for further cardiac assessment by using reliable predictors of cardiac risk would be a cost-effective way to reduce death rates after AAA surgery. Therefore, clinical evaluation of cardiac status was used as a predictor to guide further cardiac workup in patients before AAA repair was reported.

Method.—All 146 patients having asymptomatic AAA repair between 1986 and 1990 were placed retrospectively into one of three groups on the basis of their clinical evaluation. Group 1 patients had no history of myocardial infarction or angina, no congestive heart failure, and no ischemic changes on ECG. Group 2 patients had a history of myocardial infarction or class I–II angina, or ischemic changes on ECG. Patients in group 3 had congestive heart failure or class III–IV angina. Patients in group 1 had no further cardiac workup. Those in group 2 who had angina had left ventricular ejection fraction evaluation by multiple gated acquisition and were cleared for surgery by a cardiologist. Group 2 patients without angina had no further cardiac workup. Group 3 patients had coronary angiography followed by then coronary revascularization.

Findings.—The overall mortality was 4.8%, and cardiac mortality was 3.4%. Group 1 had a mortality of 1.8%, with no cardiac-related deaths. Group 2 had a mortality of 9.5%, with 8% of the deaths cardiac related. None of the patients in group 3 died. The difference between the cardiac death rates and in postoperative cardiac morbidity between groups 1 and 2 was significant. Compared with group 2, group 3 had significantly fewer postoperative myocardial infarctions. Within group 2, neither the left ventricular ejection fraction nor the finding of angina or any ST-T segment changes predicted increased cardiac-related deaths.

Conclusions.—Even mild-to-moderate cardiac symptoms, such as those seen in group 2, should undergo a more aggressive cardiac assessment, including dipyridamole thallium scans and/or coronary angiography. Patients with clinically severe coronary artery disease seem to benefit from previous coronary bypass. These patients should therefore be evaluated before AAA repair with coronary angiography.

▶ In contrast to the conclusions of this article, several recent studies have shown that low rates of cardiac morbidity and mortality can be achieved in patients undergoing aortic surgery without extensive preoperative cardiac evaluation. In addition, cardiac evaluation in patients with peripheral vascular disease often leads to coronary angiography and prophylactic coronary revascularization, which is expensive, of unproven value, and not without risk. Although some patients who require aortic reconstruction likely benefit from preoperative cardiac evaluation, determining who these patients are remains very difficult.—J.M. Seeger, M.D.

Comparison of Cardiac Morbidity Rates Between Aortic and Infrainguinal Operations: Two-Year Follow-Up
Krupski WC, Layug EL, Reilly LM, Rapp JH, Mangano DT, and the Study of Perioperative Ischemia Research Group (Univ of Colorado, Denver; Univ of California, San Francisco)
J Vasc Surg 18:609–617, 1993   140-94-14-5

Objective.—Two-year data on cardiac risk are available for 53 patients having major abdominal vascular operations and 87 having infrainguinal procedures.

Results.—Hospital mortality was 9% for patients having aortic surgery and 7% for those having infrainguinal vascular procedures. The surviving patients were followed for a median of approximately 2 years. Fatal myocardial infarction occurred in 4% of the aortic group and 16% of the infrainguinal group. The respective figures for nonfatal infarction were 2% and 5%. One patient in the aortic group and 3 having infrainguinal procedures were admitted with unstable angina during follow-up. The overall rate of adverse cardiac outcomes was 8% in patients having aortic surgery and 25% in those having infrainguinal vascular procedures. Multivariate analysis showed that, in both groups, adverse outcomes correlated with a history of diabetes and with definite coronary artery disease.

Conclusion.—An adverse cardiac outcome is likelier in high-risk patients having infrainguinal vascular surgery than in those having aortic surgery, chiefly because of more frequent diabetes and coronary artery disease in the former group.

▶ Long-term as well as perioperative cardiac complications are significantly more common in patients undergoing infrainguinal bypass procedures, and this is particularly true in patients with diabetes mellitus requiring femoral distal bypass. Such patients may be candidates for aggressive cardiac follow-up and treatment, although the efficacy of this approach remains to be proven. Regardless, it appears that in such patients, their tibial artery disease is reflective of their coronary artery disease.—J.M. Seeger, M.D.

Axillofemoral Bypass With Externally Supported, Knitted Dacron Grafts: A Follow-Up Through Twelve Years

El-Massry S, Saad E, Sauvage LR, Zammit M, Davis CC, Smith JC, Rittenhouse EA, Fisher LD (Hope Heart Inst; Providence Med Ctr, Seattle; Univ of Washington, Seattle)

J Vasc Surg 17:107–115, 1993   140-94-14–6

Background.—Axillofemoral bypass is an accepted approach to patients having an infected aortofemoral graft or hostile intra-abdominal conditions, but its use in high-risk patients who are markedly limited by aortoiliac occlusive disease remains controversial. Thrombectomies may be needed at frequent intervals to maintain graft function, and the rate of infection is relatively high.

Series.—Seventy-nine consecutive axillofemoral bypass graft operations were done on 77 patients who had conditions that made an abdominal procedure prohibitively risky. In a majority of cases, the graft had an axillounifemoral configuration.

Results.—Operative mortality was 5%. There were no graft-related deaths during a mean follow-up of 42 months. The primary patency rate was 78% at 5 years and 73% at 7 years, and it did not change subsequently. Neither the graft configuration nor the patency of the superficial femoral artery influenced patency rates, but patients treated for disabling claudication had a somewhat higher patency rate than those who underwent surgery for limb salvage. Actuarial survival at 10 years was 23% compared with 72% for a concurrent group of patients having aortofemoral bypass surgery.

Conclusion.—The externally supported, knitted Dacron axillofemoral bypass graft may be an appropriate treatment for patients with severe aortoiliac disease who require revascularization but are at high risk from abdominal surgery.

▶ The role of axillofemoral bypass in the treatment of aortoiliac disease remains controversial. This paper advocates a conservative approach of using this procedure only in high-risk patients, and it reports very good long-term results with such an approach. Whether external support of the grafts is the primary factor in achieving these results remains to be determined, however.—J.M. Seeger, M.D.

Iliac Arteries: Reanalysis of Results of Balloon Angioplasty
Johnston KW (Univ of Toronto)
Radiology 186:207–212, 1993   140-94-14–7

Objective.—The results of percutaneous transluminal balloon angioplasty (PTA) of the iliac artery were reviewed in 667 patients who were among 984 originally having the procedure for arterial occlusive disease. Criteria for success included at least one grade of symptomatic improvement and improvement in the ankle-brachial pressure ratio, Doppler waveform, or treadmill exercise test.

Results.—Three fourths of 82 occluded iliac arteries were patent at 1 month. The predicted 3-year success rate for PTA of a single iliac occlusion was 66%, but that for occlusion with a tandem lesion was only 17%. For 313 common iliac angioplasties, the success rates were 97% at 1 month, 68% at 3 years, and 60% at 5 years. In 209 external iliac angioplasties, the predicted 3-year success rate was 57% for men but only 34% for women. In 58 PTAs of both common and external iliac stenoses, 73% of patients with good runoff and 30% of those with poor runoff had a good outcome at 3 years. The rate of serious complications was 4%, and mortality was 0.3%. Surgery was required in 1% of cases.

Conclusion.—Iliac PTA has a significant role in the management of occlusive disease and should be seriously considered if the estimated chances of long-term success are good.

Is Iliac Angioplasty Indicated in the Treatment of Critical Limb Ischemia?
Hartnell G, Wakeley C, Wyatt M, Horrocks M (Univ of Bristol, England; Bristol Royal Infirmary, England)
J Intervent Radiol 7:101–103, 1992   140-94-14–8

Background.—Reported results of percutaneous balloon angioplasty (PTA) of iliac artery stenoses in patients with intermittent claudication are favorable. Some studies, however, have included patients who, at present, would not be considered to have critical limb ischemia. Other studies have failed to define the criteria for chronic critical ischemia.

Patients.—Forty-nine iliac angioplasties were performed over a 7-year period in 45 patients with critical lower extremity ischemia. In addition to persistently recurring pain at rest that necessitated analgesia for longer than 2 weeks or gangrenous changes in the foot or toes, the patients had absent palpable pulses or an ankle systolic pressure below 50 mm Hg.

Results.—Successful radiologic results were achieved in 38 of 49 angioplasties, and symptomatic improvement persisted after 1 week in 24 instances. Eight of these patients required a further procedure. Seventeen remained improved after 1 month, but 4 required amputation. Seventeen patients who failed to improve at 1 week required a further procedure. Seven of these patients were improved at 1 month, 7 were unchanged, and 7 required amputation.

Conclusions.—Iliac angioplasty may succeed initially in patients with critical ischemia of the lower extremity, but long-term patency rates are poor and many patients require further intervention. Either surgical revascularization or combined angioplasty and surgery may be a better approach to these patients.

▶ Selection of patients with symptomatic peripheral vascular disease for treatment with balloon angioplasty must be based on an understanding of the likelihood of long-term success of the procedure rather than a "try it and see" approach. These 2 articles (Abstracts 140-94-14–7 and 140-94-14–8) demonstrate that iliac artery balloon angioplasty can be valuable in patients with peripheral vascular disease, but only if proper patient selection is utilized.—J.M. Seeger, M.D.

Stenting of the Iliac Arteries With the Palmaz Stent: Experience From a Multicenter Trial
Palmaz JC, Laborde JC, Rivera FJ, Encarnacion CE, Lutz JD, Moss JG (Univ of Texas, San Antonio)
Cardiovasc Intervent Radiol 15:291–297, 1992   140-94-14–9

Objective.—Experience with balloon-expandable intraluminal stenting of the iliac arteries was reviewed in 486 patients having a total of 587 Palmaz stent procedures during a 4-year period. Eighty-one patients had bilateral iliac stent placements. The mean follow-up was 13 months, and 201 patients had follow-up angiography an average of 8½ months after stent placement.

Results.—Ninety-one percent of patients had a good clinical outcome after 1 year; 84% at 2 years; and 69% at 43 months. The angiographic patency rate was 92%. The mean ankle-brachial index rose from 0.62 to 0.8 shortly after treatment, and it remained at 0.8 at last follow-up. Both poor distal runoff and diabetes had adverse effects on the clinical outcome. Procedural complications occurred at a rate of 10%.

Conclusion.—The balloon-expandable stent is an effective and safe approach to treating atherosclerotic disease of the iliac arteries.

A Comparison Study of Self-Expandable Stents vs Balloon Angioplasty Alone in Femoropopliteal Artery Occlusions
Do-dai-Do, Triller J, Walpoth BH, Stirnemann P, Mahler F (Univ of Bern, Switzerland)
Cardiovasc Intervent Radiol 15:306–312, 1992   140-94-14–10

Introduction.—The initial use of the vascular stent supported the device's application in maintaining immediate vascular patency after percutaneous transluminal (balloon) angioplasty (PTA) and in preventing restenosis. In the femoropopliteal artery, however, restenosis often occurred if the blockage measured 3 to 5 cm. Results of a comparative, controlled prospective study of self-expandable stents were presented in an attempt to prevent late restenosis in femoropopliteal occlusions 3 cm or longer.

Methods.—Patients undergoing balloon PTA either received additional stent implantation or PTA alone (controls). The occlusions underwent guidewire traversing before the balloon dilatation. Twenty-six patients with femoropopliteal occlusions ranging from 3 to 18 cm comprised each group.

Technique.—All patients underwent the same treatment, except that controls had an 8F introducer sheath inserted into the femoral artery. The stent was attached to a 7F delivering catheter via an invaginated double membrane. Retraction of this membrane causes the stent to expand to full diameter. Because of additional expansion after 24 hours or more, the stent ends overlap by about 1.5 cm to prevent any delayed separation.

Results.—All patients had successful PTA or PTA plus stent insertion. Thrombosis of the stent requiring catheter thrombolysis occurred in 5 of the 26 test patients within 1 to 10 days of implantation. All 5 were successfully reopened. The PTA-alone patients experienced 6 reocclusions during the first 6 months postsurgery and 4 blockages occurred after 6 months. After 12 months, the PTA plus stent insertion group had a secondary patency rate of 69%, whereas the PTA-alone group showed a patency rate of 65%.

Conclusion.—Whether using a stent in addition to PTA or not, a patency rate of approximately 67% could be achieved one year after the surgery. Early and late rethrombosis continue to pose problems for a successful PTA outcome.

▶ Use of metallic, endoluminal stents to improve early and long-term results of balloon angioplasty is increasing. These 2 articles (Abstracts 140-94-14–9 and 140-94-14–10) demonstrate that although stenting may be a valuable adjunct to iliac artery balloon dilatation, stenting of superficial femoral arteries does not seem to improve results. Rather, significantly more interventions were required to achieve equal patency when stents were inserted after SFA angioplasty. The exact role of endoluminal stents in the treatment of peripheral vascular disease is still evolving; however, once again, initial enthusiastic reports of the value of new endovascular procedures must be viewed with a "jaundiced eye" until these procedures are fully evaluated.—J.M. Seeger, M.D.

Infrainguinal Reconstruction for Patients With Chronic Renal Insufficiency

Whittemore AD, Donaldson MC, Mannick JA (Brigham and Women's Hosp, Boston)
J Vasc Surg 17:32–41, 1993   140-94-14–11

Background.—Infrainguinal arterial reconstruction provides 5-year graft patency rates approaching 80% in patients with occlusive peripheral vascular disease. However, the outcome in patients with varying degrees of chronic renal insufficiency is less certain.

Methods.—Fifty-six patients seen in the past 15 years with a serum creatinine level exceeding 2 mg/dL underwent 70 autogenous vein bypass operations. Thirty-one others had a total of 42 primary major amputations. Most reconstructed extremities were treated for salvage; about half required infrapopliteal bypass.

Results.—Operative mortality was 17% in patients having amputation and 11% in those having reconstructive surgery. The respective 5-year survival rates were 9% and 40%, a significant difference. Reconstruction resulted in a cumulative 5-year limb salvage rate of 80%, a primary graft patency rate of 74%, and a secondary patency rate of 77%. Both limb salvage and survival rates were lower for diabetic patients. No patient undergoing dialysis lived beyond 3 years, but these patients had a 2-year limb salvage rate of 76%.

Conclusion.—Infrainguinal reconstructive surgery in patients with chronic renal insufficiency provides limb salvage and graft patency rates comparable to those achieved in patients whose renal function is normal. They do, however, have a higher risk of perioperative death and reduced overall survival. Diabetics and patients requiring maintenance hemodialysis have the poorest outlook.

▶ Although the postoperative complication rate is high, the good long-term graft patency and limb salvage reported in this study appear to justify lower extremity arterial reconstruction in patients with renal insufficiency who are not dialysis-dependent. In contrast, the poor limb salvage and patient survival rates in those patients who are undergoing dialysis and have diabetes or other serious medical problems suggest that lesser procedures, such as angioplasty or even amputation, may be more appropriate.—J.M. Seeger, M.D.

A New Look at Intraoperative Completion Arteriography: Classification and Management Strategies for Intraluminal Defects

Marin ML, Veith FJ, Panetta TF, Suggs WD, Wengerter KR, Bakal C, Cynamon J (Montefiore Med Ctr/Albert Einstein College of Medicine, New York)
Am J Surg 166:136–140, 1993   140-94-14–12

	Classification of Intraluminal Defects
0	No visible abnormality in the graft or runoff vessels
I	Minimal defects in graft or runoff vessels consisting of round lucencies (air bubbles) or valve leaflets
II	Moderate defects in the graft or runoff vessels consisting of uniform smooth tapering (up to 90% of the luminal diameter); irregular intraluminal filling defects ($<60\%$ of the luminal diameter); or incomplete or faint graft opacification
III	Severe defects in the graft or runoff vessels consisting of irregular intraluminal filling defects ($>60\%$) and complete cutoff of graft or outflow artery opacification

(Courtesy of Marin ML, Veith FJ, Panetta TF, et al: *Am J. Surg* 166:136–140, 1993.)

Background.—Although completion arteriography is the gold standard for postoperative assessment of bypass grafts, the significance of and management strategies for various intraluminal filling defects are not clear. To clarify the relationship between these angiographic irregularities and vein graft patency, intraluminal defects occurring after infrapopliteal vein bypass were classified.

Methods.—The study included 78 patients undergoing infrapopliteal reversed vein bypass graft. Standard completion arteriography including proximal and distal anastomoses was performed. Images were graded on the basis of intraluminal filling defects (table). Postoperative bypass patency was monitored by frequent physical examination, pulse volume recordings, and duplex ultrasonography.

Results.—Thirty-nine arteriograms showed no visible abnormality; 6 showed minimal defects. Eighteen bypasses with grade II intraluminal defects improved with nonsurgical treatment. Irregular filling defects were treated with injection of 40 to 60 mL of papaverine; some patients received later a 250,000-nit urokinase infusion. All of these bypasses were improved at follow-up arteriography. One-month and 1-year patency rates with grade I and II defects were comparable to patency rates for grafts that did not have defects. One-month and 1-year patency rates with grade III defects were significantly worse despite aggressive surgical correction. Runoff vessel patterns did not differ significantly between groups.

Conclusion.—Repeat completion arteriography is an indispensable component of bypass surgery. Grade I or II defects seen at arteriography need only minimal intervention. The full extent of a grade III defect, however, may not be revealed at arteriography.

▶ The quality of the vein used for infrainguinal bypass and the technical perfection of the bypass significantly influence short- and long-term graft patency. Therefore, it is critical to carefully inspect both the vein and the completed bypass using the best available techniques before completing an infrainguinal reconstructive procedure.—J.M. Seeger, M.D.

Does Correction of Stenoses Identified With Color Duplex Scanning Improve Infrainguinal Graft Patency?
Mattos MA, van Bemmelen PS, Hodgson KJ, Ramsey DE, Barkmeier LD, Sumner DS (Southern Illinois Univ, Springfield)
J Vasc Surg 17:54–66, 1993   140-94-14–13

Objectives.—Because graft thrombosis continues to be the chief factor in early and late failures of infrainguinal grafts. Whether this practice resulted in better graft survival when infrainguinal bypass stenoses detected by color duplex scanning were corrected was determined.

Methods.—A total of 462 color-flow duplex scans were obtained in 170 extremities bearing infrainguinal autogenous vein bypass grafts in a 39-month period. The 115 men and 55 women in the study had a mean age of 67 years. Grafts were evaluated within 3 months of surgery, after 6 and 12 months, and then annually. A doubling of flow velocity at any point, compared with that just above or below, was taken as evidence of hemodynamically significant (50% or greater) narrowing.

Results.—A total of 110 stenoses were found in 62 extremities. Nine involved native vessels; 30, the anastomoses; and 71 were in the graft itself. Three-fourths of stenoses were detected in the first postoperative year. Twenty-four altered grafts were revised, most often by vein patch angioplasty or interposition vein grafting. Occlusion developed in 8% of the revised grafts; in 26% of unrevised grafts with positive scan findings; and in 9% of grafts with negative scan findings. Ninety percent of scan-negative grafts remained patent at 1 year, and 83% after 2–4 years. Among the positive revised grafts, 96% remained patent at 1 year and 88% at 2–4 years. In contrast, only 66% of unrevised grafts with positive scans remained patent at 1 year, and 57% at 2–4 years. Occlusion was not predicted by a flow velocity less than 45 cm/second or by the ankle/brachial index.

Conclusion.—When an infrainguinal autogenous vein graft has a velocity ratio of 2.0 or above on color duplex scanning, secondary revision can be expected to prolong graft patency. Less severe lesions may be followed by repeat scanning at shorter intervals.

▶ Based on the results of this and several other recently reported studies, routine surveillance of vein grafts using color duplex scanning appears to be appropriate, as these stenoses can be easily detected using this technique, allowing timely repair and potentially improving long-term graft patency.—J.M. Seeger, M.D.

A Prospective Study of the Clinical Outcome of Femoral Pseudoaneurysms and Arteriovenous Fistulas Induced by Arterial Puncture

Kent KC, McArdle CR, Kennedy B, Baim DS, Anninos E, Skillman JJ (Beth Israel Hosp, Boston)
J Vasc Surg 17:125–133, 1993   140-94-14–14

Objective.—Spontaneous thrombosis of femoral false aneurysms (FAs) and arteriovenous fistulas (AVFs) has been described, but its frequency remains uncertain. A prospective study therefore was undertaken to document the natural history of FA and AVF.

Methods.—Sixteen patients with a femoral FA and 6 with an AVF induced by percutaneous arterial puncture underwent duplex sonographic study and were then monitored by serial scans, either in hospital or on a weekly basis as outpatients. Indications for surgery include doubling of the size of an FA; the development of symptoms; and a patent lesion more than 2 months after diagnosis.

Results.—Nine of the 16 FAs closed spontaneously, as did 4 of the 6 AVFs. Although FAs larger than 1.8 cm in diameter more often had to be repaired, 2 small aneurysms remained patent and 2 large ones closed spontaneously secondary to thrombosis. Three of 7 patients requiring repair had received anticoagulation continuously, but none of those whose FAs closed spontaneously were receiving anticoagulation at the time this occurred. Thrombosis did not correlate with the length of the neck of the FA, velocity in the aneurysmal cavity, or velocity of flow in the AVF.

Conclusions.—At least one third of FAs secondary to arterial puncture will require operative repair. Repair is indicated in patients who receive continuous anti-coagulant therapy. Patients with an FA less than 1.8 cm in diameter may safely be discharged. Patients with an AVF do not require repair unless the lesion enlarges or symptoms and signs develop.

▶ Complications of femoral artery catheterization are commonly seen, and the natural history of these problems, as described in this article, should be helpful in determining which lesions need immediate surgical repair and which will resolve without intervention.—J.M. Seeger, M.D.

Long-Term Results of Venous Reconstruction After Vascular Trauma in Civilian Practice

Nypaver TJ, Schuler JJ, McDonnell P, Ellenby MI, Montalvo J, Baraniewski H, Piano G (Univ of Illinois; Cook County Hosp, Chicago)
J Vasc Surg 16:762–768, 1992   140-94-14-15

Objective.—Many major trauma centers have adopted a more aggressive approach to the repair of venous injuries, emphasizing repair rather than ligation. Some aspects of venous reconstruction (VR) remain controversial, however, and its natural history in terms of patency and clinical outcome after vascular trauma remains to be established. A long-term follow-up study was done to define the physiologic results and patency of venous repair of the extremities.

Patients.—The study sample comprised 32 patients who underwent VR for vascular trauma to the upper or lower extremity and were available for long-term follow-up. All but 1 was male (mean age, 29 years). Eighty-one percent of the injuries were in the lower extremity, and 88% resulted from gunshot or laceration/stab wounds. Fifty-six percent of injuries were managed by lateral venorraphy, 22% by interposition grafting, 12.5% by patch repair, and 9.5% by end-to-end repair. The mean follow-up was 49 months, with noninvasive venous evaluation consisting of Doppler ultrasonography, impedance plethysmography, photoplethysmography, and color-flow duplex scanning (CFDS).

Results.—Of 17 patients who underwent postoperative venography, 8 had documentation of patency and 9 of thrombosis. At follow-up, there were only 2 cases of significant clinical edema. Venous refilling time, assessed by photoplethysmography, was 35 seconds in the injured extremity vs. 37 seconds on the uninjured side. Ninety percent of VRs were patent according to standard CFDS criteria. All 8 repairs that were patent on venography remained patent, and 8 of 9 of those with early thrombosis were patent on CFDS.

Conclusions.—Venous reconstruction of venous injuries to the extremities appears to give good long-term results. Morbidity is minimal, long-term patency is good, and venous competence is maintained. The natural history of these repairs appears to consist of local thrombus absorption and recanalization.

▶ This report confirms previous observations that despite early thrombosis, of more than one half of venous repairs for trauma, long-term venous patency is achieved in a high percentage of patients (90% in this study). In addition, the long-term results were good, with significant edema occurring in only 2 patients who had extensive thrombosis develop. Whether venous repair contributed to the extensive thrombosis seen in these 2 patients and whether similar long-term results could have been achieved with simple ligation rather than repair remain to be determined.—J.M. Seeger, M.D.

Advances in the Treatment of Phlegmasia Cerulea Dolens

Hood DB, Weaver FA, Modrall JG, Yellin AE (Univ of Southern California, Los Angeles)

Am J Surg 166:206–210, 1993   140-94-14-16

Background.—Phlegmasia cerulea dolens (PCD) is a potentially lethal form of deep venous thrombosis in a lower extremity, characterized by pain, swelling, and cyanosis of the involved extremity. A significant percentage of patients have rapid progression of the thrombotic process to gangrene, amputation, and death. Various treatment regimens have been proposed, but the relative value of specific therapeutic approaches remains uncertain. Experience with treating this disorder was reviewed.

Patients.—During a 10-year period, 9 women and 3 men aged 34–74 years were treated for PCD involving 18 lower extremities. Six patients had bilateral disease. Eleven patients had associated conditions known to predispose to thrombotic events, including previous placement of a bird's nest vena caval filter in 2 and malignant disease in 8. Three patients had venous gangrene in 4 extremities on admission. All patients were initially treated with bedrest, extremity elevation, fluid resuscitation, and high-dose systemic heparin therapy.

Outcome.—Five patients with PCD in 9 extremities had complete resolution of all symptoms with the initial treatment regimen. One patient who had to discontinue heparin therapy because of heparin-induced thrombocytopenia was switched to dextran and oral warfarin. She had gangrenous toes and later had a transmetatarsal amputation. Two other patients did not respond to heparin therapy and required catheter-based delivery of urokinase, which gave marked clinical improvement. The remaining 4 patients died at 1–10 days after initial evaluation.

Conclusions.—Phlegmasia cerulea dolens can be treated with a regimen of bedrest, extremity elevation, fluid resuscitation, and aggressive systemic anticoagulant therapy if the condition is diagnosed early. Patients who fail to respond to this treatment approach should be given selectively administered thrombolytic therapy. Venous thrombectomy should only be used when thrombolysis is contraindicated.

▶ Phlegmasia cerulea dolens is an uncommon but devastating complication of lower extremity venous thrombosis. The approach to this problem presented in this article is conservative but is associated with good results. As the authors point out, this problem can usually be managed medically, but fasciotomies can be useful in selected patients, whereas venous thrombectomy is seldom necessary.—J.M. Seeger, M.D.

Vena Tech-LGM Filter: Long-Term Results of a Prospective Study

Crochet DP, Stora O, Ferry D, Grossetête R, Leurent B, Brunel P, Nguyen JM

(Hôpital G et R Laënnec–CHR Nantes, France)
Radiology 188:857–860, 1993   140-94-14–17

Objective.—Inferior vena cava (IVC) filters have been widely used to prevent pulmonary embolism (PE) in patients with thromboembolic disease. Percutaneously placed devices have been in use since 1984, but there have been few long-term follow-up studies. The long-term efficiency and tolerance of the Vena Tech-LGM filter were evaluated prospectively.

Patients.—The study population consisted of 142 patients with deep venous thrombosis who underwent successful percutaneous insertion of the Vena Tech-LGM filter. Follow-up examinations were scheduled every 2 years. Each control visit included a physical examination to identify symptoms of PE, a plain frontal film of the abdomen to monitor filter migration, and Doppler ultrasonography to assess IVC patency.

Results.—During follow-up, 53 patients (37.3%) died of causes unrelated to thromboembolic disease. None of the patients were lost to follow-up. Thirteen of the 150 scheduled follow-up examinations (8.7%) could not be done because of poor patient health. During follow-up, PE was suspected in 5 patients (3.5%), 4 of whom had patent filters. After 2 years of follow-up, there had been 16 retractions (18.4%), 15 distal migrations (17.3%), 1 proximal migration in the IVC (1.1%), and 1 tilt (1.1%). Actuarial patency rates were 92% after 2 years, 80% after 4 years, and 70% after 6 years. The clinical status of the lower extremities deteriorated over time, but the decline was unrelated to filter patency.

Conclusions.—The percutaneously placed Vena Tech-LGM filter effectively prevents PE and has a long-term patency of 70%. No deleterious effects were recorded during 2–6 years of follow-up.

▶ Multiple intracaval devices to prevent pulmonary emboli have been developed and marketed. Unfortunately, the long-term results from careful clinical evaluation of these devices, such as reported in this article, are limited.—J.M. Seeger, M.D.

Perioperative Morbidity in Patients Randomized to Epidural or General Anesthesia for Lower Extremity Vascular Surgery
Christopherson R, Beattie C, Frank SM, Norris EJ, Meinert CL, Gottlieb SO, Yates H, Rock P, Parker SD, Perler BA, Williams GM, the Perioperative Ischemia Randomized Anesthesia Trial Study Group (Johns Hopkins Med Insts, Baltimore, Md; Johns Hopkins Univ, Baltimore, Md; VA Med Ctr, Portland, Ore)
Anesthesiology 79:422–434, 1993   140-94-14–18

Background.—Studies comparing mortality and morbidity after surgery performed with either regional and general anesthesia have been conducted in various populations, with varying results. In a randomized, prospective study, epidural (EA) and general (GA) anesthesia–analgesia regimens were compared in patients undergoing lower extremity revascularization for atherosclerotic peripheral vascular disease.

Methods.—One hundred patients received either EA followed by epidural analgesia or GA with subsequent intravenous patient-controlled analgesia. Monitoring included continuous electrocardiography from the day before surgery through the first 3 postoperative days, and subsequent serial ECGs and cardiac enzyme determinations. Morbidity also was determined at hospital discharge and at 1 and 6 months.

Results.—Mortality and major cardiac morbidity rates did not differ between the treatment groups. Cardiac ischemia occurred in 35% of patients after EA and in 45% after GA. Perioperative cardiac ischemia was a significant predictor of major cardiac morbidity: Seven of the 40 patients with ischemia had major morbidity, compared to only 1 of 60 without ischemia. Significantly more GA patients than EA patients required regrafting or embolectomy before discharge. A similar, nonsignificant trend was observed for amputations of the foot or leg. Regression analysis revealed GA as the only risk factor significantly related to regrafting or embolectomy.

Discussion.—A clinical recommendation regarding use of EA vs. GA is not possible because major cardiac morbidity occurred equally in both groups. The higher prevalence of graft occlusion with GA may be related to depression. Epidural anesthesia preserves cardiac output and also enhances arterial inflow and venous emptying in the lower extremities.

Conclusion.—In this population, carefully managed regimens of EA followed by epidural analgesia or GA followed by intravenous patient-controlled analgesia did not differ in overall mortality, major cardiac morbidity, or myocardial ischemia. Any difference between the anesthetics was most pronounced immediately after surgery. Inadequate tissue perfusion was more prevalent with GA, often necessitating early repeat surgery.

▶ Although it has been suggested that regional anesthesia decreases cardiac stress in patients who are undergoing vascular reconstructive procedures, this does not seem to be the case. However, epidural anesthesia does appear to reduce the risk of postoperative graft occlusion, a surprising but most welcome benefit.—J.M. Seeger, M.D.

Vascular Laboratory Cost Analysis and the Impact of the Resource-Based Relative Value Scale Payment System
Fillinger MF, Zwolak RM, Musson AM, Cronenwett JL (Dartmouth-Hitchcock Med Ctr, Lebanon, NH)
J Vasc Surg 17:267–279, 1993   140-94-14–19

Objective.—The actual cost of noninvasive vascular laboratory studies was compared with reimbursement under Medicare Part B and also with reimbursement under current resource-based relative value scale (RBRVS) guidelines.

Methods.—The cost of operating the authors' laboratory was calculated, and national costs were estimated for small- and large-model vascular laboratories. Reimbursement under Medicare Part B was determined for each Current Procedural Terminology code from average allowances and national case volumes in 1990.

Results.—The technical costs for laboratory time ranged from $143 to $173 per study hour. Fixed costs for personnel, equipment, and facilities were the major components of laboratory expenses, and variable costs such as billing accounted for most of the rest. Costs were lowered for large laboratories that allocated their equipment more efficiently. In a laboratory, the continued use of depreciated equipment lowered costs to $127 per hour.

Projections.—Estimates of technical reimbursement with RBRVS were $82/hr nationally and $80/hr locally. The respective global reimbursement figures, including professional services, were $116/hr and $110/hr. Based on 1990 case volumes, the RBRVS system will lower national global reimbursement by at least 35% compared with the previous Medicare Part B system. Technical reimbursement is expected to decline by 27% nationally, and professional reimbursement by 52%. Technical reimbursement will be from 37% to 54% below actual costs, and global reimbursement will be 13% to 34% under technical costs, even if operating efficiency is optimized.

Implications.—This analysis applies only to outpatients, and a case mix including inpatients will lower reimbursement further since only the professional part will be allowed. The new RBRVS system may ultimately make noninvasive vascular testing less available to elderly patients.

▶ Physiologic and ultrasound imaging studies of the vascular system have become essential in the diagnosis and treatment of peripheral vascular disease. This article points out that recent changes in reimbursement may mean limited availability of these studies, which can only decrease the quality of care for elderly patients with peripheral vascular disease.—J.M. Seeger, M.D.

Warfarin in the Prevention of Stroke Associated With Nonrheumatic Atrial Fibrillation

Ezekowitz MD, for the Veterans Affairs Stroke Prevention in Nonrheumatic Atrial Fibrillation Investigators (Yale Univ, West Haven, Conn)
N Engl J Med 327:1406–1412, 1992   140-94-14-20

Background.—Experience in treating deep vein thrombosis and other states suggests that low-intensity warfarin anticoagulation is as effective as more intense treatment for preventing thromboembolism, and it also causes less bleeding. In a prospective, randomized, double-blind study, low-intensity warfarin was compared with placebo in men with chronic atrial fibrillation of nonrheumatic origin.

Methods.—The occurrence of cerebral infarction, cerebral hemorrhage, and death was monitored in 571 male veterans of all ages who had documented atrial fibrillation, 46 of whom had previously had cerebral infarction. Warfarin was given to prolong the prothrombin time ratio by 1.2 to 1.5.

Results.—Cerebral infarction occurred at an annual rate of 4.3% per year in those patients receiving placebo who did not have a past history of stroke; the annual rate was 0.9% per year in warfarin-treated patients. A 79% reduction in risk was evident with warfarin therapy. The annual rate of all events in patients older than age 70 years was 79% less in warfarin-treated patients. The risk of death not preceded by a cerebral end point was reduced by 31% in the warfarin group.

Conclusion.—Low-level anticoagulation with warfarin can prevent cerebral infarction in patients—even elderly patients—with nonrheumatic atrial fibrillation, while not producing an excessive risk of major bleeding.

▶ This study and several others have clearly demonstrated the usefulness of low-intensity coumarin in preventing stroke in patients with atrial fibrillation, which is a common problem in elderly patients with peripheral vascular disease.—J.M. Seeger, M.D.

Subject Index*

A

Abdomen
closure
in severe trauma with visceral edema, 93: 90
towel clip of skin, 93: 92
inability to close because of visceral edema, 93: 85
intra-abdominal infection
critical, planned reoperation and open management, 93: 114
relaparotomy in, planned, 93: 115
study, of surgical infection society, management techniques and outcome, 94: 107
intra-abdominal pressure increase, effect on blood flow, 93: 92
surgery
decreasing carbohydrate oxidation and increasing fat oxidation in, growth hormone for, in total parenteral nutrition, 94: 201
enteral feeding after, immediate, weight loss decrease and wound healing improvement due to (in rat), 93: 191
wound dehiscence in, 93: 180
trauma
autotransfusion of potentially culture-positive blood in, 93: 98
closure in visceral edema, 93: 90
massive, delayed gastrointestinal reconstruction after, 94: 89
penetrating, antibiotic duration in, 93: 100
penetrating, cephalosporin in, 93: 100
penetrating, laparoscopy to evaluate, 93: 89
penetrating and blunt, comprehensive algorithm for, 93: 107
penetrating and blunt, septic morbidity after, enteral vs. parenteral feeding in, 93: 101
severe, abdominal wall reconstruction after, tissue expanders for, 93: 96
wall reconstruction after severe trauma, tissue expanders for, 93: 96
Ablation
of Barrett's esophagus epithelium, squamous mucosa restoration after, 94: 242
Abscess
"undrained," of multiple organ failure, and gastrointestinal tract, 94: 103

Academic
medicine, and Health Security Act, 94: 10
role models, women surgeons as, 94: 12
Achalasia
esophagomyotomy in, thoracoscopic, 93: 215
pneumatic dilatation for, causing esophageal perforation, surgical repair, 94: 253
Acidosis
in critical injury, 93: 93
Acute illness
of medical patients, mortality and hypomagnesemia, 94: 52
Adenocarcinoma
in Barrett's esophagus with high-grade dysplasia, 93: 214
colorectal polyps containing, endoscopic polypectomy or colectomy, 93: 306
esophageal, and Barrett's esophagus, 93: 215
invasive, and colorectal polyps, lymph node metastases risk in, 93: 303
lung, *ras* gene mutations as prognostic marker, 93: 428
rectal
preoperative radiotherapy and surgery for, 93: 312
surgical adjuvant, radiotherapy, 5-fluorouracil and semustine in, 93: 315
rectal and rectosigmoid, preoperative radiotherapy in, 93: 314
Adenoma
parathyroid, found after neck dissection, 93: 169
solitary, causing hyperparathyroidism, different surgical regimen results, 93: 166
Adenomatous polyposis (*see* Polyposis, familial adenomatous)
Adenopathy
hilar, clinically staged ipsilateral, in lung cancer with radiotherapy, 94: 451
Adenosine
monophosphate, cyclic, beta adrenergic receptor stimulation impairment of, in septic shock, 94: 39
triphosphate depletion, pulmonary endothelial cell, due to intestinal ischemia-reperfusion injury, 94: 37
Adhesion molecules
endothelial, expression in kidney transplant, 94: 141

---

* All entries refer to the year and page number(s) for data appearing in this and the previous edition of the YEAR BOOK.

513

Author Index

A

Abdullah KM, 226
Abe Y, 433
Abner AL, 339
Abou-Azama A-M, 331
Abramson D, 92
Abramson JE, 112
Acuff TE, 465, 474
Adams DB, 280
Adams MB, 140
Addiss DG, 272
Adzick NS, 236, 237
Afdhal NH, 273
Agnew DK, 20
AhChong AK, 316
Ainslie N, 425
Akbari CM, 110
Åkerström G, 152
Alasio L, 406
Albain KS, 456
Albelda SM, 217
Albertine KH, 43
Albertson S, 224
Alexander JW, 70, 194
Alexander RW, 226
Alfieri S, 376
Alibegovic A, 171
Allen RP, 461
Alling DW, 48
Allred EN, 330
Alm T, 302
Almond PS, 138
Altavilla G, 490
Althaus U, 475
Amadori D, 379
Amalric R, 334
Ames FC, 422
Anbazhagan R, 351
Anderson MC, 280
Andrade S, 47
Andreassian B, 156
Andrus CH, 2
Angeletti CA, 442
Anninos E, 506
Anscher MS, 345
Ansel JC, 222
Anthony JP, 434
Antman KH, 485
Antonyshyn OM, 430
Appel S, 209
Araneo BA, 66
Arbuckle P, 132
Arends J-W, 187
Argilés JM, 206
Armitage JM, 135
Asoh H, 460
Assendelft A, 453
Attie JN, 167, 406
Auf'M'Kolk M, 90
Aufses AH Jr, 289

B

Babyn P, 311
Baccino FM, 206
Bacher JD, 48
Bachulis BL, 79
Bäckman L, 128
Bagby GJ, 206
Baim DS, 506
Bains MS, 472, 481
Bakal C, 503
Bakamjian V, 482
Baker C, 81
Bakker A, 361
Bakker WH, 287
Balch CM, 391, 425
Baldock G, 36
Baldwin BJ, 414
Ball DW, 159
Ballard DJ, 495
Balsara ZN, 296
Banks SM, 48
Baraniewski H, 507
Barba L, 137
Barbul A, 196
Baredes S, 409
Barie PS, 107
Barker DE, 84
Barkmeier LD, 505
Barkun AN, 270
Barkun JS, 270
Barnhill R, 391
Bartlett RH, 32
Bartoli C, 406
Bartolucci AA, 391
Bates T, 351
Bättig U, 28
Baudet EM, 134
Bauer TW, 444
Baylin SB, 159
Beale R, 36
Beard CJ, 487
Beart RW Jr, 299
Beattie C, 509
Beauchamp RD, 188
Beck DJ, 197
Beegle PH Jr, 428
Beekhuis H, 260
Beger HG, 390
Beinfield M, 343
Belkin M, 496
Bellantone R, 376
Belluco C, 331
Benfell K, 203
Benfield JR, 456
Bengtson BP, 414
Benini E, 323
Benito E, 355
Bensard DD, 476
Benya RV, 256
Berenson MM, 242
Bergstrahl EJ, 154
Berling DP, 129
Bernard A, 156

Berne T, 137
Bevilacqua P, 330
Biester TW, 1
Bigini D, 442
Bihari D, 36
Binns GS, 264
Birnbaum EH, 304
Bjøro T, 201
Blackstock W, 345
Blanc-Jouvan F, 489
Bland KI, 197
Blane CE, 298
Bleichrodt RP, 260
Blinman TA, 88
Bloom GP, 110
Blumenson LE, 482
Bode BP, 197
Bonfanti G, 379
Booth B, 104
Boracchi P, 323, 379
Borah GL, 427
Böttcher K, 381
Boutron MC, 356
Bowers CM, 476
Boyett JM, 347
Bozzetti F, 379
Braghetto I, 257
Brathwaite CEM, 95
Breeden M, 224
Bremner CG, 251
Bremner RM, 251
Brennan MF, 153, 157, 401
Brennan TA, 22
Bret P, 470
Broemeling LD, 226
Brones MF, 75
Bross DS, 21
Broughan TA, 347
Brouillet J-P, 327
Browder W, 277, 292
Brown AC, 307
Brown AE, 106
Brown AJL, 113
Brown DH, 416
Brown LF, 223
Browne BJ, 140
Bruining HA, 287
Brummer R-JM, 187
Brunel P, 508
Bryan CS, 100
Bryant JL, 170
Bucalo B, 214
Buchi KN, 242
Büchler M, 390
Buhr HJ, 160
Bulas DI, 86
Bülow S, 302
Burdiles P, 257
Burke JF, 72, 100
Burkhard TK, 296
Burleson DG, 68
Burstin HR, 22
Burt M, 153, 446
Burt ME, 472, 481

567

We've read
236,287
journal
articles
(so you don't have to).

The Year Books–
The best from 236,287 journal articles.

At Mosby, we subscribe to more than 950 medical and allied health journals from every corner of the globe. We read them all, tirelessly scanning for anything that relates to your field.

We send everything we find related to a given specialty to the distinguished editors of the **Year Book** in that area, and they pick out *the best*, the articles they feel *every practitioner in that specialty should be aware of*.

For the **1994 Year Books** we surveyed a total of 236,287 articles and found hundreds of articles related to your field. Our expert editors reviewed these and chose the developments you don't want to miss.

The best articles–condensed, organized, and with personal commentary.

Not only do you get the past year's most important articles in your field, you get them in a format that makes them easy to use.

Every article that the editors pick is condensed into a concise, outlined abstract, a summary of the article's most important points highlighted with bold paragraph headings. So you can quickly scan for exactly what you need.

In addition to identifying the year's best articles, the editors write concise commentaries following each article, telling whether or not the study in question is a reliable one, whether a new technique is effective, or whether a particular trend you've head about merits your immediate attention.

No other abstracting service offers this expert advice to help you decide how the year's advances will affect the way you practice.

With a special added benefit for Year Book subscribers.

In 1994, your **Year Book** subscription includes a new added benefit. Access to **MOSBY Document Express**, a rapid-response information retrieval service that puts copies of original source documents in your hands, in a little as a few hours.

With **MOSBY Document Express**, you have convenient, *around-the-clock-access to literally every article* upon which **Year Book** summaries are based. What's more, you can also order journal articles cited in references—or for that matter, virtually any medical or scientific article that can be located. Plus, at your direction, we will deliver the article(s) by FAX, overnight delivery service, or regular mail.

This new added benefit is just one of the enhanced services that makes your **Year Book** subscription an even better value—it's your key to the full breadth of health sciences information. For more details, see **MOSBY Document Express** instructions at the beginning of this book.